Research and Discovery in Medicine

RESEARCH AND DISCOVERY IN MEDICINE

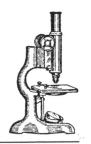

CONTRIBUTIONS FROM JOHNS HOPKINS

A. McGehee Harvey, M.D.

A. McGehee Harvey

The Johns Hopkins University Press

Baltimore and London

Copyright © 1976, 1977, 1978, 1979, 1980, 1981 by The Johns Hopkins University Press
All rights reserved
Printed in the United States of America

The Johns Hopkins University Press, Baltimore, Maryland 21218
The Johns Hopkins Press Ltd., London

Library of Congress Cataloging in Publication Data
Harvey, A. McGehee (Abner McGehee), 1911-
    Research and discovery in medicine.

    1. Johns Hopkins University. School of Medicine—History—Addresses, essays, lectures. 2. Johns Hopkins Hospital—History—Addresses, essays, lectures. 3. Medical research—Maryland—Baltimore—History—Addresses, essays, lectures. 4. Medical scientists—Maryland—Baltimore—Biography—Addresses, essays, lectures. I. Title.
[DNLM: 1. Education, Medical—History—Maryland. 2. History of medicine—Maryland—Biography. 3. Research—History—Maryland. W 20.5 H341r]
R747. J62H38   610'.7207526   81—47647
ISBN 0-8018-2723-X   AACR2

Contents

List of Illustrations

Preface

Research, as a principal concern of medical schools and their associated hospitals, received an important stimulus with the opening of The Johns Hopkins Hospital. At that time, John Shaw Billings commented on the widespread hope and expectations that the new Johns Hopkins Institutions would endeavor "to produce investigators as well as practitioners, to give to the world men who cannot only sail by the old charts, but who can make new and better ones for the use of others."

The Johns Hopkins Hospital opened its doors in 1889, and The Johns Hopkins School of Medicine began the instruction of its first class a little over four years later in October 1893. Thus the history of these two great institutions has paralleled that of the century in which the greatest progress has been made in the advance of medical science and the treatment and prevention of the diseases affecting man. Early members of the hospital staff and the medical school faculty played a major role in bringing the new scientific approaches and the new era of experimental medical science to this country from Germany. From 1889 onward Baltimore was the site of revolutionary change in medical education, important contributions to the medical sciences, and the evolution of a new member of the medical team who has come to occupy a position interposed between the basic scientist and the practicing physician—the clinical scientist or clinical investigator.

Welch, Mall, and others on the original faculty stressed the importance to medicine of science, of scientific methods, or scientific thinking and techniques of expression. They recognized the need for laboratories and strove to provide career opportunities for talented young men motivated to become full-time medical scientists. It has been said that Welch's greatest contribution to medical education was his insistence on the importance of the medical sciences.

Members of the Johns Hopkins medical community made vital contributions to many of the outstanding medical research accomplishments of the past century, including the development of chemotherapy in the treatment of infectious diseases, the development of an effective vaccine against poliomyelitis, the emergence of cardiac surgery, and the evolution of cell culture as an important technique for medical research.

In addition, many students, both undergraduate and postgraduate, migrated to other institutions where they established themselves as outstanding teachers and made important contributions to medical knowledge. Examples include the conquest of yellow fever, pioneer work in virology, research on the peripheral circulation, studies of the pituitary gland, and on such important diseases as tuberculosis, scarlet fever, and malaria.

This volume represents a continuation of the essays which appeared in 1976 in a volume entitled *Adventures in Medical Research*.

Acknowledgments

I am indebted to the *Maryland Medical Journal* for permission to reproduce the article entitled "William Osler and Medicine in America: With Special Reference to the Baltimore Period" (Md. State Med. J., 25 (10): 35, 1976) and to the Pergamon Press, publisher, and Dr. David Earle, editor, for permission to reprint the article entitled "Clinical Investigation of Chronic Diseases: Its Successful Pursuit in an Outpatient Setting" (J. Chron. Dis., 33: 529, 1980).

My deep appreciation goes to Patricia King and Carol Bocchini for their expert help in editing these essays. My thanks to those who contributed material or helped in the review of these essays is expressed at the end of each article.

Research and Discovery in Medicine

Research and Discovery in Medicine

1.

William Osler and Medicine in America: With Special Reference to the Baltimore Period

EARLY YEARS

Whatever rank the 20th century may assign to William Osler in the medical roll call of the 19th, it is certain that he was the outstanding figure of the profession, both in this country and abroad. He represented not only the older type of clinician who was above all else a great observer, but also the newer generation whose advances were in the main noteworthy because of the application of the methods of science to the study of human disease. William Osler stood at the gateway of the newer world of medicine and added to his wide clinical knowledge a familiarity with the basic sciences. He made a lifelong career of teaching medicine to students, house officers and physicians in practice, and the achievement of which he was proudest was that he taught at the bedside and popularized this technique which still dominates medical education today.

Osler's American period extends from his birth in the parsonage at Bond Head in upper Canada on July 12, 1849, to the time of his departure for Oxford in May, 1905. He was the eighth of nine children, of whom at least five led lives of great distinction. His early education was gained in the schools at Bond Head, Dundas, Barrie, Weston and Trinity College, during which time he was greatly influenced by a naturalist, the Reverend Arthur Johnson, and a physician of diverse interests, Dr. James Bovell, whose name Osler constantly scribbled on his notes and in his books throughout his prolific literary career.

Osler received his undergraduate medical education in Toronto and Montreal, where he came under the influence of Dr. R. Palmer Howard and other leading medical men. During his first graduate studies in Europe, he profited most by his work in experimental physiology under Sir John Burdon-Sanderson, whom he was to succeed some 34 years later as Regius Professor of Medicine at Oxford. While in Europe, he came in contact with the prominent clinicians and pathologists of the day in England, Scotland, Germany and Austria.

On his return to Montreal in August, 1874, as lecturer in the Institutes of Medicine (which included physiology and pathology), his consuming passion for books, which grew over the years, was becoming clearly evident.

Reprinted from the *Maryland State Medical Journal* **25**(10): 35, 1976.

In 1875, Osler was put in charge of the smallpox ward in the Montreal General Hospital, his first clinical appointment. His accurate observations on the early rash in smallpox led to the first publication on the subject in English. For his services on this ward, he received $600, which he used to purchase 12 French microscopes to aid him in the teaching of normal histology to his students. An interesting anecdote of the period tells of an encounter with an elderly man on the street. Osler gave him some money and his overcoat. The old gentleman died two weeks later and willed the coat back to Osler who had not had enough money to buy another in the meanwhile.

After Osler's arrival, a renaissance began at McGill of which he was the moving spirit. Dr. Palmer Howard had something of the insight that was so marked a quality in Daniel Coit Gilman, the first President of Johns Hopkins—the ability to pick out promising men when they were still quite young. When Osler made his first address to the students, the rules of life that he urged upon them as physicians were his own and never changed with the passing years: 1) You must always be a student, 2) You must treat the man as well as the disease, and 3) The poor you have always with you and you must consider them beyond all others.

He quoted Sir Thomas Browne: "No one should approach the pinnacle of science with the soul of a moneychanger." In spite of all the time involved in preparing lectures and doing his many other chores, he took on voluntary work in the pathological laboratory. Although visiting physicians and surgeons were supposed to perform their own autopsies, they gradually began to look to Osler, who eagerly assumed the task.

During the April, 1877, recess, Osler spent a week in Boston. While there he listened to a recitation on anatomy by Oliver Wendell Holmes. It gives meaning to the history of American medicine to look back a full century at the vista of Holmes at the age of 68 standing on the lecture platform while looking up at him from the audience was young William Osler, aged 28. As Reid, in her biography of Osler, has written: "The sweet, kindly face of the old man and the dark, glowing one of the youth mirrored much the same ideals. Holmes was the greater writer and his humor was the deep-seated humor of genius. Osler was the greater physician and his whimsical humor and boyish fun were more on the surface. But these two were singularly alike in spirit . . . listen to a part of Oliver Wendell Holmes' lecture delivered in 1867:

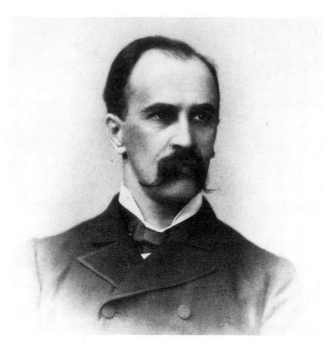

Fig 1. Osler as a young man. The McGill Period.
From the Archives, Medical and Chirurgical Faculty of Maryland

'A medical school is not a scientific school except just so far as medicine itself is a science. On the natural history side, medicine is a science; on the curative side, chiefly an art. This is implied in Hufelands' Aphorism: "The physician must generalize the disease and individualize the patient.'" And compare with the expression in Dr. Osler's address, *Teacher and Student.* 'The practice of medicine is an art, based on science. Working with science, in science and for science, it has not reached, perhaps never will, the dignity of a complete science with exact laws like astronomy and engineering.' And as a rubric to his *Principles and Practice of Medicine,* he quotes the words of Plato, "And I said of medicine that this is an art which considers the constitution of the patient and his principles of action and reason in each case."

In 1878, Osler was appointed physician to the Montreal General Hospital. Later, as registrar of the medical school, Osler met the entire student body as they were admitted. His memory for names and faces was uncanny; he was loved by the students, who were greatly stimulated by his personal touch, which extended to his close work with them on the medical wards of the hospital.

Dr. Osler believed that the use of too many drugs was one of the great errors of the day. He was fond of saying that Hahnemann had done more good than anyone else in the profession because he had shown that the natural tendency of disease was toward recovery. In his first bedside manual for the instruction of students, he wrote the following motto from Froude: "The knowledge which a man can use is the only real knowledge which has life and growth in it and converts itself into practical power. The rest hangs like dust above the brain, or dries like raindrops off the stones."

In 1881, the great International Medical Congress—perhaps the greatest medical meeting ever held—took place in London under the Presidency of Sir James Paget. The epoch-making event of the Congress was Pasteur's account of the anthrax test inoculation that he had made and the discussion on vaccination in relation to "chicken-cholera" and "splenic fever." These earthshaking experiments opened the door of preventive medicine through which the entire medical world was to follow in the next decade.

Also it was at this meeting that Koch received worldwide attention for his laboratory techniques which had so much to do with the recognition of the specific bacterial cause of most of the infectious diseases in the ensuing years. There were, too, violent discussions on spontaneous generation. Pasteur believed that life comes only from life and his view was supported by a distinguished group including Lister, Koch, Tyndall, Huxley, Darwin and Charcot, among others. However, he had a number of opponents, including Bastian, and Englishman who was the chief proponent of the belief that germs could develop spontaneously in diseased tissues.

Osler did not enter into the discussion and dismissed it in his report back to Canada with the casual statement that "there was an abundant discussion of germs in the pathological section." It was many years before Osler fully appreciated the importance of the bacterial theory of the origin of infectious diseases. While at the Congress, Osler gave his important paper on endocarditis and it was here that Dr. Samuel Gross, Jr. met Osler and became entranced with his knowledge and personality. It was Gross who wrote back to Philadelphia recommending that Osler be the major candidate to succeed Tyson as Professor of Medicine there.

Later, when Tyson wrote to Osler asking if he would accept the Chair of Medicine in the University of Pennsylvania, Osler told his confidantes that the temptation was too great and he had decided to reply in the affirmative. This seemed a broader field for the development of this extraordinary young man who had made such a tremendous impression in Montreal, a contribution summed up by his biographer, Harvey Cushing: "During the short span of years since his McGill appointment, he had stirred into activity the slumbering Medical-Chirurgical Society; he had founded and supported a students' medical club, he had brought the medical school into relation with the university, he had introduced the modern methods of teaching physiology, he had edited the first clinical and pathological reports of a Canadian Hospital, he had recorded nearly a thousand autopsies and made innumerable museum preparations of the most important specimens, he had written countless papers—many of them ephemeral, it is true—but most of them on topics of live interest for the time and a few of them epoch-making; he had worked at biology and pathology, both human and comparative, as well as at the bedside; he had shown courage in taking a smallpox ward, charity in dealing with his fellow physicians in and out of his own school, generosity to his students and fidelity to his tasks and his many uncommon qualities had earned him popularity unsought and of a most unusual degree."

Thus, all of the groundwork had been laid for the future development of this engaging young Canadian who was for the next few decades to occupy the center stage in the rapidly evolving heroic age of scientific medicine.

THE PHILADELPHIA PERIOD

In a city in which the members of the medical profession were so closely knit, there was an avalanche of protest in Philadelphia over Osler's selection to succeed Tyson as Professor of Medicine. And though he had the backing of Weir Mitchell and Samuel Gross who had largely determined his appointment, it would have been difficult for him in spite of his early fame from the Montreal days to succeed easily in the city of Brotherly Love had he been a man of lesser talent. Osler recorded the story of his "inspection" by Weir Mitchell: "Dr. Mitchell cabled me to meet him in London as he and his good wife were commissioned 'to look me over,' particularly with reference to personal habits. Dr. Mitchell said there was only one way in which the breeding of a man suitable for such a position in such a city as Philadelphia could be tested: 'Give him cherry pie and see how he

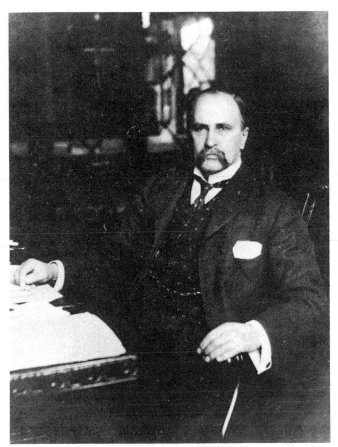

Fig 2. Osler in 1905: The Baltimore Period.
From the Archives, Medical and Chirurgical Faculty of Maryland

disposes of the stones.' I had read of the trick before and disposed of them genteely in my spoon—and got the Chair."

His actual plunge into the Philadelphia pool was so ably and so gracefully done that he quickly became very popular. His engaging personality was an important asset, but the dominant factor that made him successful was in the words of a student: "He was up—that is, he knew his subject and how to teach what he knew . . . His first class was an eye-opener. In it he frolicked in enthusiastic delight and in a few moments had every man interested and avid for more. Every new specimen that he came to at autopsy, and every interesting manifestation of disease in the living was to him a treasure and just as Leidy saw in every flower and stone and bone, and worm and rhizopod, an inner beauty, so Osler, to change my metaphor, was as the light-hearted child who, finding a field of daisies, shouts his delight so exaltingly that all of the other children become interested and gleeful and shout with him. Osler did more than any other man of his day in this city to teach all men that the study and pursuit of disease is a pursuit that a properly trained mind can follow with as keen enjoyment and uplift as an artist can study great pictures or a musician can hear great masters."

Osler took part in every aspect of the medical life in Philadelphia with one exception—he never engaged to any significant degree in private practice. It was the dead house at the old Blockley with a crowd of students around him that he spent a major portion of his time. In 1870, the University of Pennsylvania moved from the city of Philadelphia to property adjoining the Blockley Hospital and a few years later erected a hospital of its own at that site. One could leave the university hospital by the rear and enter Blockley enclosure through a gate in the old wall. Near this gate stood a little red building, a halfway house to the Potter's field. Blockley had at that time over 2,000 patients with all manner of maladies and the opportunity for postmortem studies was extraordinary. The diener soon saw Dr. Osler's enthusiasm and whenever an examination was waived they would at once inform Osler who, at the earliest possible moment, collected his students and marched to Blockley to make an autopsy. This method of teaching pathology was an innovation which was enthusiastically received by the students.

While in Philadelphia, Osler published 39 papers covering a variety of aspects of clinical medicine. The three greatest clinicians in America at the time—Austin Flint, Edward G. Janeway and William Osler—felt their success was due to their grounding in Pathology. Dr. Osler, the greatest of the three, kept up his pathological work during the entire Philadelphia period.

After four busy years in Philadelphia, rumors began to circulate concerning a call to the new school in Baltimore. The final blow fell when William Pepper on Oct. 3, 1888 received the following letter from Osler: "I have received a definite offer from the Johns Hopkins authorities and have determined to accept it. I will leave with great regret. You have been like a good, kind

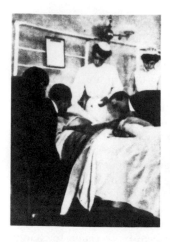
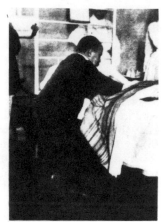
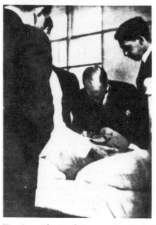
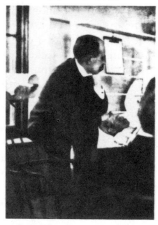

Fig 3.   The Baltimore Period: Snapshots of Osler at the bedside.
From the Archives, Johns Hopkins Medical Institutions

brother. There need be no hurry about any official action."

Clearly Osler had been just as important a ferment in Philadelphia as he had been in Montreal, and again there was a deep feeling of regret concerning his leaving in the hearts of all of his friends, colleagues and students. However, as before, it appeared that Baltimore offered him the most significant opportunity of his life as "the opening of The Johns Hopkins Hospital in 1889 marked a new departure in medical education in the United States. It was not the hospital itself, for there were many larger and just as good; it was not the men appointed, as there were others quite as well qualified; it was the organization. For the first time in an English-speaking country, a hospital was organized in units—each one in charge of a Head or Chief."

Perhaps what appealed to Osler most was that in Philadelphia and Montreal the universities were part of a community and had developed over the years strong traditions of their own. They were to some extent under political control. However, in Baltimore the new university was entirely independent and was able to break new ground. By his association with it in an important role,

Osler could realize his own ideals of what a medical school should be. The years in Philadelphia, built on the foundation in Montreal, had deepened his understanding of the science and of the art of medicine.

THE BALTIMORE PERIOD: OSLER AS CHIEF OF THE MEDICAL CLINIC

The opening of the Medical Clinic at The Johns Hopkins Hospital in 1889 created an opportunity for significant advances in both the science and the art of medicine. The time corresponded to the floodtide of natural science. Biology, physics and chemistry were advancing rapidly and medicine was ready to apply this new knowledge to the study of disease in man. A series of special divisions of medical science including anatomy, histology, embryology, physiology, physiological chemistry, pharmacology, pathological anatomy, bacteriology and physiology were being developed. For the first time, these new branches were to be taught by men who gave up their whole career exclusively to this effort. Such resources were to serve as a foundation upon which a great superstructure of clinical science might be built.

The position offered to William Osler was that of the Professorship of Medicine at The Johns Hopkins University as well as the appointment as Physician-in-Chief to the new Johns Hopkins Hospital. This was a unique situation, for there was to be created a well endowed hospital designed to be an integral part of the medical school of an endowed university and funds were provided for salaries of the leaders of the clinics as well as for the chiefs of other university departments, a situation quite different from that which prevailed in the "proprietary medical schools" of the time.

At last a medical school was to be organized as part of a true university. Another important aspect was that a basic responsibility of this new university in all of its departments was to be an interest in original research as well as competent instruction. There were to be distinguished investigators in the university itself with men such as Martin and Brooks in Biology and Physiology, Roland in Physics, Remsen in Chemistry and Welch in Pathology. A basic criterion for appointment was to be a capacity for personal research and the ability to stimulate others to engage in fruitful research. This was considered as important as the ability to teach and to organize in adding up the assets of candidates for the professional chairs of the university.

The hospital planned by John Shaw Billings was to offer better facilities for the organization and conduct of clinical work than any that had hitherto been constructed in the United States. Thus, in the search for the men to occupy the clinical chairs, great value was placed on native ability and experience to match up with these unusual opportunities. The Chair of Medicine was generally conceded to be the most important one, and for this Professorship the university and hospital as it turned out made the right appointment when they chose William Osler.

Osler entered upon work in Baltimore with an enthusiasm that stimulated everyone. He began to organize his department promptly, selecting a group of young men as assistants and soon set an example in practice, teaching and investigation that was contagious. Here Osler had the opportunity to put into practice all of his previous training and experience in Montreal, in Europe and in Philadelphia.

For him, the welfare of the patients who presented themselves in the clinic for diagnosis and treatment came first; next, consideration of how undergraduate and graduate students could best be taught; and finally came the desire that every opportunity for contributing to the advancement of knowledge of internal medicine should be eagerly seized. Here, for the first time in Osler's clinic, a variety of diverse elements were synthesized into a harmonious whole. It represented a new form in teaching, practice and research which was excellent for the time, yet plastic enough to allow for remolding with the passage of time.

The Johns Hopkins Medical School did not open until 1893. Four years were thus available for perfecting the organization of the wards, the outpatient department, the laboratories, the staff, the records, the library, the hospital, the medical society and the care of patients in the hospital before the function of teaching undergraduates was added. Courses for postgraduates were, it is true, offered during this period, but the numbers involved were small and the work was not therefore burdensome.

First and most important in the success of the new clinic was the arrangement for a graded staff, particularly for a graded full-time resident staff, among whom the responsibility of the work was divided, not according to a "military plan," but rather in the manner of the so-called "composite functional type" of organization. The Professor of Medicine, though giving most of his time to the work of the clinic, lived outside the hospital, as did the Associate Professors who "visited" the wards, the outpatient department and the laboratories. The Resident Physician, the Assistant Resident Physicians and the medical Interns lived in the hospital and were in close contact with the work always by day, and as far as was necessary, also by night.

This resident staff of the clinic consisted of two parts: one, a lower resident staff constituted by the medical Interns appointed for a single year, usually on graduation with high standing from the medical school and, two, an upper resident staff made up of the Resident Physician and several Assistant Resident Physicians, usually men of exceptional promise, men who already had been hospital Interns and who were willing to serve a more prolonged resident service, often of several years' duration, in order to secure the best possible groundwork for the "higher walks" of internal medicine.

This upper staff was chosen partly from the lower staff, and in order to prevent "inbreeding," from members of the resident staffs of hospitals in other medical centers. The position of Chief Resident Physician, which carried with it large responsibilities and opportunities,

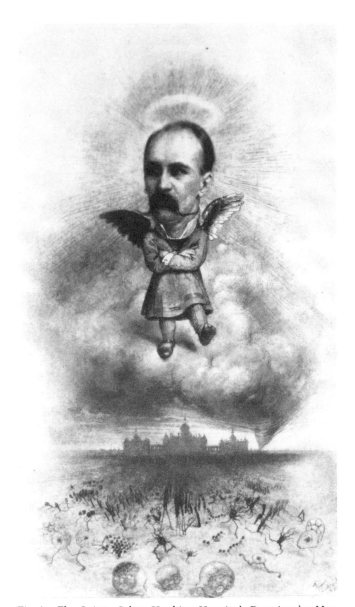

Fig 4. The Saint—Johns Hopkins Hospital. Drawing by Max Brödel.
Courtesy of Mrs. Charles Austrian

was a prize to be won only by men of exceptional ability, extensive experience and favorable promise. Those occupying this position in Osler's time included Henery A. La Fleur (1889–91), William S. Thayer (1891–98), Thomas B. Futcher (1898–1901), Thomas McCrae (1901–04), and Osler's last Resident, Rufus I. Cole (1904–06). The careers of these men during their terms of service and later illustrate on the one hand the wisdom of Osler, who selected them, and on the other the growth-promoting influence of the duties and authority attached to the office.

Such an upper resident staff supported by interns and senior students, besides forming a full-time group of enthusiastic young internists for development under ideal conditions, afforded an excellent working force for

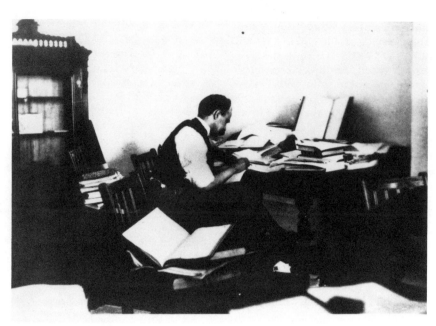

Fig 5. "Osler in Labor; A Book Is Born."
From the Archives, Johns Hopkins Medical Institutions

carrying on the routine of the wards, laboratories and outpatient department; this left the Physician-in-Chief and his visiting associates largely free for planning, standardizing, supervising and controlling the practice in the clinic; for teaching and for promoting original inquiries.

This system of "residency training" was soon adopted throughout the country and perhaps has had as great an influence on the development of America's outstanding position in the world of medicine as any other single event.

A second important feature of Osler's medical clinic was the introduction of more systematic courses of instruction in the practical methods of gathering data regarding disturbances of structure and function in the sick than had before that time been customary. The importance of careful history-taking and of accurate physical diagnosis had been, it is true, generally recognized; but the machinery of instruction in these forms of information accumulation had been inadequate in the vast majority of medical clinics and one of the first efforts of the new clinic consisted in planning and installing a better organization for this purpose.

The most distinctive advance made in instruction in technique was, however, the establishment of a systematic course in the application of the laboratory methods of chemistry, physics and biology to the study of patients. Students in their third year of medical school were not only taught the principles of these methods, but for two or three afternoons throughout the year were thoroughly drilled in the practical aspects of these methods, so that, when the course had been completed, each student had attained a real skill in the use of all the more important ways of examining clinically the blood, the stomach juice, the feces, the urine and the cerebrospinal fluid. Of the many contributions Osler made, the devel-

opment of the clinical laboratory and the thorough education of students in clinical laboratory work before entering upon their duties in the medical wards was one of the most important advances.

A third distinctive feature of the organization in Osler's clinic was the arrangement by which each medical student became for a considerable period a member of the group that did the day-to-day care of the patients in the hospital. Thus, each student in his third year, after having had instruction in history-taking and in the elements of clinical diagnosis, assisted, under the supervision and control of instructors, in recording histories and in making physical examinations in the outpatient department.

More important still, through the fourth year of the course, each third of the class acted successively for three months as "clinical clerks" in the medical clinic, giving their whole time to the medical wards. Thus, the medical staff was reinforced during the entire school year by 30 student assistants who under the eye of the resident staff took the histories of all new patients, assisted the interns in the making of the first physical examination, made all the clinical laboratory tests on these patients and accompanied their Chief on morning rounds.

On these rounds, the clinical clerk gave orally an epitome of the findings in the patient, watched the process of examination used by the Professor and participated at the bedside in discussion of the important aspects of the case. The student looked up recent articles on the subject and reported them at later ward rounds, followed the patient to the operating room if surgical procedures were indicated, watched the effects of the treatment employed in each patient assigned to him and kept in touch with him during convalescence at his home.

The knowledge that the history he registered and the results of the laboratory tests he made would become a part of the permanent records of the hospital, the feeling of responsibility he had when he realized that the diagnosis made and the treatment instituted were based in part upon facts accumulated by him, the personal relationship established between students and professor at the hospital and on delightful Saturday nights at the professor's home at One W. Franklin Street—all this combined to make the time of the clinical clerkship in Osler's clinic a period of rich experience and of intense stimulation never to be forgotten by any who passed through it.

The main teaching event of the week was the Saturday morning clinic in the Amphitheatre, where all the students of the 3rd and 4th years, the whole resident staff, and many visiting physicians of the hospital, physicians of the town and medical men from a distance were assembled. The clinical clerk was asked to tell this audience briefly from memory, unaided by notes, the main points of the history of the patient and to report upon the important laboratory and other findings.

The pupil-teacher thus grew accustomed to facing a large audience and to thinking and speaking on his feet, an admirable preparation for some of the contingencies of later professional life. All of these new approaches that Osler introduced now seem quite commonplace, but at that time they were revolutionary in scope, and the fact that they are still incorporated as principal features of current teaching programs indicates the enormity of Osler's contribution to clinical medicine and to medical education.

Osler understood human nature and loved it, despite its faults and its frailties. No chief ever secured in greater measure the good will and loyalty of his staff. Though he could be firm on occasion, he rarely found need to act as a strict disciplinarian. He was always cognizant of the good qualities of those about him, and, though not blind to their defects, he had learned that great lesson of successful management—that for most subordinates, a word of appreciation is of far greater value as a stimulus to good work than a volume of carping criticism. He possessed to an extraordinary degree the capacity of making you feel that he was interested in you and your personal welfare; to come into contact with him meant for most, the birth of a genuine affection for him.

OSLER'S INTEREST IN MEDICAL SOCIETIES AND OTHER ACTIVITIES

Wherever Osler went, he was active in organizing societies, encouraging his associates and assistants to work for the common good as well as for their own individual advancement. Osler played a role in the organization of the Association of American Physicians, the Laennec Society for the Study of Tuberculosis, the International Association of Medical Museums and many others. He founded in 1905 the Interurban Clinical Club that brought young internists from several Eastern sea-

board cities into very fruitful cooperation. He played a key role in organizing the Johns Hopkins Medical Society, the first meeting being held on Oct. 22, 1889.

A week later, the Journal Club—similar to the foreign periodical clubs that Osler had organized in Montreal and Philadelphia—was started. The object was to keep the staff informed of the work being done in every branch of medical science throughout the world. Current literature was reviewed, book notices written and many other subjects discussed with great enthusiasm. President Gilman was quick to recognize the importance of what was happening, and through his effort and that of others, the first number of the *Johns Hopkins Hospital Bulletin* was issued in December, 1889. Since that time the bulletin has been most important in bringing the work of the Hospital and the School of Medicine before the medical world. The Historical Club was also established at the same time, the prime movers being Drs. Osler, Billings and Welch.

Only those who knew Osler well could appreciate how much he missed the fine library of the College of Physicians in Philadelphia. In Baltimore, the Library of the Medical and Chirurgical Faculty was crumbling into disuse. At that time it possessed only a few hundred volumes which were kept in the basement of the Maryland Historical Society. The very mention of them "made one think of mold and dust." Osler volunteered to be on the Library Committee, and served on it vigorously until he

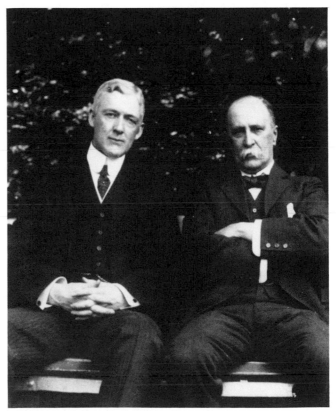

Fig 6. Osler with his successor as Professor of Medicine at Johns Hopkins, Lewellys F. Barker.

departed for England in 1905. It was largely through Osler's efforts that the Library came to life. He secured for it good quarters and increased its contents from the few hundred volumes to more than 15,000, helped to support it with his time and effort, as well as financially, and succeeded in getting a trained librarian.

Even after he left Baltimore, he maintained an interest in this Library. This was quite typical of the man. Everywhere he went he became completely dedicated to improving the local library, including the one at McGill, the Surgeon General's Library in Washington, the Johns Hopkins Hospital Library and numerous others. Throughout his life, he had a deep interest in books, and this aspect of his career was commented on by Dr. Welch as follows: "It may, I think, be safely predicted that history will preserve Osler's fame as a serious and scholarly student of medical history and as a bibliographer as only second to his repute as a great clinical teacher. Possibly being based more upon written record than upon tradition, it may be more enduring. But his interest in this matter arose not only from the mind, but from the heart. He was a passionate lover of books."

"It is hard for me," Osler wrote, "to speak of the value of libraries in terms which would not seem exaggerated. Books have been my delight . . . and from them I have received incalculable benefits. To study the phenomena of disease without books is to sail an uncharted sea; while to study books without patients is not to go to sea at all."

OSLER'S TEXTBOOK: THE PRINCIPLES AND PRACTICE OF MEDICINE

From September, 1890, to January, 1892, William Osler devoted most of his time to writing the *Principles and Practice of Medicine*. He was then 41 years old. Essentially uninterrupted periods of time were available to him since the hospital was operating smoothly under the guidance of his competent assistants, and the medical school had not yet opened because of the financial difficulties resulting from the failure of dividend payments from the Baltimore and Ohio Railroad in which much of the endowment of The Johns Hopkins University was invested. This task got underway in full swing in January, 1891.

Osler's textbook is credited with a major role in directing Rockefeller philanthropy into the field of research and education in medicine and public health. This came about through the activities of a layman, Frederick T. Gates, a Baptist minister who was one of Rockefeller's main advisers. Gates recalled the sequence of events as follows: "In the early summer of 1897, my interest in medicine was awakened by a . . . Minneapolis boy (Edon O. Huntingdon, a student at the College of Physicians and Surgeons at the time who had been in Gates' congregation in Minneapolis) who, in his loneliness in New York, used often to spend his weekends with us in Montclair. I determined as a result of my talks with this enthusiastic young man to make myself more intelligent on the whole subject of medicine, and at his suggestion I bought a copy

of Dr. Osler's *Principles and Practice of Medicine* . . . I read the whole book without skipping any of it. I speak of this not to commemorate my industry or intelligence, but to testify to Osler's charm, for it is one of the very few scientific books that are possessed of high literary quality. There was a fascination about the style itself that led me on and having once started, I found a hook in my nose that pulled me from page to page . . . until the whole of about a thousand large and closely printed pages brought me to the end . . .

"When I laid down this book, I began to realize how woefully neglected in all civilized countries and perhaps most of all in this country, has been the scientific study of medicine . . . it became clear to me that medicine could hardly hope to become a science until it should be endowed, and qualified men could give themselves to uninterrupted study and investigation on ample salary, entirely independent of practice."

Gates took this idea to Rockefeller and what has come out of it is common knowledge to all of us. It was a landmark in the development of the heroic age of modern medicine.

When the call to Oxford to become the Regius Professor came in 1905, Mrs. Osler urged her husband to accept it, knowing that the strain of the life in Baltimore had become altogether too great for Osler to bear much longer. His three valedictory addresses are among his most memorable productions. In them he reiterated his belief that scientific advances of the first rank must be made by the young or comparatively young men. He extolled the pleasures of the "student life" and urged the promotion of "unity, peace and concord" among the members of our profession. No physician who has dwelt among us more than William Osler deserves to be classed among the "immortals." His memory will be cherished during the generations to come.

(Dr. Osler was knighted by King George V on June 21, 1911, thus becoming Sir William Osler. He died on Dec. 23, 1919. Today, Med-Chi's Osler Hall and Towson's Osler Drive are named after him.)

REFERENCES

1. Barker, LF: Osler as Chief of a Medical Clinic. Johns Hopkins Hosp. Bull., 30: 189, 1919
2. Barker, LF: Osler in America: with Special Reference to the Baltimore Period. Can Med Assoc J, 33: 353, 1935
3. Cole, R, Welch, WH, McCrae, T: Special Meeting of the Johns Hopkins Historical Club, Presentation to the Hospital of Memorial Plaque of Sir William Osler. Bull Johns Hopkins Hosp, 41: 19, 1927
4. Cushing H: The Life of Sir William Osler. (2 vols.) Oxford: Clarenden Press, 1925
5. Harrell, GT: Osler's Practice. Bull. Hist. Med., 47: 545, 1973
6. McCrae, T: The Influence of William Osler on Medicine in America. Can Med Assoc J, 10: 102, 1920
7. Reid, EG: The Great Physician: A Short Life of Sir William Osler. New York: Oxford University Press, 1931
8. Thayer, WS: The Osler Clinic. Bull Johns Hopkins Hosp, 52: 101, 1933

2.

Henry Mills Hurd: The First Superintendent of The Johns Hopkins Hospital and the First Professor of Psychiatry

INTRODUCTION

Accounts of the early days of Johns Hopkins have been dominated by the achievements of the four doctors who organized the hospital departments: Osler in medicine, Halsted in surgery, Kelly in gynecology, and Welch in pathology. Another physician who played a very important role in the success of the hospital and the medical school was Henry Mills Hurd. Without his administrative skills, the four doctors would not have been able to accomplish so much. Henry Mills Hurd (Fig 1) set up an innovative type of hospital organization. He took the responsibility of establishing and maintaining the publications of the hospital including the *Bulletin of the Johns Hopkins Hospital* and the *Johns Hopkins Hospital Reports*. It was he who, with his great tact and ability to pull all of the various elements together effectively, was in large measure responsible for the phenomenal success of The Johns Hopkins Hospital and later the medical school in all of its relationships with the hospital. Possessing rare skill as an organizer, broad culture, literary attainments of high order, a thorough medical training, and a keen knowledge of men enabled him to make the institutions work smoothly and efficiently, both individually and together.

HURD'S PRE-BALTIMORE PERIOD

Henry M. Hurd was born on May 3, 1843 at Union City, Branch County, Michigan. His father, a pioneer physician, came to Michigan in 1834. Worn out by laborious practice amid the hardships of pioneer life in a malarious country, he died at the early age of 39. Hurd's mother remarried in 1848 and in 1854 the family moved to Galesburg, Illinois. In 1858 Hurd entered Knox College, where he spent two years. He then devoted a year to teaching in general studies and in 1861 entered the junior class of the University of Michigan, graduating in 1863. In the same year he began the study of medicine with his stepfather, who was a physician. Hurd attended lectures

Reprinted from the *Johns Hopkins Medical Journal* **148**: 135, 1981.

at the Rush Medical College and at the University of Michigan and graduated from the department of medicine and surgery of the University in 1866. The year following graduation he spent in New York in study and in hospital work. He then moved to Chicago where he did general practice for two years.

In 1870 he was appointed assistant physician to the Michigan Asylum for the Insane at Kalamazoo and entered that field of special medical practice in which he achieved much distinction. After eight years as assistant physician at the Asylum, he became assistant superintendent. On the opening of the Eastern Michigan Asylum at Pontiac in 1878, he became its first superintendent, a position which he occupied for 11 years. He was active in the Association of Medical Superintendents and it soon became evident that he had rare skills as an organizer and teacher.

During his period as superintendent of the Eastern Michigan Asylum many innovations occurred in the field of psychiatry: abolition of the use of restraints on patients, employment of the insane, extension of the system of night nursing, development of the "cottage plan" and introduction of home comforts into the dull, unattractive institutional life of previous years. Of all of these important changes he was an enthusiastic advocate. Henry M. Hurd contributed as much as anyone in that generation of alienists in the United States to the rapid growth of progressive methods in the care of the insane and the rapid advances in American psychiatry. His philanthropic instincts, his compassion and his keen insight into the needs of the insane, coupled with his skills as a physician, made him an ideal asylum superintendent. His personal enthusiasm for the work infused in his staff the same tireless energy which he exhibited, unified them and created an outstanding institution. It was these rare qualities that led to his appointment as the first superintendent at Johns Hopkins.

In 1881 Hurd visited Europe for travel and investigation of psychiatry on the European continent. His writings on various aspects of mental medicine grew in volume and were of a high order. Numerous papers appeared in the *American Journal of Insanity* and were well

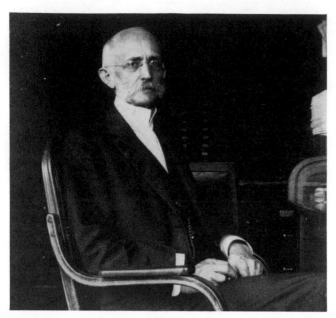

Fig 1. Henry Mills Hurd—Superintendent, The Johns Hopkins Hospital, 1889–1911 and Professor of Psychiatry, The Johns Hopkins University School of Medicine, 1889–1911.

From the Alan M. Chesney Medical Archives, The Johns Hopkins Medical Institutions.

received. His annual reports as superintendent of the Eastern Michigan Asylum were written in a masterly and finished style and clearly indicated the later skills he showed as editor of the *Bulletin of the Johns Hopkins Hospital* and the *Johns Hopkins Hospital Reports.* Hurd was a vice president of the 9th International Medical Congress. One of his most scholarly presentations was his presidential address in 1889 before the Alumni Association of the Medical Department of the University of Michigan on "The Mental Hygiene of Physicians."

HIS PUBLICATIONS RELATING TO PSYCHIATRY

During Hurd's period in Michigan he wrote about various aspects of the insane and their management. In 1881 he published a paper on "Recent Judicial Decisions in Michigan Relative to Insanity" and in 1882 "A Plea for Systematic Therapeutical, Clinical and Statistical Studies" in which he carefully analyzed the methods employed in the various asylums and clearly pointed out where improvements might be inaugurated: "Much of the present statistical information contained in the published reports of the institutions for the insane is unsatisfactory. There are tables enough, but they lack uniformity, precision in statement and practical utility . . .

"In this earnest plea for more systematic, therapeutical, clinical and statistical inquiries, I would not be understood as criticizing the thorough work now done in connection with asylums. I merely attempted to point out the necessity for further progress and have suggested methods which would tend to increase the efficiency of asylum work." In 1882–83 Hurd's publications

included "Practical Suggestions Relative to the Treatment of Insanity" and "The Treatment of Periodic Insanity."

At a convention held in Pontiac in January 1883 Hurd gave an address on "The Hereditary Influence of Alcoholic Indulgence upon the Production of Insanity." His views, published almost a century ago, are of interest:

> I have endeavored to show that inebriety in parents is a frequent cause of insanity in their children. Because drunkenness produces a transient insanity, even in a healthy brain; chronic drunkenness produces organic brain disease, bringing in their train impairment of the memory, inactivity of the reason, a weakening of the will, and a loss of the natural affections; also moral perversions and vicious propensities, and finally unmistakable diseases of the mind and nervous system—all of which are capable of transmission in children.
>
> That the children of inebriet parents inherit diseases such as epilepsy, hysteria, chorea and idiocy, or if not actual diseases, nervous systems which are abnormally responsive to every form of disturbing influence and are easily disoriented.

In 1883 Hurd discussed his views concerning the responsibilities of the State for the care of insane patients in an article entitled "Future Provisions for the Insane in Michigan":

> I would reiterate the conviction that it is the duty of the state to continue to care for her insane in the state asylums: that no consideration of false economy should prevent her from doing everything which can be done for the comfort and restoration of every insane person. If he requires the restraint and seclusion of an asylum for the dangerous insane he should have it. If he requires curative treatment in a hospital, or suffers from a form of disease which calls for constant nursing, he should have that. If his welfare would be promoted by giving him labor, the liberty of home and a manner of life nearly resembling that of a private family he should receive them. No money should be wasted upon buildings, surroundings or care. Sufficient, however, should be expended to render each unfortunate as comfortable as his condition will permit. Anything less than this is unworthy of a great state like Michigan.

It was in June of 1889 that he was offered the position of director of The Johns Hopkins Hospital. When Hurd came to Baltimore to visit the hospital, one of the trustees from the Eastern Michigan Asylum at Pontiac came with him with the intention of urging Hurd to decline the invitation. After this trustee had met the Johns Hopkins trustees and had visited the hospital, he turned to Hurd and said: "My object in coming with you was to see that you returned to Michigan but I've changed my mind. If they offer you this position and you do not accept it you will make the mistake of your life."

THE BALTIMORE PERIOD

Hurd was appointed superintendent of The Johns Hopkins Hospital in June 1889 (Fig 2) and assumed his duties on August 1, at which time President Gilman, who had acted as director of the hospital since the preceding

July 2, 1889

My dear Dr. Hurd,

I was very glad to get your telegram yesterday just before the Executive Committee met, and today we shall herald your appointment. Mr. King has been absent from home most of the time since you were here and it is quite possible that a letter from you has reached him, or is waiting for him. In any case the others of us are eager to let it be publically known that you are coming. Allow me now to express once more the satisfaction that this appointment gives to all who are acquainted with it— and let me say to Mrs. Hurd and to you that I am sure you will find Baltimore a delightful residence. It will give Mrs. Gilman and me the greatest pleasure to be of service to you when you come. I have been lodging in the Hospital for a week and have become familiar with its works and ways. Now I hope soon to go away and Dr. Osler will have control during July. As far as possible, we have deferred until your arrival—*Regulations*. We want you to make the rules, in accordance with your best judgment.

Yours with high regards,

Daniel C. Gilman

Fig. 2.   Letter of Hurd's appointment as Superintendent of The Johns Hopkins Hospital.
From the Alan M. Chesney Medical Archives, The Johns Hopkins Medical Institutions.

February and Dr. John Shaw Billings who had been medical advisor to the Board of Trustees for 12 years, terminated their connection with the hospital. Now Hurd would have his opportunity to display his talents in a hospital for patients suffering from a broad variety of ailments rather than simply mental ills. Hurd was destined to establish in his new position not only a unique new hospital in terms of organization and functional efficiency, but also the most harmonious relationship between the hospital and the new Johns Hopkins University School of Medicine, which opened its doors four years later.[1] His wise counsel, his broad viewpoint and his tact in large measure were responsible for the continuous cordial and close relations that were established between the medical school and the hospital. Hurd's standard of excellence in the preparation of his annual reports was outstanding and the history of The Johns Hopkins Hospital is succinctly reported in this yearly record. In these reports, one has a carefully constructed record of the events which took place as the hospital evolved into the renowned institution that it became. The staff that Hurd worked with was innovative (Fig 4).

HURD'S ANNUAL REPORTS

The First Report

Hurd submitted his first report (for the period May 1889–January 31, 1890) on the initial 7½ months of the hospital's function. First he discussed the organizational

[1] Hurd was also made Professor of Psychiatry in October 1889 (Fig 3).

Oct. 12, 1889

Dear Sir,

At a meeting of the Trustees held on Monday last you were invited to hold a professorship in the University while you continue in your present station at the Hospital. The title affixed to the resolution was "Professor of the Treatment of Mental Diseases," but I understand from you that Psychiatry would be more suitable and I will ask that the minute be so amended. It was not expected that any salary would be attached to the office.

Yours Sincerely

D. C. Gilman
Pres. JHU

Dr. H. M. Hurd, Superintendent,
Johns Hopkins Hospital

Fig 3.   Letter of Hurd's appointment as Professor of Psychiatry.
From the Alan M. Chesney Medical Archives, The Johns Hopkins Medical Institutions.

structure which differed in some essential features from that of other general hospitals in the United States:

The service was divided into three distinct departments: medical, surgical and gynecological, each under a responsible chief with continuous service. These chiefs were non-resident but arrangements were made for them to give as much time to the work of the hospital as the patient needs and other responsibilities demanded [Fig 4].

Each department had a responsible resident physician who had a long and varied experience in a general hospital and was abundantly able to fill the place of the chief of the department whenever he was absent. Each resident physician had a staff of assistants who gave aid in case taking, surgical operations, clinical notes, examination of laboratory specimens and dispensary work as well. The resident and assistant resident physicians, surgeons and gynecologists were resident in the hospital.

The dispensary had a chief who directed and arranged the work of the different departments, and each department in turn was under the special direction and control of a responsible head who took care of the work and had continuous service. Each head of the dispensary department had as many assistants as the proper work of his department required.

The nursing work of the hospital was under the charge of the superintendent of nursing, who also acted as the principal of the training school. She had the responsibility of the management of the nurses' home and the instruction of nurses. She selected and accepted the probationers, prescribed courses of study and arranged duties. In essence, she supervised all nursing work.

The purchase and delivery of provision and the cooking, distribution and serving of food were placed in the hands of a purveyor, L. Winder Emory, who was made responsible for all of these duties.

The care of the rooms and buildings and the oversight of the work of the laundry were the responsibility of the matron who was charged with the duty of purchasing bedding, dry goods, clothing, house hold and laundry supplies. In addition to these various individuals, there was a comptroller of accounts who supervised the receipt

HOSPITAL STAFF.
Superintendent:
HENRY M. HURD, M.D.

Physician:	*Resident Physician:*
WILLIAM OSLER, M.D.	HENRY A. LAFLEUR, M.D.

Assistant Resident Physicians:

HARRY TOULMIN, M.D.,	D. MEREDITH REESE, M.D.

Surgeon:	*Resident Surgeon:*
WILLIAM S. HALSTED, M.D.	F. J. BROCKWAY, M.D.

Assistant Resident Surgeon:
GEORGE E. CLARKE, M.D.

Gynecologist and Obstetrician:	*Resident Gynecologist:*
HOWARD A. KELLY, M.D.	HUNTER ROBB, M.D.

Assistant Resident Gynecologists:

W. W. FARR, M.D.	A. L. GHRISKEY, M.D.

Pathologist:	*Associate in Pathology:*
WILLIAM H. WELCH, M.D.	W. T. COUNCILMAN, M.D.

Assistant in Bacteriology and Hygiene:
ALEXANDER C. ABBOTT, M.D.

OUT-PATIENT DEPARTMENT.
Chief of the Dispensary:
WILLIAM S. HALSTED, M.D.

1. *Department of General Medicine:*
   WILLIAM OSLER, M.D.
2. *Department of Diseases of Children:*
   WILLIAM OSLER, M.D., and W. D. BOOKER, M.D.
3. *Department of Nervous Diseases:*
   WILLIAM OSLER, M.D., and H. M. THOMAS, M.D.
4. *Department of General Surgery:*
   W. S. HALSTED, M.D., assisted by J. M. T. FINNEY, M.D.
5. *Department of Genito-Urinary Diseases:*
   W. S. HALSTED, M.D., and JAMES BROWN, M.D.
6. *Department of Gynecology:*
   H. A. KELLY, M.D., assisted by HUNTER ROBB, M.D.
7. *Department of Ophthalmology and Otology:*
   S. THEOBALD, M.D., and R. L. RANDOLPH, M.D.
8. *Department of Laryngology:*
   JOHN N. MACKENZIE, M.D.
9. *Department of Dermatology:*
   R. B. MORISON, M.D.

MISS ISABEL A. HAMPTON, *Superintendent of Nurses and Principal of the Training School.*

L. WINDER EMORY, *Purveyor.*
MISS RACHEL A. BONNER, *Matron.*

STANLEY HUTCHINS, *Comptroller of Accounts.*

Fig 4. Staff, Johns Hopkins Hospital, 1889. First Report of the Superintendent of The Johns Hopkins Hospital from May 15, 1889 to January 31, 1890, The Johns Hopkins Press, 1890, p. 4.

of money and the payment of bills; an apothecary, who purchased medicines and prepared and delivered prescriptions; a supervisor of grounds who looked after all the outside work; and an engineer who had the care and oversight of the engines, boilers, filters, pumping apparatus, machinery, warming and ventilating apparatus, water tanks, sewers, water closets, laboratories, steam cooking apparatus, water, gas, electrical and steam distribution.

Upon the opening of the hospital in May 1889, Welch had already been appointed pathologist, William Osler physician-in-chief and William S. Halsted acting surgeon and chief of the dispensary; Henry A. LeFleur was resident physician and Dr. F. J. Brockway, resident surgeon; with H. A. Toulmin, assistant physician and George E. Clark assistant surgeon. In June, Howard A. Kelly was appointed gynecologist and obstetrician and Hunter Robb, resident gynecologist. Hurd pointed out that Gilman's services as an organizer had been of great value. By an unusual occurrence of events, it was possible for him to bring the university idea into hospital management and to give to the inauguration of the hospital enterprise a breadth and liberality which it might have lacked had it been exclusively organized by a purely hospital officer.

Beginning on January 6, 1890, courses of postgraduate instruction in medicine, surgery and gynecology were inaugurated. Daily lectures were given in the clinical amphitheatre and clinics in medicine, surgery and gynecology were given three times a week, utilizing the wealth of clinical cases afforded by the hospital and the dispensary.

On September 1, 1889 the hospital formally assumed responsibility for the pathology laboratory under the direction of Dr. Welch; the work of the laboratory had previously been carried on under university auspices, although the medical school had not opened. The clinical laboratory was under the direction of William Osler. Analyses of blood were available not only for routine determinations of its constitution, but also "to ascertain the presence of malarial or other organisms and parasites." In addition, there was a hygienic laboratory which was equipped and made ready for practical work under the direction of Billings and Abbott. During the first year its work was confined to meteorological observations, the study of ventilation, the analysis of ground air and the bacterial examination of water.

The nurses' training school was formally opened in October 1889 and a full report of this occasion was published in the first number of the *Johns Hopkins Hospital Bulletin* (December 1, 1889). After a short address by the president of the Board of Trustees, Mr. Francis T. King, Miss Isabel Hampton, the superintendent of nurses, spoke at length on "The Aims of the Johns Hopkins Hospital Training School for Nurses." She was followed by Dr. Hurd who took as his theme "The Relation of the Training School for Nurses to the Johns Hopkins Hospital." In his address, Hurd spoke of the influence of The Johns Hopkins Hospital as follows:

From its inception in the mind of its founder and the subsequent elaboration of the idea by the trustees so wisely chosen by him—during the preparation of its plans and in the whole course of its erection—from the first foundation stone to the last tile upon the roof it has constantly been fulfilling its mission. It has all along stimulated hospital construction to an unprecedented degree. From a personal knowledge of hospitals east and west, I do not hesitate to say that there's not a single hospital in this broad land which has not felt the influence of its construction, either directly or indirectly, or has not been energized by its example to make more perfect provision for the care and treatment of sick people. It has taught hospitals the practical application of the laws of hygiene to heating, ventilation, house drainage, sewerage and hospital construction in general. It has commanded attention to the importance of sunlight and air space and to the absolute necessity of an abundant supply of pure air to each individual—a supply properly tempered to meet the varying conditions of summer heat and winter cold. The cardinal principle of the hospital has been to give the sick the most perfect hygienic surrounding attainable in a city. It has so prepared the way for better provision for the comfort of the sick, whether rich or poor, that the public now demand it. So great in fact has been the force of its example for good, I do not hesitate to say that had the hospital never received or treated a single patient, the work it has already accomplished in showing the way to better hospital construction would have fully justified the expenditure of every dollar spent.

The Second Report

In his report for 1890 (for the year ending January 31, 1891) Hurd referred to the work of the hospital among the poor of Baltimore and emphasized the fact that care must be taken to see that people who are financially able should not be given free treatment.

It is evident, however, that some persons who apply for gratuitous advice and prescriptions in the dispensary and free beds in the hospital are not objects of charity and should not receive the benefits of the institution. . . After a careful review of the whole subject I am strongly of the opinion that the time has come when an arrangement should be made with the Charity Organization Society of Baltimore whereby all suspected cases may receive a prompt investigation. It demoralizes any man to receive as a gift what he is able to pay for wholly or in part. . . In addition to the evil effect upon the community of indiscriminate charity there is also danger of doing injustice to the profession of medicine, which numbers among its members so many persons actively engaged in charitable work. Neither the hospital nor dispensary should interfere with the sources of support of these men by affording free medical or surgical treatment to those who can pay for it.

In this report Hurd also made reference to the training school for nurses. "Each month demonstrates the value and necessity of the work of the training school for nurses. The school is developing a new field of usefulness for the young women of Baltimore and Maryland and is growing in popular favor. The dignity and the importance of the profession of nursing were never so well appreciated in this community as now."

The Third Report

In his report for 1891 (year ending January 31, 1892) Hurd describes the graduation of the first class of nurses. Among them were Mary E. Gross (Mrs. John M.T. Finney); Georgie M. Evans, who became superintendent of the Garfield Hospital, Washington, D.C.; M. Adelaide Nutting, who became superintendent of nurses in the Johns Hopkins training school and then professor in the teacher's training school at Columbia University, New York City; and Susan C. Reed (who became the wife of William Sydney Thayer).

The Fifth Report

In his report for 1893 Hurd described the ward for black patients: "The colored ward of which mention was made in the last report has also been erected during the year and is now ready for the reception of patients. It consists of two stories surmounted by a half story." Hurd also referred to important changes in the library which was one of his principal interests:

The opening of the medical school and the increased demand for medical books on the part of medical students have rendered it desirable to pay special attention to the library of the hospital. Miss Thies who has received a careful training in the Enoch Pratt Free Library has accordingly been employed at the joint expense of the university and hospital to catalog and arrange the collections which have grown rapidly during the year. . . . It seems eminently proper to refer to the great advantages which the medical officers of the hospital and the students in our medical courses have derived from the proximity of the library of the Surgeon-General's Office. The enlightened policy of this library, whereby valuable books of reference otherwise unobtainable are loaned to the hospital under satisfactory guarantees against loss, cannot be too highly praised.

The Sixth Report

In the report of 1894 reference was made to several important new developments. It was decided by the trustees, after a thorough consideration of the subject by the medical board, to organize a pathological department and to give it an equal standing in the medical staff by appointing a resident pathologist and an assistant resident pathologist. Dr. Simon Flexner, associate in pathology in the medical school, was appointed resident pathologist and L.F. Barker, associate in anatomy, was appointed assistant resident pathologist. This was the first instance where similar officers were appointed with staff standing in connection with any hospital in the United States.

The outpatient-obstetrical service was placed under the immediate charge of Dr. J. Whitridge Williams, the associate in obstetrics in the medical school, who was appointed assistant obstetrician to the Johns Hopkins Hospital. George W. Dobbin became an additional assistant in the gynecological department to be responsible for this work in the dispensary and in attending patients in their homes.

It was during this year that Miss Isabel Hampton, who had been superintendent of the training school for nurses since its opening, tendered her resignation. Miss M. Adelaide Nutting, who had been her assistant for the previous two years, was made acting superintendent and on December 1 appointed superintendent and given leave of absence for eight months, from February 1, to visit other hospitals and training schools in this country and Europe.

In the report for 1894 one finds also the first reference to the Colored Orphan Asylum: "By the will of the founder of the hospital, the erection and maintenance of a colored orphan asylum was enjoined, and provision was made for its support out of the income of the hospital. A tract of land on Remington Avenue and King Street was purchased as a permanent site for the Johns Hopkins Colored Orphan Asylum and the children were removed to their new home."

In the report of 1896 Hurd made reference to the new clinical laboratory: "By an unexpected gift of $10,000 from a generous donor whose name we are not privileged to mention it has been practicable to erect a large and convenient clinical laboratory for the use of the hospital and medical school between the amphitheatre and the dispensary. This portion of the building which was formerly one story in height has now been raised to three stories and the additional room furnishes ample accommodation for medical classes."

Also in the 1896 report Hurd mentions the gift of Mr. William Wallace Spence of a reproduction of Thorwaldsen's Statue of Christ: "One of the most noteworthy and appropriate gifts which the hospital has ever received is a reproduction of Thorwaldsen's celebrated Statue of Christ, by Stein of Copenhagen, which has been placed in the rotunda through the liberality of William Wallace Spence of Baltimore." A full account of the exercises held at the unveiling of this statue appeared in the *Bulletin of the Johns Hopkins Hospital* for January 1897.

The Eighth Report

The report for 1897 contained the details of a most interesting landmark in the history of the institutions. In that year the first class of the Johns Hopkins University School of Medicine received their degrees and the 12 students who stood highest in their class were eligible for positions in the hospital. Dr. Hurd, in his report, spoke as follows:

> Beginning with the first of September 1897 twelve members of the graduating class of the Johns Hopkins Medical School are in future to be appointed resident medical officers. These positions are divided into three groups and serve four months in each department of hospital service, the service being determined by lot. In this manner each resident medical officer secures four month's service in medicine, surgery and gynecology.
>
> In addition to these resident medical officers, the resident physician, surgeon and gynecologist each is supplied with a first and second assistant who are appointed from those who have had previous hospital experience. The working of this plan has thus far been satisfactory.

In accordance with this arrangement the following named persons were appointed resident medical officers: Dr. G. L. Hunner, J. F. Mitchell, O. B. Pancoast, L. P. Hamburger, Thomas R. Brown, E. L. Opie, R. P. Strong, W. G. MacCallum, W. S. Davis, I. P. Lyon, C. A. Penrose and Mary S. Packard. The rotation system was abandoned after a few years.

Also in this annual report Hurd listed the scholarships and honorable mention in the training school for nurses. He spoke as follows: "The experience of another year has demonstrated the feasibility and desirability of extending the course of training of nurses from two to three years. The changes in the course of study have enabled nurses to spend more time in learning the fundamental branches of their work and the shortening of hours of duty has enabled them to bring greater freshness and vigor of mind to their studies and regular duties. The result has been to improve the standard of nursing and to give a greater state of efficiency to the school than it has previously had."

The Twelfth Report

In 1901 Hurd mentioned a substantial addition to the public gynecological ward: "During the year, in order to furnish additional accommodations for patients recovering from gynecological operations and to secure facilities for an examining room and a laboratory in connection with this ward, Dr. Kelly with great liberality gave to the hospital the sum of $10,000. The sum has been expended in building on the north side of the public gynecological ward a large two-story annex which affords accommodation for 12 patients."

The Fourteenth Report

The report of 1903 (for the year ending January 31, 1904) was a very important one. On February 7, 1904 the annual income for the hospital was decimated as a result of the great Baltimore fire. (As it often requires six months to assemble the data of the preceding year, the annual report appeared about the middle of the following year. Hence the Baltimore fire of February 1904 was mentioned in the report for 1903.) Hurd addressed himself to the Board of Trustees of The Johns Hopkins Hospital as follows:

> Gentlemen, The close of the past year has been marked by the most serious calamity which has befallen the hospital during its existence. On the morning of February 7 almost before it had been possible to sum up the results of the operation of the previous fiscal year which closed February 1, a general conflagration swept over the city of Baltimore and proved most disastrous to the real and lease-hold property of the hospital. During the fire 64 stores, warehouses and office buildings, widely scattered in the business portion of the city representing an assessed valuation of more than a million and a quarter dollars, were destroyed, entailing a loss of income for at least two years of about $120,000. A portion of this loss was made up by insurance. In accordance, however, with the policy of the hospital, an insurance had not been secured against a total loss, but merely for a sum which had been deemed sufficient to provide for rebuilding in case of partial destruction by fire. The results, however, prove that such insurance was wholly inadequate to repair the effects of a widespread calamity and a loss of capital funds of between $300,000 and $400,000 resulted."

For several weeks thereafter great anxiety was felt lest it should become necessary to curtail seriously the work of the hospital by closing wards and cutting down the staff of nurses and employees. However, through the generosity of Mr. John D. Rockefeller, of New York, who had familiarized himself thoroughly with the work of the hospital, its financial standing, and its loss of income and capital, a half million dollars had been placed at the disposal of the trustees to repair these losses and to enable the work to go on without diminution. Never was assistance more timely to the institution.

That same year brought another generous donation to the hospital: "Through the liberality of Mr. Henry Phipps of Pittsburgh, the sum of $20,000 has been given to the trustees of the hospital to increase the facilities of the outpatient department for the study and treatment of tubercular patients. It was the wish of the donor that one-half of this sum should be used to construct a separate dispensary for tubercular patients so as to render it possible to segregate these from other patients [Fig 5]. It was his further wish that the remaining $10,000 should be so invested that the income may serve to promote special work and investigation."

The Fifteenth Report

In his report of 1904 Hurd was able to describe the new clinical building: "The amphitheatre and surgical building to which reference was made in the last report were completed and made ready for occupancy in October 1904. The basement of the building has been fitted up for a genito-urinary clinic under the charge of Dr. H. H. Young."

The new surgical building and clinical amphitheatre were formally opened on October 5, 1904. Ap-

propriate addresses were made by Henry D. Harlan, president of the Board of Trustees; Dr. Lewis A. Stimson of New York; Dr. T. Clifford Allbutt of Cambridge, England; Dr. A. Jacobi of New York; and Dr. D. C. Gilman, ex-president of the Johns Hopkins University. At the unveiling of the tablet in memory of Dr. Jesse W. Lazear who lost his life while serving on the Yellow Fever Commission of Walter Reed, addresses were made by Dr. James Carroll of the United States Army, another member of that commission and by Dr. William S. Thayer.

Also that year the new Phipps Tuberculosis Dispensary was opened with appropriate ceremonies on the 21st of February. Short addresses were given by Mr. Henry Phipps, Dr. William Osler, Dr. H. M. Biggs of New York City and Dr. Henry Barton Jacobs, president of the Laennec Society, a society for the study of tuberculosis. Mr. Phipps subsequently gave $5,000 to be used for the purchase of books and apparatus and for the endowment of the dispensary.

The Sixteenth Report

In the report of 1905 Hurd refers to the fact that the departure of Professor Osler wrenched the heartstrings of the Hopkins family: "In May last Dr. William Osler, who had filled the position of physician-in-chief to the hospital since its opening in 1889, resigned to accept the position of professor of medicine at the University of Oxford. This closed a most faithful, efficient and active service on the part of Professor Osler covering a period of 16 years." Hurd then referred to the fact that to fill the vacancy occasioned by this resignation, Dr. Lewellys F. Barker of the University of Chicago, once an intern and later a resident pathologist in the hospital and for several years a teacher in the medical school, was appointed physician-in-chief and Dr. William S. Thayer, for many years resident physician at the hospital and former associate in medicine, was appointed associate professor. It

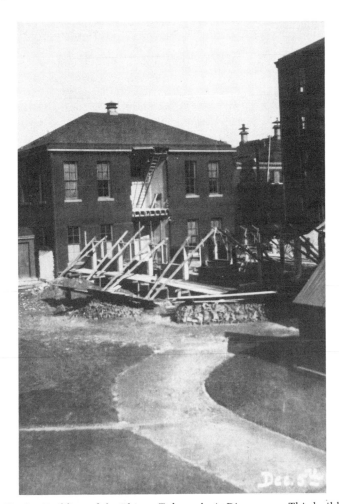

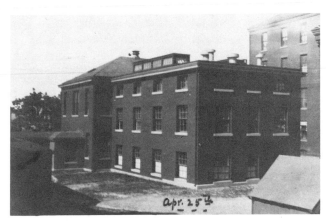

Fig 5. Building of the Phipps Tuberculosis Dispensary. This building, located on Monument Street next to the Pathological Building, occupied the area where there were stables for horses originally. In October, 1908 Mr. Phipps authorized an addition to the Tuberculosis Dispensary. This addition took the form of a three-story building extending south from the original two-story structure. The work started on May 30, 1908 and was completed on April 30, 1909. **A.** Photograph taken on December 5, 1908. **B.** Photograph taken on April 25, 1909.

was made clear in a letter written to Lewellys F. Barker on March 4, 1905 that his appointment was not entirely pleasing to Osler:

> The faculty seems to be unanimous in favor of you as my successor. You may have heard something from Welch about this, as I was not at the meeting and only heard last eve of the action. Naturally I was placed in a most awkward position. Thayer has done so much 1st class work and is such a good fellow that it seemed cruel to pass him by; but the general feeling was not towards him in the faculty or on the Hospital board and while I might have perhaps forced it, had I felt more strongly, everything came round to a choice between you and [George] Dock [Professor of Medicine at the University of Michigan School of Medicine]. I suppose the governors will act shortly. The important thing will be to make Thayer comfortable and you can help in this. He has behaved splendidly and we must do everything possible for him. This is only a preliminary note—there will be hosts of things to confer about . . . I am taking Plato's advice and sitting under a wall until the storm is over. . . .

OTHER NEW BUILDINGS

During Hurd's term as superintendent of the hospital, many capital improvements were made. In 1905, by the will of the late Mrs. Harriet Lane Johnston of Washington, a home for invalid children from the State of Maryland had been established with an ample endowment to be known as the Harriet Lane Home for Invalid Children of Baltimore City. The trustees of the home deemed it wise to establish a working relation between the proposed institution and some well-organized hospital. After careful consideration on the part of the trustees of The Johns Hopkins Hospital and of the Home for Invalid Children, an arrangement was made whereby the Home was placed as a children's hospital for medical and surgical cases upon the grounds of The Johns Hopkins Hospital. The hospital agreed to provide a site for the building free of charge, furnish heat and light and assume the maintenance and nursing of the children at a specified price. The Home was to remain under the charge of the Board of Trustees as established by its founder and an agreement was made to ensure a harmonious relationship between the two institutions.

In the Superintendent's Report for 1906, which was made by Rupert Norton in Dr. Hurd's absence, he described the Marburg bequest. Mr. William A. Marburg, Mr. Albert Marburg, Mr. Theodore Marburg and the Misses Marburg gave to the hospital a sum of $100,000 in memory of their brother, the later Charles Marburg. The money was expended in the erection of a four-story private ward called the Marburg. This building enabled the hospital to handle more private patients than had hitherto been possible and it served this function until 1976 when the new Nelson wing was dedicated.

In June 1908 Mr. Henry Phipps gave the money for the erection of the Phipps Psychiatric Clinic, representing the largest gift that the hospital had received since its opening. The trustees were able to secure Dr. Adolf Meyer of New York as director of the new Phipps Clinic. In his report for 1910, Hurd made the following statement in regard to the development of the psychiatric department: "The professor of psychiatry, Dr. Adolf Meyer, has been appointed psychiatrist to the hospital and although the psychiatric clinic is not ready for occupation, Dr. Meyer has been able to do very effective work in connection with the hospital wards and the outpatient department. It seems fortunate that prior to the opening of the Phipps Psychiatric Clinic it has been possible to utilize his services in connection with various charitable agencies in Baltimore. There is reason to anticipate when the clinic is opened that these relations may be productive of great good by promoting cooperation with the clinic on the part of many charitable organizations."

DR. HURD AND HIS RELATION TO THE HOSPITAL STAFF

When The Johns Hopkins Hospital opened, there was no medical school from which to draw interns, and they consequently were continually recruited from all parts of the United States and Canada. This system had many advantages. Nearly every man came from a different school. They compared notes, told one another of the methods in vogue in the school or hospital from which they had come, and thus each man soon became fairly familiar with what was being done in medicine over all the country.

Some of these interns had had several years of training or by instinct immediately dropped into line. There were others, young and immature, who needed careful and persistent supervision. Dr. Hurd was a past master in stimulating the house men to do their best. As Cullen put it: "He did not mollycoddle them in the least. This good old state of Maryland is celebrated for its Maryland or beaten biscuits and it is a well known fact that the more they are hammered in the making the better they are. Dr. Hurd, with his keen perception, soon learned this fact and he applied the principle to good purpose in his training of these men."

Hurd, who interviewed the incoming group of interns, had a very apt story which he related on that occasion. He recalled these sessions as follows:

> When the men who had been selected for the position of interns at the Johns Hopkins Hospital out of the first graduating class of the Johns Hopkins Medical School (1897) came on duty, they found an organization for their work which had already been in successful operation for about eight years. They were bright enterprising students who were peculiarly receptive to all new ideas and much inclined to adopt them with little regard to their bearing upon the former routine of hospital service. As all were men of marked ability some of the innovations which they wished to inaugurate were improvements without doubt and made for better service, but the general effect of their combined action caused confusion and a lack of coordination in the different departments. In fact since the changes of hours of duty and general methods of work caused so much trouble, it was felt that some steps were needed to check a similar individualism on the part of equally active and zealous young men who were to enter hospital service in succeeding years. After the interns for the coming year had been appointed I called them into

my office for a friendly talk about their duty and without referring to the embarrassments of the past year, I rehearsed the tale of the small boy who while on his way to school trudging through the deep snow was overtaken by a gentleman, in a fine turnout with a dashing span of horses, who kindly asked him to ride with him. The invitation was joyfully accepted and the boy was soon making fine progress when the idea occurred to him that the driver of the horse was not driving them properly. He knew that he could drive them much better and suggested a transfer of the reins to him in order that he might display his superior skill. To his great surprise and discomfort the host stopped his sleigh and gravely, but decidedly, informed him that an invitation to ride did not carry with it the privilege of driving and that he might get out if he thought otherwise. I added that it gave the management of the hospital much pleasure to know that they were willing to ride with us during the coming year and I felt sure that such a journey together would be of great service to them and to the hospital, but I deemed it my duty to say frankly that the management of the hospital must do the driving and would continue to do so in the future as it had in the past."

OTHER INNOVATIONS

Dr. Hurd was very instrumental in starting journal clubs at The Johns Hopkins Hospital and published an article on the subject in the *American Journal of Insanity* for 1892. In this article, he gave an enthusiastic evaluation of such clubs and detailed how they should be conducted. He felt that the work must be made obligatory and a part of the regular routine of the institution, not being pushed aside by any trivial matters. The same rule which governed excuses from any regular professional duty should govern all absences from the journal club.

A definite hour, reasonably certain to be free from interruption, should be selected and rigidly adhered to. Such an hour should not be at the close of an exhausting day's work. The proceedings should be informal and free discussion should be encouraged. The journals studied should have the widest possible range, including French, German and Italian journals.

The work should be thoroughly supervised by the superintendent of the hospital or some person whom he might select. Whoever took charge of the club should prepare himself to sum up each subject and present its practical bearings upon the better study or the better treatment of patients.

Hurd listed the advantages of such a journal club: first, it develops a spirit of professional study among the members of the hospital. The spirit of investigation and inquiry is easily lost unless special efforts are made to develop it. This is particularly true where routine duties constantly press themselves upon the attention. Second, it provides for a systematic acquisition of knowledge by division of labor and the least possible waste of time on the part of each person concerned. Hurd pointed out that this was an age of cooperation in literary work. Library and subject catalogs were undertaken by associated laborers and the enterprises which would be impossible to an individual became practical to the many. He mentioned the success of H. H. Bancroft's gigantic historical enterprises. The work which he finished with the aid of collaborators would have consumed 400 years of individual effort. The medical literature was becoming so vast that each student could not read the good, the bad and the indifferent. The grain should be winnowed before it was gathered into storehouses. Third, it supplies a common field of study where the members of the staff may meet for contact of mind with mind. It also affects the readier training and more rapid integration of new members of the staff. Young men came to the hospital fresh from medical schools with a keen zest for scientific work. This should be stimulated and habits of regular study of what is going on in research should be acquired as speedily as practical. The journal club also contributes materially to the unification of the staff which may have been brought together from different schools of medicine.

In addition to all his other duties, Hurd personally answered all inquiries addressed to the hospital, as illustrated by the following interesting letter:

Your letter of 12th (Oct. 12, 1892) is received. This Hospital is provided with two classes of wards. The Open or Public wards where a large number of patients are received for treatment in adjoining beds in the same room. In these wards the rates for non-resident patients are $5.00 per week.

In our private wards, where each patient has a single room and the luxuries and comforts of a first class hotel, a definite price is fixed for each room. These prices vary from $15.00 to $35.00 per week, depending on the size of the room, location etc.

These charges do not include the services of an Eye, Ear, Throat or Skin specialist nor do they include the expense of a surgical operation. No consultation fee is charged for patients who come to the Hospital. Patients, however, who merely come for consultation only are referred to the heads of our different departments at their offices in the City. For example, in case of diseases of women, reference is made to Dr. H. A. Kelly, 905 N. Charles St.; in Surgery, Dr. W. S. Halsted, corner Dolphin St. and Eutaw Place; and in Medicine, including nervous trouble, Dr. W. Osler at the Mt. Vernon Hotel.

I think your better way will be to write me definitely as to your wife's symptoms and I can then say, whether in my judgment she will need to stay in the Hospital and if not who she shall consult in connection with the staff. . . .

Hurd also performed many chores for the convenience of the senior staff, as illustrated by this letter to him from Halsted:

Cashiers, July 23, 1892
Dear Dr. Hurd: Will you kindly send to Annandale No. 1, Vol. I, of the J.H. Bulletin and also my fasciculus in the 2nd vol. of the Hospital Reports? I am very sorry to contribute so often to your labors.

Very sincerely yours,
Wm. S. Halsted

P.S. If you should think of it sometime will you allow your clerk to send me ½ doz. small sheets of blotting paper. We are 35 miles from a store and none of us can raise a blotter. W. S. H.

During his period as superintendent, Hurd remained an active contributor to the literature. In 1892 he published an article on postfebrile insanity. After discussing the subject in detail, he recorded three cases that had occurred in The Johns Hopkins Hospital: one after laparotomy for removal of diseased ovaries; another following pneumonia, and a third during convalescence from typhoid fever. Hurd wrote a number of articles on various aspects of medical education, including "The Relation of Hospitals to Medical Education," which appeared in the *Boston Medical and Surgical Journal*, and "Laboratories in Hospital Work" in the *Bulletin of the American Academy of Medicine*. He also gave many talks and wrote a number of papers on hospital organization and management. For example, on February 17, 1897 he addressed the training school for nurses at the Hospital of the University of Pennsylvania:

> I cannot resist the temptation to say a word respecting the improvements which have been made in the hospital construction during the past 30 years. These improvements I believe to be largely due to the experience of the Crimean War in Europe and of the Civil War in America. The first gave us training schools for nurses and trained nurses and the latter improved hospital construction. . . . The most noteworthy improvement in hospital construction has been in the direction of better sites for buildings which are no longer crowded into narrow dingy streets with unpleasant surroundings and amidst insalubrious and unsanitary conditions, but a place in open squares, in commanding situations, where sunlight and fresh air can freely come upon their joyous and health giving mission. The buildings themselves are more scattered and sickness and suffering are diluted by differentiation and segregation rather than concentrated by piling one ward upon another. Special efforts have been made in the construction of wards to provide for heating, ventilation, the isolation of infectious, harmful, or offensive patients and for all sanitary needs. Laboratories for the investigation of disease have been built and fitted with instruments of precision for the more accurate and scientific study of disease processes. . . . The best method of keeping the torch of knowledge lighted is to pass it along from hand to hand; hence I have little sympathy with those who deplore the use of hospital wards as means of instruction. They should be used for the training of nurses and for the instruction of medical students and by their very use for these purposes their efficiency for the cure of disease will be augmented. . . . If I were asked to indicate the best machinery for hospital government I should say a Board of Trustees to be sovereign and responsible for the whole institution; a medical board to advise the trustees in all medical matters; a chief executive officer to be known as director, secretary or superintendent, whose duty it should be to coordinate and supervise all other departments; a purveyor to look after food supplies; a matron to supervise the household and a superintendent of nurses to have charge of the training school and the nurses.

Dr. Hurd continued his interest in psychiatry and at a meeting of the Gynecological and Obstetrical Society of Baltimore on December 13, 1898 he presented a paper on "The Postoperative Insanities and Undetected Tendencies to Mental Disease." His remarks were of general interest:

> Postoperative insanity may be considered a complex affair comprising symptoms which may differ in cause, manifestation, course and termination. There would seem in fact to be little ground for the use of the term were it not for the existence of infectious processes accompanied by delirium or prolonged depression. In other words, if an operation is free from septic infection in a case destitute of any tendency to insanity, there can be no ground to think that the operation per se produces mental disease or that the insanity is postoperative in the sense that the operation bears a causative relationship. There are disturbing factors, it is true, in connection with surgical operations which may be competent to produce an insanity . . . But the insanity which they produce can only be considered postoperative in point of sequence rather than of causation. It is unquestionable that the prolonged use of anesthetics like ether, chloroform, or nitrous oxide has produced excitement, delirium, mental confusion and often prolonged mental alienation without the accompaniment of any operation whatever. Instances are also not at all uncommon where following an operation excitement has followed the local application of iodoform, the installation of atropia or the administration of the salicylate of soda, and where notwithstanding the surgical operation, the symptoms of insanity subsided wholly upon the withdrawal of the intoxicating agent.
>
> Similarly we may have mental symptoms following an operation clearly ascribable to shock, loss of blood, excessive exhaustion from the fatigue of a constrained and unnatural position, long continued vomiting from an anesthetic, or abstinence from food owing to anorexia. There may also be a poisoning of the blood and consequent interference with proper cerebration from defective action of the kidneys, due wholly to the withdrawal of water by the mouth lest it may excite vomiting after an abdominal operation; or the anesthetic may have caused a temporary nephritis with accompanying loss of kidney function. These and similar causes which are not surgical in character, but are necessarily an accompaniment of a surgical operation, may produce insanity which cannot in any manner be differentiated from actual postoperative insanity due to infection.

Dr. Hurd had an intense interest in promoting proper facilities for the care of the insane. In 1902 he was made chairman of the section on neurology and psychiatry of the Medical and Chirurgical Faculty of Maryland. At a meeting of the section held November 14, 1902, he took for his subject the future policy of Maryland in the care of her insane. He had carefully studied the situation in Baltimore and in the various counties and found that Maryland was far behind the times. At a meeting of the faculty in 1897, a symposium on the state care of the insane had been arranged. The papers read on that occasion brought forth much resentment on the part of the state authorities. Hurd, in his 1902 address, pointed out what had been accomplished in the interim, but also stated in no uncertain terms that in many places throughout the state the conditions were still deplorable. He did not generalize as is so frequently done, but was specific, mentioning the institutions at fault and indicating how these appalling conditions should be rectified. His concluding paragraph, addressed to the medical profession, was quite apt for the occasion:

> Those who have read the recently published life of Pasteur (every physician ought to read it) must have been impressed by the fact that in the mind and life of this wonderful man scientific knowledge was invariably regarded as the handmaiden of humanity. In the height of Pasteur's interest in the study of ferments, which opened the way to our present antiseptic surgical methods, he turned aside from his chosen work for five years to study the diseases of silk worms, because of the suffering of the people in certain portions of France consequent upon the destruction of the silk industry. His subsequent studies in puerperal fever, charbon, chicken cholera, plague and hydrophobia were inspired by a similar notion; to use his own words, "to give the heart its share in the progress of science." We may not be able to imitate Pasteur in scientific achievement and in broad and vivifying generalization from isolated scientific facts, but we can imitate with broad humanity and his desire to ameliorate the lot of the unfortunate. We can at present do no greater service to humanity and the commonwealth than to use our professional influence and personal effort to promote the hospital treatment of acute cases of insanity and appropriate state care for the insane poor of the chronic class.

One of Hurd's most interesting papers was on psychiatry as a part of preventive medicine, published in the *American Journal of Insanity* in 1908–09: "The object of preventive medicine being to lessen the burdens of mankind by obviating preventable diseases, it is deemed appropriate at this time to inquire in what manner the experience of those who are familiar with the problems of psychiatry may be utilized to assist in this good work. It needs no elaborate demonstration to show the evils of insanity and the heavy public and private burdens which it entails upon every community. Next to alcoholism it is probably the most potent cause of pauperism and dependence."

Hurd's conclusions are particularly interesting:

> The methods of rendering the teachings of psychiatry more effective to prevent disease should be: 1) to instruct children in the school the art of healthy and useful living. Teaching should be more thorough and not restricted to fit one to get on in the world, but rather to inculcate ideals which will give him a conception of the prime importance of self control and moral rectitude. It also should include a knowledge of the dangers of immorality and intemperance; 2) to use the newspapers and the special reports of officers of institutions for the insane and defective classes, to scatter broadcast a knowledge of the laws of bodily and mental health, and the best means of preventing the development of mental disorders; 3) to give better recognition of psychiatry in the curriculum of every medical school, so that physicians may become familiar with the diagnosis and treatment of insanity. To this end psychopathic hospitals should be established to give clinical instruction, so that the family physician may recognize insanity, may be able to scrutinize carefully the

mental condition of neurotic children and may give wise advice upon all educational problems.

Hurd had certain ideas in hospital management that were well ahead of his time. In referring to the purchase of hospital supplies, he mentioned a method that had given splendid results: "A very obvious form of cooperation is for all the hospitals of the city to adopt a common standard of ordinary everyday supplies and to arrange for their purpose through a common purchasing agent.

"In the city of New York also an attempt has been made with very gratifying success to establish a hospital bureau, which is a central supply bureau under a purchasing agent whose duty it is to make contracts for gauzes, cottons, surgical instruments, rubber goods, furniture, fixtures, bedding, blankets and the like. These supplies are purchased in large quantities according to a definite standard of excellence and at the lowest market prices."

Probably one of the most interesting articles that Dr. Hurd wrote was entitled "The Site of The Johns Hopkins Hospital," read as a paper before The Johns Hopkins Hospital Historical Club in December 1910 and published in the *Johns Hopkins Nurses' Alumni Magazine* for April 1911.

> A plat of the site of the Johns Hopkins Hospital which was prepared to facilitate the sale of the property to the late Johns Hopkins has recently come to light among the records of the hospital and an examination of the survey has suggested to me that it would be interesting to all persons connected with the hospital to see it and to learn something of its previous history [Fig 6].
>
> The site of the hospital has been used for hospital purposes for somewhat over 100 years. A general hospital was established on this site in 1797 or in the early part of 1798. In an old report it is spoken of as a beautiful site upon a hill, about a mile from the city of Baltimore. When I came here 21 years ago, the town extended but little to the east of the hospital and most of the neighboring streets have been opened since the present site was selected. In 1808 the old hospital was leased to a firm of physicians, Dr. Smythe and Dr. Mackenzie. In 1834 it was used as a lunatic asylum, later called the Maryland Hospital for the Insane [Fig 7].

From Hurd's paper one learns that at one time the town of Joppa on the Gunpowder River was larger than Baltimore and that from this town there was a brisk trade in tobacco, many ships sailing from Joppa to England. The old Joppa Road ran from Joppa through Baltimore to Annapolis. It crossed the present hospital grounds a few feet north of the present Administration Building. A house that faced on the Joppa Road existed until June 1919. The Joppa Road crossed the present Monument Street going northward and westward between Bond and Caroline Streets. In 1836 land was bought by the hospital on the north of the Joppa Road and this once busy main thoroughfare was closed.

Among the books written by Dr. Hurd is one which

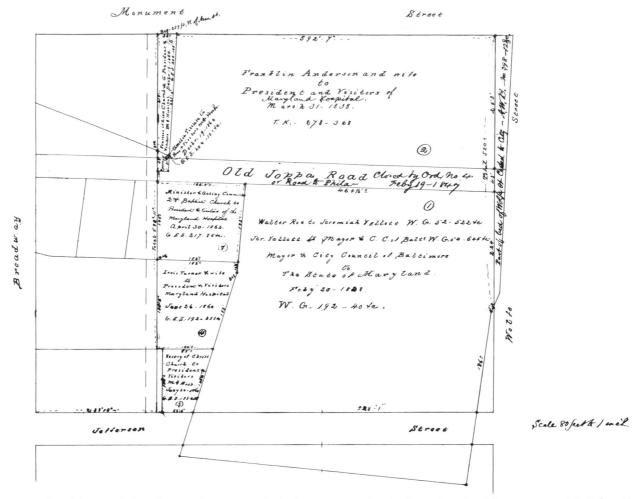

Fig 6.   A plat of the site of The Johns Hopkins Hospital which was prepared to facilitate the sale of the property to Mr. Johns Hopkins.
From the Alan M. Chesney Medical Archives, The Johns Hopkins Medical Institutions.

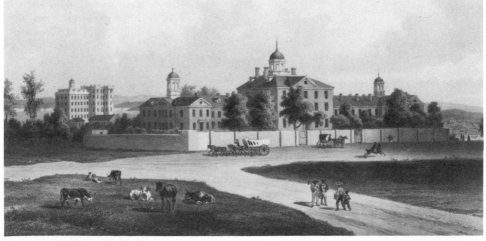

Fig 7.   The Maryland Hospital for the Insane which occupied the site where The Johns Hopkins Hospital now stands. In an old report it is spoken of as a beautiful site upon a hill about a mile from the city of Baltimore.
Reprinted from Hurd HM: The site of the Johns Hopkins Hospital. Johns Hopkins Nurses Alumnae Magazine 9: 5, 1910–1911.

he edited with John Shaw Billings entitled *Hospitals, Dispensaries and Nursing.* The International Congress of Charities, Correction and Philanthropy was held in Chicago, June 12 to 17, 1893. Section 3 was devoted to the hospital care of the sick, training of nurses, dispensary work and first aid to the injured. Dr. John Shaw Billings was chairman and Dr. Henry M. Hurd secretary of this section. Miss Isabel A. Hampton was chairman of the subsection on nursing. Many valuable papers were read in the section and it was clearly evident that the addresses should be published, but the necessary funds were lacking. Billings and Hurd came to the rescue and at their own expense published, and also edited, the large volume of over 700 pages. This splendid publication contains much of interest to Baltimoreans, not only on account of the many valuable papers, but also because Baltimoreans contributed in no small measure to the success of the Congress. Dr. Hurd gave a paper entitled "Description of the Johns Hopkins Hospital." After detailing the gift of Johns Hopkins and speaking of the plans in the building of the hospital, he described the institution in detail, giving numerous illustrations. The picture that had the most appeal was one of the isolation ward, with the old boardwalk extending from the northern exit of this building over to the steps of the pathological building. One can easily visualize those going from the hospital to the laboratory in rainy weather, turning up their coat collars and sprinting rapidly over to the pathological department.

Hurd's most important literary effort was as editor of four volumes on the institutional care of the insane in the United States and Canada. At the sixty-sixth annual meeting of the American Medico-Psychological Association held in Washington, D.C. in May 1910, Hurd gave an address entitled "A History of Institutional Care of the Insane in the United States and Canada." This paper was published in the *American Journal of Insanity* in 1910. In the course of his address Dr. Hurd said:

> The movement to write a history of the Association and its work had its origin at the Baltimore meeting in 1895, when Dr. Powell of Georgia presented a very interesting outline of the "rise and progress of a vast system of charities in the 15 commonwealths of the south," with detailed accounts of institutions in Virginia, North Carolina and Georgia. It was evident from the interest which was then excited that much had been done by similar foundations in all the states of the union and from this conviction grew the original resolutions subsequently presented by Dr. J. W. Babcock of Columbia, South Carolina. These resolutions were considered and favorably acted upon, and a committee was appointed, but nothing seems to have come of it, although progress had been reported from time to time, and an effort had been made to stir up the general sentiment in favor of completing the work. For this and other reasons, although not aware of any special personal fitness for the work, I did not feel at liberty to decline the appointment made at the Cincinnati meeting of which by the way I learned for the first time in June last at Atlantic City. Since that time I have made an intermittent effort to organize the work and collected such material as I could find.

In his concluding paragraph Dr. Hurd said the following: "I've taken the liberty to embody the substance of this paper in a resolution which I now offer to ascertain the will of the Association in the matter of the publication of the book. I should be glad to have it modified, revised, or in any way changed so as to bring out more completely the wishes of the Association in the matter. I am not wedded to any theory of publication, or any form of work. I am anxious that the work go on with as much rapidity as possible. It is equally important, however, that the work be done thoroughly, so then in the future all may know who in the past contributed to the success of an important philanthropic movement."

Volumes 1, 2 and 3 of this stupendous work appeared from the Johns Hopkins Press in 1916 and volume 4 in 1917. These four volumes contain in all 2,926 pages.

Volume 1 is historical in character. It gives a clear account of the Association of Medical Superintendents of Institutions for the Insane from 1844 to 1893 and of the American Medico-Psychological Association from 1893 to 1913. It then described what the *American Journal of Insanity* had accomplished. Volumes 2 and 3 and part of volume 4 are devoted to a detailed description of the institutions for the care of the insane in the United States and Canada. In each article is a detailed list of the medical personnel of the institution from its beginning to the time the volume appeared, so that the previous activities of any man who has devoted his life to psychiatry can be readily followed.

These volumes brought forth much praise. *Science* for July 28, 1916, in reviewing Volume 1 which was written in its entirety by Hurd, said:

> This is one of the few works in the English language in which the history of a separate branch of medicine has been exhaustively treated. ... The present volume, although it professes to deal only with the general history of institutional care of the insane on this continent, is, in reality, an exhaustive history of American psychiatry in all its phases and is therefore likely to remain the authoritative work on the subject for an indefinite period. ...
>
> Dr. Hurd modestly regards this work as a source book for the historians of the future but it is undoubtedly a permanent history which may be extended, but will hardly be duplicated. The chapters are complete in themselves, the book is well illustrated and the style is charming in its simplicity, sobriety and its traces of delicate humor.
>
> It must be remembered that during the immense amount of labor entailed in the preparation of these volumes Dr. Hurd had been greatly troubled with his eyes. It was only his indomitable will that continually spurred him on to the completion of these labors that were a fitting climax to his many successful years of hospital directorship.

HURD'S RESIGNATION

In Hurd's report for 1911 the following appeared: "In May 1911 Dr. Henry M. Hurd resigned from the superintendency of the hospital to become secretary of the Board of Trustees and Dr. Winfred H. Smith, general medical superintendent of Bellevue and Allied Hospitals in New York, was appointed his successor.

"Dr. Hurd was the first superintendent of the hospital and held the office for 22 years. Dr. Hurd's wise administration, his high ideals, his example and his readiness at all times to give of his knowledge to others have contributed largely to the general development of hospitals throughout the country."

Thus, this extraordinary man, the first professor of psychiatry and the first superintendent of the hospital, although not robust maintained an astounding input into his routine duties as superintendent and vigorously pursued his interest in the psychiatric problems of the day. He also found time to spearhead the journal club, to edit the hospital publications and to author an informative series of annual reports of the activities of the hospital. Much of the credit for the success of the hospital and its relationship with the school of medicine must be given to Henry Mills Hurd.

ACKNOWLEDGMENTS

I am grateful to Dr. Huntington Williams for his help in the preparation of this article, and to Patricia King for her editorial assistance.

REFERENCES

1. Cullen TS: Henry Mills Hurd: The First Superintendent of the Johns Hopkins Hospital. Baltimore, The Johns Hopkins Press, 1920

2. Hurd HM: Journal club. Am J Insanity 48: 372, 1891–92

3. Hurd HM: Postfebrile insanity. Md Med J 27: 661, 1892

4. Hurd HM: Hospital organization and management. Address before the Training School for Nurses of the University of Pennsylvania, February 17, 1897. Univ M Mag Phila 9: 488, 1896–97

5. Hurd HM: The postoperative insanities and undetected tendencies to mental disease. Am J Obstet 39: 331, 1899

6. Hurd HM: The future policy of Maryland in the care of her insane. Md Med J 46: 45, 1903

7. Hurd HM: A history of institutional care of the insane in the United States and Canada. Am J Insanity 67: 587, 1910–11

(For Hurd's complete bibliography see the *Bulletin of the Johns Hopkins Hospital* 30: 370, 1919.)

3.

Amebic Dysentery Gets Its Name: The Story of William Thomas Councilman

INTRODUCTION

One of the innovations of the new Johns Hopkins University was the recruitment of professors from other universities rather than locally. Thus of that remarkable group of men who composed the early faculty of Johns Hopkins, few were natives of Maryland. However, one native Marylander achieved great distinction in medicine—William Thomas Councilman.

Councilman was born on a busy farm which straddled the Reisterstown turnpike not far from Baltimore. Throughout his life he retained fond memories of his childhood and considered himself fortunate that his early years were passed in such an environment. There he learned to plow, "to swing a cradle," to bind sheaves and to do other things that were unforgettable, "like the gathering of spring simples." Councilman frequently recalled his childhood experiences in later-year addresses:

> The earliest of my childhood recollections is being taken by my grandfather when he set out in the first warm days of early spring with a grubbing hoe (we called it a mattock) on his shoulder to seek the plants, the barks and roots from which the spring medicine for the household was prepared. If I could but remember all that went into that mysterious decoction and the exact method of preparation, and with judicious advertisement put the product upon the market I would shortly be possessed of wealth which might be made to serve the useful purpose of increasing the salaries of all pathologists ... But, alas! I remember only that the basic ingredients were dogwood bark and sassafras root, and to these were added blood root, poke and yellow dock. The medicine benefitted my grandfather I have every reason to believe, for he was a hale, strong old man, firm in body and mind until the infection came against which even spring medicine was of no avail. That the medicine did me good I well know, for I can see before me even now the green on the south hillside of the old pasture, the sunlight in the strip of wood where the dogwood grew, the bright blossoms and the delicate pale green of the leaf of the sanguinaria, and the even lighter green of the tender buds of the sassafras in the hedgerow, and it is good to have such pictures deeply engraved in the memory.

Councilman was sent off to school at St. John's College, Annapolis, which he left at the age of 16 and for the next 6 years "led an independent existence, raised side whiskers, considered himself a very ripe individual and did pretty much as he chose." He confessed frequently in his later years that he was always something of a rebel and disinclined to do anything which did not interest him. However, at the age of 22 he decided to follow in the footsteps of his father, a country doctor "who had never lost the childish desire to find things out by observation and the test of experiment." He entered the University of Maryland Medical School, which at that time was a 2-year course consisting largely of a series of lectures. The dissecting room provided the contact with "nature" for which he yearned, and the form and structure of the body soon excited his curiosity. The farm provided an excellent opportunity to satisfy this sudden stimulus and beginning with the mole, he proceeded to make a comparative study of the skulls of all available animals until the collection finally threatened to crowd him out of his bedroom. He became so engaged with this project that he neglected his second-year course of lectures; thus it was perhaps somewhat of a blessing that one day during his absence one of his small nephews "with a good business head" sold the whole collection for a few pennies to an itinerant bone merchant. Deprived of this engrossing project, he returned to attendance at his lectures, qualifying in March of 1878 "to exercise the art of medicine, which he had so laboriously learned, for the advantage of the public."

It was at this time that he first discovered that The Johns Hopkins University was a new sort of institution which had what was called a laboratory.

> I vaguely knew of the Johns Hopkins University but not a great deal about it. It had opened in 1876 and Huxley came on to give the opening address; my father drove in from the country and heard this address and came back and told us what an impression it had made on him. . . . There seemed something remarkable about the opening of this university. . . . Martin, Rowland, Brooks, and Remson were young men and as young men they felt no hampering traditions. Traditions may be very important, but they can be extremely hampering as well, and whether or not tradition is of really much value I have never been certain. Of course, when they are very fine they do good. But it is very difficult, of course, ever to repeat the conditions under which good traditions are formed, so they may be and are often injurious. So the Johns Hopkins University started without traditions and started with young men, full of vigor and enthusiasm as its leaders. The university at its beginning made provision for 20 fel-

Reprinted from the *Johns Hopkins Medical Journal* **146:** 185, 1980.

lowships, each fellow being paid $500; and the idea of going to a university and being paid for it made an impression.

HIS START WITH HENRY NEWELL MARTIN

Henry Newell Martin permitted Councilman to join his small class in the biological laboratory for the next three months (April to June, 1878). Councilman was completely thrilled with the informal spirit of the place and with the method of teaching through observation and experiment. That summer he became assistant to the quarantine officer, bought a cheap microscope with his first small earnings, and began with its aid to study such histological preparations as he could find time to make in the intervals of his routine work. That autumn Martin offered him the assistantship in physiology for the following year and Councilman believed that his "cup was overflowing." For the first paper he ever wrote, an experimental study of inflammation of the cornea, he was given a prize of $100 and with this encouragement made the final decision to embark upon biology as a career. However, this decision had hardly been made when a more attractive opportunity appeared. During the summer months of the 3 years following his graduation he worked partly at the Marine Hospital and partly at the Bayview Asylum (the city almshouse and hospital) which led to an interest in pathology. He came to the conclusion that in order to learn his subject properly he must go abroad, which his frugal savings permitted him to do.

He could scarcely have gone abroad to study at a more appropriate time, for almost daily new discoveries were being made and new methods developed. German medicine in 1880 was approaching its peak under the stimulus of the new cellular pathology of Virchow and the identification of pathogenic bacteria, both of which were greatly advanced by the increasing use of analine dyes in the study of tissues and microorganisms. His longest sojourn was in Vienna under pupils of the great Rokitansky. He also spent a profitable period with von Recklinghausen in the new school at Strasbourg. Councilman was studying under Cohnheim and Weigert at Leipzig when in April 1882 the exciting news came of Koch's discovery of the tubercle bacillus.

On March 2, 1883, after his return from his first venture abroad, he wrote the following letter to Professor Martin:

> Dear Sir: I propose to go to Germany again this spring and thought that while there I might prove useful to you in the following manner. In view of the fact that pathological material is extremely abundant there and here owing to the infrequency of autopsies correspondingly scarce, I would propose to collect a quantity of specimens illustrative of pathological conditions, to be used in teaching when the medical department is added to the university and to serve as the nucleus of the future pathological museum. It would be my idea to collect only such specimens as were typical of the chief pathological changes in the various organisms and to form complete sets of specimens showing the changes of different stages of disease. In a year a better collection could be made

than would be possible here in 10 or 12. . . . Most respectfully, W. T. Councilman

Henry Newell Martin sent this letter to Mr. Gilman, the president of the university, with the following note attached: "I think this suggestion of Dr. Councilman's worthy of consideration. There is no pathological museum in Baltimore and we must have one at the Johns Hopkins Medical School. To build it from the start with such scanty material as can be obtained in this country, where permission to make a postmortem is nearly always refused by the friends of hospital patients, could take years. . . ." On the same day Martin wrote a more formal letter to President Gilman as follows:

> Dear Sir: I send you herewith a note from Dr. Councilman endorsed by a few words from me on its back. I write now to suggest that if the Trustees accept Dr. Councilman's offer it had better be on a business footing and not as a present from Dr. Councilman of his time or to the university. In view of the near opening of the medical school it seems to me very desirable to keep clear of any entanglements which might arise from being under obligations to this or that promising and energetic young man. I am not at all sure that Dr. Councilman would not be the best teacher of pathological anatomy we could get. He has a thorough knowledge of his work, has been student and assistant in physiology and knows our plan of work in the departments the university already organized. So I am not in any way desirous to interfere with his chance should the Trustees determine to appoint an instructor in pathological anatomy in the medical school. So far as I am at present advised I doubt if we could get a better man. But I think a better man might turn up, and that it would be unfortunate in that case to have Dr. Councilman in a position to say that he had a claim on the university for gratuitous services during a year or more in collecting specimens for it. I would therefore suggest that $500 be appropriated for expenditure by Dr. Councilman in the purchase of alcohol, glass bottles, etc. for the preservation and display of specimens and that $250 or $300 additional be given him for his services during a year in collecting and putting up pathological specimens. In this way he would have received his pay for the work done and the university would be under no actual and constrictive obligation to him. I remain yours very truly, H. Newell Martin

On April 9, 1883, Martin again wrote to Gilman:

> Since receiving your communication I have made the following arrangements with Dr. Councilman on behalf of the university: 1) Dr. Councilman who proposes to go to Europe this month is to collect typical specimens of the more common pathological changes found in various diseases and properly preserve them so that they may be used afterwards as museum specimens; 2) On the first of September next Dr. Councilman will send me a statement of the sum of money which he has expended up to that day in the purchase of alcohol and other preservative reagents and in the purchase of proper vessels for the preservation of the specimens which he has obtained and of such other expenses as he has been put to directly in the obtaining and preservation of the specimens; 3) On my receiving the above statement the treasurer of the university will send at my request to Dr. Councilman such sum not exceeding

$500 as Dr. Councilman has expended in obtaining and preserving the specimens above referred to; and in addition $200 as compensation to Dr. Councilman for his work in obtaining and preserving the specimens. 4) If $500 has not been expended by Dr. Councilman in the collection and preservation for the University of typical pathological specimens on September 1, 1883 then Dr. Councilman will continue to collect such specimens and from time to time send to me a statement of the necessary expenses incurred. On my forwarding a statement of these expenses to the treasurer of the university he will forward the amount to Dr. Councilman provided that the sum total of all expenses for the collection and preservation of specimens spent apart from Dr. Councilman's personal services should not exceed $500; 5) Dr. Councilman will pack the specimens so that they may be forwarded safely to the university and send them to Baltimore; the university to pay freight, insurance, etc., etc.; 6) On his return to the United States Dr. Councilman will mount the specimens for exhibition—the university providing the necessary jars and so forth and he will also prepare and deliver to the university a descriptive catalog of the specimens. When the specimens are all mounted and the catalog delivered the treasurer of the university will pay to Dr. Councilman the further sum of $50. I have the honor to remain yours faithfully, H. Newell Martin

There is appended at the bottom of this letter the following: "The above is a correct statement of the agreement made by me with Dr. Martin. W. T. Councilman." It is interesting to see how much of the details of the day-to-day conduct of the university crossed Gilman's desk. On February 29, 1884 Martin made the following recommendation to President Gilman:

Dear Sir, I beg leave to recommend that Dr. William Councilman be appointed temporarily on the biological staff for the remainder of the present year as instructor in pathological anatomy and that he be permitted to receive under my supervision a limited number of graduates in medicine as pupils. I have sounded out Dr. Councilman on the subject and found that he would like such work and would consider $250 as adequate compensation. I know that there is a demand in the city among the younger physicians for such instruction and guidance in the study of pathological anatomy as Dr. Councilman is competent to give. I've had several applications recently from some of our brightest young physicians for opportunities such as I suggest, but have had to refuse them . . .

Councilman spent much of that second period in Europe with Hans Chiari, a man of his own age whom he had first known in Vienna and who then held the chair of pathology in Prague. From this place under the date of July 16, 1883, a certain "correspondent" W.T.C. sent off to the *Medical News* an entertaining letter concerned mainly with climate and food:

One misses ice-water and our various cooling appliances very much; it is possible, with a good deal of trouble, to get a glass of water with a few pieces of dirty ice in it, but it always seems to excite so much surprise, alarm, and horror in the spectators that one has to seek out a secluded corner of the restaurant to drink it. I do not know which they regard as the worst, drinking ice-water or eating raw tomatoes. Now, I am very fond of the latter,

and always eat them when I can; but from seeing a crowd around my part of the room every day, I begin to have some suspicion that the proprietor uses me as an advertisement, and that crowds come daily to see the great American tomato-eater. Ice-water especially seems to be regarded as a deadly poison, the cause of all the dyspepsia in America.

THE FIRST OF THE "WELCH RABBITS"

Councilman, in his final address to the students at Harvard in 1921, had the following to say about this period of his life:

I came back from Europe very full of all of the things which I had learned and with a more or less definite idea of . . . practicing medicine. But I put off later and later the putting up of a sign showing that I was willing to serve, and finally never put it out because it seemed to me there were so many other interesting things to do. And as long as one saw the possibility of doing these interesting things without actual starvation, there is no question of the choice and there should never be a question of the choice. I reasoned that if worse came to worse I had a few acres of good land on which I could raise all the food I required and something over. . . . But I never had to resort to agriculture for a living. I speak of this because at that time there seemed to be no possibility of earning a living by teaching pathology and Welch in New York and I were probably the first two men in the country who tried it. I rather think Dr. Welch took the greater risk because he had not my agricultural resources, though a training and mental capacity far greater than mine.

After his return from Europe in 1883, Councilman engaged in a variety of enterprises: doing the autopsies at Bayview, teaching in the two local medical schools, helping John S. Billings prepare his *National Medical Dictionary*, writing articles for encyclopedias, and for a year serving as physician to the Baltimore City coroner. This position paid him $300, but it "tied him down too much to places and dates" and "being of a rather roving disposition" he "did not care to be at a certain place at a certain time." So he surrendered the job to another physician who had, according to Councilman, "greater political pull." Meantime, Welch came to Baltimore and on October 9, 1885 wrote the following letter to President Gilman:

Dear Sir, In recommending the reappointment of Dr. W. T. Councilman as associate in pathology I wish to say a word as to the efficiency and faithfullness with which he has performed the duties of his position during the past year. By securing the appointments as pathologist to the Bayview Hospital and as one of the Coroner's physicians to the city he is able to control a large pathological material and thereby has obtained many valuable specimens for the university.

With much sacrifice of time and convenience he has remained in the city throughout the past summers in order to make required daily visits to the Insane Asylum of Bayview, the control of which it is desirable to retain for the university.

Dr. Councilman's thorough training and experience in pathology, his high aims and his great enthusiasm in the pursuit of his specialty make his services of the greatest value to the pathological department of the university and have secured for him the esteem and appreciation of the medical faculty. In view of his services and of the great demand which they make upon his time I would suggest that his reappointment be accompanied by an increase of salary.

His appointment was renewed in October 1885 at a salary of $1250.

Thus, one of Welch's first moves after his appointment as professor of pathology was to make Councilman a member of his staff, which proved to be a very wise choice indeed. In June of that year Welch outlined to Gilman his plans for beginning systematic instruction the following year. He was to teach pathological histology in collaboration with Councilman. Demonstrations of gross pathological specimens and methods of postmortem examinations were to be given by Councilman alone and Welch himself was to give lectures on the general pathology of fever and a course in bacteriology. Without Councilman's ability to secure the pathological material needed for these courses, it would have been impossible to conduct them. Councilman purchased a tricycle in which to transport specimens across the city from Bayview to Johns Hopkins and he had "occasional accidents which even got into the newspapers." It was clearly a relaxed and stimulating laboratory in which he worked. In those years the Baltimore Orioles won the pennant three successive times. "We are the champions" Welch wrote to his sister, "and everybody here is fully aware of the fact that I have attended most of the games and have become an enthusiast, even a crank, on the subject." Welch's stout figure became familiar to the rooters in the grandstand. Between innings he would correct the proof of the *Journal of Experimental Medicine*, but once the play had resumed, he was all attention, continually scribbling on a complicated diagram he held on his knee. Welch had invented a system for keeping a record of every play which he considered far in advance of any then in existence, and he could not have been more proud of a major scientific discovery. A mine of baseball lore, he knew everyone's batting average and the most personal facts about the players. Daily he compared form with performance and he was delighted when Baltimore won.

It amused Welch no end to make out that he went to the games reluctantly. "Councilman," he wrote to Flexner, "returned Saturday, wildly enthusiastic about baseball all of the time and dragging me out daily to see the game." Councilman described the intimacy that existed among that early group of workers in the newly erected pathological laboratory which he had joined with Welch in 1886.

Councilman was described as being of choleric temperament, optimistic and buoyant. He stuttered a little, Harvey Cushing having described his speech as "his engaging hesitancy of speech." Councilman also had command of a choice line of expletives, being able to laugh, and swear, on occasion most heartily, both at himself and at the world. Barker remembered walking into the laboratory one hot day in summer and seeing Councilman peering through a microscope with a sheet of sticky flypaper over his bald head as a protection from flies.

Unlike many religious bodies, the men of Johns Hopkins had the example of Welch, Osler and Halsted (but not Kelly) to show that clothes and food and drink did not have to be put down but could be integrated into their professional lives; that fullness of being was no crime against their calling. Eating and drinking were simply pretexts for letting the life of the hospital go on out of hours. When Councilman was caught in an error he would say, "B-b-boys, l-l-let's go over to the ch-ch-church," and everybody would run across to Hanselmann's Bar—"the church"—at the corner of Wolfe and Monument Streets, and the shop talk would go on over the beer. Here Hanselmann had once run his hand over Halsted's head and cried out, "You have not approximately lost your hair," and Halsted had turned red and angry.

To prepare himself for the opening of the medical school, Councilman decided to go abroad for another year of study. Clearly his interest in medical education was deep. The proposition that Councilman be involved in the teaching of anatomy came after a discussion he had with Dr. James Cary Thomas (a University trustee). Thomas talked the matter over with Welch and on January 13, 1888 Welch wrote the following letter to the Executive Committee of the Board of Trustees of the Johns Hopkins University:

Gentlemen: At the request of Dr. James Cary Thomas I write to say that the appointment of Dr. W. T. Councilman as assistant or associate professor of anatomy would be in my judgment a judicious one.... The capacity which he has already shown as student instructor and investigator give assurance that he would perform satisfactorily the rights of the new position now in view. It is ... manifestly desirable that ... he should be able to devote some time to a more minute study of normal anatomy ... and especially to the great improvements in the methods of teaching the subject. This work can be done far better in Germany than in any other place. If therefore it can be arranged that he can spend some time there before beginning his new work in case of his appointment it would be of distinct advantage to himself and to the university.

Councilman wrote the following letter to President Gilman on February 2, 1888:

At your request I take this opportunity to call attention to some of the defects relating to the usual methods of teaching human anatomy in the medical schools of this country and to make certain suggestions concerning the proper method in my opinion of studying and teaching the subject which lies at the foundation of any scheme of medical education.

In consequence of the short term of study required to obtain a medical degree in this country too little time is devoted to the study of anatomy, and on account of the large size of the classes in the better equipped schools sufficient opportunity is not afforded for personal instruction. Instruction is carried on to a disproportionate extent by purely didactic lectures and not enough by demonstration and actual dissection. As little or no preliminary education is required for admission to most of the medical schools, the students have not that knowledge of embryology and of comparative anatomy which is essential to a proper understanding of the laws of human anatomy. Dissociated from these branches of knowledge the study of human anatomy loses much of its interest and becomes hardly more than the dry rehearsal of a mass of unconnected facts. The great exponents of anatomical teaching of the present day, such men as Gegenbauer, His, Kolliker and Waldeyer, recognize this fact and base their teaching of human anatomy upon a knowledge of embryology and comparative anatomy.

I should propose therefore in teaching human anatomy to make the course rather a continuation of the instruction which most of the men will already have had in embryology and comparative anatomy. The lectures would embrace descriptive and topographical anatomy but, to teach the details of anatomy the most reliance would be based on work in the dissecting room which should be careful and painstaking and carried on under the personal supervision of the teacher. There should be kept on hand a supply of bones and preparations of the more difficult dissections for the use of the students. I should expect that original work in mammalian embryology, in histology and in the connection between normal and pathological anatomy would be carried on. In connection with the place I would desire a leave of absence from April 1, 1888 until the fall of 1889. This time I would spend in the European laboratories. My object in this

would be to study thoroughly the manner of instruction in the different universities, to know the principal teachers of anatomy and by study under them to learn their ideas and aims. In addition to this I wish to learn the different methods which are in use for preserving bodies, making preparations and so forth. In a word the details of anatomical technique. Further I desire to perfect myself in anatomy for although the character of my work renders me familiar with human anatomy I wish to study further embryology and comparative anatomy. In accepting the position I wish to feel that I am in everyway capable of filling it.

On February 11 a minute was adopted by the Executive Committee: "The Executive Committee is willing to nominate Dr. Councilman without increase of salary to be associate professor of anatomy until otherwise ordered by the Board and to give him leave of absence for a year from the university continuing his salary, provided that he make arrangements to have his present work continued. This might be considered as a sabbatical year with salary." Thus, Councilman had a dual appointment when the medical school opened and this experience was of great benefit both to the school and Councilman's future career (Fig 1).

COUNCILMAN'S RESEARCH ON MALARIA

The prevalence of malaria in Italy and North Africa stimulated early work by French and Italian observ-

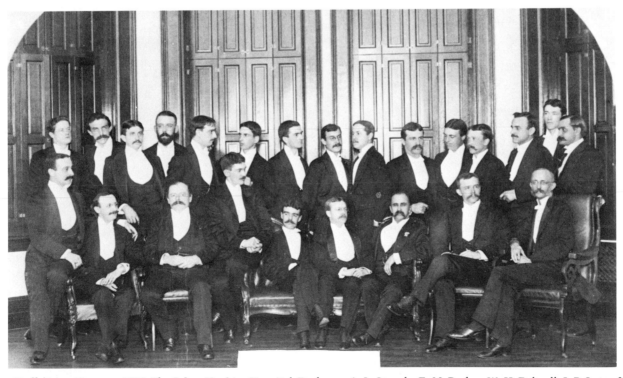

Fig 1. Staff dinner, January 1892, The Johns Hopkins Hospital. Back row: A. L. Stavely, E. M. Parker, W. H. Baltzell, J. P. Lotsy, W. W. Russell, J. Hewetson, T. S. Cullen, A. Hoch, E. Van Ness, J. M. T. Finney, W. S. Thayer, H. Phippen, J. G. Clark, L. F. Barker, F. R. Smith. Front row: G. H. F. Nuttall, S. Flexner, W. T. Councilman, A. A. Ghriskey, A. C. Abbott, H. Robb, W. Osler, H. A. Kelly, H. M. Hurd.
From the Alan M. Chesney Archives, The Johns Hopkins Medical Institutions.

ers. Reports of the work in Europe had hardly appeared before enthusiastic young physicians in the United States began to study the subject in those regions of the Eastern Seaboard where the disease was prevalent, one of which was Baltimore. Much of this work was done, however, in a spirit of confirming or disproving those foreign observations which were the subject of active controversy. Councilman and Abbott described in meticulous detail the lesions in two patients dead of "comatose malaria." They pointed out the intense pigmentation of the organs in the small cerebral vessels choked with hyaline masses as if they were outlined in ink. They discussed the controversy as to a bacillary or protozoal cause for the disease and, like many early writers, ended up by begging the question: "We confess our inability to say what these hyaline bodies are."

In the same year Councilman presented a critical discussion of the whole subject at the spring meeting of the Association of American Physicians: "What the real nature of this body is—whether it is a parasite and the cause of malaria . . . time and further investigation will show." In the discussion, Osler said: "I am not prepared to give a positive opinion as to the nature of these bodies. They look to me more like vacuoles or areas of hyaline transformation than definite organisms." Then George M. Sternberg, who had worked in Baltimore in the laboratory of Newell Martin, spoke as follows: "I have seen the body in question and have observed its ameboid movements in the blood of a patient with intermittent fever in the Santo Spirito Hospital at Rome, and also in that of a patient in the Bayview Hospital at Baltimore." Councilman, commenting further after this discussion, said: "I cannot think that these bodies are vacuoles (as suggested by Dr. Osler). The staining is too definite. As Dr. Sternberg has said, they also contain pigment granules which would rather speak against their vacuolar nature. With regard to the remarks of Dr. Sternberg, I have no doubt that Laveran did see the motile bodies he described and I have never supposed that they were the result of changes in the blood corpuscles or could have been produced by them."

It gradually became evident that there was a class of cases in which the blood contained only the small hyaline ameboid bodies with perhaps a few fine granules of pigment, associated, often, with the large ovoid and crescentic bodies of Laveran, while in some cases only the latter forms were to be found. Councilman, in 1887, was the first to hint at the practical diagnostic value of this fact. He said: "The character of these bodies varies in different forms of the disease. Although they seem in rare cases to run into one another, still, in general, we can say that where the plasmodia inside the red corpuscles[1] are seen the patient has intermittent fever, and where the crescentic or elongated masses are found he has either some form of remittent fever or malarial cachexia. . . . We are not only enabled to diagnosticate the disease as such, but in most cases the particular form."

[1] He refers here to the large pigmented, probably tertian forms.

Sternberg reviewed the literature, describing confirmatory observations of his own, and was one of the first to accept the parasites as the cause of malaria. In later studies Osler observed the parasites and not only related them to malaria but discussed in detail their diagnostic value (Fig 2).

COUNCILMAN'S WORK ON AMEBIC DYSENTERY

William Osler in 1890 was the first observer in the United States to describe amebae in dysentery and liver abscess: "Dr. B, age 29, resident in Panama for nearly 6 years . . . had a chronic dysentery . . . He began to have an irregular fever with occasional chilling sensations and sweats, to lose flesh, and to have a very sallow complex-

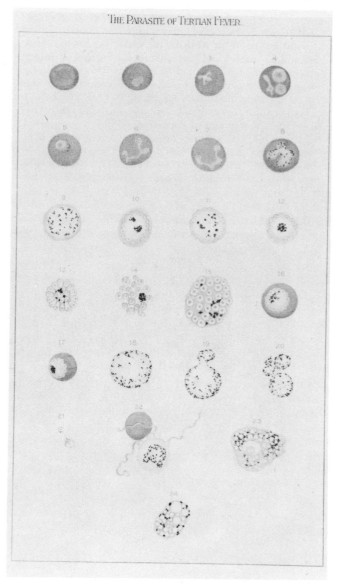

Fig 2.   The parasites of tertian fever. Drawn by Max Brödel. The drawings were made with the assistance of the camera lucida from specimens of fresh blood.
Reprinted from Thayer WS: Lectures on the malarial fevers. New York: D. Appleton and Co, p 313, 1897.

ion ... He had six or eight mucoid stools with traces of blood daily." The liver abscess was diagnosed and evacuated surgically. Osler found in the pus "in large numbers the amoebae which Kartulis had described ... The material was taken at once to the pathological laboratory where Professor Welch and Dr. Councilman confirmed the observation ... After the operation the dysenteric symptoms did not abate in the slightest; he continued to have from 8 to 16 movements daily." Osler then gave a detailed description of the amebae, drawings of which were reproduced in an article by Stilwell. Osler concluded: "It is impossible to speak as yet with any certainty as to the relation of these organisms to the disease. The subject is deserving of extended study and a point of special interest will be determination of their presence in the endemic dysentery of this country."[2]

Shortly after this report Henry A. LaFleur (Osler's first resident physician) reported a case of dysentery in a sailor on a steamship sailing between Baltimore and the Caribbean "in which the Amoeba coli had been found in the stools, and exhibited the living parasite under the microscope." The patient had been in the tropics in 1880. A third case soon followed, reported by Charles E. Simon. The patient had been in the West Indies in 1883 but was quite well when there. He developed diarrhea and cough, and "on the day of admission the expectoration was noticed to be a peculiar rusty, reddish-brown color, purulent and resembling anchovy sauce. Actively moving amebae were found in it, a fact which at once called attention to the bowels and to the liver ... Our attention would never have been called to his actual condition by the character of the stool. As they looked perfectly healthy, with simply adherent mucus, we should probably have regarded the case as a pleurisy."

Thus the atmosphere at Johns Hopkins was ripe for the work of Councilman and LaFleur. After these three case reports, there were various confirmatory reports of the presence of amebae in dysentery and in liver abscess. These were all carefully reviewed by Councilman and LaFleur. Their monograph of some 150 pages was stimulated by the cases from the Johns Hopkins Hospital and was a landmark in the study of the subject. "In this article we propose to consider a disease which is characterized by definite pathological lesions, and is separated not only by its destructive pathological anatomy, but also by its etiology and clinical history from other affections of the intestines with which it has hitherto been classed under the general name of dysen-

tery." Thus Councilman and LaFleur were the first workers who unequivocally defined amebic dysentery as a specific disease and gave it a specific name. They also renamed its causal agent Amoeba dysenteriae. Councilman and LaFleur gave a detailed description of the parasites and emphasized the presence in them of red blood cells, "as many as six or eight having been seen in a single amoeba," as well as describing the appearance of dead amebae stained by a variety of techniques (Fig 3). They reported some 15 cases of amebic dysentery and gave a classic clinical analysis of every feature of the disease. The section in their monograph on hepatic abscess is especially important, pointing out the frequency with which this complication develops in patients who have had no evidence of overt dysentery. Thus, later studies really added little to their definitive analysis. As to therapy they spoke as follows: "Ipecacuanha was administered in case VIII after the manner recognized by surgeons in India," and in other cases "quinine was given by mouth, on theoretical grounds rather than from empirical evidence as to its value." Clysters of quinine as well as of bichloride of mercury, 1 to 5,000 or 1 to 3,000, were employed in two cases and each injection was retained for 10 to 15 minutes. "Results achieved are not brilliant but warrant a more extended trial. This much can be said, that quinine injections do destroy amoebae in the contents of the bowel, but whether they reach and destroy the amoebae in the tissues is an open question." One of the outstanding features of this monograph is the section in which the pathological lesions are described in brilliant detail. The writers concluded that the amoebae produced a necrosis of tissue and exercised a solvent effect on the intercellular substance. "The ulceration is produced by infiltration of the submucous tissue and necrosis of the underlying mucous membranes, the ulcer in consequence having the undermined form. Frequently in addition to the ulcers there is infiltration of the submucous tissue without ulceration (Fig 3). In all of these lesions, unless complicated by the action of bacteria, there is absence of the products of purulent inflammation. These abscesses (of the liver) differ in their anatomical features from those produced by other causes. The chief difference is found in the absence of purulent inflammation, the abscess being caused by necrosis, softening and liquefaction of the tissue. In these liver abscesses the amoebae are not associated with any other organism. This is the form of dysentery which has been commonly called tropical dysentery." There are numerous reproductions of microscopic sections of the lesions and colored drawings of stained amoebae showing their structure in this excellent monograph (Fig 4).

The following year Councilman gave a paper on dysentery before the Association of American Physicians. At that time his study was based on 34 cases which had been found in 320 autopsies at the Johns Hopkins Hospital. He divided the dysenteries into simple or catarrhal, diphtheritic, and amebic. The last is distinguished from the others not only by the anatomical differences in the lesions, but also by the broader difference of a definite etiology. (Shiga did not isolate his bacillus from cases of

---

[2] On March 20, 1890, Osler wrote to Musser in Philadelphia as follows: "We have been much excited over Kartulis' amebae which we have found in a liver abscess from a case of dysentery—a doctor from Panama. They are most extraordinary and striking creatures and take one's breath away at first to see these large amebae—10 to 20 times the size of a leukocyte—crawling about in the pus. The movements are very active and in one case kept up for 10 hours. I get a fresh stock of pus from the drainage tube everyday so if you could run down some eve, we could look for the creatures in the morning. Keep an eye on your Blockley dysenteries as it would be most interesting to find similar bodies in our dysenteries."

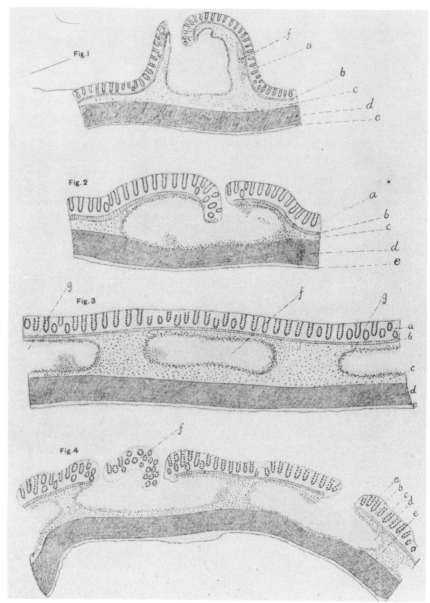

Fig 3.   Histological sections through amebic ulcers in the colon.
Reprinted from Councilman WT and LaFleur HA: Amebic dysentery. Johns Hopkins Hosp Rep 2: 395, 1891 (Plate I)

dysentery until some 15 years later. It was on a trip to the Philippines made by Flexner and Barker at the end of the Spanish-American War [1899] that Flexner isolated his species of *Bacillus dysenteriae* from cases of bacillary dysentery occurring in the Philippines at that time.) Councilman goes on to describe in detail these different forms of dysentery and among them clearly are cases of bacillary dysentery. The conclusions that he drew from this study were as follows:

> From the various inflammations of the large intestine which form the anatomical lesions of dysentery we can separate one distinct form, both clinically and anatomically, which is produced by amoebic dysentery.
>
> The other inflammations of the colon appear independently or in the course of other diseases. It is probable that they may be due to a number of causes. It is at pres-

ent not possible to distinguish in them a characteristic lesion which we can regard as due to the action of a single cause.

> Our endeavors both clinically and pathologically should be mainly in the direction of ascertaining whether there are other diseases due to definite etiological factors, the anatomical lesions of which are found among the catarrhal and diphtheritic inflammations of the colon.

PROFESSOR OF PATHOLOGY AT HARVARD

As the years passed Councilman became Welch's right hand man, doing most of the autopsies and conducting the business end of the Department of Pathology in a most effective way.

Harvard tried to entice both Osler and Welch to come to Boston and assist in a reorganization of the

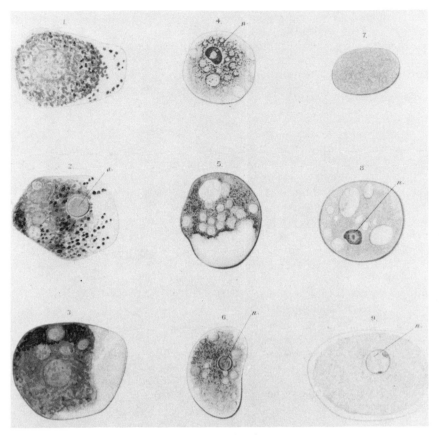

Fig 4.   Drawing of amebae as they appeared under the microscope.
Reprinted from Councilman WT and LaFleur HA: Amebic dysentery. Johns Hopkins Hosp Rep 2: 395, 1918 (Plate VII)

medical education program at Harvard. This offer came in the year 1892, just before the medical school opened here, and at a time in which both had become quite restless because of the difficulties involved in securing the funds to get the medical school going; nevertheless, they both refused. However, Welch saw an opportunity for his close associate Councilman and recommended him for the position. In 1892 Councilman was appointed Shattuck Professor of Pathology at Harvard. This was the first time that a professor had been appointed from outside the city of Boston. On May 21, 1892 Councilman wrote to the president of the Board of Trustees of the Johns Hopkins University as follows: "Having accepted the position of professor of pathology in the medical school of Harvard University I beg leave to tender my resignation as associate professor of anatomy. At the same time I wish to express to you my deep sense of gratitude for the advantages I have enjoyed in my connection with the university. These advantages have not only been in the means and encouragement given me for advancing my knowledge in the work which I have chosen, but also in the privilege of being a co-worker in furthering the high ideals of the university. I trust that sufficient of the spirit of the Johns Hopkins University has entered into me that I can carry it into my new field of work."

Councilman taught for 30 years in the Harvard Medical School, which profited greatly by his ferment. During this period, he continued active in several time-consuming investigations. As depicted by his friend Harvey Cushing, he loved to play, but when once "on a scientific quest he pursued it relentlessly and virtually lived with his problem." Although his published papers dealt with many timely subjects, he was more keenly interested in stimulating the work of his associates and pupils than in studies carried out himself. Most of his later work was done in collaboration with his outstanding disciples: "On epidemic cerebrospinal meningitis" (1898) with F. D. Mallory and J. H. Wright; "Studies of 220 fatal cases of diphtheria" (1900) with F. D. Mallory and R. M. Pierce; "A syllabus of pathology for students" (1904) with F. D. Mallory; and the several important studies on variola and vaccinia (1891–92) were subsequently brought together (1904) in a monograph under the names of his several co-workers, G. B. Magrath, W. R. Brinckerhoff, E. E. Tyzzer, E. E. Southard, R. L. Thompson, I. R. Bancroft, and G. N. Calkins.

After the opening in 1913 of the Peter Bent Brigham Hospital, to which he was appointed Pathologist-in-Chief, his routine responsibilities greatly enlarged; most of his time from then on was consumed in the hospital and the departmental protocols of those days are models of thoroughness (Fig 5). These routine-filled days served to accentuate his love of the outdoors and his interest in horticulture. Cushing speaks of this interest as follows: "Disturbed by the architecturally un-adorned exterior of the new hospital, he personally selected, planted, and during his odd hours, cultivated the well-chosen variety of rambler roses that still sur-round it; and when so engaged nothing gave him greater delight than for passersby to mistake him for the official gardener. He had a gift of making things grow and was forever planting and tending shrubs and flowers some-where. One of his chief joys was the Arnold Arboretum and his knowledge of every shrub and tree in that mar-velous place was scarcely exceeded by that of his greatly admired friend, Charles S. Sargent the director. He was, in the broadest sense, a naturalist and all things in-terested him."

Councilman's interest in the unfamiliar flora of other regions and his fondness for travel in order to study them firsthand was made possible in 1916 when he ac-companied the Rice Expedition to the Amazon and, in 1923 when he was invited to join temporarily the staff of the Peking Union Medical College, at which time he took the opportunity to travel around the world. On relin-quishing his chair and with it his hospital position, Councilman merely shifted his attention from the dis-eases of man to those of plants. One of his last printed

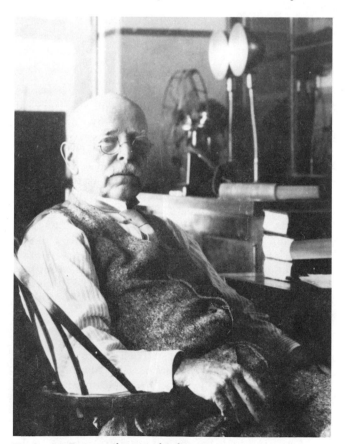

Fig 5. W. T. Councilman in his later years.
From the Alan M. Chesney Archives, The Johns Hopkins Medical Institutions

papers issued from the Arnold Arboretum was the result of a microscopic study of the relation of the fungi of its essential humus to the root system of *Epigaea repens*. As befitted its place of publication in the *Proceedings of the National Academy of Sciences*, it was a detailed presenta-tion of a novel and little-studied subject couched in sci-entific terms.

In 1912 The Johns Hopkins University awarded Councilman the honorary M.A. degree. He wrote from Boston on March 23 to Professor Remsen as follows: "I wish to express my great appreciation of the honor which the university has so unexpectedly conferred upon me. I shall never forget the joy and work and the inspiration of the early days when I first knew the university, and we know there has not been, nor will there be, any departure from the early ideals."

Remsen replied on March 25: "I thank you for your letter of the 23rd just received. A diploma will be sent to you as soon as we get the blanks. This will probably be in a few days. We wanted you on our rolls, and now we have you there."

On May 13, 1915 a dinner was held at Baltimore's Belvedere Hotel in honor of Dr. Councilman. On that oc-casion a portrait, which had been subscribed to by his friends and painted by Mr. Seyffert, was presented to Mrs. Councilman.

"Councilman went through life observing, study-ing, recording and speculating on things small and on things large, but always with consuming interest in the quest that engaged him and living up to his maxim that the chief happiness lies in work. When uprooted from his warm and fertile Maryland soil and transplanted to the rugged shores of Puritan New England, there must have clung to him some of the essential native humus which guaranteed more than a precarious footing. Though 'deeply engraved on his memory' was the bursting springtime of his boyhood home, he came to appreciate no less the beauties of a slower year's awakening. So it is suitable to leave him—engrossed in the study of the tiny Mayflower and vigorously championing its right to sur-vive."

Thus, a native Marylander became a member of the original medical school faculty and made significant contributions to new knowledge in the field of infectious diseases. He was one of the early members of the faculty to be chosen for a position of leadership in another uni-versity. Councilman's successful career at Harvard high-lights one of the principal contributions of Johns Hopkins—the population of the faculties of other schools with outstanding teachers and contributors to medical care, teaching and research.

ACKNOWLEDGMENTS

I wish to express my appreciation to Dr. Thomas B. Turner, Patricia King and Sondra Love for their help in the preparation of this vignette.

REFERENCES

1. Councilman WT: A contribution to the study of inflamma-tion as illustrated by induced keratitis. Prize essay of the Balti-

more Academy of Medicine. Baltimore: J. Murphy and Company, 1880. (Reprinted from J Physiol 3: 76, 1880–82)

2. Councilman WT: A letter from Prague. (Dated July 16, 1883, signed "W.T.C.") Med News 43: 160, 1883

3. Councilman WT: Preliminary notes on the study of malarial blood. Md State Med J 15: 441, 1886

4. Councilman WT: Certain elements found in the blood in cases of malarial fever. Trans Assoc Am Physicians 1: 89, 1886

5. Councilman WT: Further observations on the blood in cases of malarial fever. Med News 50: 59, 1887

6. Councilman WT: The malarial germ of Laveran. Am Public Health Assoc Rep 13: 224, 1888

7. Councilman WT: Some further investigations on the malarial germ of Laveran. Md State Med J 18: 209, 1887–88. Also, Boston Med Surg J 119: 436, 1888

8. Councilman WT: Neuere Untersuchungen über Laverans Organismus der Malaria. Fortsch d Med 6: 449, 500, 1888

9. Councilman WT: Dysentery. Boston Med Surg J 127: 1, 1892

10. Councilman WT: Dysentery. Trans Assoc Am Physicians 7: 113, 1892

11. Councilman WT: An anatomical and bacteriological study of forty-nine cases of acute and subacute nephritis with special reference to the glomerular lesions. Med Surg Rep Boston City Hosp 8.s: 31, 1897

12. Councilman WT: An anatomical and bacteriological study of acute diffuse nephritis. Am J Med Sci 114: 23, 1897

13. Councilman WT: Acute interstitial nephritis. J Exp Med 3: 393, 1898. Also, J Boston Soc Med Sci 2: 189, 1897–98 and Trans Assoc Am Physicians 13: 300, 1898

14. Councilman WT: A lecture delivered to the second-year class of the Harvard Medical School at the conclusion of the course in Pathology. December 19, 1921. (Last lecture as a teacher of undergraduates in medicine). Privately printed.

15. Councilman WT: The root system of epigaea repens and its relation to the fungi of the humus. Proc Natl Acad Sci 9: 279, 1923

16. Councilman WT and Abbott AC: A contribution to the pathology of malarial fever. Am J Med Sci 89: 416, 1885

17. Councilman WT and LaFleur HA: Amebic dysentery. Johns Hopkins Hosp Rep 2: 395, 1891

18. Councilman WT and Lambert RA: The Medical Report of the Rice Expedition to Brazil. Cambridge: Harvard University Press, 1918

19. Councilman WT, Magrath GB and Brinckerhoff WR: A preliminary communication on the etiology of variola. J Med Res 9: 372, 1903

20. Councilman WT, Magrath GB and Brinckerhoff WR: The pathological anatomy and histology of variola. J Med Res 11: 12, 1904

21. Councilman WT et al.: Studies on the pathology and on the aetiology of variola and of vaccinia. J Med Res 11: 1, 1904

22. Councilman WT and Mallory FB: Pathology syllabus. Copyright, 1899

23. Councilman WT, Mallory FB and Pearce RM: A study of the bacteriology and pathology of two hundred and twenty fatal cases of diphtheria. J Boston Soc Med Sci 5: 139, 1900

24. Councilman WT, Mallory FB and Wright JH: Epidemic cerebrospinal meningitis and its relation to other forms of meningitis. A monograph published as a report of the State Board of Health of Massachusetts, Boston, 1898. Also, J Boston Soc Med Sci 2: 53, 1897–98

25. Councilman WT, Mallory FB and Wright JH: Epidemic cerebrospinal meningitis. Am J Med Sci 115: 251, 1898. Also, Phila Med J 1: 937, 1898

26. Councilman WT and Strong RP: Plague-like infections in rodents; summarized report. Trans Assoc Am Physicians 36: 135, 1921

27. Cushing H: The Life of William Osler. London: Oxford Univ Press, Volume 1, p 326, 1926

28. Cushing H: Biographical memoir of William Thomas Councilman, 1854–1933. Science 77: 613, 1933

29. Flexner S and Flexner JT: William Henry Welch and the Heroic Age of American Medicine. New York: Viking Press, p 254, 1941

30. LaFleur HA: Demonstration of amoebae coli in dysentery. Bull Johns Hopkins Hosp 1: 91, 1890

31. Osler W: The hematozoa of malaria. Br Med J 1: 557, 1887

32. Osler W: On the amoeba coli in dysentery and in dysenteric liver abscess. Bull Johns Hopkins Hosp 1: 53, 1890

33. Simon CE: Abscess of the liver, perforation into the lung; amoebae coli in sputum. Bull Johns Hopkins Hosp 1: 97, 1890

34. Sternberg GM: The malarial germ of Laveran. Med Rec 29: 489, 517, 1886

35. Stilwell GG: Amoebiasis: Its early history. Gastroenterology 28: 606, 1955

4.
Johns Hopkins and Yellow Fever:
A Story of Tragedy and Triumph

INTRODUCTION

It is generally recognized that the demonstration that yellow fever is transmitted by mosquitoes is one of the greatest achievements of modern medical science. The credit for this demonstration belongs to the Yellow Fever Board of which Major Walter Reed, Surgeon, U.S. Army, was president, and James Carroll, Jesse Lazear and Aristides Agramonte were members. This Board was sent to Cuba in 1900 on the recommendation of George M. Sternberg, then Surgeon-General of the Army. What is not generally known is that all of these men, with the exception of Agramonte, had a close association with The Johns Hopkins Medical Institutions.

Johns Hopkins decreed in his will that the University and Hospital should cooperate in the promotion of medical science. Consequently, President Daniel Coit Gilman and the original faculty gave much thought to postgraduate medical education and in the premedical course a thorough foundation was provided by a special program of instruction in physics, chemistry, and biology. Many of those who trained in these laboratories in Baltimore were later to make distinguished contributions to medical science.

The importance of these early laboratories was emphasized by Henry Sewall, who was awarded his doctoral degree in physiology under Henry Newell Martin:

> The precious influence of those early days of halting development is attested in the careers of many who there first tested the exultant freedom of scientific thought. Councilman was one of those pupils and often has he eagerly acknowledged his debt to Martin for kindling and shaping his early ambitions ... Later, Sternberg, just winning his spurs in bacteriology, was cordially given the run of the laboratory and there developed some of the essential researches on which his scientific reputation rests. And, incidentally, it may be remarked that, in my belief, the vast uplift which the medical and hygienic standards of the government medical service has witnessed in the past quarter century has been chiefly due to the influence of the biological departments of the Johns Hopkins University, first through the stimulus given by Martin and later by the precious association enjoyed by workers with Welch. There was illustrated the very ideal of pedagogy in which the soul of the teacher combined with the soul of the pupil and charged it with a force which irresistibly impelled to the search for revelation in Nature. It may well be doubted whether without this teaching there would have been as we know them in person or in memory, a Reed, a Carroll, a Gorgas or a Lazear. Without this teaching it is probable that yellow fever would have remained a mysterious miasm and the attempt to trench the continent at Panama would have been a disastrous failure.

THE DEPARTMENT OF BIOLOGY

Prominence was given to biology because of its fundamental relation to medicine. Henry Newell Martin, the first professor of biology, was familiar with the best methods employed in the physiological laboratories in England and on the continent. A pupil of Michael Foster, professor of physiology at Cambridge, Martin had also had an important relationship with T. H. Huxley and under Huxley's direction had prepared a famous *Textbook on Practical Biology*, published in 1876. Martin was the first to take the degree of doctor of science in physiology at Cambridge, while at the same time qualifying in medicine in London.

In 1874 the call to America came. At Johns Hopkins, Martin was free to teach and do research in physiology in accordance with his own personal training. In University Circular #9 a description of the graduate instruction and opportunity for research in the department of biology was given. A few key areas of biology and physiology were emphasized to begin with and the best facilities possible were provided for their study. The university allowed the student to select his plan of study from one of several schedules described in the university catalog. Among the subjects which could be taken up after preliminary work in physics and chemistry was biology and its study was recommended to those preparing themselves for the study of medicine.

Martin was actively involved in stimulating research among those interested in physiology. The degree of his success is attested to by the outstanding students in his department including William T. Councilman, Henry Sewall, William Henry Howell, John J. Abel, W. T. Sedgwick, T. H. Morgan, Ross G. Harrison and Frederic S. Lee.

Reprinted from the *Johns Hopkins Medical Journal* **149**: 25, 1981.

[1] Sewell H: Henry Newell Martin. Bull Johns Hopkins Hosp 22: 327, 1911.

The first course offered in the laboratory was one in general biology following the lines of the textbook by Huxley and Martin. The personnel of the first class was drawn chiefly from the more ambitious students of the University of Maryland and the undergraduates of that school. Among those who attended these lectures given by Henry Newell Martin in 1881 was Walter Reed, later of yellow fever fame. At that time, Reed was the surgeon at Fort McHenry. He lived with his wife and only child at the Carrollton Hotel in Baltimore, which was referred to by H. L. Mencken as the "Gourmet's Delight."

In 1884 the new laboratory of biology, a four-story building of 80 by 54 feet, was opened. It contained large rooms for general and undergraduate work and separate work rooms for advanced students or those engaged in physiological or morphological research; a small museum of comparative anatomy; as well as special rooms for chemical physiology, electrophysiology, microphotography, myograph work and advanced histology.

THE DEPARTMENT OF PATHOLOGY

In 1884 William Henry Welch accepted the professorship of pathology in the new Johns Hopkins University. Since the pathological laboratory was under construction and would not be available until 1886, Welch set out for further study in Europe. The new science of bacteriology was evolving at a rapid pace and Welch recognized its significance. With Frobenius in Munich, he learned the techniques of bacteriology and also worked with von Pettenkofer who stimulated his interest in public health and hygiene. Acting on Koch's advice, Welch then went to Goettingen to work with Flugge who contributed greatly to Welch's bacteriologic background. This was followed by several weeks of working under Koch himself.

In September 1885 Welch returned to Baltimore to begin his activities in a temporary laboratory on the top floor of the new biology building. Soon he occupied the building on the hospital lot that had originally been intended as a "deadhouse" but was converted according to his specifications to house a laboratory of experimental medicine as well.

Welch's laboratory was a beehive of activity and had a tremendous influence on the progress of medical research in the United States. Many important investigators had their early experience in this laboratory including W. T. Councilman, William S. Halsted, Franklin P. Mall, A. C. Abbott, Simon Flexner, L. F. Barker, and George Nuttall.

In 1891 Walter Reed returned to Johns Hopkins for training, working this time under Welch.[2] James Carroll, after graduation from the University of Maryland in 1891, came to Welch's laboratory where he remained for two years, receiving training in pathology and bacteriology. George M. Sternberg also did bacteriological work in Welch's laboratory.

[2] Reed's period with Welch was interrupted for several weeks for temporary duty at Fort Keogh in Montana during the Battle of Wounded Knee.

THE CLINICAL LABORATORY

The clinical laboratory was organized by William Osler after the opening of The Johns Hopkins Hospital. This laboratory was under the direction of Jesse Lazear during the period in which he was an assistant resident in medicine (1895–97).

GEORGE MILLER STERNBERG

George M. Sternberg (Fig. 1) was a fellow by courtesy in the department of biology under Henry Newell Martin in 1880–81. On his return in 1884, he was again a fellow by courtesy in biology, and after 1886 utilized the facilities for bacteriology developed by Welch.

Sternberg was born at Hartwick Seminary, Otsego County, New York on June 8, 1838. At an early age he began the study of anatomy and physiology under Dr. Horace Lathrop of Cooperstown, New York. He attended his first course of medical lectures during the winter of 1859–60 at Buffalo. Later he entered the College of Physicians and Surgeons in New York City, receiving his M.D. degree in 1860. He then practiced medicine in Elizabeth City, New Jersey until the outbreak of the Civil War.

On October 19, 1865, Sternberg married Miss Louisa Russell, daughter of Robert Russell of Cooperstown, New York. She joined her husband at Fort Harker, Kansas in the spring of 1867 and on July 15 died in a cholera epidemic. Sternberg remarried in 1869, his second wife being the daughter of Thomas Thurston Pattison, a prominent pioneer in Indiana, who had settled

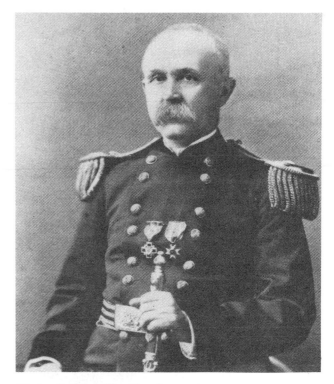

Fig 1.   George Miller Sternberg
Courtesy of the National Library of Medicine.

earlier on the eastern shore of Maryland. Sternberg's experience in the Army brought him in contact with several epidemics of yellow fever and by 1875 he was an authority on the subject. Sternberg had yellow fever in 1875. To recuperate he was granted a leave of absence for six months and on November 9, 1875 he and his wife sailed for Europe.

While at Fort Walla Walla in 1878, Sternberg began experiments to determine the practical value of commercial disinfectants, a line of work with which his name henceforth became conspicuously identified.

On April 18, 1879 Sternberg returned to Washington and was detailed for duty with the Havana Yellow Fever Commission of the National Board of Health. It was during this commission's existence that Sternberg attempted to find the causative organism of yellow fever in the blood of patients suffering from the disease. Many of the photomicrographs he made at that time won commendation from experts. In fact, Sternberg was the pioneer in bacteriology in the United States: there were no other workers in pure bacteriology in this country when he entered the field. He failed to find the causative organism, of course, but recognized that greater progress must be made in the new science of bacteriology before definite conclusions regarding the causative organism of yellow fever could be made.

In February 1881 Sternberg discovered a pneumococcus which was recognized as the pathogenic agent of lobar pneumonia and which he found to be constant in his own sputum. This microorganism was identical with one described by Pasteur in 1881. Thus priority, in accordance with the usual rules, belongs to Pasteur. Both Pasteur and Sternberg found that this bacillus produced bacteremia in inoculated animals. Further experiments that he made in the biological laboratory of The Johns Hopkins University fully confirmed his results.

On August 10, 1881 Sternberg was ordered to Fort Mason in California. Here he established, at his own expense, a laboratory for biological research and there in 1881 photographed the tubercle bacillus discovered by Professor Robert Koch earlier in the year.

On November 27, 1883 Sternberg addressed a letter to Surgeon-General Robert Murray of the U.S. Army indicating that he earnestly desired to devote his time to scientific and literary work and especially to microscopical and experimental studies relating to the etiology of infectious diseases.

An order came in April 1884 transferring Sternberg to the Department of the East. Shortly after his arrival in the East, Sternberg was detailed as Attending Surgeon and Examiner of Recruits at Baltimore. The following is quoted from the biography of Sternberg written by his wife, Martha L. Sternberg:

> We rented a prettily furnished house and as I was fortunate in my domestic arrangements our new home was most enjoyable. Baltimore is a charming city with excellent libraries, good universities, and a fine school for training in classical music (Peabody Institute), which has served to educate the citizens generally in a demand for a higher class of music. Science is well supported. The Johns

Hopkins University is a mecca for students and advanced workers in the sciences, higher education, and medicine.

In March 1885, Sternberg demonstrated for the first time in America at The Johns Hopkins University the living motile plasmodium of malaria discovered by Laveran in 1880. The demonstration was made from freshly drawn blood of a patient suffering from malarial fever and the ameboid movements of the plasmodium in the interior of the red blood corpuscles were plainly visible. In the next year he introduced the bacillus of typhoid fever to the American medical profession in a paper presented to the Association of American Physicians. . . .

In 1886 we made a trip to Berlin in order that Dr. Sternberg might have the opportunity of knowing personally Professor Koch and perhaps have the opportunity to work in his laboratory. While working in Koch's laboratory, this distinguished investigator naturally referred to Sternberg's discovery of the pneumococcus and the fact that he had first found the organism in his own mouth. Sternberg volunteered to demonstrate the germ from his saliva. On his return from the laboratory he was somewhat absorbed in thought and when I asked him the reason he confided: "How dreadfully I would feel if I lost that germ in the meantime from my mouth and could not demonstrate a thing that I have written and talked so much about." He need have had no concern as he performed the experiment most satisfactorily.

After his return from Europe, Sternberg was informed that he had won the "Lomb Prize" for his long and faithful work on the practical value of disinfectants. These experiments, begun in 1878 at Walla Walla, Washington, were continued in Washington, D.C. and were completed in the laboratory of The Johns Hopkins University. They were the culmination of studies undertaken as chairman of a committee of the American Public Health Association which had made an appropriation for such investigations. The results were published in full in the *Transactions* of that association for 1888.

In the early part of 1887 Sternberg was assigned to do experimental work in South American countries and gave up his Baltimore house in preparation for these new duties. The investigations which he conducted in Havana in the summers of 1888 and 1889, and in Decatur, Alabama in the autumn of 1888, and pathologic research in the laboratories of The Johns Hopkins Hospital during the intervals between visits to infected localities, formed the basis of Sternberg's final *Report on Etiology and Prevention of Yellow Fever* published by the Government Printing Office in 1890.

In 1890 Sternberg was assigned as medical purveyor at San Francisco. It was while there that he completed his monumental work on bacteriology, a volume covering 900 pages and giving an extensive account and systematic classification of microorganisms describing more than 500 species, including 158 pathogenic varieties. Walter Reed commented on the book in the following letter:

Headquarters Department of Dakota,
St. Paul, Minn., March 28, 1893

Dear Doctor:

Please accept my heartiest thanks for the cultures which arrived in good shape, a few days ago. I should be very glad to give more of my time to bacteriology, but, alas, my dear doctor, when most interested I must stop for practical things, so that I can only do the merest "dabbling." I have your new work, which was sent to me on special requisition. How an Army medical officer, in the midst of daily routine work, could have written so excellent and so exhaustive a work, I can't understand. . . .

> Sincerely yours,
> Walter Reed

On May 30, 1893 Sternberg was made Surgeon-General of the Army.

Very soon after becoming Surgeon-General, Sternberg recommended the establishment of the Army Medical School in Washington, D.C., which was accomplished by General Order No. 51, Adjutant General's Office, June 24, 1893.

On May 23, 1900 Sternberg wrote the following letter to the Adjutant-General of the Army:

> I have the honor to recommend that Major Walter Reed, Surgeon, U.S. Army, and Contract Surgeon James Carroll, U.S. Army, be ordered to proceed from this city (Washington, D.C.) to Camp Columbia, Cuba, reporting their arrival and instructions to the commanding officer of the post.
>
> I also recommend the organization of a medical board with headquarters at Camp Columbia for the purpose of pursuing scientific investigations with reference to the infectious diseases prevalent on the Island of Cuba and especially of yellow fever.
>
> The Board is to be constituted as follows:
>
> Major Walter Reed, Surgeon U.S. Army; Contract Surgeon James Carroll, U.S. Army, and Contract Surgeons Aristides Agramonte and Jesse W. Lazear, U.S. Army. . . .
>
> The Board should act under general instructions which will be communicated to Major Reed by the Surgeon-General of the Army."

When Sternberg retired from the Army at age 64, a distinguished list of physicians attended a testimonial dinner in New York City, the proceedings of which were recorded in the *Medical News* for June 21, 1902. At this dinner Dr. William H. Welch said that Sternberg was the pioneer worker in bacteriology in this country; he had been compelled to acquire the technique from reading and the entire world knew how he had perfected a technique equal to that of the best. He had made many important discoveries, his work on disinfection and disinfectants standing as a monument alone. Also, as the first worker to isolate the microorganism of pneumonia, he had gained renown and his work with yellow fever would stand forever.

Sternberg in reply said the following: ". . . but while I met with a serious disappointment in my failure to discover the yellow fever germ, I have the satisfaction of knowing that my research has cleared the way for the subsequent demonstration by Reed and his associates of the method by which this disease is transmitted from man to man. . . ."

WALTER REED

Walter Reed (Fig 2) was born in Gloucester County, Virginia on September 13, 1851. In 1886, at age

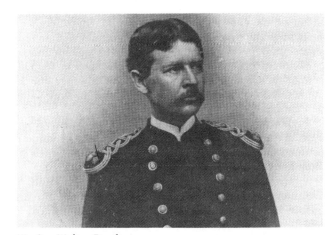

Fig 2. Walter Reed
Courtesy of the National Library of Medicine.

15, Reed attended a private school in Charlottesville kept by Mr. Abbot, a graduate of the University of Virginia. He remained there for two sessions and then entered the university by dispensation, as he was only 16. In spite of his youth, his work was always good and he held a high place in all of his classes. Since he had two brothers at the university, and his father's means were limited, he soon realized he could not take the entire course. He applied, therefore, to the faculty, in person, to be certified in the studies he had pursued, but this request was refused on the ground that he was underage. He then inquired whether he would be allowed to take the degree of doctor of medicine if he could pass the examinations. To this the faculty silently assented, thinking that it was a safe promise, for the undertaking appeared to be an impossibility. Reed at once began his medical studies and graduated nine months later in the summer of 1869, standing third in his class—the youngest student ever graduated from the medical school in Charlottesville.

A few months after graduation, he matriculated at the Bellevue Hospital Medical College where he completed the requirements for the M.D. degree one year later.[3] He was attached then to several of the hospitals in New York and Brooklyn, including the King's County Hospital where he was an intern. Later he was appointed physician to one of the poorest districts in Brooklyn which brought him in daily contact with all the misery arising from poverty and vice in a large city, an experience which affected him deeply. Reed attracted the attention of Dr. Joseph C. Hutchison, then the leading physician and surgeon in Brooklyn, and through his influence Reed was appointed one of the five inspectors on the Brooklyn Board of Health while still 22 years of age. He was quite disillusioned by the incompetence of the physicians with whom he came in contact.

In 1874 he abandoned the idea of general practice

---

[3] Although Reed fulfilled the work required for the M.D. degree at 18 years of age, it was a school rule that the candidate had to be 21 years of age. When he reached age 21 he did not have the $25.00 to pay for the diploma which, though dated that year, was not awarded until the commencement held after he was 22. There is a note by Austin Flint, Jr. to this effect in the old school records. (Personal communication, William B. Bean)

and decided to enter the Army as a surgeon, one of his reasons being his desire to pursue scientific research. Another was the need to possess an assured competency as soon as possible in order that he might seek Miss Emilie Lawrence's hand in marriage. The stress of taking the highly competitive examinations had a deleterious effect on his health for a temporary period, but in February 1875 he passed his examinations brilliantly and in the following June received his commission as assistant surgeon with the rank of First Lieutenant. After assignment to a station in New York harbor,[4] he was ordered to Arizona. This led to speeding up the arrangements for his marriage, which took place on April 25, 1876. After four challenging and rugged years in the West, Reed was ordered east again and promoted to the rank of Captain.

In 1881 he was stationed for a brief period at Fort McHenry, Baltimore, and while there made use of the opportunity to attend Henry Newell Martin's lectures on physiology at The Johns Hopkins University. Reed's exposure to Martin was his introduction to the world of modern scientific research.[5]

In 1882 Reed was transferred to the Department of the Platte and was stationed in western Nebraska. In 1887, after five years in Nebraska, Reed was ordered to Mount Vernon Barracks, Alabama. In 1889 he began to feel keenly that he needed time and opportunity for study, in order to keep abreast of advances in medical research. He applied, therefore, for a leave of absence, stating his reasons for doing so and the advantages to himself and others that he hoped to gain from it. The Army replied that if he would pay the salary of a contract surgeon to fill his place he might go. This was a bitter disappointment, but fortunately for only a short time. The old order in Washington was just then giving place to the new, and sufficient interest was manifested in 1890 to ensure Reed's appointment as Attending Surgeon and Examiner of Recruits in Baltimore with permission to pursue some line of professional work at The Johns Hopkins Hospital, at that time, just opened to physicians for graduate courses in clinical medicine, surgery, and pathology.

[4] He was stationed at Willet's Point (now Fort Totten), which is just past the end of the east-west runway at LaGuardia Airfield.

[5] Provision was made for special students. The number of medical men, for example, who entered for a course of instruction in histology or animal physiology was quite large and each year several students from medical schools in the city were admitted to study in the laboratory. In accordance with the general principle of the University, to be chary of its honors but liberal of its benefits, such persons though not candidates for a degree were willingly received when circumstances, such as the time which could be given to this work, showed that it was likely to be profitable. A systematic course of instruction for students who had not matriculated and who did not intend to take the B.A. degree was opened to those who intended thereafter to study medicine and who could pass an entrance examination designed to show whether they had a fair general education. Professor Martin conducted two series of 20 demonstrations in animal physiology before a class of students from the medical schools of the city, several physicians also attending. In these, all the fundamental physiological experiments were shown.

According to Kelly, Reed consulted the superintendent of the hospital as to his best line of work and was advised to take courses in pathology and bacteriology in addition to certain clinical work in general medicine and surgery. Reed had no difficulty in obtaining the necessary permission to devote himself largely to pathology and bacteriology.

The winter of 1890–91 was one of the keenest enjoyment to Reed. After living for so many years at a distance from the scientific world and cut off from congenial companionship, he returned to both with delight. His work at The Johns Hopkins Hospital brought him into the society of cultivated scientific men, with whom his own genial nature and charming manner made him universally popular.[6] He made many warm friendships

[6] While with Welch, Reed shared a table with Simon Flexner and Reed complained in a joking way that Flexner had squeezed him right off the end of the work bench. In 1891, when Reed and Carroll were students at Johns Hopkins, the instruction in pathology and bacteriology was given in the pathological laboratory, one of the buildings of The Johns Hopkins Hospital, by Professor William H. Welch, William T. Councilman, and George H. F. Nuttall. The courses were opened to physicians and advanced students of biology. Opportunity was given for advanced work in pathology and bacteriology. The laboratory was equipped with material for investigations in pathological histology, with the necessary apparatus for work in experimental pathology, and with cultures and facilities for bacteriological work. In addition to the fresh material from the wards of the hospital, attention was paid to the pathological studies of diseases of animals for which purpose abundant material had been collected. Opportunity was afforded to witness postmortem examinations and instruction was given in the methods of conducting such examinations and of recording in proper protocols the results. Fresh material from postmortem examinations held in the pathological laboratory and elsewhere in the city were demonstrated in connection with the course in pathological histology. Two courses in the latter subject were given, one beginning early in October and the other the first of February with classes on three afternoons of the week. Microscopical sections were given to be stained, mounted, and carefully studied and drawn in addition to the study of inflammation and other subjects in general pathology and the pathological histology of the different tissues and organs of the body taken up in regular order. Written examinations consisting in the diagnosis and description of microscopical sections were held frequently during the course. Courses in bacteriology given by Welch and Nuttall began in the middle of October and the first of February. These courses consisted in practical work in the bacteriological laboratory which occupied rooms in the pathological building. The student was taught the preparation of culture media, the principles of disinfection and sterilization, methods of cultivating, staining, and studying bacteria and familiarity with the important species of bacteria, particularly those of a pathogenic nature. The general plan of instruction was that adopted in the Hygienic Laboratory in Berlin. The pathological laboratory, being upon the same grounds with the hospital and dispensary, the opportunities were convenient for combining clinical work, attendance upon operations and clinical lectures and studies in the clinical laboratory with the work in pathology. Opportunity was also afforded for practical instruction in hygiene in the hygienic laboratory under the direction of Drs. J. S. Billings and A. C. Abbott.

during this year of his life, particularly that of Professor William Henry Welch.

The following account of Reed's work at The Johns Hopkins Hospital was given by Welch to Kelly:

Dr. Reed was sent to Baltimore in October, 1890, as Attending Surgeon and Examiner of Recruits, and he remained there until the following October. The Medical Department of the University was not opened until October, 1893, but the Hospital was in full operation in 1889, and the Pathological Laboratory of the Hospital and the University had been equipped and opened for the reception of physicians and advanced students and for research since 1885. Here systematic laboratory courses were given in pathology and bacteriology, and it was here that Dr. Reed received his fundamental training in these subjects.

Reed began his work on the clinical side of the Hospital, but after a few weeks, a new Surgeon-General having in the meantime been appointed, he was able to follow his own inclination and to enter the regular courses in pathology and bacteriology in the Pathological Laboratory. I well recall with what eagerness and enthusiasm he turned his attention to the new fields of scientific medicine thus first opened to him, which from that time until the end of his life became the center of his professional interest and activity, and which he himself was destined to cultivate with such signal benefits to medical science and to the welfare of mankind.

The decade preceding the time when Reed began his practical studies at the Johns Hopkins had been a period of marvelous progress in our knowledge of infectious diseases. Upon the basis of the discoveries of Pasteur and of Koch, and particularly as a result of the new methods introduced by Koch for the cultivation and study of bacteria, there had followed in rapid succession within this period such important discoveries as those of the specific germs causing tuberculosis, cholera, leprosy, and numerous others. Pasteur had discovered methods of rendering animals artificially immune from chicken-cholera and other diseases and had devised his method of protective inoculation against rabies. . . .

While Reed took the regular courses in pathology given in the laboratory and was interested in the subject, his special object was bacteriology. . . . In the conduct of these courses there were associated with me at that time, Drs. Councilman, Abbott, Nuttall, and Flexner; and among others then engaged in research work in the laboratory I call to mind, Drs. Halsted, Lafleur, H. M. Thomas, Berkeley, W. T. Howard, Jr., Barker, Robb, Ghriskey, Randolph, Clement, Blackstein, Gilchrist, and Thayer.

Dr. Reed soon made a place for himself in this intimate group of active workers. We early recognized that he possessed unusual aptitude for the work which he had undertaken, and that he combined with excellent endowment of mind a sincere, manly, and winning personality. The friendships formed with his teachers and co-workers at this period were strong and enduring. Dr. Reed applied himself with great energy to his work in the laboratory, devoting to it daily a large part of his time and carrying it much beyond the regular class exercises. After he had acquired familiarity with technical methods, he undertook advanced and independent work. He attended postmortem examinations and sometimes conducted them; moreover, he was accustomed to study for himself pathological material and cultures which he had obtained from autopsies. He followed and profited by the various investigations which were at that time in progress in the laboratory and the Hospital, and he was a regular attendant at the meetings of the Johns Hopkins Medical Society. Drs. Abbott, Flexner and I were at that time engaged in the study of diphtheria, the toxin of which had been discovered two years previously, and the antitoxin of which was discovered by Behring in 1890. The investigations of hog-cholera made at this time by Dr. A. W. Clement and myself enabled Reed to become familiar with the hog-cholera bacillus, so that he had no difficulty later in recognizing the resemblance to this bacillus of the microorganism erroneously claimed by Sanarelli to be the cause of yellow fever. He also followed with great interest the studies of Councilman and Lafleur on amoebic dysentery, as well as investigations in the hospital on the malarial parasite.

During the latter part of his stay in Baltimore Dr. Reed was assigned, at his own request, a special subject for research. This was the microscopical and experimental study of the so-called lymphoid nodules which are found in the liver in cases of typhoid fever. He succeeded in producing these nodules experimentally and demonstrated that they originated as small foci of dead liver cells. His paper upon his subject, published in the *Reports of the Johns Hopkins Hospital*, is a valuable contribution, and it embodies the results of his first original scientific investigation.

When Reed left Baltimore in October 1891 he was well trained in pathological and bacteriological methods, he had acquired a considerable amount of experience, and he was thoroughly fitted to make the best use of such opportunities as might present themselves to add to his experience and training, as well as to undertake original investigation. . . .

In 1893, when Reed was assigned to duty as curator of the Army Medical Museum and professor of bacteriology and clinical microscopy in the Army Medical School, he at once re-established relations with the Pathological Laboratory in Baltimore. He was a frequent visitor, together with his now associate and former fellow student, Dr. Carroll, at the laboratory and he kept in touch with the men and the work there. He often attended the meetings of the Johns Hopkins Medical Society, at which he occasionally made contributions. I was often consulted by him regarding his own investigations, and his relations were likewise very intimate and cordial with Drs. Flexner, Abbott and Thayer. He talked over with me the plan of the yellow fever work to be undertaken by the commission of which he was the head, and he kept me informed by letter and by conversation of the results of this work while it was in progress.

In volume 8 of the *Bulletin of The Johns Hopkins Hospital*, there was a paper on water-borne malaria presented before the Johns Hopkins Medical Society by Rupert Norton and another on the Johnson modification of the Widal test for typhoid fever. After each of these papers Reed presented his own experience in detail. Reed also published a paper in the *Bulletin* on the association of *Proteus vulgaris* with the *Diplococcus lanceolatus* in a case of croupous pneumonia. This paper was read before the Johns Hopkins Medical Society on February 19, 1894.

MAJOR JAMES CARROLL

James Carroll (Fig 3), an Englishman born at Woolwich on June 5, 1854, intended to enter the Navy as an engineer student but at age 15, when still at a private school, emigrated to Canada. For the next few years he roughed it in the backwoods, but in 1874, at age 20, he enlisted in the U.S. Army. While serving in the far West (Department of Dakota and Fort Custer, Montana), Carroll became interested in the study of medicine.

When hospital steward William Grant, U.S. Army, first met James Carroll—then 1st sergeant of Company C, 7th U.S. Infantry at Fort Snelling, Minnesota, where they both were stationed in 1882—he recognized in Carroll the "material suitable for higher and better work than that in which he was then engaged," suggested to him the idea of studying for the position of Hospital Steward, U.S. Army, and offered "to place at his disposal certain opportunities which were then and there available for the purpose." This was a perceptive proposal on the part of Grant and a vital moment in the life of Carroll, for he promptly took advantage of the offer and made such good use of it that in the summer of 1883 he was examined by Major W. C. Spencer, Medical Corps, U.S. Army, passed an excellent examination, and was appointed hospital steward on September 15, 1883. His duties carried him to different stations in the Department of Dakota, including the post at Fort Custer, Montana, where he came under the observation and command of Captain James E. Pilcher, Medical Corps, U.S. Army.

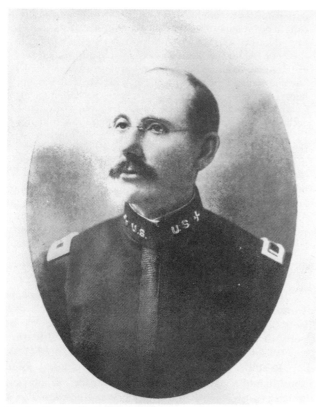

Fig 3.   James Carroll
Courtesy of Dr. Theodore E. Woodward.

From Fort Custer he took a leave of absence in 1886 and proceeded to New York City to begin the study of medicine at the University of the City of New York. On completion of his leave of absence, he returned to the Department of the Platte where he was on duty from September 1886 to February 1889. He was then ordered for duty to Fort McHenry, Maryland, where that efficient officer, himself a Marylander by birth, Captain C. B. Byrne,[7] appreciated Carroll's talents. Carroll attended lectures in medicine at the University of Maryland in 1889–90 and 1890–91, receiving his M.D. in 1891.

Carroll became deeply interested in bacteriology, which was to be of such importance to the future of medical science, and during the winters of 1891–92 and 1892–93 he took the courses in bacteriology and pathology given by W. H. Welch and his associates at The Johns Hopkins Hospital. Reed and Carroll met during the period when they were both working in Welch's laboratory.

Welch, in speaking of his laboratory in Baltimore during the period when Reed and Carroll were there, said the following: "Here his bacteriological training was acquired [Reed's]. . . . It was during this period that Carroll came to assist him. He was still a hospital steward and so subordinate to Reed, helping him in making media, assisting in experiments, and doing the simpler things. His peculiar aptitude soon became evident, however, and he was allowed to take the regular courses. . . . Carroll was very intimate with Reed and his training and reputation were due to this association. They frequently came back here together to attend lectures, two or three times a week, and kept fully in touch with the research work going on in the laboratories. . . ."

During the World's Fair at Chicago in 1893, we find Carroll assisting Captain L. A. Le Garde of the Medical Corps, himself an eminent bacteriologist. At Chicago and elsewhere, Carroll demonstrated so well his fitness for experimental work that Surgeon-General Sternberg assigned him to duty at the Army Medical Museum in Washington, where Reed was the curator. Carroll remained on duty there until assigned to Cuba in connection with the Yellow Fever Board.

Reed and Carroll had common interests as far as their scientific work was concerned and Carroll assisted Reed in the search for Pfeiffer's supposed parasite in the blood of vaccinated calves, children and monkeys done at the Columbian University (now George Washington University). In 1899 Reed and Carroll were appointed by Surgeon-General Sternberg to investigate the true nature of the *Bacillus icteroides*, which Sanarelli had erroneously concluded was the specific causative agent in yellow fever. Their work generated further interest in the study of this disease and, when an Army Medical Board was appointed in 1900 to go to Cuba to investigate the cause and mode of transmission of yellow fever, Reed was given command and Carroll became his deputy.

Carroll was appointed demonstrator in the Medical School of the George Washington (then Columbian)

[7] Byrne was the medical officer in charge at Willet's Point for most of the year Walter Reed spent there.

University in 1895 under the supervision of Walter Reed, who was then, and for many years, professor of pathology and bacteriology in this medical school. In 1903, Carroll was promoted to associate professor of bacteriology and pathology and appointed to succeed Reed as pathologist to the University Hospital. In 1905 he was promoted to a full professorship in the department of medicine and also given supervision over the students pursuing researches in bacteriology under the supervision of the Faculty of Graduate Studies.

Carroll's connection with the University included the period during which the University Hospital was created and set in operation, and the new Medical School Building was built. Dr. De Schweinitz, dean of the medical school, relied upon the judgment, special knowledge, and experience of Carroll in planning the building, and the excellent bacteriological laboratory with which the department of medicine was provided was largely due to Carroll's advice.

At the memorial session held by the Johns Hopkins Historical Club on October 14, 1907 Dr. H. H. Donnally of Washington had this to say:

> As a student in the Medical Department of George Washington University I came to know and admire Walter Reed and James Carroll, for both of whom all of the students had the highest respect. The emphasis laid by Dr. W. W. Johnston upon the importance of their courses to us as medical students was the beginning of my respect for Reed and Carroll, which grew by contact with them in the laboratory.
>
> Reed lectured to us, and model lectures they were, while after the lecture Carroll went around the room from student to student, and patiently demonstrated our specimens under the microscope. Each man received his personal attention, too, although often it was necessary to wait for it well beyond the scheduled hours, as Carroll continued as long as the men waited.
>
> Carroll's rise from a private was a great achievement. Surgeon-General Sternberg was important in James Carroll's life. He discovered James Carroll. He was his faithful friend. It was Sternberg's influence which brought Carroll to Fort McHenry, putting the study of medicine in his grasp. His claim to fame, of course, was the yellow fever work. From 1899 until his death he published 27 articles on this subject. As professor of bacteriology in the George Washington University, he was respected by faculty and literally loved by the students. Finally in March 1907 he was promoted to the rank of Major.

JESSE WILLIAM LAZEAR

Jesse W. Lazear (Fig 4) was born in Baltimore, Maryland on May 2, 1866. His earliest known ancestor, Joseph de Lazier, left France in 1682 amidst the persecution of the Huguenots. In the waters of the Kanawha in West Virginia he was scalped by the Indians. Lazear's maternal grandfather was Samuel Pettigrew, the seventh Mayor of Pittsburgh.

During his childhood, young Lazear spent much of his time at Windsor, the estate of his retired grandfather, a beautiful wooded property in the suburbs in West Bal-

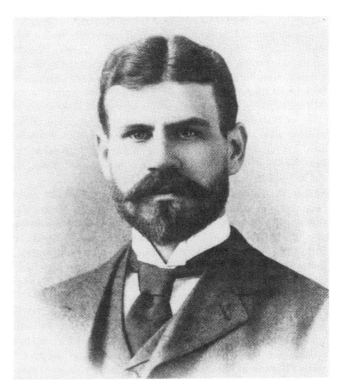

Fig 4. Jesse William Lazear
Courtesy of Dr. Theodore E. Woodward.

timore, overlooking what once had been a mill on the Gwynn's Falls. In 1881 Jesse attended Trinity Hall Academy in Washington, Pennsylvania and three years later was admitted to Washington and Jefferson College. Two years later he transferred as a sophomore to The Johns Hopkins University, matriculating in the group III course which included studies in chemistry and biology preparatory to medicine. He received his A.B. degree in June 1889. Young Lazear then entered the College of Physicians and Surgeons of Columbia University in New York, which had recently moved to new buildings on West 59th Street close to the Sloane Maternity and Vanderbilt Clinic. In those days, students who passed the entrance examination selected a preceptor. Dr. Frank Hartley was chosen by Lazear. An essential part of the educational process at that time was the private "Quiz" for which the student paid an additional fee. At the end of his first year at Columbia, Lazear went to Scotland where he registered for two courses on anatomy under Sir William Turner.

Lazear received his doctorate in medicine on June 8, 1892 at the 138th Annual Commencement of Columbia College held at the Music Hall on 57th Street and 7th Avenue. He successfully passed the competitive examination for Bellevue Hospital and became junior assistant in the department of medicine.[8]

[8] Kelly noted: "Much of Dr. Lazear's time after he was graduated in medicine was spent in research, and during his residency at Bellevue he succeeded in isolating, for the first time, the diplococcus of Neisser in pure culture from the circulating blood in a case of ulcerative endocarditis."

This was at a time when the discoveries of Pasteur and Koch had directed widespread attention to medical bacteriology and it was this field which Lazear decided to pursue. In October 1894 he and his mother sailed for Europe, where Lazear worked at the Kaiserlisches Institute until March 1895. It was during this trip that he met Mabel Houston of San Francisco, whom he later married.

From May to July 1895, Lazear attended a course on microbiological technique offered at the Pasteur Institute by Professors Emil Roux and E. Metchnikoff which consisted of lectures, laboratory observations and clinical demonstrations at the Hôtel Dieu.

At the meeting of the Medical Board of The Johns Hopkins Hospital in October 1895, William Osler recommended that Jesse W. Lazear be appointed assistant resident physician. He served in this capacity until the following August. While a member of the staff of the outpatient department at The Johns Hopkins Hospital, Lazear did much valuable work as a teacher and investigator in the laboratory of clinical pathology. At the first meeting of the Advisory Board of the Medical Faculty for the year in October 1897, Lazear was appointed an assistant in clinical microscopy. Lazear taught undergraduates in the laboratory of clinical microscopy and with Thomas B. Futcher organized a postgraduate course on clinical microscopy.

In 1896 Lazear married and began the practice of medicine in Baltimore. Holding the position of assistant in clinical microscopy in the university, much of his time was spent in research. The three years which followed were devoted mainly to the study of the malarial parasites (Fig 5). Lazear was the first in this country to confirm and elaborate on the studies of Romanovsky and others concerning the intimate structure of the haematozoa of malaria. He was, with Wooley and Thayer, the first in this country to confirm in part the work of Ross and the Italians on the mosquito cycle of the malarial parasites. Futcher and Lazear reported a new method of staining malarial parasites.

Thayer and Lazear observed a second case of ulcerative endocarditis associated with the gonococcus. In this instance, the gonococcus was obtained from the circulating blood on three occasions in pure culture, while at autopsy growths of this organism were obtained upon human blood serum agar from infected heart valves, from the heart's blood, and from the pericardium. Lazear also wrote a detailed paper on the parasites of the malarial fever, which was presented at the annual meeting of the American Medical Association in June 1900.

Early in 1900 Lazear applied for service in the U.S. Army in order to study tropical diseases in Cuba. He wrote to the Surgeon-General and forwarded a letter of introduction: "My Dear General Sternberg . . . I desire to endorse most cordially Dr. Lazear's eminent fitness for this position . . . he has already distinguished himself by valuable scientific work . . . and is an expert in clinical microscopy . . . He is now engaged in original studies on the malarial parasite which have yielded interesting results. He is a clinical man, a bacteriologist, and withall a gentleman of cultivation and agreeable personality.

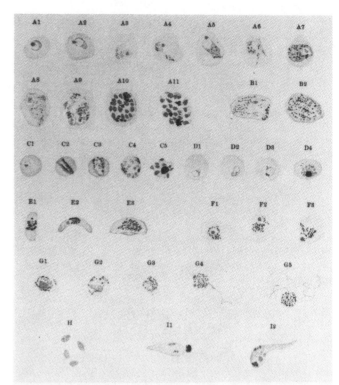

Fig 5. Plate 1 showing various forms of the malarial parasites Reprinted from Lazear JW: Structure of the malarial parasites. Johns Hopkins Hosp Rep 10:1, 1902

Signed, William H. Welch." Lazear was offered a contract as acting assistant surgeon in charge of the laboratory of Camp Columbia, Marianao, Cuba.

When Lazear arrived in Cuba, he found James Carroll and Aristides Agramonte already at work. The three were soon joined by Major Walter Reed. These four men, commanded by Reed, composed the Yellow Fever Board whose task it was to discover the cause of the epidemic fever. The Surgeon-General ordered them to begin testing the theories of Sanarelli; Surgeon-General Sternberg, on the basis of his own studies, doubted Sanarelli's claim to have found a bacillus which caused the fever. Lazear became interested in the work of Carlos Finlay, who had postulated that the fever was not transmitted by contact but by means of an intermediary. In 1881 Finlay had suggested the mosquito as the culprit but no one paid attention to his work except Lazear, who began to concentrate his efforts on verifying Finlay's hypothesis. Reed gave consent to the mosquito project and Lazear began breeding and feeding insects in the fever wards of a nearby hospital while Reed returned to Washington to complete his report on typhoid fever.

Lazear contracted yellow fever and died of the disease. He was buried in the military cemetery outside of Havana, but his remains were subsequently moved to Baltimore and interred in the Loudon Park Cemetary. A tablet to his memory was erected by his friends in the new surgical amphitheatre of The Johns Hopkins Hospital, with the following inscription written by President Eliot of Harvard University:

"In memory of
JESSE WILLIAM LAZEAR,
born May 2, 1866, at Baltimore,
Graduated in Arts at
the Johns Hopkins University in 1889;
and in Medicine at Columbia University in 1892.
In 1895-96 Assistant Resident Physician
in the Johns Hopkins Hospital.
Member of the Yellow Fever Commission in 1900
with the rank of Acting Assistant Surgeon.
He died of Yellow Fever at Quemados, Cuba,
28 of September, 1900.

With more than the courage and devotion of the soldier, he risked and lost his life to show how a fearful pestilence is communicated and how its ravages may be prevented."

THE ACCOMPLISHMENTS OF THE REED BOARD

In 1915 Aristides Agramonte wrote his version of the "inside" story of the greatest medical discovery of the twentieth century, the demonstration that yellow fever, like malaria, could be spread only by the bites of infected mosquitoes:[9]

"The whole series of events tragic, pathetic, comical and otherwise took place upon a stage made particularly fit by nature and the surrounding circumstances. Columbia Barracks, a military reservation garrisoned by some 1400 troops, distant about eight miles from the city of Havana, the latter, suffering at the time from an epidemic of yellow fever which the application of all sanitary measures had failed to check or ameliorate and finally, our experimental camp, a few Army tents, securely hidden from the road leading to Marianao, and safeguarded from intercourse with the outside world; the whole setting portentously silent and gloriously bright in the glow of tropical sunlight and the green of luxuriant vegetation.

On the morning of August 31, 1900 two members of the Commission were busily examining under microscopes several glass slides containing blood from a fellow officer who, since the day before had shown symptoms of yellow fever; these men were Drs. Jesse W. Lazear and myself; our sick colleague was Dr. James Carroll who presumably had been infected by one of our 'experimental mosquitoes.' As the idea that Carroll's fever must have been caused by the mosquito that was applied to him four days before became fixed upon our minds, we decided to test it upon the first nonimmune person who should offer himself to be bitten; this was a common occurrence and taken much as a joke among the soldiers about the military hospital. Barely fifteen minutes may have elapsed since we had come to this decision when as Lazear stood at the door of the laboratory trying to coax a mosquito to pass from one test tube to another, a soldier came walking by toward the hospital building . . . The man stopped upon coming abreast, curious no doubt to see the performance with the tubes, and after gazing for a minute or two at the insect he said: 'You still fooling with the mosquitoes doctor?' 'Yes,' returned Lazear, 'will you take a bite?' 'Sure, I ain't scared of them,' responded the man. When I heard this I turned to the soldier and asked him to come inside and bare his forearm. Upon a slip of paper I wrote his name while several mosquitoes took their fill; William H. Dean, American by birth belonging to Troop B, 7th Cavalry; he said he had never been in the tropics before and had not left the military reservation for nearly two months. Ideal conditions for a test case. Five days later when he came down with yellow fever he represented the first clear case of the disease to be produced experimentally by the bite of purposely infected mosquitoes. We sent a cablegram to Major Reed who a month before had been called to Washington upon another duty, apprising him of the fact that the theory of the transmission of yellow fever by mosquitoes, which at first was doubted so much and the transcendental importance of which we could then barely appreciate, had indeed been confirmed.

It was on the afternoon of June 25, 1900 that the four officers comprising the Commission, Major Reed, James Carroll, Dr. Jesse W. Lazear, and myself met for the first time on the veranda of the officer's quarters at Columbia Barracks Hospital. After deciding upon the first steps to be taken, it was unanimously agreed that whatever the result of our investigation should turn out to be, it was to be considered as the work of the Board as a body, never as the outcome of any individual effort; that each of us was to work in harmony with the general plan; though at liberty to carry out his individual methods of research.

On July 21 Major Reed and I investigated a series of outbreaks of yellow fever at Pinar del Rio. Of particular interest was the case of a soldier prisoner who had been confined to the guardhouse since June 6; he showed the first symptoms of yellow fever on the 12th and died on the 18th; none of the other eight prisoners in the same cell caught the infection, but one of them continued to

[9] The story of the work of the Yellow Fever Board varies with the observer. Knowing that Dr. William B. Bean had made an intensive study of the important experiments made by the Board, I asked him to carefully check the facts in this essay. He made the following comments: "Agramonte was one, as Carroll was another, who after Reed died made very strong efforts to take more credit than I believe they deserved for the yellow fever work. Everything that was done, it seems to me, derived from orders and instructions from Reed, directed officially by Sternberg and undoubtedly with much in the way of suggestions from Welch, the most clearly documented being the one on the filterable virus which had recently been described by Loeffler and Frosch for hoof and mouth disease. This led to the studies that were actually done by Carroll, but they were done according to the plans Welch suggested and Reed forwarded. Carroll's input was mainly that of a technician. Reed was working hard to get Carroll promoted. After his nearly fatal bout with yellow fever, Carroll felt that he was being mistreated and not given enough credit. He developed a profound hatred of Walter Reed as manifest in a series of remarkable letters to his wife. It is interesting to read them in parallel with the letters and information of Reed trying to get Sternberg to promote him [Carroll]."

sleep in the same bunk previously occupied by his dead comrade. More than this; the three men who handled the clothing and washed the linen of those who had died during the last month were still in perfect health. Here were the observations made earlier. The infection at a distance, the harmless condition of bedding and clothing of the sick; the possibility that some insect might be concerned in spreading the disease deeply impressed us. This was really the first time that the mosquito transmission theory was seriously considered by the members of the Board and it was decided that although discredited by the repeated failure of its most ardent supporter, Dr. Carlos J. Finlay of Havana to demonstrate it, the matter should be taken up by the Board and thoroughly sifted. As Lazear was the only one of us who had had any experience in mosquito work, Reed thought proper that he should take charge of this part of the investigation. A visit was made to Finlay, who kindly explained to us the many points regarding the life of the one kind of mosquito he thought most guilty, and ended by furnishing us with a number of eggs which laid by female mosquito nearly a month before had remained unhatched on the inside of a half empty bowl of water in his library. Much to our disappointment, Major Reed was called to Washington in order to complete his report on typhoid fever in the Army. Thus we were deprived of his able counsel during the first part of the mosquito research. He was detained longer than expected and could not return to Cuba until early in October, several days after Lazear's death.

The mosquito eggs obtained from Finlay hatched out in due time and proved to be a species called *Stegomyia fasciatus*. Lazear applied some of these mosquitoes to cases of yellow fever at Las Animas Hospital, keeping them in separate glass tubes properly labelled and everything connected with their biting being carefully recorded. The original batch soon died and the work was carried on with subsequent generations. Considering that in case our surmise as to the insect's actions should prove to be correct, it was dangerous to introduce infected mosquitoes amongst a population of 1400 nonimmune at Camp Columbia. Lazear thought it best to keep his presumably infected insects in my laboratory at the Military Hospital #1 from where he carried them back and forth to the patients who were periodically bitten. After the mosquitoes fed upon the yellow fever patients, they were applied at intervals of two or three days to whoever would consent to run the risk of contracting the disease in this way. No secret was made of our attempts to infect mosquitoes, in fact many local physicians became intensely interested. Dr. Finlay himself was somewhat chagrined when he learned of our failure to infect anyone with mosquitoes, but, like a true believer, he was inclined to attribute this negative result more to some defect in our technique than to any flaw in his favorite theory.

Although the Board had thought proper to run the same risks, if any, as those, who willingly and knowingly subjected themselves to the bites of the supposedly infected insects, opportunity did not offer itself readily since Major Reed was away in Washington and Carroll at Camp Columbia, engrossed in his bacteriological studies, came to Havana only when an autopsy was on hand. I was considered an immune ... and so time passed and several Americans and Spaniards had subjected themselves in a sporting mood to be bitten by the supposedly infected mosquitoes without causing any untoward results when Lazear applied to himself (August 16, 1900) a mosquito which ten days before had fed upon a mild case of yellow fever in the fifth day of the disease. The fact that no infection resulted, for Lazear continued in excellent health for a space of time far beyond the usual period of incubation, served to discredit the mosquito theory and the opinion of the investigators to a degree almost beyond redemption and the most enthusiastic, Dr. Lazear himself, was almost ready to throw up the sponge. Some loss of faith in the possibility that the mosquito was the vector led Lazear to relax and become less scrupulous in his care of the insects. After applying them to patients, if pressed for time he would take them with him to his laboratory at Columbia Barracks rather than leaving them at the military hospital laboratory. Thus on the 27th of August he had spent the whole morning at Las Animas Hospital getting his mosquitoes to take yellow fever blood. Among the tubes containing fed mosquitoes was one insect that for some reason or other failed to take blood when offered it. This mosquito had been hatched in the laboratory and in due time fed upon yellow fever blood from a severe case on August 15, that is 12 days before; the patient then being in his second day of illness. At that time no particular attention had been drawn to this insect except that it refused to suck blood when tempted on that morning of August 27. After luncheon that day, Carroll and Lazear were in the laboratory where the conversation turned to mosquitoes and their apparent harmlessness. Lazear remarked how one of them failed to take blood. Carroll thought he might try to feed it, as otherwise it was liable to die before the next day. This he proceeded to do. Three days later Carroll was down with the chill, thought at first due to malaria. Lazear and Agramonte were almost panic stricken when they realized that Carroll had yellow fever. They finally realized that it was the mosquito which was the culprit, making it necessary to subject that same mosquito to another test as Carroll had other possibilities of infection. This led to the inoculation of Private Dean, already described.

Fortunately, both Carroll and Dean recovered but the great tragedy was still to unfold. On the morning of August 18, Lazear began to feel 'out of sorts' and that evening suffered a moderate chill. The following day he had all the signs of a severe attack of yellow fever. Lazear revealed that while at Las Animas Hospital five days earlier, as he was holding a test tube with a mosquito upon a man's abdomen, some other insect flying about the room rested upon his hand. At first he was tempted to frighten it away but as it had settled before he had time to notice it he decided to let it fill and then capture it. Besides, he did not want to move for fear of disturbing the insect contained in his tube which was feeding avidly. He told his colleagues that although Carroll and Dean's cases had convinced him of the mosquitoes' role in transmitting yellow fever, the fact that no infection had resulted from his own inoculation before had led him to believe himself to a certain extent immune. Thursday, the 25th of September, saw the end of the life of Jesse W. Lazear which found its place upon the portals of immortality. Thus grief overshadowed a feeling of accomplishment although it was realized that two experimental cases and one accidental were not sufficient proof. In reality, only one case, that of Dean's, was beyond critical analysis. Nevertheless, a preliminary report was prepared which Major Reed returned to the States and presented before the American Public Health Association in Indianapolis on October 24.

After Reed's return to Havana in November, it became clear that another experimental camp was necessary. A site was chosen near Camp Columbia and the new site was named Camp Lazear, consisting of seven Army tents guarded by military garrisons composed of men who had been carefully selected by virtue of their previous good record and their interest in the work to be undertaken. It was here that the famous infected clothing building was set up where potentially infected yellow fever clothing, excreta from patients, and so forth were accumulated and to which the men exposed themselves for twenty consecutive days. It was in this way that the faith of the group in the mosquito theory was demonstrated, as infected clothing and excreta proved entirely harmless. In addition two others, John R. Kissinger and J. J. Moran, volunteered and in both experimental yellow fever was produced by mosquito transfer.

An important experiment done on December 21 clinched the evidence. A jar containing 15 hungry mosquitoes that had previously stung cases of yellow fever was introduced in a room divided into two compartments by a double wire screen which effectually prevented mosquitoes on one side from passing to the other. Into this room Mr. Moran, dressed as though about to retire for the night, entered and threw himself upon the bed for half an hour. During this time, two other men and Major Reed remained in the other compartment separated from Moran only by the wire screen partition. Seven mosquitoes were soon at work upon young Moran's arms and face. He then came out but returned in the afternoon when five other insects bit him in less than twenty minutes. The next day at the same hour of the afternoon, Moran entered the 'mosquito building' for the third time and remained on the bed for fifteen minutes, allowing three mosquitoes to bite his hands. The room was then securely locked but the two Americans continued to sleep in the other compartment for nearly three weeks without experiencing any ill effects. Promptly on Christmas morning Moran, who had not been exposed to infection except for his entrance into the mosquito building as described, came down with a well marked attack of yellow fever.

In addition, seven other men were subjected to the sting of the infected mosquitoes, of which five developed the disease. Two of those who came down with yellow fever had previously been exposed to the 'infected clothing building' without their becoming ill, showing that

they were susceptible to yellow fever after all. The evidence seemed to show that the mosquito could only be infected by sucking blood of a yellow fever patient during the first three days of the disease; to prove that the parasite was present in the circulating blood at that time. We therefore injected some of this fluid taken from a different case each time under the skin of five men. Four of these suffered an attack of yellow fever as a result of the injection. Thus terminated the experiments with mosquitoes which though necessarily performed on human beings fortunately did not cause a single death. On the other hand, they served to revolutionize all standard methods of sanitation and led to the elimination of yellow fever in the cities where it had previously been rampant and made it possible to construct the Panama Canal."

In 1901 William Gorgas and his associate John Guiteras, while conducting vaccine studies (suggested by Carlos Finlay) in volunteers, independent of the Reed Commission, encountered three deaths. This resulted in considerable public alarm. Reed, then in the United States, became disturbed by the exaggerated reports which reached him through the press. On August 23 he sent the following message to Carroll who was then in Cuba recruiting volunteers and conducting the clinical screening and other studies: "You say 'prospects favorable.' And this leads me to strongly advise against further experiments on humans. Our work has been too good to be marred now by a death. As much as I would like to know whether the filtrate will convey the disease, I shall advise against it." Carroll decided to act on his own initiative. The Yellow Fever Board owed the completion of their planned studies to Carroll's willingness to forge ahead. Carroll did complete the studies and showed for the first time that the causative agent present in the serum of yellow fever patients was capable of passing through a filter which excluded bacteria and that the agent in the blood was heat labile; heated blood was noninfectious for volunteers. After completing this work, Carroll, on October 24, 1901, answered a reprimand which he had received from the Adjutant General of Cuba: "I have the honor to acknowledge the receipt of letter dated October 23, 1901 prohibiting any further experimentation among United States troops or civilian employees with yellow fever serum and conveying the censure of the department commander for practicing such experiments upon Privates Hamman and Covington and permitting them to remain with their command 'under no restrictions' and beg to submit the following statement . . . I am glad to be able to report that my work is completed and I have no desire to make any further inoculations. The results are of inestimable value.

"Of thirteen persons experimented upon, Hamman and Covington are the only ones in the service of the government."

THE EXPERIMENTS SUGGESTED BY WILLIAM HENRY WELCH

In the summer of 1901, William H. Welch called Reed's attention to the experiments of Loeffler and

Frosch, in which they had demonstrated that the specific infectious agent of foot and mouth disease in cattle would pass through a porcelain filter and was, therefore, too small to be discovered by the microscope. According to Loeffler and Frosch, there were two possible explanations of this result: either the filtered lymph held in solution an extraordinarily active toxin, or the specific agent of the disease was so minute as to pass through the pores of a filter which prevents the passage of the smallest bacteria. They themselves accepted the latter explanation, since they were able in later experiments by means of the filtered lymph to convey the disease through a series of six animals, the last of which sickened just as promptly after the injection of the filtered lymph as the first of the series. Having thus determined that the microorganisms might be considered ultramicroscopic, Loeffler and Frosch offered the suggestion that, perhaps, the specific agent of some of the acute infectious diseases of man and the animals, such as smallpox, scarlet fever, measles, and so forth, might belong to the same category. The remaining members of the Army Commission, Reed and Carroll, considered that investigations carried out along the lines just suggested might throw light upon the etiology of yellow fever, and as an outbreak of the disease at Santiago de las Vegas, near Havana, in the summer of 1901 offered an opportunity of carrying on the necessary experiments, Carroll returned to Cuba for the purpose, landing at Havana on August 11, 1901. Dr. Carroll was quartered at Las Animas Hospital, where he was provided with a good laboratory and where inoculation experiments were then being made by Dr. John Guiteras. Carroll's experiments were instituted and carried out along the following lines: 1) injection of the fresh blood taken from a vein at the bend of the elbow; 2) injection of unheated and partially defibrinated blood; 3) injection of partially defibrinated blood heated for ten minutes at 55°C; and 4) injection of diluted blood previously filtered through a Berkefeld laboratory filter.

The results of these experiments showed that of seven individuals who received subcutaneously the fresh or partially defibrinated blood in quantities of 0.5 to 5 cc., six developed an attack of yellow fever within the usual period of incubation of the disease, thus demonstrating that the specific agent of yellow fever is present in the blood, at least during the first, second and third days of the attack, at which time the blood employed in the experiments was abstracted.

It also appeared that if, after blood had been injected into the non-immune subject, additional blood was at once withdrawn in considerable quantity and transferred to tubes of nutritive bouillon, no organic growth could be obtained even when a much smaller amount injected into the individual as a control sufficed to produce a severe attack of yellow fever.

It was further found that the specific agent contained in the blood was destroyed, or at any rate attenuated, by heating up to 55°C for ten minutes, so that the injection of 1.5 cubic centimeters of the heated defibrinated blood was harmless, although the injection of 0.75 cubic centimeters of the same defibrinated blood,

unheated, sufficed to induce a prompt attack of yellow fever.

Of no less interest was the fact brought out by these experiments that yellow fever could be produced by the injection of a small quantity of bacteria-free filtrate, obtained by passing the diluted serum through a Berkefeld filter. The writers concluded with the following remarks:

The production of yellow fever by the injection of blood serum that has previously been passed through a filter capable of removing all types of bacteria is, we think, a matter of extreme importance and interest. The occurrence of the disease under such circumstances and within the usual period of incubation might be explained in one of two ways, viz., first, upon the supposition that the serum filtrate contains a toxin of considerable potency; or, second, that the specific agent of yellow fever is of such minute size as to pass readily through the pores of a Berkefeld filter.

In favour of the supposition that in yellow fever an active toxin is present in the blood, may be cited the early and marked jaundice; the free haemorrhage from the mucous membranes of the mouth and stomach, doubtless due to profound changes in the capillary vessel walls; the rapid progress of the disease to a fatal termination, the advanced fatty degeneration of the hepatic cells, as well as the marked parenchymatous changes found in the kidneys. If present in the blood, this toxin would in all likelihood be found in the serum filtrate obtained from the blood, and if injected in sufficient quantity might induce an attack of yellow fever in a susceptible individual after the usual period of incubation. In this respect it would bear analogy to the production of tetanus in the human being, after the usual period of incubation of this disease, by the subcutaneous injection of a very small quantity of tetanus toxin, as reported by Nicolas, in 1893. . . .

Against the view that a toxin is present in the serum filtrate, we invite attention to the innocuousness of the partially defibrinated blood when heated to 55°C for ten minutes . . . Here the toxin, which must have been present in just the same quantity as in the serum filtrate obtained from this blood, appears to have been completely destroyed by the temperature above mentioned. Now, although certain bacteria are destroyed by this temperature, as yet we know of no bacteria toxin that is rendered inert by such a low degree of heat continued for such a short time. . . .

As a further test, and in order to determine whether the serum filtrate contained something more particulate than a soluble toxin, we availed ourselves of the opportunity of observing the effect that would follow the transference to a third individual of blood drawn from one of the patients whose attack had been occasioned by the injection of 1.5 cc. of serum filtrate. If under these circumstances it should be found that the injection of a small amount of blood was followed by an attack of yellow fever in a third individual, the evidence would point in the strongest manner to the presence of the disease in such blood, since we can hardly believe that a toxin which had undergone so great dilution in the body of the second individual would still be capable of producing the disease.

The patient who submitted to inoculation for the purpose of determining this important point was a young

American non-immune subject who was injected with 1.5 cc of serum filtrate, and then, at the beginning of the eighth day after his first inoculation, was given a subcutaneous injection of 1.5 cc of blood drawn from the venous circulation of a patient in whom the disease had followed the injection of 3 cc of serum filtrate, representing 1.5 cc of the undiluted serum. At the time of the inoculation the subject's condition was normal. After an incubation period of just twenty-four hours he developed a well-marked case of yellow fever, which ran a typical course and ended in prompt recovery. The incubation period of yellow fever in cases induced by the bite of the mosquito has been shown to vary from six days, one hour, in the longest case, to two days, thirteen hours in the shortest; while in cases produced by the injection of blood it varied from five days, two hours to one day, seventeen hours. "In view of this data," Reed and Carroll remarked, "we believe that we are justified in expressing the opinion that the source of infection in the case just described must be attributed to the injection of blood rather than to the injection of filtered serum derived from the blood and, further, that the blood contained the specific agent of yellow fever, which had, therefore, passed through the filter along with the filtrate with which the individual in this case had been inoculated."

With these experiments of Carroll's at Las Animas, the business of the Army Board came to an end and Reed's own active work in yellow fever ceased, although his interest in the subject continued for the remainder of his life. The results obtained by Carroll were embodied by the Board in a paper presented to the Society of American Bacteriologists when it met in Chicago at the end of 1901 and was published in *American Medicine* for February 22, 1902, under the title, "The Etiology of Yellow Fever: A Supplemental Note." This was the last publication issued in the name of the Board, but other interesting papers were published later by Carroll.

Howard Kelly, in his monograph *Walter Reed and Yellow Fever,* says the following: "All the reports of the Commission bear Dr. Carroll's name as well as that of Dr. Reed, and in reading them we should always bear in mind that, while the experiments were planned by the master mind of the chief, the accuracy with which they were carried out and the care by which all possible precautions were taken to exclude every source of error, are due to Dr. Carroll quite as much as Dr. Reed."[10]

General William C. Gorgas took his cue from the findings of the Reed commission and conquered yellow fever first in Havana by isolation of yellow fever patients and eradication of the responsible mosquitoes. Such work made it possible to complete the Panama Canal.

On April 24, 1901 Reed delivered an address to the 103rd annual meeting of the Medical and Chirurgical Faculty of the State of Maryland. His lecture was entitled, "The Propagation of Yellow Fever; Observations Based on Recent Researches." In that address he said the following: "That . . . I am here in the capacity of your annual speaker is due to my unwillingness even to appear disobliging to this old and honorable association of physicians, amongst whose number I find included some of my most valued friends; friends who, in years gone by, have labored so faithfully to instill into my mind the value of the scientific method, but to whom I have been able to make such small return."

On the 119th anniversary of the University of Maryland about 2000 visitors and citizens attended the unveiling of a bronze tablet in memory of Major James Carroll in the hall of the University Medical Building at Lombard and Greene Streets in Baltimore. This event was recorded in the *Maryland Medical Journal* and included a description in Carroll's own words of his inoculation by an infected mosquito on July 27, 1900.

ACKNOWLEDGMENTS

I am indebted to Dr. William B. Bean who reviewed and offered helpful criticism of this essay and to Patricia King for editing and typing the manuscript.

---

[10] During William Henry Welch's last illness, Lewellys F. Barker talked to him about a number of events in which he had been involved during his career. On April 2, 1934 the following notes about yellow fever were made: "Welch goes over the state of knowledge of yellow fever and says that Reed's studies at first were of the bacilli and other bacteria. He took little interest at first in the mosquito theory, but later became somewhat interested in Finlay, who had happened on the right mosquito. When the question of human experimentation came up, Reed felt the responsibility very keenly. He felt that if human beings were to be submitted to the test, he as head of the commission should be one, but Welch advised him against this. Carroll deserves great credit, for he developed yellow fever under strictly controlled conditions. After Reed and his group had brought the proof, Sternberg, being Surgeon-General, was inclined to take all the credit. The members of the commission had been delegated by him to study yellow fever, but as a matter of fact his suggestion had been to study the bacillus of Sanarelli. Sternberg naturally had a keen disappointment in having worked all his life to solve the question of yellow fever to find that his ideas about bacteria, etc., had all been wrong. However, he wrote an article for some magazine, not medical, in which he took all the credit. Reed was very resentful and was inclined to give up his commission in the Army, for while he remained in the Army he could not answer Sternberg, his superior. Welch advised against this and told him that he need have no fear about the credit; the articles had been published, the researches had been outlined, and the credit would go where it belonged. As a result of Welch's advice, Reed did not resign from the Army and was very glad afterwards that he had not done so."

Welch gave Sternberg full credit for creation of the Yellow Fever Board: "To the Editor: In the all too generous appreciation of my work in the editorial in The Journal, April 9, it is intimated that my advice may have led to the creation of the Yellow Fever Commission. As all that relates to the history and work of this commission is highly important, permit me to say that the credit for the creation of this commission belongs solely to General Sternberg, who had previously so completely exhausted the purely bacteriologic study of yellow fever that it was possible for the commission to follow the new direction which proved so fruitful in results.

William H. Welch"

48

Research and Discovery in Medicine

REFERENCES

1. Adami JG: The Art of Healing and The Science of Medicine: Ceremonies at the Opening of the New Medical Building. Ann Arbor: University of Michigan; p 47, 1901

2. Carmichael EB: Jesse William Lazear. Ala J Med Sci 9:1, 1972

3. Carroll J: The treatment of yellow fever. JAMA 39: 117, 1902

4. Carroll J: The transmission of yellow fever. JAMA 40: 1429, 1903

5. Carroll J: The etiology of yellow fever: An addendum. JAMA 41: 1341, 1903

6. Carroll J: Remarks on the history, cause and mode of transmission of yellow fever and the occurrence of similar types of fatal fevers in places where yellow fever is not known to have existed. J Assoc Military Surg 13: 177, 1903

7. Carroll J: A brief review of the etiology of yellow fever. NY Med J and Phila Med J 79: 241, 307, 1904

8. Carroll J: Without mosquitoes there can be no yellow fever. Am Med 11: 383, 1906

9. Carroll J: Description of his inoculation by an infected mosquito, July 27, 1900. Md Med J 51: 506, 1908

10. Del Regato JA: Jesse William Lazear. P&S Quarterly (Columbia University College of Physicians and Surgeons) 16: 10, 1971

11. Flexner S: Ceremonies held in connection with the Dedication of the William H. Welch Medical Library of The Johns Hopkins University. Johns Hopkins Hosp Bull 46: 95, 1930

12. Futcher TB: A method of staining malarial parasites. (Meeting of The Johns Hopkins Hospital Medical Society, October 17, 1898) Md Med J 9: 52, 1898–99

13. Futcher TB: A new method of staining malarial parasites. Bull Johns Hopkins Hosp 10: 70, 1899

14. Kelly HA: Walter Reed and Yellow Fever. New York: McClure, Phillips and Co., 1906

15. Lazear JW: Pathology of malarial fever, structure of the parasites and changes on tissues. JAMA 35: 917, 1900

16. Rapport S and Wright H (Eds): The inside story of a great medical discovery, Aristides Agramonte. *In* Great Adventures in Medicine. New York: The Ideal Press, 1952 (Originally published in Scientific Monthly, December 1915)

17. Reed W: Association of *Proteus vulgaris* with *Diplococcus lanceolatus* in a case of croupous pneumonia. Bull Johns Hopkins Hosp 5: 24, 1894

18. Reed W: An investigation into the so-called lymphoid nodules of the liver in typhoid fever. Johns Hopkins Hosp Rep 5: 379, 1895

19. Reed W: The propagation of yellow fever; observations based on recent researches. Med Rec 60: 201, 1901

20. Sternberg GM: An inquiry into the modus operandi of the yellow fever poison. New Orleans Med Surg J 3: 1, 1875

21. Sternberg GM: A study of the natural history of yellow fever and some remarks upon the treatment based upon the same; with cases and tables of observation upon the temperature and urine. New Orleans Med Surg J 4: 638, 1877

22. Sternberg ML: George Miller Sternberg, A Biography. Chicago: American Medical Association, 1920

23. Thayer WS and Blumer G: Ulcerative endocarditis due to the gonococcus; gonorrheal septicemia. Bull Johns Hopkins Hosp 7: 57, 1896

24. Thayer WS and Lazear JW: A second case of gonorrheal septicemia and ulcerative endocarditis with observations upon the cardiac complications of gonorrhea. J Exp Med 4: 81, 1899

25. Unveiling of the Tablet to Jesse W. Lazear. Bull Johns Hopkins Hosp 15: 387, 1904

26. Welch WH and Clement AW: Remarks on hog-cholera and swine plague. (Delivered before the 1st International Veterinary Congress of America. Chicago, Ill., October 20, 1893; Phila., 1894, p. 37, volume 8) Vet J and Ann Comp Path Lond xxxix: 235, 324, 1894; also see Papers and Addresses by William Henry Welch, Baltimore 2: 86, 1920

5.
The Influence of William Stewart Halsted's Concepts of Surgical Training

INTRODUCTION

The concept of prolonged periods of training in specialty services in a university-affiliated hospital originated in Germany. It was introduced into this country when The Johns Hopkins Hospital opened in 1889. The Medical Board of the Hospital asked Drs. Osler, Halsted and Kelly to present their views as to the best method to follow in the appointment of interns. In response, Osler presented a report dealing with the larger question of resident physicians and interns. The first paragraph read as follows:

The Resident Physician. It would be well to use for this officer the term First Assistant at the Medical, Surgical and Gynecological Clinics respectively. Ultimately we should look forward to having Second Assistants, as at the German Clinics. These men should, as now, be salaried. They should be selected with the greatest care by the Staff, with the approval of the Medical Board and of the Trustees. They should be appointed annually, and it is expected that these men will remain for an indefinite period, so long in fact as they do their work satisfactorily.

Perhaps the one special advantage which the large German hospitals have over corresponding American Institutions, is the presence of these highly trained men who remain in some cases 3, 5, or even 8 years and who, under the Professor, have control of the clinical material.[1]

Osler's recommendations were accepted, but the innovative method of training for surgery implemented by Halsted attracted so little attention that 15 years later Halsted thought it appropriate to state the following in an address at Yale University: "Although we now have in the United States several (five or six) moderately well endowed medical schools with a university connection, the problem of the education of our surgeons is still unsolved.... Here I may be permitted to instance conditions which evolved in a natural way at the Johns Hopkins Hospital, where the plan of organization of the staff differs from that which obtains elsewhere in this coun-

try.... It was our intention originally to adopt as closely as feasible the German plan, which, in the main, is the same for all the principal clinics of the German universities. The house surgeon, or first assistant, as he is called in Germany, is selected, after several years of service, from a number of well-tried assistants. There is no regular advancement from the bottom to the top of the staff."[2] An important reason for the slow appreciation of the value of this method may be found in the status of surgery in the 1890s and early 1900s. This can be described as unscientific and purely empirical. Any licensed doctor was allowed to operate. A knowledge of anatomy was deemed far more important than knowledge of surgical technique. Dexterity and rapidity in operating were the hallmark of greatness. An additional factor was the retiring manner of Halsted, who made no effort to actively promote or to publicize his school of surgery.

HALSTED'S OBJECTIVES

The residency training program for surgery which William Stewart Halsted (Fig 1) inaugurated at The

[1] Chesney AM: The Johns Hopkins Hospital and the Johns Hopkins University School of Medicine: A Chronicle. Volume 1. Baltimore: The Johns Hopkins Press, 1943, p. 161.

Reprinted from the *Johns Hopkins Medical Journal* **148:** 215, 1981.

[2] Halsted WS: The training of the surgeon. Bull Johns Hopkins Hosp, 15: 267, 1904; see pp. 271–272. Halsted appended the following footnote: "The surgical staff consists of nine men, eight internes and one externe. The externe is an assistant in surgical pathology, he attends operations whenever it seems desirable in order to do with a clearer understanding the pathological work, to take charge of and describe the pathological material obtained at operations and to keep in touch, for his own benefit, as well as for the sake of the surgical department, with the clinical work. Four of the internes serve for one year, only the honor men of each class at graduation being entitled to these positions; but the *permanent staff*, so-called, consists of four men, the house surgeon and three in line of preferment. Men from any part of the country, if they have had the proper training, are eligible for the permanent positions. Great care is exercised in the filling of the vacancy on the permanent staff, which occurs once in two or three years, and advancement is not guaranteed to the appointee. The House Surgeon's term of service is still optional. The assistants are expected in addition to their ward and operating room duties, to prosecute original investigations and to keep in close touch with the work in surgical pathology, bacteriology and, so far as possible, physiology."

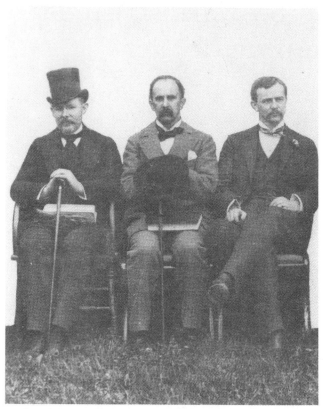

Fig 1.   Left to right, William S. Halsted, William Osler, Howard
A. Kelly. Dr. James S. Mitchell, a member of the first class to
graduate from The Johns Hopkins University School of Medicine (1897), took a picture of the staff of The Johns Hopkins
Hospital at the time of his graduation. This picture is an enlargement made from Dr. Mitchell's photograph.
From the Alan M. Chesney Medical Archives, The Johns Hopkins Medical Institutions.

Johns Hopkins Hospital in 1889 was not only the original
program of its kind in this country, but was unique in its
primary purpose and continued to be so for many years.
It was Halsted's objective to establish a school of surgery
which would eventually lead to the dissemination
throughout the world of those principles of surgery and
attributes of the surgeon which he considered essential.
It was his farsighted purpose to establish a residency
training program which, in his own words, would develop "not only surgeons but surgeons of the highest
type, men who will stimulate the first youth of our country to study surgery and to devote their energy and their
lives to raising the standards of surgical science." The
cardinal features of Halsted's program were: 1) close association of the resident with the professor; 2) harsh
competition for the top position; 3) indefinite tenure; 4)
responsibility for the total care of all charity patients; 5)
teaching of the housestaff; and 6) participation in
research.

The great benefits accruing from such a long period of discipline with responsibility in an institution devoted to teaching and investigation had to be demonstrated before interest was aroused and imitation began.
The system spread mainly through the men who had par-

ticipated in the original program. The first surgical residency in a private hospital was initiated by Dr. J. M. T.
Finney, Sr. at the Union Protestant Infirmary in Baltimore. In 1907 Stephen T. Watts left Baltimore to be professor at the University of Virginia and organized a three
year residency there. In 1912 Cushing went to the Peter
Bent Brigham Hospital in Boston and introduced a duplicate of the Baltimore program in which he had been
resident from 1900 to 1903. In the next decade Gatch did
the same in Indianapolis; McClure in Detroit; Goetsch in
Brooklyn; and Brooks in Nashville. In 1922 Heuer and
Reid instituted a superb residency at the Cincinnati General Hospital. Thus, it took over 30 years to have approximately 10 Halsted-type surgical residencies, but by
1939 the American Medical Association directory listed
203.[3] It was Halsted's aim to train teachers and investigators and not merely competent operating surgeons.

The importance of Halsted's efforts can only be
appreciated when one considers the situation that
existed at the turn of the century and in the early 1900s.
Good teachers of surgery were in very short supply. For a
number of reasons, it was very difficult to attract the
outstanding surgeons of that era to accept chairs of
surgery. The salaries were poor; the renowned surgeons
carried on their work in hospitals which were not connected, for the most part, with university centers; and
the successful surgeons of that generation were not disposed to pass on to others their hard earned skills acquired under, to say the least, very difficult conditions.
Research and the practice of surgery were almost completely separated and among the surgeons in practice
then there was very little exchange of knowledge and
extremely little intellectual stimulation. The acquisition
of skill in surgery at that time was a matter of personal
drive and most surgeons were essentially self-taught.

THE RESIDENCY STRUCTURE
UNDER HALSTED

Halsted's resident staff usually consisted of three
assistant resident surgeons and one resident surgeon who
were carefully selected on the basis of their ability and
promise of future development, regardless of where they
had received their education and training although the
majority were medical graduates of Johns Hopkins.
There was no set length of time required to complete the
residency, nor was there any orderly succession to it. In
the final selection of the chief resident, Halsted emphasized originality, capacity for independent thinking,
a real interest in teaching others, and adequate surgical
skill. During the 33 years in which he supervised his system of surgical training, he appointed 17 chief residents.
The average length of time spent by most of the men as
resident was between 2 and 2½ years, although Joseph
Colt Bloodgood remained for 4½ years and Mont Reid for
3½ years. Out of these 17 men, 7 professors of surgery
emerged, 1 surgeon-in-chief of a hospital, 1 professor of

---

[3] Most of these were residencies in name only and merely
designated a year or more after an internship devoted entirely to
surgery.

clinical surgery, 3 associate professors of surgery, 1 instructor of anatomy, and 4 private practitioners in surgery. Fifty-five men served under Halsted as assistant resident surgeons, remaining on the staff for periods ranging from one to three years, with an average of about 1½ years. This group was also of high caliber as indicated by their subsequent attainments, both academically and professionally. Special mention should be made of these men that Halsted directed into special fields including Frederick H. Baetjer in roentgenology, William S. Baer in orthopedics, Hugh H. Young in urology, and Samuel J. Crowe in otolaryngology. Eleven of the 17 resident surgeons trained by Halsted instituted residency training programs of their own. From these training programs have come a second generation of resident surgeons trained in the Halsted tradition, many of whom have also had successful academic careers and in turn trained others.

Halsted's trainees represent a rather heterogeneous group as far as their subsequent careers are concerned. This essay will attempt to document this variable course which they followed and will illustrate the broad impact which they had on American surgery. To illustrate the breadth of influence, the careers of five of his residents, one of his assistant residents, and one of his interns will be depicted.

JOSEPH COLT BLOODGOOD

Early in the career of Joseph Colt Bloodgood (Fig 2), his fourth resident surgeon, Halsted suggested that he should undertake in a more systematic manner than had hitherto been done the study of all tumors and other tissues removed at operation. Thus, surgical pathology was the first specialty established in the surgical department and Bloodgood was the first of a group of young men invited by Halsted to develop one of the surgical specialties.

Joseph Colt Bloodgood, or "Bloody," as he was generally called, was born in Milwaukee, Wisconsin on November 1, 1867 and received the B.S. degree from the University of Wisconsin in 1888. Three years later he obtained his M.D. degree from the University of Pennsylvania. He served as resident physician in the Children's Hospital in Philadelphia for a year before coming to Baltimore in 1892. He was appointed assistant resident surgeon in May 1892. In November 1892 he visited European clinics and hospitals and returned to be resident surgeon of The Johns Hopkins Hospital, a post which he held from June 1893 to October 1897. On his return from Europe in June 1893, Bloodgood had with him a microtome for cutting frozen sections and a firsthand knowledge of how to stain them. Active work in surgical pathology began soon after his return; all tissues from the operating room were prepared and studied in a room in Dr. Welch's laboratory and a record was made on the hospital history. Bloodgood had appointments in the School of Medicine from 1895 until his death on October 22, 1935. In 1907 Bloodgood was appointed surgeon-in-chief of the St. Agnes Hospital in Baltimore.

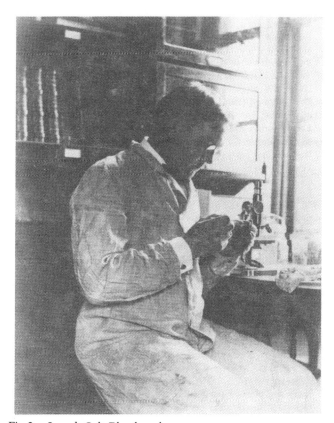

Fig 2. Joseph Colt Bloodgood.
From the Alan M. Chesney Medical Archives, The Johns Hopkins Medical Institutions.

He was an instructor in surgery (1895–97), associate (1897–1903), associate professor (1903–27), clinical professor (1927–32), and finally adjunct professor (1932–35).

In 1924 Bloodgood was made vice president of the American Surgical Society. He was a fellow of the American College of Surgeons and member of the editorial board of the *American Journal of Cancer*.

In 1912, when Theodore Roosevelt was campaigning for the presidency as candidate of the Progressive Party, he was shot and wounded by a political fanatic at Milwaukee. Bloodgood, who happened to be visiting relatives there, assisted in the diagnosis and treatment of the wound.

Bloodgood had a very important role in the development of surgical pathology in this country. However, the facilities he was given for this work were quite meager. An example of the shoestring nature of this laboratory in the early days is the following letter written by Bloodgood to Dr. Halsted on October 28, 1908:

> I would consider it a great favor if you would bring the following matter before the Advisory Board ... Dr. Lambert of New Orleans and Dr. Thomas of Texas, who were postgraduates in my department last year, are with me again this year ... These men are unusually well trained and with their help I've been able to improve the technique of frozen sections and the entire technique of the sectioning and staining of tissues hardened in Zenkers ... During the summer I found it impossible to train Frank any further in technical matters and for this reason

I offered Drs. Thomas and Lambert their board and lodging at my house during the summer for their help in the laboratory. It proved so successful that I let Frank go and asked these two men to remain with me during the year. Dr. Thomas is willing to give half his time for $5 a week, the amount given me by the university and I told Dr. Lambert that I would be responsible for his expenses and living for the year. I requested Dr. Hurd to give Dr. Lambert his meals in the hospital which does not seem unreasonable for his aid in the pathological reports for the surgical histories and I should like to request the university to give me, in addition, $5 a week for Dr. Lambert for his assistance in maintaining the laboratory and aiding in teaching . . .

I need also help in teaching. On Wednesday afternoons from October to May . . . I have a class of 71 students. At the present time, I am following this method of teaching: "There is, first for half an hour for the entire class a demonstration in the lecture room, then a group of ten meet me in one of the smaller rooms for a special demonstration; a group of five meet Dr. Thomas for instruction in the methods of freezing and cutting sections for immediate microscopic study, and a group of five meet Dr. Lambert for instruction in the newer methods of preparation of sections and preservation of museum specimens. The remainder of the class—51—work in the three larger rooms where there is prepared for them a demonstration. . . . On three mornings a week at 8:00 there are demonstrations of fresh material to the elective group of fourth year students and on Friday afternoon a demonstration to the elective group of third year students. In addition, there are demonstrations everyday to postgraduate students. In addition, one evening every two weeks will be devoted to a demonstration with the projection apparatus. Although I am in the laboratory on Tuesday from 8 to 12 and Wednesday and Friday afternoons from 1 to 5 and short intervals on other days, it is essential to have a well-trained man in the laboratory all the time. He must be prepared to make frozen sections, to keep a careful record of all material received, look after the preparation of museum specimens, and the hardening of blocks of tissue in the carrying out of the techniques for their sectioning and training . . ."

Dr. Lambert at the end of the year returns to New Orleans to organize a department of surgical pathology at the University of Tulane in connection with Dr. Matas' surgical department. Dr. McGlannan, who is my associate in surgery at the St. Agnes Hospital . . . has been following my work in the surgical pathological laboratory for five years, first as a postgraduate student, then as a voluntary assistant and this year he's helping me in demonstrations. I should recommend his appointment as voluntary assistant . . . I am requesting from the university an additional appropriation of $250 a year.

Bloodgood was provided with the help and the funds requested.

Bloodgood was an untiring worker. For the remainder of his life he spent every hour he could spare from private practice working in his laboratory, teaching undergraduate and postgraduate students, and studying cancers of the breast, bone tumors and many other pathological conditions. In reporting the results of operations for the cure of cancer of the breast from June 1889 to January 1894, Halsted noted: "Thanks to the most per-

sistent efforts of my house-surgeon, Dr. Joseph C. Bloodgood, the results of the operations have been obtained in all but two cases." In his paper on adenocarcinoma of the breast Halsted, in discussing case IV, said: "In a note on the macroscopic appearance of a section through the middle of the tumor, Dr. Bloodgood emphasizes the fact that on pressure of the tumor a number of long, very fine, soft cylinders were extruded from the cut surface." In the same publication, when discussing his radical operation for breast cancer, Halsted noted: "Dr. Bloodgood was, I believe, the first to demonstrate the advantages of completing the cleaning out of this postero-internal subscapular region by the suprascapular route." To add further to his praise of Bloodgood's work Halsted, in an article on hernia, remarked: "If our operation for the radical cure of inguinal hernia has improved, it is due in no small measure to the arduous (follow-up) labors of Dr. Bloodgood."

Dr. Halsted was not prone to be overenthusiastic about the talents of his pupils. While resident surgeon, Bloodgood operated on a man with disease of one testicle. Unfortunately, when the patient came out of ether, it was discovered that the healthy testis had been removed by mistake. The angry patient promptly sued Bloodgood only to learn that his lawsuit was invalid because the surgeon was acting as an agent of the hospital. He thereupon sued the hospital. The trial was long and bitterly fought, but the decision was finally rendered in favor of the defendant. Halsted had been called as a witness to the surgical ability of Bloodgood. The rest of the yarn can be told in Bloodgood's own words: "After the trial, Halsted and I left the courthouse together and started to walk down St. Paul Street. He put his hand on my arm, stopped me and said: 'Now, Bloodgood, I said some very fine things about you at the trial, but, of course, you understand we had to win the case.'"

In the course of time, Bloodgood accumulated a large collection of tumor biopsy specimens which he used to advantage in the instruction of both undergraduate and postgraduate students. This activity led him naturally into the cancer field. In spite of this important activity in surgical pathology, Bloodgood could not admit his private patients to The Johns Hopkins Hospital.[4]

During his early career, Bloodgood had a major interest in operations for hernia, publishing a technique

[4] In the early days of the hospital, the privilege of admitting one's private patients was restricted to the senior members of the visiting staff. This policy forced the younger members, many of whom were graduates of the school and just beginning to make a name for themselves in practice in Baltimore, to establish connections with other hospitals in the city to which they might take their private patients. Examples are the intimate association of Dr. J. M. T. Finney with the Union Protestant Infirmary, later the Union Memorial Hospital; of Dr. Thomas S. Cullen with the Church Home and Infirmary; and of Dr. Bloodgood with St. Agnes Hospital, all to the good of these institutions but perhaps to the detriment of Johns Hopkins at the same time (Bernheim BM: The Story of the Johns Hopkins. New York: McGraw Hill Book Co., Inc., 1948, pp. 142−152). The policy in time gave rise to what Bernheim has aptly called "secondary

for transplantation of the rectus muscle in certain cases of inguinal hernia in which the conjoined tendon is obliterated. In 1899 he published his observations on 459 cases of hernia in The Johns Hopkins Hospital treated from June 1889 to January 1899. In this monograph, there was special consideration of 268 cases operated on by the Halsted method and the transplantation of the rectus muscle. Early in his career he became interested in tumors of the bone, both benign and malignant, and published an excellent summary of the features of these tumors based on a study of some 370 cases.

In 1891 von Recklinghausen published his treatise upon the diseases of bone in which several maladies, formerly confused, were separated and described. Osteitis fibrosa cystica was recognized as a distinct clinical entity. Some of the earliest and most valuable contributions on this subject were made by Bloodgood. He pointed out the differential diagnosis between this disease and central giant cell tumor and demonstrated that central giant cell tumor is a benign lesion, for the relief of which mutilating operations were not necessary.

Bloodgood's first publication on bone disease was in 1902 and dealt with his examination of 42 cases of bone tumor. By 1929 his laboratory at Johns Hopkins handled more than 3,000 cases of bone disease, studying the biopsies for diagnosis. By that time, the total specimens examined in the surgical pathology laboratory had grown from 1 in 1889 to 40,000 in 1929. Bloodgood's award of the Gold Medal by the Radiological Society of North America in 1929 was made for his pioneering work in surgical pathology and the study of bone diseases, both benign and malignant, and their diagnosis by x-ray and by use of the microscope. At that time, only 18 persons had received this medal, including Madame Curie of France.

As time passed, Bloodgood became immersed in education of the public and of physicians in the prevention and treatment of cancer. With a view toward arousing greater public awareness of the need for cancer research, a small group of physicians (James Ewing, Howard C. Taylor, Thomas S. Cullen, Frank F. Simpson, and Joseph C. Bloodgood) met in New York City in May 1914 and drew up plans for a new society "to disseminate

---

medical centers" in Baltimore which may have served to deflect from The Johns Hopkins Hospital a degree of financial support which could have been most helpful. Later on the policy was relaxed, perhaps because more facilities for taking care of private patients in the hospital became available. After the great Baltimore fire of 1904, the trustees issued an announcement to the Associated Press "of the disaster which had befallen the hospital, and the great curtailment of income by reason of the burning of its warehouses." The superintendent was also instructed "to issue a notice to the heads of all departments asking for the exercise of the most careful economy in all expenditures," and, "in order to promote the private work of the hospital," he was "authorized to admit the patients of Drs. Bloodgood, Cushing and Young to the private wards." Obviously this last mentioned action was taken to increase the institution's income (Minutes of the Board of Trustees of The Johns Hopkins Hospital, Volume 1, page 439).

knowledge concerning the symptoms, treatment and prevention of cancer, to investigate conditions under which cancer is found, and to compile statistics in regard thereto." This new organization was the "American Society for the Control of Cancer." Its primary objective was to put information about cancer into a language understandable by the lay public. Many young men interested in cancer were attracted to Bloodgood's laboratory. Many of them contributed greatly to cancer control after receiving their stimulation from Bloodgood. Charles F. Geschickter, who received his M.D. degree from Johns Hopkins in 1927, worked in Bloodgood's laboratory for a number of years before becoming Professor of Research Pathology at Georgetown University School of Medicine. Murray M. Copeland, a classmate of Geschickter's at Johns Hopkins, was also associated with the laboratory during its very active period while Dean Lewis was Professor of Surgery. Copeland later became Professor of Surgery and Vice-president of the University Cancer Fund, the University of Texas and the M. D. Anderson Hospital and Tumor Institute.

Through his educational work related to the prevention and treatment of cancer, Bloodgood soon became widely known. He was a frequent speaker at medical association meetings, both in this country and abroad, where he visited hospitals and clinics, discrediting fraudulent cures and emphasizing the necessity of early diagnosis and research relating to the cause and prevention of cancer.

In 1928 the Garvin Fund was given to Johns Hopkins to support the work of Bloodgood. Francis P. Garvin, president of the Chemical Foundation, provided $10,000 for additions to the laboratory and $10,000 a year for each of the next five years for the support of research. Bloodgood devoted these funds to the study of human cancer, particularly to the use of dyes and stains in its early diagnosis. The demand for a more certain method of identifying cancer in its earliest stages was the result of a long educational campaign instituted by Thomas S. Cullen of Baltimore nearly 20 years previously. At that time, it was comparatively easy to diagnose a case of cancer. As a rule, patients did not consult a physician until the disease had reached a stage where the difference between a malignant and a harmless growth was obvious to even the inexperienced eye. Because they came too late, little could be done for most of the patients with cancer. Cullen urged that people who had the least suspicion of harboring a cancerous growth should consult an expert at once. A nationwide campaign of education along that line followed with the cooperation of the American Medical Association. As a result, patients with suspicious lesions began to come for examination much earlier and it became difficult to tell the difference between a malignant and a benign growth by sight and touch alone. The microscope became the instrument employed for diagnosis and biopsies became everyday events. As earlier and earlier stages of cancer were seen, even the histological sections became difficult to interpret.

Bloodgood was one of the pioneers in advocating

the use of postgraduate courses to make more available the latest developments in this field. Annually he held such a course for surgical pathologists. He also made full use of the press and radio to advance his ideas. In 1930 he published a paper which had behind it the full authority of The Johns Hopkins University, Dr. Joseph S. Ames, the president, having approved it in advance. Bloodgood explained that his request for Ames's approval marked inauguration of a new policy of his surgical pathology laboratory, a policy designed to serve as a model for future statements emanating from medical centers on matters of vital importance to the public. Public statements concerning cancer, where there is danger of misleading the public by giving it inaccurate information or raising false hopes, not only would gain in authoritativeness by having the official support of an institution but would be more certain not to endanger the public health in any degree, according to Bloodgood.

By 1930 there was growing evidence that, to a significant degree owing to the evangelistic work of Bloodgood, physicians could diagnose cancer better than they could 15 years previously. In one of his three-day conferences for surgical pathologists, Bloodgood put their skills at diagnosis to the test. The majority of the pathologists in 1930 apparently made the correct diagnoses of the microscopic slides shown them while the majority in 1915 did not. At this conference all the doctors agreed on every definite case of cancer and all agreed on every definite benign tumor. The disagreement was entirely on borderline cases. This implied better security to the patient facing an operation for possible cancer.

Dr. Bloodgood's untiring efforts in the field of cancer and its prevention and early treatment were recognized in an editorial in *The Baltimore Sun* on October 24, 1935:

> The death of Dr. Joseph C. Bloodgood removes another of the group of eminent physicians whose names are permanently associated with Johns Hopkins and with this city as a great medical center and it does more. It removes a man of singular devotion. For years Dr. Bloodgood gave without stint of his training, his energy, and his financial resources in the war on cancer. He gave, indeed, all that he could give and sought untiringly for more to give. He pressed the war on every front, including that of popular education, and no undertaking was too big and no detail too small for his attention if he saw in it hope of guarding humanity against the dreadful malady. There were times when his zeal outran that of his associates. No matter; he pressed on and on. The members of his profession will know how to pay tribute to his distinguished work, but the public may be permitted its tribute to a man in whom the physician's passion for healing dominated all else in life and work.

GEORGE JULIUS HEUER

George Julius Heuer (Fig 3) was born in Madison, Wisconsin on February 6, 1882. In 1903, shortly after his graduation from the University of Wisconsin, he began the study of medicine at Johns Hopkins.

Heuer related an experience as a medical student

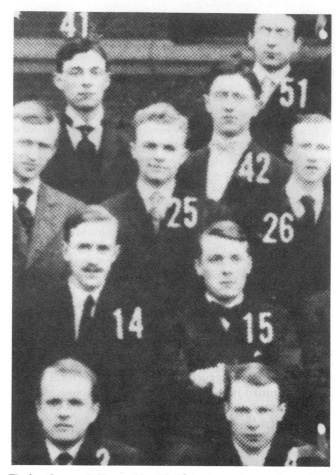

Fig 3.   George J. Heuer (No. 25). This picture is an enlargement made from a photograph of the Class of 1907 of The Johns Hopkins University School of Medicine.
From the Alan M. Chesney Medical Archives, The Johns Hopkins Medical Institutions.

illustrating Halsted's approach to the examination of the patient. For his oral quiz in surgery Heuer had three patients to examine, one of whom had a sarcoma of the tibia. Heuer looked at the patient, was pleased that he could make a diagnosis, and passed on to the remaining patients upon whom he spent more time. When called into Halsted's office, he entered with a feeling of confidence. Looking at his card to verify Heuer's name, Halsted said: "Heuer, what do you suppose caused the lengthening of that man's leg?" "I was at a complete loss for I had not noticed that it was longer and therefore had not thought to measure it. Halsted said: 'Did you measure the leg?' And I confessed I had not. 'Why we (editorial) spent twenty minutes measuring the leg,' he said, whereupon he rose, opened the door and ushered me out of his office. No other questions, and my despair may be imagined. I confirmed the fact that the patient had been seen by several members of the senior surgical staff. None had noticed the lengthening of the tibia; none had measured it. They had been content, as I had been, with the diagnosis of sarcoma, a diagnosis which to Halsted was so self-evident that he did not even question a medical student about it."

Heuer graduated with honors in 1907 and was appointed house officer on the surgical service at The Johns Hopkins Hospital. In Heuer's intern year, Harvey Cushing often demanded his services and he spent a good deal of time giving anesthetics for, or assisting Cushing in, his brain operations. The illness of John F. Ortschild during that year resulted in Heuer's transfer to the private service at a time when Hugh Young was establishing his record of 125 perineal prostatectomies without an operative fatality. These patients required a great deal of Heuer's time and between Young and Cushing, both very demanding individuals, there was little opportunity for Heuer to assist Halsted in the operating room. Having been given in September 1908 the choice of serving as Cushing's special assistant in neurosurgery or as an assistant resident on Halsted's staff, Heuer had chosen the former and spent one entire year in neurosurgery. In September 1909 it appeared that his surgical training at Johns Hopkins was at an end, for he did not accept the position Halsted had offered, and it had been filled, leaving no vacancies on the resident staff. But later in the year the resignation of Louis Reford gave Heuer the opportunity of continuing his training under Halsted. Heuer always felt that he owed his good fortune in returning to Halsted's staff in part to Dr. Henry Hurd. Under a crotchety exterior, Hurd sheltered a very kindly nature. When Heuer was out of a job Hurd called him to his office, questioned him about his hopes for a career in surgery, and told him he might live at the hospital until something turned up. In Heuer's experience he did many kind deeds for young men about the hospital, few of which ever became known.

When Heuer returned to Halsted's service, John W. Churchman was resident surgeon and Charles M. Remson first assistant resident. Heuer followed these men and succeeded to the residency in surgery in September 1911.

Heuer was Halsted's thirteenth resident serving for three years (1911–14). His diagnostic ability and technical skill at the operating table so completely won the admiration of Halsted, of the senior surgeons on the visiting staff, and of his associates on the house staff that in 1914 he was made associate professor of surgery of The Johns Hopkins University and associate surgeon of the Hospital.

During his 7 years on the surgical resident staff of The Johns Hopkins Hospital, Heuer became proficient in several branches of surgery including neurological, abdominal, and thoracic surgery. When Cushing moved to Harvard in 1912, Halsted asked Heuer to take over the neurosurgical work of the hospital in addition to his other duties in general surgery and in the Hunterian Laboratory. Just before World War I, Halsted arranged an exchange of assistants with the professor of surgery at the University of Breslau. Heuer was appointed an exchange professor in Kuttner's clinic in Breslau, sailing for that city in early June 1914. Due to the onset of the war, Heuer's stay in Breslau lasted only 6 weeks. However, he was given a free rein to examine patients and was given charge of one of the surgical wards. In the operating room, tincture of iodine was painted on the patient's skin and a cotton glove was worn over the rubber glove, a practice which Heuer deplored because the double gloving led to clumsiness. When general anesthesia was administered, drop ether was the choice; no endotracheal methods were used. The surgeons there were not really interested in anesthesia and as a matter of necessity a great deal of the surgery was done with local injection of 1/2 percent novocaine. The practice undoubtedly influenced Heuer in his later preference for local anesthesia.

Following his stay in Breslau, Heuer returned to Baltimore and was immediately made a Captain in the Medical Corps of the American Expeditionary Forces. The Johns Hopkins Medical and Surgical Unit was organized under the direction of Dr. John M. T. Finney. Heuer was chief surgeon in Evacuation Hospital #10. The unit was busy in France caring for acute war casualties. Heuer left eight handwritten volumes and about 500 card indices of his own cases. In later life, Heuer loved to talk about his experiences in France during World War I, deploring the fact that the lessons learned were not taken full advantage of in postwar surgery. During his stay in France, he maintained an active correspondence with Halsted. Heuer complained that no appreciation was shown for his conscientious efforts to do a good job by either a pat on the back or a promotion. Halsted offered little encouragement: "It must be a source of satisfaction that you have not been overrewarded for your achievements. It is mortifying to receive undue recognition and undeserved advancement." During his stay in Europe Heuer formed a close association with Dr. Eugene Pool of New York, the beginning of a relationship between the two men which entered a new phase when Heuer assumed the chair of surgery at the New York Hospital some 14 years later.

Following discharge from the army as a Major in February 19, 1919, Heuer returned to Johns Hopkins expecting to be named chief of the neurosurgical service. He was, however, disappointed to learn that this appointment had been given to a later Halsted resident, Walter Dandy. That Halsted had a higher regard for Dandy's ability is evidenced from a letter written to Heuer during the war in which he stated that "if Dandy goes we shall be up a tree."

From 1919 to 1922 Heuer remained at Johns Hopkins, holding the title of associate professor of surgery. In 1920 Halsted requested the well-known Philadelphia surgeon, W. W. Keen, to endorse Heuer for membership in the American Surgical Association, a request to which Keen readily agreed. There was a close personal relationship between Heuer and Halsted evidenced by their correspondence and the frequency with which Heuer was entertained at Halsted's home, both at Baltimore and at High Hampton, North Carolina. Heuer had a silver cigarette case suitably inscribed which was presented to him by Halsted as a token of his esteem and affection. For Heuer and Mont R. Reid, Halsted had a very special affection and trust. It was to these two that Halsted turned when he had to undergo his final operation. A letter written to Professor René Leriche, the great French surgeon, in January 1922 sums up Halsted's esteem for Heuer's competence as a surgeon: "I am quite despondent at the loss of Heuer [Heuer had just assumed his new post at Cincinnati]. He covers the whole field of surgery better than anyone in the United States. He operates beautifully, tranquilly and honestly." Cushing was not given to praising his colleagues unless he thought them very worthy of it. He had these words to say of Heuer when he was a visiting surgeon at the Peter Bent Brigham Hospital in 1932: "An inspiring teacher and clinician, he instills the utmost confidence in his patients. His skill, resourcefulness and composure put him in a class by himself as an ace of operating surgeons."

Heuer's zeal for original investigation took root early. His first scientific publication appeared in the *Bulletin of The Johns Hopkins Hospital* in 1906, one year before receiving his M.D. degree. Its title was "The Pancreatic Ducts in the Cat." Next came written discourses on distemper and then the development of the lymphatics in the small intestine of the pig. He published several papers while a resident, on neurosurgical subjects, some co-authored with Harvey Cushing and Walter Dandy. His publications were always scholarly and carefully edited. William DeWitt Andrus, also a Johns Hopkins graduate, who was associated with Heuer for many years at Cincinnati and at Cornell, relates that following a review by Halsted of one of Heuer's early writings copies of Webster's *Dictionary* and Quiller-Couch's book on the art of written English were returned along with many penciled notations on the manuscript. When Heuer went to Cincinnati, he made up his mind that it was to be his primary task to set up a surgical residency outside the Baltimore perimeter which would be patterned after his own training with Halsted. He was to find that the introduction of Halsted's training program elsewhere would tax all his resources and patience.

The Professorship of Surgery at Cincinnati

The surgical chair at Cincinnati was first offered to Dandy, who declined. Heuer was next approached and talked with Dandy about the position. Heuer was strongly tempted to go and decided to leave the decision up to Halsted. He had been for so long a part of the Baltimore scene and Halsted relied on him to such an extent that he was reluctant to leave him. Halsted expressed pleasure at the glad tidings which he said were at the same time distressing to him: "I . . . had difficulty in considering the Cincinnati proposition unselfishly . . . I have leaned on you so long and your loyal and capable support has been such a delight to me that I can hardly even yet regard the situation fairly . . . To me it seems a fine and rare opportunity aside from possible handicaps of which, of course, I am ignorant." Then followed some advice: "Before accepting you should stipulate that your voice must have great weight in the choosing of the faculty, otherwise you might have endless conflict with men whose views are antagonistic—who could surpass you in political intrigue. You operate so well and cover the

operative field so completely that I feel the natural career for you is the operating table . . . But surely you should be a teacher. The constant combat with students is a great stimulus and the surgeon should encompass himself with incentives less he become merely a performer of routine."

In 1922 Heuer became the first occupant of the Christian R. Holmes[5] Chair of Surgery at Cincinnati and thus came his opportunity to set up a surgical residency in a major medical center. To assist him Heuer recruited a group of Johns Hopkins trainees including Mont Reid, Bill Andrus, Nick Carter, Max Zinniger, and Ralph Bowers. Heuer and Reid were to be full-time clinical teachers. To make this arrangement possible, the Carnegie Foundation provided $250,000 on a matching basis for endowment of the full-time plan. At this time, outside of Baltimore, only the system of postgraduate instruction in surgery offered at the Peter Bent Brigham Hospital in Boston was comparable in scope. Heuer endeavored to include as many of the local surgeons as possible in the activities of his department. He had great difficulty in getting funds to run his department but his public support was substantial and he had a favorable press. One Cincinnati daily paper ran the following editorial: "Heuer is today rendering . . . the community a great service in his care of patients at the Cincinnati General Hospital but the university Board has not made good its side of the contract. It has been prevented largely by the opposition who . . . want the medical college maintained as a narrow gauge, provincial institution. Heuer has not been accorded the facilities he was promised. The school cannot afford, if it expects to amount to anything, to limit itself in appointments to Cincinnati men."

Professor of Surgery at Cornell

After 9 years in Cincinnati, the Board of Governors of the New York Hospital selected Heuer to be chief of

[5] The history of modern medical education in Cincinnati centers largely around Christian R. Holmes. He built upon a rich medical tradition which began in the Ohio Valley under the dynamic leadership of Daniel Drake. Christian R. Holmes saw the possibilities of bringing the Cincinnati General Hospital and the University School of Medicine together in a closely integrated unit. Under his influence and leadership the campaign to build a new city hospital was conducted successfully. In 1909 two rival schools, the Medical College of Ohio and the Miami Medical College, had united as the College of Medicine of the University of Cincinnati. This was housed in the new college building in Cincinnati with its fine hospital. The first two years of the medical school were headed by a group of young scientists devoting their full time to the teaching of medicine. The first step to extend this plan into the clinical years was taken when Roger Morris, a Johns Hopkins graduate, was appointed professor of medicine and became a salaried member of the university faculty. At this point, World War I intervened and further development was delayed until 1920, when the Rachford Professorship in Pediatrics was established. In 1920 Kenneth Blackfan, Howland's perennial resident in pediatrics at Johns Hopkins, was brought to Cincinnati to be the new professor of pediatrics.

surgery at their institution. The recommendation for the appointment was made by G. Canby Robinson, who had been at Johns Hopkins and knew of Heuer's work there. Robinson had maintained contact with Heuer at Cincinnati, visiting there in 1924 on an inspection tour of full-time departments. The position in New York had first been offered to Evarts Graham who declined. A formal letter was sent by the Governors of the New York Hospital and the Trustees of Cornell University to Heuer on November 12, 1930, appointing him to the position of surgeon-in-chief, stipulating that the appointment would be effective July 1, 1931. Heuer consulted Pool before accepting in order to determine whether the surgical profession in New York would be less hostile than in Cincinnati. Heuer was apparently given the impression that there would be a minimum of resistance to a residency program but there turned out to be a great deal of enmity on the part of the incumbents. Preston Wade, who had been on the surgical staff since 1925 and had recently retired as surgical chief, was under the impression that Heuer really did not care what the old staff thought of him and did nothing to make the old guard feel like receiving him with open arms.

Heuer had many obstacles to overcome in establishing a Halsted-type pyramidal residency training program in New York City as he had in Cincinnati, but he was able to surmount most of them with the able assistance of his dedicated lieutenants.

Heuer was not the first to introduce the Halsted concept of training to New York City, although he did pioneer in setting up a full scale formal residency. Allen Whipple had previously organized an informal training program at the Presbyterian Hospital in New York. In 1921 Whipple assumed the Valentine Mott Chair of Surgery at Columbia and although he had no formal training under Halsted, he espoused the principles of the Halsted school. In 1928, four years prior to the installation of the New York Hospital residency, Whipple designated four advanced trainees on the surgical service. They were not labelled as residents but were called fellows. George H. Humphries in his summary of the department of surgery (1928–53) of the Presbyterian Hospital wrote: "These first fellows and their successors during the next eight years worked in the wards, clinic and research laboratories in a way comparable to our present resident." Whipple emphasized that he did not call the men "residents" because he wished to initiate a program with as little prejudice as possible. In 1936 the program was changed to a three year residency but it was not until after World War II that the residency training period was lengthened to five years.

Perhaps among the surgical residents of Halsted, the one who made the greatest contributions to perpetuation of the Halsted school of surgery was George Heuer. When Heuer began his professorship at Cincinnati the residency system, while well established at Johns Hopkins and a few other university clinics, was looked upon as impractical, if not undesirable for other hospitals. It was felt that such a system was adaptable only in a rather narrow academic atmosphere and unsuited to the

situation in the ordinary city hospital, for example. This constituted a challenge which Heuer accepted with enthusiasm, and to many his greatest contribution was his demonstration that the residency system was not only practical under quite diverse circumstances, but that it produced results in the care of patients and in operative mortality which surpassed those of other types of organization for training.

In 1935, participating in a symposium on the teaching of surgery sponsored by the American Surgical Association, Heuer presented a paper entitled "Graduate Teaching of Surgery in University Clinics," in which he traced the spread of such teaching throughout the country and analyzed its status at that time. He concluded: "The study shows that . . . there are still lacking sufficient opportunities to meet demands of men seeking a higher degree in surgery and to meet the needs of the country in respect to trained surgeons." This symposium gave impetus to the founding of the American Board of Surgery and Evarts Graham credits the stimulation of Heuer's address on this occasion with a large share in bringing this about.

Except for a maintained interest in stimulation of young investigators and an occasional appearance to demonstrate an operative method, Heuer, in his later years, was not very active in the experimental laboratory. His earlier work on pneumonectomy in dogs, with particular reference to the healing of the bronchial stump, was fundamental, however, and so exhaustive that little, save minor alterations, of the technique have been added since it appeared. He stimulated others to study the effects of removal of the lung on the remaining pulmonary tissue from both the anatomic and functional standpoint.

George Heuer was probably the best living exponent of the meticulous surgical technique first introduced into American surgery by Halsted; certainly he improved upon it. His greatest interest was in the training and development of young surgeons. The idea that surgical patients could be entrusted to the care of residents without any increased danger was difficult for the profession and the public to accept. Everybody realized that Heuer stood among the top surgeons of the world in technical ability. The fact that such an excellent operating surgeon could champion a program in which the residents did much of the surgery helped greatly to win converts to the Halsted concepts of residency training. One could safely assume that a surgeon of Heuer's skill would not be willing to turn over the care of surgical patients to residents unless they were fully qualified to do the work.

MONT ROGERS REID

Mont Reid (Fig 4) died prematurely on May 11, 1943. Rarely has a man so universally won the affection of his fellow citizens that, during his final illness, those in higher walks of life should have awaited daily reports of his progress; that telephone operators, taxi cab drivers, hotel clerks, and newsstand attendants should have in-

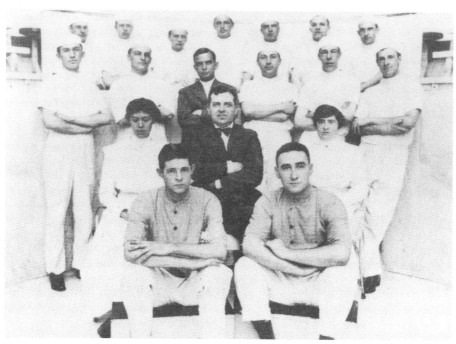

Fig 4.   Mont R. Reid (far left in 3rd row from bottom). The two in civilian dress are Richard H.
Follis (middle of 2nd row from bottom) and Walter E. Dandy (directly behind Follis).
From the Alan M. Chesney Medical Archives, The Johns Hopkins Medical Institutions.

quired how he fared; that churches should have invoked special prayers for his recovery; that on his death the flag on the City Hall of Cincinnati should have been flown at half mast for one not connected with the government; that civic organizations should have attended his funeral services in a body; that the American Surgical Association meeting at the time in Cincinnati should have interrupted its scientific program to do him honor—these are but a few of the indications of his extraordinarily successful career as a surgeon.

Born on a farm near Oriskany, Virginia on April 7, 1889, he obtained his elementary education largely from his father, who acted as schoolmaster for his seven children. Reid attended the Daleville Normal School for two years then entered Roanoke College, from which he graduated with the A.B. degree in 1908. He entered The Johns Hopkins University School of Medicine in the fall of that year, and on graduating in 1912 was appointed an intern in surgery under Halsted. The following year (1913–14) he was an assistant resident in pathology after which he returned to surgery and held the position of assistant resident surgeon from 1914 to 1918.[6] In 1918 he was appointed resident surgeon, a post he occupied for three years. Following this, he was an associate surgeon

of the hospital until his departure in 1922. He was successively instructor in pathology, instructor in surgery, and associate in surgery in the medical school.

In 1922 Reid accompanied George J. Heuer to the newly organized department of surgery at the University of Cincinnati Medical College. It was due in no small measure to Reid's loyalty, sound judgment, and winning personality that the department of surgery there underwent its successful development. In 1925 he was appointed visiting professor of surgery to the Peiping Union Medical College of China and spent a year there. He returned a victim of malaria which, for a time, considerably impaired his health.

In 1931, with Heuer's departure for Cornell, Reid was appointed professor of surgery and director of the surgical service of the Cincinnati General Hospital. Reid's long training under Halsted, whose principles and methods of surgery but few of his pupils better understood or more closely followed, made him a careful, meticulous surgeon of unusually sound judgment. As a teacher, he was not a brilliant lecturer nor an inspiring master of the clinical method of instruction. However, at the bedside his kindness to patients, his attention to the salient facts of the history, his careful physical examination, his critical interpretation of clinical data, his sound techniques in the operating room, and his good medical judgment were a great example to students, both undergraduate and advanced.

Reid was particularly interested in the surgery of the thyroid gland and contributed importantly to that subject. He was also concerned, as was his distinguished mentor Halsted, with the fundamental principles of

[6] Halsted planned to let Reid leave the service without being chief resident, and had appointed Ernest G. Grey. Grey offered to wait 6 months in order to give Reid a chance to be resident. Just before the time arrived, Grey died in the great influenza epidemic. Halsted's cold objectivity and impersonal attitude, shown in his willingness to bypass Reid, reveals one of his personality characteristics.

surgery such as the healing of wounds and the control of infection.

During his period at Johns Hopkins, he conducted his outstanding experimental work on vascular surgery, including such studies as the effect of arteriovenous fistulae upon the heart and blood vessels, the changes in the vessel wall and in the heart following partial occlusion of the thoracic aorta and inferior vena cava with a metallic band, the surgical treatment of angina pectoris as well as clinical studies on abnormal arteriovenous communications both acquired and congenital. For these studies, Reid was the first recipient of the Rudolph Matas Award, which was conferred in 1934. As one of his avocations, Reid accompanied Roy Chapman Andrews on his expedition into Mongolia.

Under the leadership of Heuer and Reid, the department of surgery at Cincinnati became known throughout the country as one of the outstanding clinics for graduate surgical training. Under Reid research continued to be an important part of his expanded department although he always gave first priority to clinical training, insisting that every member of his resident staff be first a thoroughly experienced surgeon.

In 1939 Reid was offered the professorship at Johns Hopkins, but two powerful factors offset his temptation to accept. The first was his deep love for Cincinnati and its medical school; the second was the fact that he had developed a school of surgery in Cincinnati which was as fine as in any institution. He did, however, prepare a comprehensive memorandum of what was needed to reorganize the surgical department in Baltimore. Reid worked tirelessly to develop the facilities needed at Cincinnati and unfortunately died before the results of his efforts were fully completed. After his death, a fund was raised as a tribute to him known as the Mont R. Reid Fund, to assure a continuance of the high standards achieved by the University of Cincinnati Medical College during his years there.

ROY DONALDSON MCCLURE

Roy Donaldson McClure (Fig 5) was born in Belbrook, Ohio on January 17, 1882. He received his A.B. degree from Ohio State University in 1904 and his M.D. from Johns Hopkins in 1908. At Ohio State University he became fast friends with Charles F. Kettering, who became director of research at General Motors and a world famous inventor. This close friendship lasted all of McClure's life. McClure studied at the University of Prague for one semester in 1906. He was a voluntary assistant to Alexis Carrel at the Rockefeller Institute, 1907–08; house surgeon at the New York Hospital, 1909–11; and resident surgeon at The Johns Hopkins Hospital, 1912–16. In 1916, in collaboration with Frank Sladen, a Johns Hopkins trained internist, he organized and became surgeon-in-chief of the Henry Ford Hospital. He was a member of the Subcommittee on Surgical Infections and the Subcommittee on Burns of the National Research Council. He served as a major in the Medical Corps, U.S. Army, 1918–19, commanding Evacuation

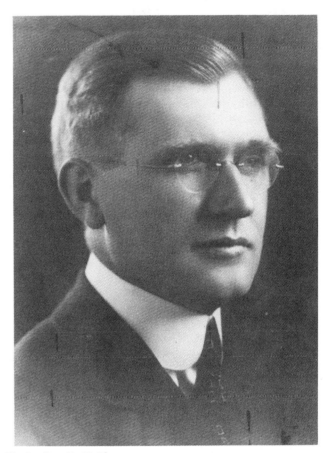

Fig 5. Roy D. McClure.
From the Alan M. Chesney Medical Archives, The Johns Hopkins Medical Institutions.

Hospital #33 AEF. He was a governor of the American College of Surgeons from 1935 to 1938, and a founder and first president of the Central Surgical Association, 1940–41.

McClure was personal physician to Mr. Henry Ford for many years. In November 1932 he performed an emergency appendectomy on Mr. Ford, then 69 years of age. The appendix was both gangrenous and strangulated and the case was so rare that medical literature had recorded only 20 like it.

McClure had a prominent role in the early experiments on blood vessel suture and transplantation of organs while with Dr. Carrel. He was one of the first to perform a blood transfusion by direct blood vessel suture between donor and patient. He helped to perfect a standard treatment for burns. After World War II, with Kettering's assistance, he developed a valuable warning device for use during operations—a photoelectric eye that recorded changes in the oxygen content of the blood. He made many contributions to surgical technique and to the effective use of drugs in pre- and postoperative care. Thyroid and breast surgery were his special interests. At the time of his retirement, he had performed almost 30,000 major operations. He was surgeon-in-chief of the Ford Hospital from 1916 to 1951. He died on March 31, 1951.

McClure related in a letter to Alan M. Chesney on
June 13, 1947 his early experience at The Johns Hopkins
Medical School. He came in close contact with Halsted as
a first year student since most of that year (1904–05) was
spent by McClure in the Hunterian Laboratory. He had
been given the option by William H. Howell, then dean,
of taking a full year's credit for previous studies, but on
his father's advice he decided to spend this time in the
laboratory rather than enter the second year class. He
was given the position as autopsy pathologist in the fall
of 1905 and W. G. MacCallum assigned him to the then
new Hunterian Laboratory where he "swept out the
shavings and sawdust" and started his "experimental
work on the heart. . . . Halsted, Osler and Cushing all
became greatly interested in this and would stand by and
watch the four pins on our kymograph change their
levels as we produced any one of the different lesions."
The paper of MacCallum and McClure on the mechanical
effects of experimental mitral stenosis and insufficiency
appeared in the *Bulletin of The Johns Hopkins Hospital.*
Experimental stenosis was readily produced by applying
a screw clamp with arm guarded by rubber tubes, by
passing a suture about the atrioventricular ring, or by
introducing a distensible balloon through the atrial appendage. The immediate result was the lowering of the
systemic arterial pressure and elevation of the pressure
in the pulmonary arteries and in the pulmonary veins
and left atrium. The pressure in the systemic veins was
little, if at all, elevated unless there arose an insufficiency
of the right ventricle or, with the dilatation of the right
ventricle, relative insufficiency of the tricuspid valve.

Insufficiency of the mitral valve was easily produced experimentally by means of a hook with blunt
point and special cutting edge, this made in such a way
that the outer surface was smooth and round so that only
thin structures such as the chordae tendineae and valves
were reached by the knife edge. The hook was introduced
through the left atrial appendage into the left ventricle
where the valves and chordae could be cut to the desired
extent. Cannulas connected with a mercury manometer
having been adjusted in various parts of the circulatory
system, the one designed to record the pressure in the left
atrium was quickly tied into the aperture in the atrial
appendix on the removal of the hook.

McClure published other papers while working in
the Hunterian. One on pancreatic atrophy in a dog following impaction of calculi in the duct appeared in the
Bulletin of The Johns Hopkins Hospital in September 1907.
This was a report of a condition found in the pancreas on
autopsy of a dog in which the duct of Wirsung was
blocked by concretions. In December of the same year
another paper by McClure and H. F. Derge represented
an extension of Mall and Halsted's studies of intestinal
reversal.

In the *Bulletin of The Johns Hopkins Hospital* for
March 1917 McClure and George Robert Dunn published
their article entitled "Transfusions of Blood: History,
Methods, Dangers, Preliminary Tests, Present Status,
and Report of 150 Transfusions."

EMILE HOLMAN

Emile Holman was born in Moberly, Missouri on
August 12, 1890, the son of the Reverend and Mrs. F. H.
Holman. The family moved to California while he was
still a youngster and Holman received his B.A. degree
from Leland Stanford University in 1911. He began by
majoring in mathematics but soon changed to the department of education. He was David Starr Jordan's
(President of Stanford University) secretary for three
years after graduation. (Holman had taken classes in
typing and shorthand at his uncle's business college in
order to help earn his way through school.)

Holman's interest in medicine began when, while
Jordan's secretary, he took a course in anatomy. At Jordan's suggestion, Holman successfully applied for a
Rhodes Scholarship. In 1914 Holman accompanied Jordan on a trip to the Balkans. After a visit of three months
they reached London just at the start of the First World
War.

After putting the Jordans on the boat back to the
U.S., Holman entered St. John's College, Oxford, taking
the course in physiology which enabled him after two
years to take the final examination for his second B.A.
degree. The third year of his Rhodes scholarship was
spent as a casualty house surgeon at the Radcliffe Infirmary. This advanced clinical work enabled him to enter
the fourth year at The Johns Hopkins University School of
Medicine, from which he received his M.D. in 1918. At the
time Holman was at Oxford, Sir Charles Sherrington was
professor of physiology. Holman recalled a student session with Sir William Osler at which he presented a veteran from the war who had sustained a gun shot wound
of the thigh, producing an arteriovenous fistula in the
groin. Although the patient had cardiac symptoms, Sir
William was not convinced that the fistula had anything
to do with their development and the patient was discharged without operation. Later Holman realized
Osler's deficient knowledge of the functional changes resulting from an arteriovenous fistula.

It was largely through Holman's meeting with
Osler that he went to Johns Hopkins, but he had an
example to stir him on in Wilburt C. Davison. Davison, a
Rhodes Scholar from Princeton, who later became the
first dean of the Duke University Medical School, went to
Johns Hopkins and after one year received his M.D. degree. Davison was Holman's tutor while he was at Oxford. Holman's first year at Oxford was interrupted by a
brief period with the Commission for Relief in Belgium
organized by Herbert Hoover in the early months of the
First World War. Twelve Rhodes Scholars were the first
Americans to go to Belgium to supervise the distribution
of food.

Holman's first year after graduation from Johns
Hopkins was spent in the Hunterian Laboratory for Surgical Research. Halsted accepted him largely on Davison's recommendation. Halsted had offered Davison an
internship in surgery because of his unusual knowledge
of the use of Dakin's solution in infections as he had seen

it applied in England. Unfortunately, a serious complication followed Halsted's operation on Franklin P. Mall for gallstones. It was generally reported that the operation lasted for 3 hours. A severe infection of the abdominal wall occurred which threatened to cause disruption of the wound. It was decided to use Dakin's solution in the infected wound. Necropsy revealed general peritonitis and a perforation of the small intestine in the area of "dakinization," which may or may not have contributed to the fatal sequence of events.

Holman became a great admirer of Halsted and in his interview with Peter Olch told many interesting anecdotes about his mentor.

According to Holman, René Leriche, the great French surgeon who visited Baltimore early in his career, was greatly impressed with Halsted's operative technique. Leriche said years later: "I had been trained in the feats of surgery. I was schooled in the tradition of the ancients who considered the surgical performance a magnificent act of prestidigitation, and I had no other ambition than to be a rapid surgeon doing things daringly. I saw a man who was careful to avoid trauma, careful in the extreme, very sparing of the patient's blood, concerned about perfect tissue reconstruction. It was a dazzling revelation. In a split second I realized my error. A real revolution took place in my mind. In three days I had gone through the experience of a great revolution. When I returned home I was a new man. I felt as if I had lived near the surgical heir of Claude Bernard."

In reminiscing about Halsted, Holman spoke as follows:

Before Halsted's day, surgery everywhere was a bloody ordeal based largely on speed and brevity of operation. German surgeons in the latter part of the 19th century enjoyed a remarkable preeminence largely because of the sheer daring of their extensive, but often blood-letting, exploits. Their surgical ambitions knew not the deterrent of compassion. When Sir Frederick Treves (1853–1923) returned to London from a tour of surgical clinics in Germany, he wryly reported that "German surgeons approach an operation on the canine principle of savage attack." To such traumatic practices, Halsted's approach was the exact antithesis. He laid the greatest stress on the gentle handling of tissue, on the avoidance or complete control of hemorrhage, on the strict observance of absolute asepsis, and on the accurate reapproximation of divided tissues. To these concepts should be added his scholarly approach to every patient who came under his care, his thoughtful consideration of every aspect of the surgical disorder before him. Time passed unnoticed as he studiously mulled over in his mind the best possible attack upon the particular problem in hand. One may recall the famous statement by Charles Mayo after visiting Halsted's clinic that "He had never before seen the upper part of an incision heal before the lower part was closed." In his personal life Halsted was just as perfectionistic. Though living in Baltimore, he sent his pictures to Keppler, the art dealer in New York, to be framed. His shoes were custom-made in London from leather especially approved by him. His suits and ties were tailored in London from personally selected goods and silks. His hosiery came from Scotland; his linens from France. He had dozens and dozens of dress shirts which he wore as needed, to be taken along to Europe each summer for laundering in London or in Paris. When entertaining at dinner he personally went to the market to select the food and the wine and supervised the laying of the tablecloth which was ironed after being accurately placed on the table. He trusted no one but himself to prepare the after-dinner coffee which was made in the Turkish manner from finely ground coffee in a long-handled brass cup, unbelievably strong. Dr. Heuer, following an illness, spent a few days of convalescence in the Halsted home where he was embarrassed by Dr. Halsted's insistence, patrician though he was, on selecting the pieces of wood destined to make a fire in Heuer's room. Only hickory and white oak properly aged would do. One of Mrs. Halsted's chores was to comb the woodyards of Baltimore for hickory and white oak.

Cushing, as a young assistant surgeon, had just arrived from Boston where, with considerable fanfare and histrionics, amputation of the breast was usually accomplished in 19 minutes flat. A case of mammary carcinoma from Cushing's ward was sent to the operating room. To Cushing's consternation, four hours passed before the patient returned to the ward. Halsted arrived just before the patient to find Cushing poised, syringe in hand, ready to administer some strychnine. "And pray what good will that do?" asked Halsted. "She must be in great shock," replied Cushing. To his amazement, when the patient arrived after the four hour ordeal, her pulse was 80 and she was not in shock at all. This was Cushing's first lesson in the importance of complete hemostasis and once learned was never to be forgotten.

According to Gatch, Halsted was afraid of Cushing. Cushing treated him like a doormat; criticized him to his face. If Halsted came to the operating room while Cushing was operating, Cushing would turn his back to him and pay no attention to him. Among other liberties, Cushing concealed cases from Halsted so that he might operate upon them himself. One day Halsted walked into the operating room to find Cushing operating upon a patient whom he had examined, and upon whom he had expected to operate. Somewhat agitated, he left the operating room, headed for the office of the superintendent, but once there he hesitated, turned and left the hospital. The next day Cushing was relieved of his duties as resident surgeon, but was advanced to be an associate on the surgical staff, in which capacity he would no longer be in control of cases on the ward. Halsted's intention the day before, fortunately suppressed, was to fire Cushing."

Harvey Cushing, a faculty associate for 13 years and in his early years as surgical resident at Hopkins and an impatient and caustic critic of Halsted, accurately sensed his character and probably assuaged his own conscience in a very sympathetic note published in *Science* shortly after Halsted's death:

A man of unique personality, shy, something of a recluse, fastidious in his tastes and in his friendships, an aristocrat in his breeding, scholarly in his habits, the victim for many years of indifferent health, he nevertheless was one of the few American surgeons who may be considered to have established a school of surgery comparable in a sense to the school of Billroth in Vienna. He had few of the qualities supposed to accompany what the world regards as a successful surgeon. Overmodest about his work, indifferent to matters of priority, unassuming, having little interest in private practice, he spent his medical life avoiding patients, even students, when this was possible, and when health permitted, working in clinic and laboratory at the solution of a succession of problems which aroused his interest. He had that rare form of imagination which sees problems and the technical ability combined with persistence which enabled him to attack them with the promise of a successful issue. Many of his contributions, not only to his craft but to the science of medicine in general, were fundamental in character and of enduring importance.

Holman (Fig 6) was resident surgeon under Halsted from September 1921 until June 1923. He had been an assistant resident surgeon for the previous two years.

After Halsted's death in September 1923, Finney was placed in charge but was so busy with his private practice that he turned the work in the Johns Hopkins surgical department over to Dr. Robert Miller, one of Halsted's former residents. Miller was very critical of everything Halsted had done and spoke freely about it to the staff, thus creating a conflict between himself and the residents. After a year, Holman took a position with Cushing at the Peter Bent Brigham Hospital, where he was put in charge of the general surgical wards under John Homans, David Cheever and Elliott Cutler which was excellent experience for him. Cutler soon left to become chief surgeon at the Lakeside Hospital in Cleveland and Holman accompanied him there.

While Holman was in Cleveland, he worked in the laboratory with Claude Beck (a graduate of Johns Hopkins), as Cutler gave him little responsibility on the wards.

After a year at Western Reserve, Holman returned to California. Ray Lyman Wilbur, on a trip to Washington via Cleveland, asked Holman to get on the train with him at Cleveland and travel to the next station. During that short trip he offered Holman the professorship of surgery at Stanford.

Holman immediately set out to improve the student teaching by giving them personal responsibility in the examination and treatment of patients according to the plan he had seen at Johns Hopkins. Different ideas of operating were also introduced and safety was stressed instead of speed. Gentleness in the handling of tissues was taught both in the hospital operating room and in the experimental laboratory. Work in the experimental laboratory was encouraged, and a course in animal surgery was developed.

Holman worked daily in the experimental laboratory, resulting in some interesting discoveries on the effects of arteriovenous fistulas of different sizes in different locations.

Holman was visiting professor of surgery at the Peking Union Medical College where Harold Loucks, a missionary surgeon, was professor. Loucks had established a residency system modeled on the Johns Hopkins plan and he wanted that residency system established on a firm basis. While there Holman studied the physiological effect of removing enlarged spleens. He observed that the blood pressure would rise and the pulse rate would slow just as they did after the excision of a large arteriovenous fistula.

While still in Baltimore, Holman studied post-stenotic dilatation, particularly the localized dilatation of the aorta beyond a coarctation and the occasional lo-

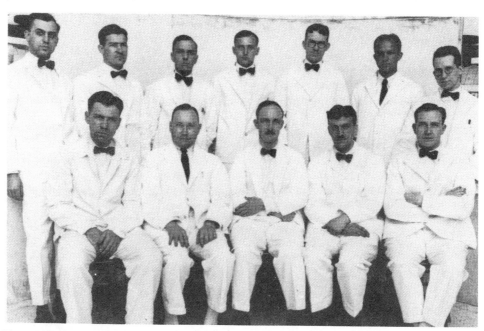

Fig 6. Emile Holman (front row, center). Others in the photograph: Front row, left to right, W. F. Rienhoff, John H. Kite, Emile Holman, Karl Schlaepfer, Jay McLean; top row, F. L. Reichert, P. B. MacCready, R. W. Telinde, W. M. Firor, J. D. Hart, S. W. Egerton, M. M. Zinniger.

calized dilatation of the subclavian artery beyond a cervical rib. In 1916 Holman presented a scholarly review of 716 cases of cervical rib, 65 percent of which were associated nerve symptoms only, 30 percent with nerve and vascular symptoms, and 5 percent with vascular symptoms only. In 27 of these an aneurysmal enlargement was observed.

He took the problem to the experimental laboratory where he and Mont Reid produced partial constriction of the terminal aorta in dogs, which was followed in about 25 percent by mild poststenotic dilatation. He suggested that the abnormal whirlpool-like play of the blood in the relatively dead pocket just below the site of obstruction and the lowered pulse pressure were the chief factors concerned in production of the dilatation. Later at Stanford, Holman did many other fascinating experiments employing a pump run by a small motor which simulated the mammalian heart exactly in driving fluid continuously, hour after hour, day after day, through a recycling circulatory system, in which system he studied the physiologic basis for cardiac dilatation.

Holman became interested in skin grafting while at Johns Hopkins by an experience with a small child who was run over by a truck, denuding one leg almost completely of its skin. To recover this area it was decided to take the skin of the mother instead of skin from the patient, who was just three years old. He transplanted 300 grafts from the mother; 150 at the first operation and 150 at a second. These grafts took and appeared to be spreading over the leg when suddenly they began to disappear and the patient developed an exfoliative dermatitis involving the entire body. It was decided that the skin they had transplanted was acting as a poison and accordingly all remnants of the transplanted dermis that remained were removed. Immediately after this, the child lost all evidence of exfoliative dermatitis and the area was ready for regrafting with the patient's skin. Complete epithelial covering of the leg occurred. In two other patients[7] he transplanted small islands of skin from three donors. Later he transplanted the second set of grafts. At the time that the second set was applied, the first had begun to disappear and to their astonishment the second set did not take at all. Thus he had discovered that the foreign protein arouses a reaction in the recipient which does not permit the further use of the same skin. This phenomenon, called the "second-set reaction to skin grafting," was described later in greater detail by Peter Medawar. At first, Holman's work received little attention. Later the Association for Transplantation recognized the importance of his contribution.

Holman later did important work on the production of intrapulmonary suppuration by secondary infection of the sterile embolic area, producing these lesions in the experimental laboratory. When an infected embolus was introduced into the jugular vein of a dog, an abscess invariably developed at the site where the embolus was held up in the pulmonary arterial tree. This same method was used in producing tuberculous abscesses of the lung in the dog. An instructive observation during these studies was the great dilatation of the bronchial artery leading to the infected area. Holman ventured an explanation on this basis for the profuse hemorrhages that occur in certain tuberculous patients, postulating destruction of the wall of the dilated bronchial artery with its systemic pressure rather than from the branches of the pulmonary artery, which have a much lower pressure.

In 1925 Holman was among the first to evince an interest in congenital anomalies of the heart and great vessels and published a classic paper on patent ductus arteriosus. He reasoned that the proper treatment of this lesion would be to close the abnormal shunt by surgical operation, but he was dissuaded from performing the operation by one of his respected medical colleagues. This unique contribution to surgery was subsequently made by Robert Gross of Boston in 1935.

The middle 1930s were for Holman vigorous and productive years. As he matured and it became clear that the residents he had trained in the Halstedian precepts were sound clinical surgeons equal in clinical competence to the outstanding senior surgeons in San Francisco, he gradually shook off the mantle of "dog surgeon," or experimentalist not to be entrusted with a practical surgical problem. By the late 1930s he had won for himself a position of trust and respect in clinical surgery. Advances in other disciplines, if understood and utilized, permitted new areas of surgical endeavor and Holman seized avidly upon each of these. With insight and skill he brought first to Stanford the radical operation for carcinoma of the rectum (Miles operation), the aseptic technique for resection of the stomach, and the resection of the scapular tip in the operation of thoracoplasty. He also introduced ligation of the patent ductus arteriosis, complete pneumonectomy for cancer of the lung, extensive decortication of the heart and great vessels for constrictive pericarditis, resection for coarctation of the aorta, the Blalock operation, the closed mitral valve operation, and he provided the stimulus which led Dr. Frank Gerbode to perform the first open-heart operation at Stanford.

Holman never applied for a federal grant-in-aid, and only after the war did he accept modest support from the Life Insurance Medical Research Fund. In World War II he persuaded Frederick L. Reichert to assume all teaching obligations at home and entered the Navy. After his initial tour of duty at Mare Island, in which he started off as a surgical intern and finished as surgical chief, he was shipped out to the Pacific Theatre, ending up in Vella la Vella. There he organized a teaching and training program for the young men, including an experimental laboratory. He began to train the young surgeons on wild animals purchased from the natives at exorbitant prices often paid from his own pocket. The compelling urge to explore the problems at hand, to seek out the truth with an alert and receptive mind characterized Holman's war experiences.

Holman's research on arteriovenous fistulas won

---

[7] Holman himself and W. M. Firor were the experimental subjects.

him the coveted Gross Prize in Surgery in 1930. In 1972 he was honored by the International Congress of thc Transplantation Society for his pioneering work in skin grafting and skin reduction. In 1952 Holman received the Rudolph Matas Award in Vascular Surgery, generally regarded as the world's highest recognition for surgery of the heart and blood vessels.

The Emile Holman Professorship of Surgery was established at Stanford in 1972 by a bequest from the estate of Dean and Louise Dart Mitchell. Holman died on March 19, 1977 at the age of 86.

In a very penetrating article entitled "Emile Holman: He Bridged the Gap Between Humanism and Science" by Victor Richards, the following anecdote appeared:

> The awe and trepidation with which we medical students at Stanford approached clinical medicine and surgery in particular was heightened by the eerie surroundings of the classroom. Holman conducted his lectures in the fifth floor amphitheatre adjoining and above the animal research laboratory in the Lane Medical Building, the old red building which stood on the corner of Sacramento and Webster Street. The odor was unpleasant and the high-pitched voice of the diener, John Kratsch, could be heard whining in the background as he vainly tried to coax and cajole the dogs into silence for the professor's lecture. The professor himself heightened our terror by bursting into the room with unbelievable energy, plunging into a discussion of shock and hemorrhage yet vividly recalling the admonition of his former professor, William Stewart Halsted, who had counseled: "There is only one weapon with which the unconscious patient can retaliate against the incompetence of a surgeon and that weapon is hemorrhage." As this theme was being developed with chilling variations an occasional cockroach would appear from the adjoining animal quarters and saunter through the lecture room. Fortunately, they beat a path between the lecture podium and the blackboard and Dr. Holman, accustomed to and unconcerned by these harmless intruders, proceeded vigorously with his exposition on shock, exterminating them while enlightening us. This quality of perseverance and, indeed, thriving in the face of adversity characterized Holman throughout his career.

WILLIS D. GATCH

Willis D. Gatch (Fig 7) was born on a farm in Indiana on October 27, 1877. His father, while a captain in the Union Army, and his uncle Dr. Charles Gatch were the first to attend President Abraham Lincoln after he was shot by John Wilkes Booth. Gatch attended Indiana University where he was elected to Phi Beta Kappa, receiving his A.B. degree in 1901. Gatch graduated from The Johns Hopkins University School of Medicine in 1907. He served on the surgical resident staff of the hospital from 1907 until 1911. In June 1908 Gatch was appointed anesthetist to the hospital. He was given simultaneously the appointment of assistant resident surgeon which he held for three years. Gatch explained his appointment to this new post: "Ether given by the open drop method was the only anesthetic used on Halsted's service prior to 1908. The preoperative administration of atropine and mor-

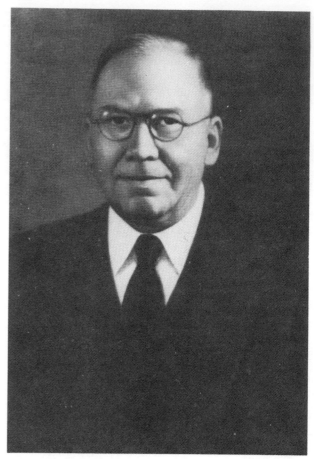

Fig 7.   Willis D. Gatch.
Courtesy of Dr. J. S. Battersby.

phine was not used. The induction was often difficult and the accumulation of mucus in the respiratory passages was dangerous and occasionally fatal. I was interested in these shortcomings while an intern, and when I became assistant resident in 1908 was appointed anesthetist in the hospital, with the understanding that I do research designed to improve anesthesia; this in addition to the ordinary duties of an assistant resident. Drs. Abel and Howell gave me advice and Dr. Hurd provided me with the equipment I needed."

Heuer described the status of anesthesia at The Johns Hopkins Hospital at the time of his internship there (1908):

> During my internship and immediately after, inhalation anesthesia was quite primitive. Dr. Halsted himself had developed local anesthesia with weak solutions of cocaine and this was not infrequently used. Chloroform was rarely employed except occasionally by Cushing. Ether was the anesthetic of choice and in my early days was administered by the interns. As interns we were taught anesthesia by the operating room orderly, Owen. He gathered us around him, demonstrated the administration of ether on patients, and told us the significant facts regarding the patient's respiration, the size and mobility of the pupils, and the lid reflex. Ether was administered with a cone made of pasteboard and covered with

oiled silk and a towel. In the apex of the cone was a sea-sponge on which the ether was poured. It was a barbarous method. After the patient had been strapped to the operating table the cone, containing usually a strangling dose of ether vapor, was clapped over his nose and mouth. There was often a period of struggle before the patient succumbed to the ether vapor; and during this period of struggling orderlies, doctors and nurses might have to cling to arms and legs to keep him on the operating table. Owen was adept in renewing the ether in the cone. Watching the patient's respiration he snatched the cone from the face during expiration and had the sponge soaked with ether and the cone back in place over the patient's face before inspiration began. This technique we all tried to master.

During my early years Dr. Halsted was highly dissatisfied with the method of administering inhalation anesthesia. He tried to get men on his resident staff interested in anesthesia, and from time to time had an assistant resident instead of an intern administer the anesthetic to the patient he was operating upon. Finally Gatch came along as a member of the resident staff. Nitrous oxide-oxygen anesthesia was just being introduced, and Gatch became interested in anesthesia and devised one of the early machines for administering nitrous oxide-oxygen anesthesia. The cone method of giving ether was replaced by the "open drop" method. Cushing began to employ a trained anesthetist in his private cases; and the trained nurse anesthetist appeared in the operating rooms, Miss Margaret Boise being the first. With these developments and with further perfection and extension of the use of local anesthesia, all of which occurred during my period at Hopkins, anesthesia at the hospital was vastly improved."

(George J. Heuer was an assistant resident surgeon at the same time as Willis D. Gatch, from September 1908 to October 1911.)

One of the results of Gatch's research was to make practical the use of nitrous oxide-oxygen anesthesia. In a paper published in the *Journal of the American Medical Association (JAMA)* in 1910, he reported on a method of administering these gases which was simple, cheap and effective. As nitrous oxide and oxygen were expensive and could be obtained only in heavy cylinders, he reasoned that it would lessen the cost if one used them repeatedly instead of wasting them after one inhalation. He demonstrated that nitrous oxide, with oxygen, could be successfully given by a simple and easily portable apparatus, that rebreathing to a moderate degree was harmless, that in many cases rebreathing was beneficial as it caused increased depth of respiration, swelling of the pulse, a rise of the blood pressure, and a rise of temperature. It seemed probable to him that all but the last of these results were attributable to the action of carbon dioxide. In a second article in the *JAMA*, Gatch concluded that rebreathing, when properly regulated and when the oxygen supply was ample, was harmless and could be put to valuable use. He stated that if one could prevent anoxemia, overconcentration of vapor, and too great a depth of anesthesia, one could obviate most of the serious objections to the closed method of giving ether. He described a method of ad-

ministering nitrous oxide and, if necessary, ether with oxygen by the method of rebreathing. Its chief advantages in his view were: 1) the rapidity and pleasantness with which anesthesia was established; 2) the ease with which any depth of anesthesia could be secured; and 3) the prevention to a very large extent of postanesthetic vomiting, pulmonary complications, and abdominal distention.

During Gatch's period as assistant resident, it was the general practice to place the patient in the upright position for the treatment of peritonitis and a number of devices were used for this purpose. The essential principle of these devices was elevation of the knees, whereby the trunk, when elevated, was prevented from slipping downward. The simple plan of putting a pillow under the knees, however, was ineffectual as the support was too yielding. Baldwin suggested the use of an ordinary rocking chair. Allaben had described a backrest on the principle of a "double inclined plane." Gilliam advocated the use of a steamer chair. Finally, McGuire advised elevating the head of the bed and using an adjustable seat to keep the patient from slipping downward. None of these methods really solved the problem. One day while Gatch was wrestling with a 200-pound patient trying to get him into the upright position, he conceived the idea of a special bed for the purpose. His initial model consisted of an oblong frame of stout boards, to the upper surface of which were hinged free movable flaps. The frame was of the exact length and width of a standard ward bed, on the springs of which it was intended to rest. Figure 8 shows the relative length of these flaps and the plan of elevating or lowering them. To cover the bed he first used a mattress hinged at the points of bending but found that an ordinary "Ostermoore" mattress if strapped down would bend as much as necessary. The straps were sewn to the undersurface of the mattress at a point about 6 inches from the edge so as to allow the covers to be tucked in between mattress and strap. Such a bed could be made inexpensively by any carpenter. While in use in a Detroit hospital, Gatch's bed was seen by Henry Ford. The result was the invention of a crank-and-screw arrangement to adjust the bed.

The reason Dr. Gatch left Johns Hopkins and later became resident in surgery at Washington University in 1911 was not that he had not been promised the residency but because of an unfortunate incident that occurred. He was making rounds with Halsted on a private patient in Marburg and she said: "Oh, professor, don't let that man ever dress me again. He was so rough he just pulled that dressing off." When they walked out of the room, Halsted said: "Gatch, I thought I taught you to be gentle." Gatch's reply used words which were offensive to Halsted who promptly said: "Gatch, you will not be my resident if you use language like that." That story was told originally by Dr. Dandy and Gatch confirmed it a number of years later to W. M. Firor. Just before the old surgical building was torn down, they found in the attic the instruments Gatch had devised, including his gas machine. Unfortunately, they were later destroyed.

In 1912, after a year at Washington University in

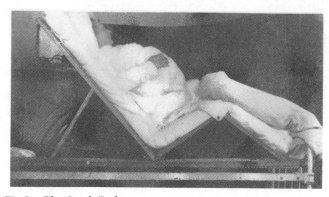 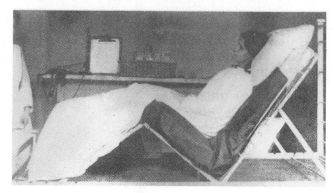

Fig 8.   The Gatch Bed.
Reprinted with permission, from Gatch WD: The sitting posture; its postoperative and other uses. Ann Surg, March 1909. Figs. 1 and 2, after p. 412.

St. Louis, Gatch established himself in the practice of surgery in Indianapolis and joined the faculty of the newly organized Indiana University School of Medicine. His research interests continued, and he established a research laboratory in which he and Frank Mann, later of Mayo Clinic fame, did experimental work on shock. His drive to do research and his strong clinical orientation led to major contributions to the surgical literature, one of which was an accurate way of measuring blood loss at the time of an operative procedure. Additional studies included those on bowel obstruction, cholecystitis, several innovative operative procedures, and an interest in cancer surgery.

In January 1928 Gatch was appointed head of the department of surgery at Indiana University. He restructured the residency training program from one of an indefinite length, but seldom more than one year's experience, to a Halsted type of program including three years' surgical experience with increasing responsibility and a research laboratory year as well.

In 1932 Gatch was appointed dean of the Indiana University School of Medicine, and during this period many changes occurred at the medical center. A new clinical building was dedicated in 1936. Clinical clerkships were inaugurated, there was an increase in student enrollment, a full-time faculty program was instituted, and many new departments including psychiatry, bacteriology, pathology, plastic surgery, neurosurgery, and medical art were established. Gatch retired from his deanship in 1946 and from the departmental chairmanship at the age of 70. He continued a vigorous practice of surgery and participated in the education of residents at the St. Vincent and Methodist Hospitals until his incapacitating illness developed in 1960. The surgical pavilion of the University Hospital was named the Willis D. Gatch Surgical Pavilion in his honor.

Gatch was an inquiring scholar, a provocative teacher, a skilled surgeon, and a strong and tireless administrator who contributed greatly to the development of the Indiana University School of Medicine.

There were many amusing stories about Gatch. One day while working late with a patient he asked the nurse to call his wife and tell her that he would be home

for dinner soon. His wife replied to the nurse: "You tell Dr. Gatch he has already had dinner."

BARNEY BROOKS

Born in Jackson, Texas on December 17, 1884, Barney Brooks (Fig 9) spent his boyhood years on his father's cattle ranch. He received the B.A. degree from the University of Texas in 1905 and in 1911 was graduated from The Johns Hopkins University School of Medicine. Life was simple on the plains and at times quite lonely. Initiative and ingenuity were required of everyone. His father believed in work and everyone learned to do his share, including his son Barney. Thus, a sense of responsibility was established early in Brooks and he developed rapidly in mind and body. The four years in college nearly depleted the money available and for the next two years he taught high school science in Texas to earn enough money to continue his education. It was here that he learned to love the role of the teacher. In medical school Brooks ranked fifth in his class. The first four in the class chose medical internships so that Barney had the opportunity to intern under William Stewart Halsted (1911–12).

Halsted did not offer him an assistant residency so Brooks joined the staff at the Barnes Hospital and the newly reorganized Washington University School of Medicine. His first two years there were spent in the field of investigative surgery. His most outstanding research during this period concerned regeneration of bone and intestinal obstruction. Unitl 1915 there was much confusion and disagreement concerning the symptomatology and pathology of intestinal obstruction. Brooks demonstrated that in intestinal obstruction, a toxin of bacterial origin is formed and that normal intestinal mucosa will not absorb this toxin. In addition, he pointed out that the presence or absence of strangulation and the portion and length of intestine involved influence the rate and degree of mucosal damage which in turn determines the rapidity of absorption of toxin.

In 1882, two years before Brooks was born, Volkmann described a paralysis and contracture in muscles which followed the application of a constricting bandage

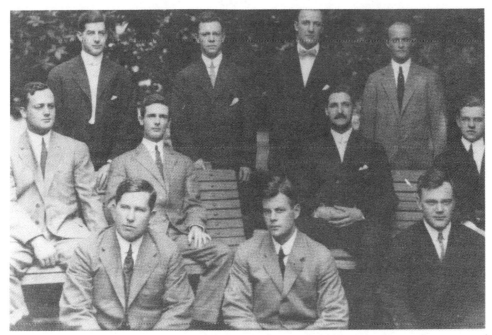

Fig 9. Barney Brooks (top row, first on the right). This picture is of the members of the Pithotomy Club, Class of 1911, Johns Hopkins University School of Medicine. Left to right, top row, C. C. Hartman, W. H. Licht, E. Stillman, Brooks; middle row, P. R. Sieber, Sr., L. C. Spencer, J. R. Miller, J. A. C. Colston; bottom row, W. N. Dunn, O. Kinsey, Jr., F. R. Crawford.

to an extremity and expressed the opinion that the cause of this condition was obstruction of the arteries. Through the years, many observers agreed with this interpretation but others attributed the phenomenon to damage to nerves, inflammatory reaction and the formation of toxic products. In 1922 Brooks demonstrated experimentally that the initial stimulus was mechanical due to increasing pressure resulting from an open artery and an occluded vein. As a consequence, degeneration of muscle fibers and complete fibrosis developed which converted the muscle and surrounding tissues into a fibrous mass characteristic of the deformity described by Volkmann.

From 1914 to 1916 Brooks was busy in his residency at Barnes Hospital. Upon completion of this training, he was offered a position in the department of surgery at Washington University, which he accepted. In August 1916 he married and within the next year the United States entered World War I. Brooks was put on the preferred list of faculty members and thus remained in St. Louis during the war. During this period in St. Louis he organized a surgical pathology laboratory and a course in surgical pathology, which served as a model for other institutions around the country.

In 1924 Brooks became the first to perform arteriography on patients by the injection of sodium iodide into the femoral artery. Prior to that time, there had been no satisfactory way of determining the location and extent of arterial occlusion in the extremity of a living patient. This new advance added a great impetus to improvement in the diagnosis of vascular disorders. Brooks planned his experimental work on a logical basis and was very meticulous in carrying it out. He displayed an

ability to grasp the basic facts in any problem and his conclusions reflected a mind which was both disciplined and profound. Two years after Brooks left Johns Hopkins, Halsted approached Joseph C. Bloodgood excitedly one day (a rare mood for Halsted). He called Bloodgood's attention to an excellent study carried out by a surgeon named Brooks in St. Louis. Halsted wondered if they should not try to get this Brooks to come to Johns Hopkins. At this point, Bloodgood reminded him that Brooks had been a surgical intern at Johns Hopkins just two years before.

From 1912 to 1925 Brooks ascended the ranks in the department of surgery at Washington University from assistant resident to associate professor. In 1925 other institutions expressed an interest in Brooks as professor of surgery and head of the department in their school, among them the University of Minnesota and Vanderbilt. Brooks chose the position offered him at the latter institution. In 1925 the new Vanderbilt Hospital had just been opened and the medical school was in a state of reorganization. Brooks had helped direct the reorganization of the department at Washington University and thus was fully experienced for the undertaking at Vanderbilt.

At Vanderbilt he maintained a wide interest in all fields of surgery, continuing to contribute in the laboratory and clinically in terms of establishing sound principles of surgery. His studies included the effects of pressure and variations in temperature upon living tissues and other studies stimulated interest in the problems of the surgical treatment of elderly patients. He was among the minority who advocated subtotal gastrectomy during a period when simple gastrojejunostomy was the widely accepted method of treating duodenal ulcer surgically.

In 1942 he was elected president of the Southern Surgical Association. The subject of his presidential address was psychosomatic surgery, a phase of the subject which he pioneered. The former dean of Yale University School of Medicine wrote Dean Leathers of Vanderbilt of his enlightenment on this subject saying: "I did not know there was any surgeon in the world who knew patients had a psyche." Brooks was not only a gifted experimentalist and a great teacher, but also attracted excellent young men whom he trained for outstanding positions in surgery.

He had a unique knack of stimulating a medical student in such a way that what he learned was never forgotten. At Brooks' clinics students were called down to the floor of the amphitheatre for questioning about the case being presented. This undoubtedly created great inner stress, the student suffering from rapid pulse and respiration, but every moment on the floor was endowed with meaning and these clinics were an outstanding educational experience. When asking a question Brooks had a characteristic way of setting his jaw, looking directly at the student, and waving his hand toward him while he waited for an answer. When the answer came back loaded with extraneous information, Brooks would interject, "My goodness man, I ask you for the biscuits and you pass me the gravy."

In December 1944 the surgical house staff at Vanderbilt gave a surprise dinner in celebration of Brooks' 60th birthday. Over 120 guests were in attendance. After dinner several brief speeches were made. Alton Ochsner spoke as follows: "In the fall of 1918 I transferred to Washington University from the University of South Dakota, after having completed my first two years of medicine in that institution. There was never a more unsophisticated and greener individual than I was when I matriculated at Washington. The very first exercise that I attended was a diagnostic clinic which was conducted by Dr. Brooks. The case which was presented was one of acute hematogenous osteomyelitis and those ... who have heard Dr. Brooks hold a clinic can easily realize how impressed I was by that presentation. The orderly chronological development of the facts about the case made a condition about which I knew nothing appear so simple that I realized here was a teacher who had ... few, if any, equals."

Brooks died on March 30, 1952. He was succeeded by H. William Scott, Jr., a Harvard graduate, who had his surgical training under Alfred Blalock at Johns Hopkins. In January 1953 Evarts A. Graham, professor of surgery at Washington University in St. Louis, gave the first Barney Brooks Memorial Lecture on the relation of cigarettes to bronchogenic carcinoma.

There are countless other examples of the pervasive influence which the Halsted school of surgery has had on the development of modern surgical care in this country. This influence has been exerted not only through those who trained directly under Halsted, but, in turn, by those trained by his numerous pupils. This process of multiplication continues and its effects on the current status of surgery and the surgical specialties knows no bounds, whether one is concerned with patient care, education, or research.

ACKNOWLEDGMENTS

I wish to thank the following for supplying me with material for this essay: J. S. Battersby, W. J. Daly, Claire Still, and R. H. Kampmeier; to Dr. W. M. Firor for his critical review of the manuscript and Dr. Peter Olch for making his oral history of Emile Holman available. I am grateful to Patricia King for her help in editing and typing the manuscript.

REFERENCES

1. Allaben JE: Intestinal perforation in typhoid fever; its diagnosis and surgical treatment. JAMA 49: 556, 1907

2. Andrus WD: George J. Heuer's contributions and his place in American surgery. Surgery 23: 321, 1948

3. Baldwin JF: The rocking chair for the Fowler position. JAMA 49: 1043, 1907

4. Beck CS and Holman E: The physiological response of the circulatory system to experimental alterations. I. The effects of intracardiac fistulae. J Exp Med 42: 661, 1925; II. The effect of variations in total blood volume. J Exp Med 42: 681, 1925; III. The effect of aortic and pulmonic stenoses. J Clin Invest 3: 283, 1926

5. Bloodgood JC: The transplantation of the rectus muscle in certain cases of inguinal hernia in which the conjoined tendon is obliterated. Bull Johns Hopkins Hosp 9: 96, 1898

6. Bloodgood JC: Operations on 459 cases of hernia in the Johns Hopkins Hospital from June 1889 to January 1899. The special consideration of 268 cases operated on by the Halsted method, and the transplantation of the rectus muscle in certain cases of inguinal hernia in which the conjoined tendon is obliterated. Johns Hopkins Hosp Rep 7: 223, 1899

7. Bloodgood JC: Method of instruction in surgical pathology. Bull Johns Hopkins Hosp 14: 220, 1903

8. Bloodgood JC: Giant cell sarcoma of bone: Report of a case of medullary giant cell sarcoma of the tibia in which the tumor was removed by chiseling without destroying the continuity of the tibia, and a discussion of the facts which justify this more conservative procedure. Bull Johns Hopkins Hosp 14: 138, 1903

9. Bloodgood JC: Importance of early recognition and operative treatment of malignant tumors. Variation of the extent of the operative removal according to the relative malignancy of the tumor. JAMA 47: 1470, 1906

10. Bloodgood JC: The conservative treatment of giant cell sarcoma with the study of bone transplantation. Ann Surg 56: 210, 1912

11. Bloodgood JC: Diagnosis and treatment of borderline pathological lesions. Surg Gynecol Obstet 18: 19, 1914

12. Bloodgood JC: Bone tumors, benign and malignant. A brief summary of the salient factors based on a study of some 570 cases. Am J Surg 34: 229, 1920

13. Bloodgood JC: The pathology of chronic cystic mastitis of the female breast, with special consideration of the blue-dome cyst. Arch Surg 3: 445, 1921

14. Bloodgood JC: Bone tumors: Sarcoma, periosteal group, sclerosing type, osteogenic—methods of diagnosis and treatment. J Radiol 4: 46, 1923

15. Bloodgood JC: What every physician should know about the breast. Arch Clin Cancer Res 1: 1, 1925

16. Bloodgood JC: Prevention, diagnosis and treatment of cancer in its earliest stages. South Med J 19: 287, 1926

17. Brooks B. Studies in regeneration and growth of bone. Ann Surg 65: 705, 1917

18. Brooks B: Studies in bone regeneration. Ann Surg 66: 625, 1917

19. Brooks B: Intestinal obstruction: An experimental study. Ann Surg 67: 211, 1918

20. Brooks B: Studies in bone transplantation: A study of a method of increasing the osteogenetic power of a free bone transplant. Ann Surg 69: 113, 1919

21. Brooks B: Pathologic changes in muscle as a result of disturbances of circulation: An experimental study of Volkmann's ischemic paralysis. Arch Surg 5: 188, 1922

22. Brooks B: Diseases of the blood vascular system of the extremities: An experimental study. J Bone Joint Surg 6: 326, 1924

23. Brooks B: Intraarterial injection of sodium iodide. JAMA 82: 1016, 1924

24. Brooks B: Ligation of the terminal abdominal aorta: An experimental study. Arch Surg 17: 794, 1928

25. Brooks B: Surgery in patients of advanced stage. Ann Surg 105: 481, 1947

26. Brooks B and Duncan GW: Effects of pressure on tissue. Arch Surg 40: 696, 1940

27. Brooks B and Duncan GW: The effects of temperature on the survival of anemic tissue. Ann Surg 112: 130, 1940

28. Brooks B and Hudson WA: Studies in bone transplantation: An experimental study of the comparative success of autogenous and homogenous transplants of bone. Arch Surg 1: 284, 1920

29. Brooks B and Johnson GS: An experimental study of the distribution of the peripheral blood flow. J Bone Joint Surg 14: 102, 1932

30. Brooks B and Johnson GS: Simultaneous vein ligation: An experimental and clinical study of therapeutic venous occlusion. Ann Surg 100: 761, 1934

31. Carter BN: The fruition of Halsted's concepts of surgical training. Surgery 32: 518, 1952

32. Gatch WD: The sitting posture; its postoperative and other uses: With a description of a bed for holding a patient in this position. Ann Surg 49: 410, 1909

33. Gilliam T: The adjustable canvas chair as an aid to the Murphy treatment of diffuse suppurative peritonitis. JAMA 51: 1133, 1908

34. Green BE, Jr: Dr. Barney Brooks, 1884–1952. Am J Surg 98: 706, 1959

35. Griswold ML, Jr: George J. Heuer, M.D.—A critical analysis of the role that he played in introducing the residency system of training. Surgery 78: 349, 1975

36. Halsted WS: The results of operations for the cure of cancer of the breast performed at the Johns Hopkins Hospital from June, 1889 to January, 1894. Ann Surg 26: 497, 1894

37. Halsted WS: A clinical and histological study of certain adenocarcinomata of the breast. Ann Surg 28: 557, 1898

38. Halsted WS: Surgical Papers. Volume 2. Baltimore: The Johns Hopkins Press, 1924

39. Halsted WS and Holman E: An end-to-end anastomosis of the large intestine by abutting closed ends and puncturing the double diaphragm with an instrument passed per rectum. Bull Johns Hopkins Hosp 32: 98, 1921

40. Harrison TR, Dock W and Holman E: Experimental studies in arteriovenous fistulas: Cardiac output. Heart 11: 337, 1924

41. Heuer GJ: Surgical experiences with an intracranial approach to chiasmal lesions. Arch Surg 1: 368, 1920

42. Heuer GJ: Dr. Halsted. Johns Hopkins Hosp Bull (Suppl.) 90: 47, 1952

43. Heuer GJ and Andrus WD: The alveolar and blood gas changes following pneumonectomy. Bull Johns Hopkins Hosp 33: 130, 1922

44. Heuer GJ and Dandy WE: A report of seventy cases of brain tumor. Bull Johns Hopkins Hosp 27: 225, 1916

45. Heuer GJ and Dunn GR: Experimental pneumonectomy. Bull Johns Hopkins Hosp 31: 31, 1920

46. Heuer GJ and Holman E: Observations on the position and movements of the diaphragm following injuries to and surgical procedures upon the thorax: An experimental study. Med Bull Univ Cinn 2: 1, 1923

47. Holman E: The physiology of an arteriovenous fistula. Arch Surg 7: 64, 1923

48. Holman E: Protein sensitization in isoskingrafting. Surg Gynecol Obstet 38: 100, 1924

49. Holman E: Experimental studies in arteriovenous fistulas. I. Blood volume variations. Arch Surg 9: 822, 1924

50. Holman E: Experimental studies in arteriovenous fistulas. III. Cardiac dilatation and blood vessel changes. Arch Surg 9: 856, 1924

51. Holman E: The etiology of the postoperative pulmonary abscess. Ann Surg 83: 240, 1926

52. Holman E: Arteriovenous fistula: Dilatation of the artery distal to the abnormal communication. An unusual feature experimentally explained. Arch Surg 18: 1672, 1929

53. Holman E: The significance of temporary elevation of blood pressure following splenectomy, with particular reference to the role of the spleen as a regulator of the circulation. Surgery 1: 688, 1937

54. Holman E: William Stewart Halsted as revealed in his letters. Stanford Med Bull 10: 137, 1952

55. Holman E: The obscure physiology of poststenotic dilatation: Its relation to the development of aneurysms. J Thorac Surg 28: 109, 1954

56. Holman E: On circumscribed dilation of an artery immediately distal to a partially occluding band: Poststenotic dilatation. Surgery 36: 3, 1954

57. Holman E: A surgical philosopher's credo: Excerpts from the writings of William Stewart Halsted. Surg Gynecol Obstet 101: 369, 1955

58. Holman E: Sir William Osler, William Stewart Halsted, Harvey Cushing: Some personal reminiscences. Surgery 57: 589, 1965

59. Holman E: Abnormal Arteriovenous Communications: Peripheral and Intracardiac; Acquired and Congenital. Springfield, Ill: Charles C Thomas, 1968

60. Holman E: The legacy of William Stewart Halsted. Bull Am Coll Surg 54: 99, 1969

61. Holman E, Chandler LR and Cooley CL: Experimental studies in pulmonary suppuration. Surg Gynecol Obstet 44: 328, 1927

62. Holman E and Kolls AC: Experimental studies in arteriovenous fistulas. II. Pulse and blood pressure variations. Arch Surg 9: 837, 1924

63. Holman E and Mathes ME: The production of intrapulmonary suppuration by secondary infection of a sterile embolic area. Experimental study. Arch Surg 19: 1246, 1929

64. Leriche R: A tribute to Dr. Halsted. Halsted Centenary. Surgery 12: 538, 1952

65. MacCallum WG and McClure RD: On the mechanical effects of experimental mitral stenosis and insufficiency. Bull Johns Hopkins Hosp 17: 260, 1906

66. Mathes ME, Holman E and Reichert FL: A study of the

bronchial, pulmonary and lymphatic circulations of the lung under various pathologic conditions experimentally produced. J Thorac Surg 1: 339, 1932

67. McClure RD: Pancreatic atrophy in a dog following impaction of calculi in the duct. Bull Johns Hopkins Hosp 18: 332, 1907

68. McClure RD and Derge HF: Comparative surgery. XVII. A study of reversal of the intestine. Bull Johns Hopkins Hosp 18: 472, 1907

69. McClure RD and Dunn GR: Transfusions of blood: History, methods, dangers, preliminary tests, present status and report of 150 transfusions. Bull Johns Hopkins Hosp 28: 99, 1917

70. McGuire S: Treatment of diffuse suppurative peritonitis. JAMA 50: 1019, 1908

71. Murphy FT and Brooks B: Intestinal obstruction: An experimental study of the causes of symptoms and death. Arch Intern Med 15: 392, 1915

72. Reid M: The effect of arteriovenous fistula upon the heart and blood vessels: An experimental and clinical study. Bull Johns Hopkins Hosp 31: 1, 1920

73. Reid M: Partial occlusion of the pulmonary aorta and inferior vena cava with the metallic band. Observations on changes in the vessel wall and the heart. J Exp Med 40: 289, 1924

74. Reid M: Studies on abnormal arteriovenous communications, acquired and congenital. I. Report of a series of cases. II. The origin and nature of arteriovenous aneurysms, cirsoid aneurysms and simple aneurysms. III. The effects of abnormal arteriovenous communications on the heart, blood vessels and other structures. IV. The treatment of abnormal arteriovenous communications. Arch Surg 10: 601, 996, 1925 and 11: 25, 237, 1925

75. Reid M: Aneurysms in the Johns Hopkins Hospital: All cases treated in the surgical service from the opening of the hospital to January 1922. Arch Surg 12: 1, 1926

76. Richards V: Emile Holman: He bridged the gap between humanism and science. Stanford, M.D. (Fall-Winter): 9, 1968–69

77. Rogers WL and Holman E: Penetrating wounds of the chest in the Pacific area. An analysis of 180 cases. Ann Surg 124: 1076, 1946

6.
Harvey Williams Cushing: The Baltimore Period, 1896–1912

Harvey Williams Cushing, the youngest of ten children of Betsy Maria Williams and Henry Kirke Cushing, M.D., was born on the Western Reserve of Connecticut in the town of Cleveland, Ohio on April 8, 1869. His forebear, Matthew Cushing, who had settled at Hingham in the Massachusetts Bay Colony, came to this country on the ship *Diligent*, which arrived at Boston on August 10, 1638. Matthew's descendant, David Cushing, Jr., a country doctor, was the father of Erastus Cushing, M.D., Harvey's grandfather, who immigrated with a young family in 1835 to the Western Reserve.

As a youth in Cleveland, Cushing attended Central High School, where he was an outstanding student. He excelled in a unique course devised by the physics teacher in manual training, and the dexterity which Cushing learned in this course undoubtedly contributed to his success as a surgeon.

Cushing matriculated at Yale College in 1887. He appeared to be more interested in baseball and the "gym" than he was in academics, later confessing to having visited the library only once in four years. His prowess at baseball was attested to by Amos Alonzo Stagg, who pitched for Yale from 1886 through 1890. On one of his trips with the baseball team, Cushing visited the White House and met President and Mrs. Harrison (April 28, 1889). Cushing also loved to attend the circus, particularly to watch feats of muscular skill and to visit the "freaks" at the sideshow—it was Cushing who later proved how gigantism and dwarfism came to be. Despite his extracurricular fascinations, however, Cushing did decide while at Yale to direct his energies toward a career in medicine. This was partially a result of the influence of his brother, Ned, who was an intern at the Massachusetts General Hospital in 1888, but mostly because of a course in physiological chemistry with Russell Chittenden. Chittenden had a lasting influence on Cushing, as well as on a number of Cushing's classmates, including among them Elliott Joslin, who became a world renowned diabetic

Reprinted from the *Johns Hopkins Medical Journal* **138**: 196, 1976.

specialist; Graham Lusk, who took over the Department of Physiology at Yale; and Lafayette Mendel, who succeeded Chittenden in the chair of physiological chemistry at Yale.

HARVARD MEDICAL SCHOOL AND THE MASSACHUSETTS GENERAL HOSPITAL

In September 1891 Cushing entered the Harvard Medical School. There were many outstanding faculty members at Harvard at that time including Henry Pickering Bowditch, Professor of Physiology. At President Eliot's urging, Bowditch had studied abroad with Claude Bernard and Carl Ludwig, and on his return to Harvard, had established the first laboratory in the United States devoted to experimental physiology. Among the outstanding clinical instructors were John Collins Warren, Reginald Heber Fitz (of appendicitis fame), Frederick C. Shattuck, and John Homans. Maurice Richardson, with whom Cushing developed a close friendship, did much to influence Cushing's surgical thinking in those early days.

During his clinical years, Cushing served occasionally as an anesthetist and one of his first patients died under the anesthetic before a class of students at the Massachusetts General Hospital on January 10, 1893. This incident had a great emotional impact on the young medical student. He and his classmate, Amory Codman, later developed the procedure of "continuous recording" which enabled both the anesthetist and the surgeon to tell at a glance the condition of the patient as indicated by pulse and respiration. At that time there was no method available for estimating blood pressure.

By 1895, Fulton points out, much of the groundwork for Cushing's career as a neurological surgeon had been laid. For example, on April 24 of that year, William N. Conant, a patient with a compound fracture of the skull was operated on. Cushing made the following notations on the back of this man's record: "Patient had fearful hemorrhage from brain sinuses. Pulse kept along very well and finally went out all at once and could not be felt at wrist. With pressure which checked the hemorrhage the pulse finally came back a few beats at a time, as an Indian starts up from a way station, and finally became pretty regular 120–110–100." On the front of the record is another scribbled note: "Bled enormously;" and finally a follow-up note, "Waverly and discharge okay," indicating that Cushing had followed the patient to the convalescent home in Waverly near Boston and had found out that the man was ultimately discharged as well. Noteworthy in Cushing's approach are the scientific attitude, the carefully kept record with its illuminating comments, the interest already evident in neurological surgery, and the following of the patient to obtain the end result. The problems of intracranial hemorrhage and anesthesia were already fixed in his mind. They were to occupy his interest for many years to come, for neurological surgery could not be advanced until these fundamental problems had been solved.

During his student days at Harvard, Cushing began his life-long practice of keeping a diary, through which it has been possible to gain great insight into the man and his character. We learn, for example, that while a student he experienced periods of depression, as did other famous personages such as Francis Galton and Weir Mitchell, even though his work was actually going very well. Throughout medical school, while attending clinics, he routinely sketched patients in order to reinforce his learning experience. One page in his student diary shows the pained expression of a woman suffering with gallstone colic; a week later a distinguished looking sailor is depicted in respiratory distress with Cheyne-Stokes respiration. His verbal descriptions reveal his skill in catching the essence of persons, situations, and experiences.

The class of 1894 at Harvard Medical School was the last three-year class. Although the majority of students took their degrees in that year, Cushing elected to remain for a fourth year, which was spent mainly in clinical work. He was awarded the degrees of M.D. and A.M. cum laude on June 26, 1895, but he had in reality begun his formal appointment as house pupil at the Massachusetts General Hospital (MGH) in April 1895.

During his year as house pupil at the MGH, Cushing, again in collaboration with Codman, helped to inaugurate the clinical use of x rays. Roentgen's discovery of a new kind of ray had been announced in Germany on December 28, 1895. Edison, Thompson, and others commenced experimentation immediately in this country, and by February 1896 American medical journals began to carry x-ray photographs. Codman apparently spent more time with the new tube than did Cushing and eventually suffered from serious x-ray burns.

Cushing's contemporary comments on surgery at the Massachusetts General Hospital were rather pithy. John Eliot, C.B. Porter, Maurice Richardson, and William Conant were highly regarded, but others were labelled as operating by the clock. For example, on April 12, 1896 he wrote: "Not operating much, considerable sepsis in the house. No wonder, these men operate about the way a commercial traveller grabs breakfast at a lunch counter."

THE JOHNS HOPKINS PERIOD

When Cushing arrived in Baltimore in the autumn of 1896 to assume his duties as assistant resident in surgery, both the Johns Hopkins Hospital and the School of Medicine were new and vigorous institutions. Halsted was 45 years of age, Osler 47, and Cushing 27. Cushing gives us some insight into the life of a house officer in his day: "It was most disconcerting to me, after the hurly-burly of the M.G.H. to have my new Chief come, as it were apologetically, some day into ward G; ask if he might be allowed to examine a particular patient; to have him spend an hour fiddling over a patient with cancer of the breast who had recently been admitted; and then to have him depart saying he was tired and would be able to do nothing more that day. If he was sufficiently interested he might ask that he be permitted to do the operation; and if he came and did operate, so soon as the breast was removed, leaving the huge closure and skin graft to Bloodgood, he would depart with the tissues. These he would study and ruminate over for an interminable time, meanwhile tagging innumerable areas which he wished to have sectioned—a duty which devolved upon the house officer. It was incumbent upon each of us to make all the clinical, bacteriological, and pathological studies for every patient in our charge—a good system for reliable house officers, which unfortunately all are not. Due to it, a great deal of most valuable material, at the Hopkins in those days was either imperfectly worked up or not worked up at all. I personally owe to this sytem what little I know of histological pathology, and my early bacteriological studies, some of which got into print would otherwise have never been made." (Fulton, 1946)

THE FIRST X RAYS AT HOPKINS

Cushing became involved with the taking of x-rays soon after his arrival at Hopkins. He has given his own account of this experience: "No x-ray photos had been taken at the Johns Hopkins Hospital when I came down in the fall of 1896. Codman and I had been fooling with some exposures at the MGH using an old static machine, and he continued for about ten years more until they had obviously affected his physical condition. We had of course no idea of burns or ductless gland disturbances and so forth. [H.C. had brought a fluoroscope with him from Boston.] There was a large static machine in ward C in Baltimore at the time and I got a small four-inch tube and began making exposures, spending many an hour in a temporary dark room off the old amphitheatre with Rodinal as a developer. The [x-ray] prints were among the first taken with an exposure of anywhere from 20 to 30 minutes and I think fully a dozen trials must have been made. It is extraordinary that there were no burns and no personal injury. . . .and I did all the x-ray work until I became resident succeeding Bloodgood."

Cushing's first formal piece of writing involved a patient who entered the emergency room on November 6, 1896, having been shot in the neck by her bartender husband during a family brawl. The bullet had entered the cervical region and lodged in the neck (Fig. 1). She showed signs of paralysis, unilaterally, and sensory impairment on the opposite side, leading Cushing to infer that the bullet had reached the spinal cord. The old static

machine was activated and plates of the cervical spine were obtained, disclosing the bullet as lodged in the body of the sixth cervical vertebra. This was Cushing's first case of a spinal cord lesion and he made detailed sensory charts illustrating the familiar Brown–Séquard syndrome. This case was first reported at the Johns Hopkins Medical Society Meeting on May 3, 1897, and it was published in the *American Journal of the Medical Sciences* under the title, "Haematomyelia from gunshot wounds of the spine: A report of two cases with recovery following symptoms of hemilesions of the cord."

In early 1897 Cushing was chosen to succeed Bloodgood as surgical resident (Fig 2). He later wrote of this as follows: "After a year in the wards, I was offered the residency, though Bloodgood stayed on in the resident's room for another 12 months while writing his monograph on hernia. There were other candidates for the post, men who had been there longer than I, men better grounded in the fundamentals of surgery, and whom I perhaps excelled in only one thing, in operative technique. Finney and I had both been schooled in this under C. B. Porter, a brilliant technician, though from the

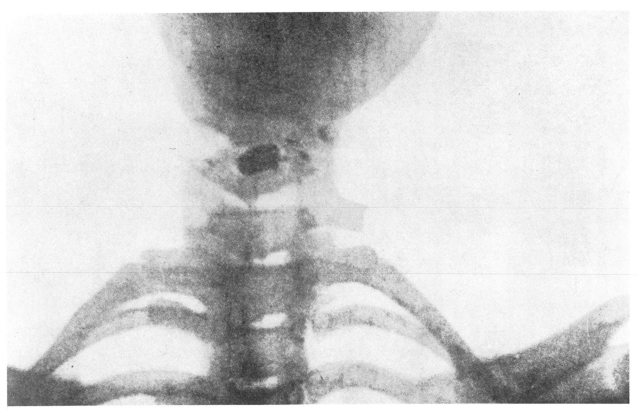

Fig 1. Bullet in the cervical spine of patient L.W. from Cushing's first paper. One of the first x rays taken (by Cushing) at The Johns Hopkins Hospital.
From the Archives Office, Johns Hopkins Medical Institutions.

Hopkins point of view not what would be called a great surgeon. Both Finney and I must have profited much from the Boston school of operating surgeons who, be it said, were most scornful of the Hopkins and its inartistic rubber-gloved methods of operating. However, to one who was familiar with the postoperative care of cases under each system, there could be no question which was superior at least from the standpoint of end results."

Stemming from his contact with Reginald Fitz in Boston, Cushing was interested in appendicitis. The new operation had been performed several times at Hopkins with unencouraging results. On September 9, 1897 Harvey Cushing operated on a patient with a ruptured appendix who died ten days later of peritonitis. Nevertheless, when Cushing himself developed the disease, although he had misgivings, he urged Halsted to operate quickly. Just before going to the operating room on September 28, 1897, he left a note in the room of his friend, C.N.B. Camac: "As I've often told patients there is a certain amount of danger in all operations, similarly some danger in getting onto a streetcar—about even they are. . . .I wrote you a small message giving you the privilege of distributing my things, books and so forth among the staff. 'Auf wiedersehen.' I hope." Cushing wrote his own case history, which was a model of directness and brevity. During his convalescence he was notified by Welch that he had been made an instructor in surgery with a salary of $100 per year.

Clinical work in general surgery occupied most of his time as an instructor, and one of his contributions was removal of the spleen for the first time in America in a patient with Banti's disease. Osler had made the diagnosis and had recommended the operation. This was the 12th case of Banti's disease listed as "cured" by splenectomy, the first dating back to Spencer Wells in England in 1851.

During Halsted's absence in the autumn of 1896, there were several operative deaths from improper etherization. Cushing began to experiment with block anesthesia produced by cocaine infiltration of the appropriate nerve trunk, a procedure which Halsted himself had been largely responsible for introducing but which for many reasons he had abandoned in his own clinic. Cushing's first major use of this procedure was an amputation at the shoulder in a boy with sarcoma of the humerus for which purpose the whole brachial plexus was successfully blocked. Later he amputated a hip and developed a successful local infiltration technique for hernia; the latter he described in a paper on cocaine anesthesia which was first communicated at the Johns Hopkins Medical Society on May 8, 1898. It was published in the *Johns Hopkins Hospital Bulletin* in August of that year. At that time, of course, Halsted's work on local anesthesia was not widely known. In a letter written later in life to Osler in which he described the circumstances surrounding his introduction of local anesthesia, Halsted described his experiments and his acquisition of the cocaine habit. Three of his assistants had acquired the cocaine habit in the course of these experiments

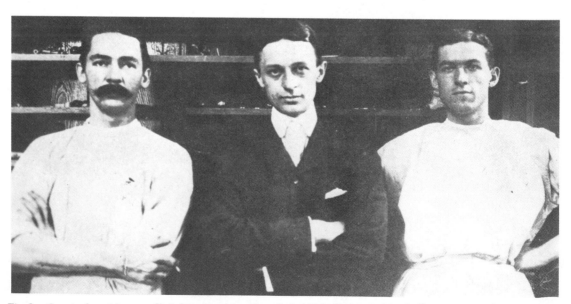

Fig 2.   Surgical resident staff, Johns Hopkins Hospital, 1899. James F. Mitchell, Harvey Cushing, and M.B. Clopton.
From the Archives Office, Johns Hopkins Medical Institutions.

in which they injected their own nerves; all died without recovering from the habit. Cushing was not aware of any of this when he was in Baltimore and when Welch told him after Halsted's death, Cushing reproached himself for having been so impatient with Halsted in the early days. In a biographical sketch written in 1922, Cushing said of Halsted: "A man of unique personality, shy, something of a recluse, fastidious in his taste and in his friendships, an aristocrat in his breeding, scholarly in his habits, the victim for many years of indifferent health, he nevertheless was one of the few American surgeons who may be considered to have established a school of surgery comparable, in a sense, to the school of Billroth in Vienna. He had few of the qualities supposed to accompany what the world regards as a successful surgeon. Overmodest about his work, indifferent to matters of priority, caring little for the gregarious gatherings of medical men, unassuming, having little interest in private practice, he spent his medical life avoiding patients—even students, when this was possible—and, when health permitted, working in clinic and laboratory at the solution of a succession of problems which aroused his interest. He had that rare form of imagination which seized problems, and the technical ability combined with persistence which enabled him to attack them with promise of a successful issue. Many of his contributions, not only to his craft but to the science of medicine in general, were fundamental in character and of enduring importance..." Although Halsted and Cushing had great admiration and respect for each other, their relationship had none of the warmth and affection of Cushing's relationships with Osler and Welch.

Few know of the great interest which Cushing developed in bacteriology in 1898 and 1899. His experiences with typhoid and his pioneer work on the surgical handling of typhoid perforations did much to crystallize his interest. His work in the bacteriological field in 1899 brought him into touch with such leaders in this area as Theobald Smith and Walter Reed, and almost carried him to the Philippines where Flexner was sent with Lewellys Barker on a government mission arising from the American occupation of Manila.

In all, Cushing completed four years "in the house" under Halsted. He was given a freer rein than other men would have been given in the same circumstances. This was largely because he proved himself capable of carrying the responsibility but perhaps even more because the "Professor" was in poor health and was seldom at the clinic. In Cushing's own words: "I saw relatively-little of him during my three years as resident, less and less as he perhaps began to feel that I might be entrusted with

the bulk of the routine work. A great deal of this was of course major surgery and the assistance was very poor. There was at that time a rotation service for house officers who were only on surgery for four months; and as Young soon was sidetracked into urology, there was no one with any experience to give anesthesia for prolonged cases like breast cases or for serious conditions such as intestinal strangulations and the like. It was owing to this that I took up local anesthesia without getting much moral support from the 'Professor.' I little realized at the time the reasons for this. . .We sometimes went out of town with him to operate, less often in private houses in Baltimore. An operating trunk was prepared for these occasions and a large part of the staff would go along—most elaborate performances they were, for which he charged prodigious fees."

The year 1900–1901 was spend abroad, an experience which proved most valuable to Cushing. In planning his trip, he gave first place to study with men whose interests were neurological and physiological, including Kocher, Kronecker, Horsley and Sherrington. After an unnerving experience watching Horsley's operation on a woman in which he cut the Gasserian ganglion, Cushing decided that the refinements of neurologic surgery could not be learned from Horsley. Much more rewarding, he believed, was the time spent with Sherrington.

When he returned to Baltimore in the fall of 1901, he joined forces with two close friends, both bachelors, Thomas B. Futcher and Henry Barton Jacobs. They moved into Three West Franklin Street next door to the Oslers. They were promptly given latch keys to the Osler household and with this intimacy for nearly four years, it is not surprising that Cushing's biography of Osler contained so much personal material.

Although Cushing long followed the advice of his mentor, Vesalius, who had insisted that he who would marry a wife must not study medicine for there was not time enough for both, in 1902 he married Katherine Crowell after a courtship of some 10 years. He and his bride lived at Three West Franklin Street for the next six years, the one remaining bachelor latch-keyer, T.B. Futcher, staying on as a member of their household.

IMPORTANT RESEARCH CONTRIBUTIONS

In the ensuing years in Baltimore, Cushing, in addition to specializing in neurosurgery, made three highly important contributions to medicine and general surgery: one, his clinical studies on blood pressure; two, the extension to the surgical clinic of Ringer's and Locke's studies on physiological saline;

and three, the establishment of the Hunterian Laboratory for Experimental Surgery.

INTRODUCTION OF THE SPHYGMOMANOMETER

Cushing's experimental work in Kronecker's laboratory in Berne had been largely concerned with the regulation of blood pressure, particularly in relation to pressure within the skull. He learned that the level of blood pressure reflects an animal's physiological condition. If during a surgical procedure the pressure should fall unduly, it indicates that the animal's condition is poor. As related, Cushing and Codman had introduced "ether charts" during their years at the Harvard Medical School so that the anesthetist could record the patient's pulse and respiration at regular intervals during an operation. When Cushing saw the Riva–Rocci sphygmomanometer during a visit to Pavia, Italy, he quickly recognized that it was an essential for anesthetists during a surgical procedure. As soon as he returned to Baltimore, he developed a new anesthesia chart and insisted that blood pressure readings be taken during all operations. His first report in the *Annals of Surgery* for September 1902 was titled "On the avoidance of shock in major amputations by cocainization of large nerve trunks preliminary to their division: with observations on blood pressure changes in surgical cases." In December 1901, while at a meeting in Cleveland, Cushing told George Crile about the new blood pressure apparatus and the advantages of it over the Gaertner instrument which Crile was then using. William T. Councilman, who also attended the meeting, overheard the conversation and later invited both Crile and Cushing to a special meeting to be held in Boston on January 19, 1903. The title of the Boston program was "Consideration of blood pressure." Crile spoke first on "My observations on the methods of control in the blood pressure," and then Cushing spoke on his "Blood pressure observations." The papers were discussed by such important Bostonians as William T. Porter, James M. Jackson, and Richard C. Cabot. As a result of the program, a printed circular was sent in February 1903 to all members of the Department of Surgery at Harvard requesting that a committee be formed to consider the "importance of blood pressure observations in surgical diagnosis and treatment." This committee after long deliberation decided that the skilled palpating finger was of greater value clinically for determination of the state of the circulation than any pneumatic instrument. However, despite this imperceptive appraisal of Cushing's recommendations, medical men throughout the country began to take an active interest in blood pressure determination. Crile's book on blood pressure appeared in the autumn of 1903 and the world promptly forgot about the Harvard committee's mistake.

Henry K. Beecher, the distinguished anesthetist, described these anesthesia records in a paper published in *Surgery, Gynecology and Obstetrics* in 1940. In this paper, Cushing's long letter of 1920 to Dr. Washburn, the hospital superintendent, in which their early experiences are described is reprinted. The early anesthesia charts stand historically as one of the principal American contributions to surgical techniques.

Cushing later wrote (April 1930), at the request of Ralph Major, the following remembrance of these events: "I brought the first Riva–Rocci apparatus to this country from Pavia in 1901 when I came back to Hopkins from my year abroad and introduced it into the Johns Hopkins clinic where Briggs and Cook subsequently modified it and got it put in a box. The original apparatus was of course simply homemade, and was perhaps as good as any of the more recent ones...But I am not so sure that the general use of the blood pressure apparatus in clinical work has *done more than harm*. Just as Floyer's pulse watch led to two previously unknown diseases, tachycardia and bradycardia, so the sphygmomanometer has led to the uncovering of the diseases of hypertension and hypotension, which have vastly added to the number of neurasthenics in the world." There is an amusing incident connected with all of this: "An inexperienced student nurse, who had heard vaguely about the blood pressure cuff, was substituting as an anesthetist; at a tense moment in the operation she was suddenly told to take a pressure reading. A few minutes later Cushing felt something tugging at his pants' leg, only to discover that the student nurse was putting the pneumatic cuff on him." (Fulton, 1946)

PHYSIOLOGICAL SALINE SOLUTION

Sidney Ringer demonstrated that so-called "physiological salt solution," consisting of sodium chloride added to distilled water, was inadequate for preserving excised tissues. Ringer discovered this when his laboratory assistant, rather than making up the solution for his experiments from distilled water, used London tap water. The tap water worked at a time when Ringer was having trouble maintaining normal function in his excised tissue preparations. Ringer, instead of chastising the assistant, analyzed the tap water and found that it contained other ions in addition to sodium and chloride. These findings were described in a series of papers published in the English *Journal of Physiology* beginning in 1880. The full significance of Ringer's studies was not appreciated until Jacques Loeb's observations appeared in this country in 1900.

Harvey Cushing first drew attention to the importance of these discoveries to clinical medicine when he published an article entitled "Concerning the poisonous effect of pure sodium chloride solutions on nerve-muscle preparations" in October 1901 in the *American Journal of Physiology*. Cushing perfused the hind-leg vessels of a frog with solutions of differing ionic content demonstrating that when pure sodium chloride (0.7%) was used, the capacity of the muscle to respond to stimulation of its nerves was abolished. If potassium chloride and calcium chloride (0.03 to 0.06%) were added, the irritability of the muscle was restored and it once again responded to nerve stimulation. Cushing concluded that solutions of saline administered to human subjects should have a carefully balanced ionic content. Many years later (1935), Elliott C. Cutler, Cushing's successor in the chair of surgery at Harvard, wrote to Cushing concerning this early work as follows: "The curious part of this whole story is that no one has really worked upon this matter seriously since your publication, a matter which I am going to bring someday to Walter Cannon's attention at our lunch at the Brigham."

Cushing gave credit to Kronecker for suggesting that he work on this problem. He noted that in 1902 he wrote a "pot-boiler" for Cohen's system of physiological therapeutics on saline irrigations and infusions in which he gave a formula of sodium chloride 0.9%, calcium chloride 0.026%, potassium chloride, 0.01%. Looking back, this potboiler of Cushing's is a much clearer statement of the problem than any offered by the other textbooks of that period.

FIRST LABORATORY OF EXPERIMENTAL SURGERY

One of Cushing's major contributions to American surgery was the organization of the "old Hunterian"—the first experimental surgical laboratory developed in this country which served as a model for those established at other medical schools. The functions of the laboratory were first described in a paper entitled "Instruction in operative medicine, with the description of a course in the Hunterian Laboratory of Experimental Medicine." According to W.M. Firor, the erection of the laboratory grew out of a need for space for teaching third year students. In a letter to Dr. Welch, Dr. Halsted said: "I should be sorry to have it forgotten that I initiated the operative course on animals. Courses in experimental surgery were given to the first class in their third year (1895). One of the inducements offered to Cushing to return to us was the transference of these courses to him." Thus, the laboratory was used for a course in practical animal surgery for junior medical students in which they carried out on animals many of the more important procedures used in general surgery. As a result, many of the students were led into various phases of physiological and surgical research.

The first classes in operative surgery were held in the corner room on the first floor in the Woman's Fund Anatomy Building, which later became the laboratory of Dr. Florence Sabin. Dr. Mall needed this room, and in 1903 Dr. Cushing requested the trustees to erect a small, inexpensive building in which to conduct his classes. The request would likely have been granted but for the financial loss suffered by the university in the great fire of February 1904. When his request was turned down, Cushing solicited the aid of friends and was promised $5000. However, the trustees declined the offer, believing the sum insufficient for the construction of a building in conformity with those already in existence. Late in 1904, MacCallum and Cushing joined forces and their further appeal to the trustees brought positive results. The trustees voted $15,000 for the erection of the building which was completed in the summer of 1905 (Figs. 3 and 4). Half of the space was allocated to pathology and the other half to surgery. Cushing favored naming the laboratory after Magendie, but it was pointed out that Magendie's name was anathema to the antivivisectionists in Baltimore. Welch suggested John Hunter's name and the laboratory became known as the Hunterian Laboratory for Experimental Medicine. "It was a good solution to the problem of a suitable name, but it mystified Baltimoreans who thought the term had reference to pointers, retrievers, and setters."

The new laboratory had three main goals: the teaching of students, the practice of veterinary medicine, and research (Figs. 5 and 6). Cushing emphasized that the unique feature in the course in operative surgery was making the exercise simulate as far as possible the actual performance of surgery on a hospitalized patient. This included the writing of a history, the keeping of an anesthesia chart, the writing of operative and postoperative notes, and the performance of a complete postmortem study. This method of teaching the principles of surgery was just as revolutionary as Osler's bedside instruction in medicine.

For many years the Hunterian provided a haven for dog fanciers who brought their pets to it for treatment. This experience in the natural diseases of canines is illustrated by the first three sets of paper that were issued by the laboratory under the

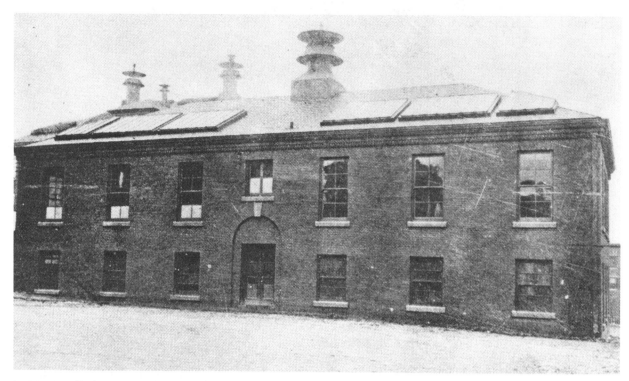

Fig 3.   East front of the Hunterian Laboratory.
From the Archives Office, Johns Hopkins Medical Institutions.

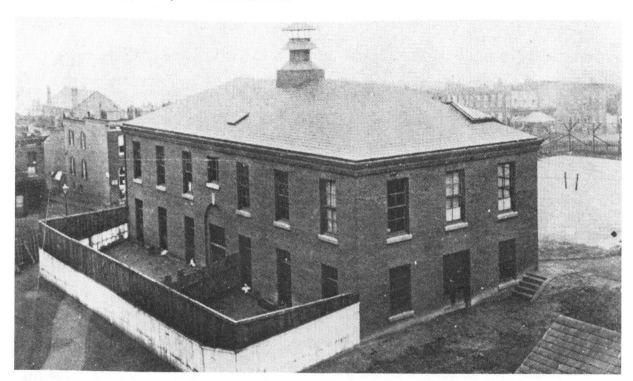

Fig 4.   Hunterian Laboratory: View from the Anatomical Building.
From the Archives Office, Johns Hopkins Medical Institutions.

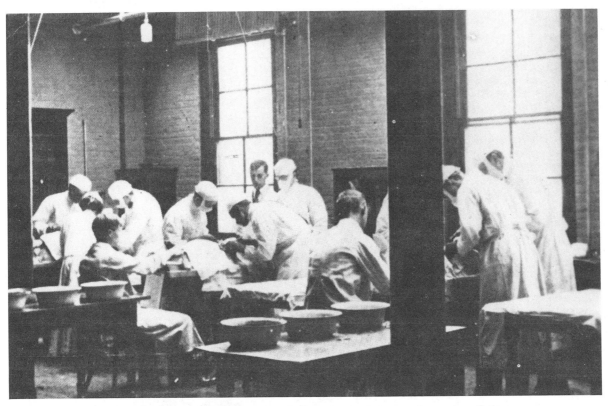

Fig 5.   Classroom scene. Cushing's course in operative surgery for third year students of medicine.
From the Archives Office, Johns Hopkins Medical Institutions.

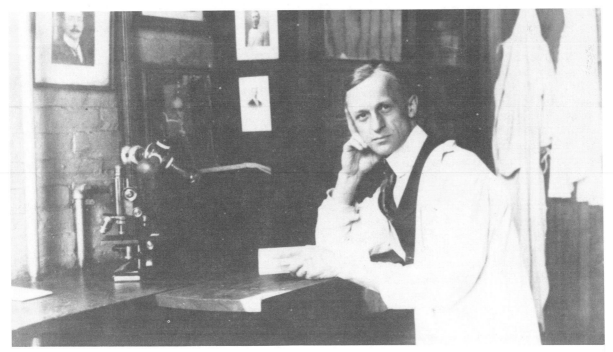

Fig 6.   Harvey Cushing at his laboratory desk in the Hunterian (1907).
From the Archives Office, Johns Hopkins Medical Institutions.

title, "Comparative Surgery." The observations made on the diseases of dogs led to efforts to reproduce some of these diseases in normal animals as models for the study of analogous diseases in human beings. This effort is well illustrated by the opening sentence in a paper by Cushing and Branch: "We wish to mention briefly some attempts which have been made in the Hunterian Laboratory to reproduce chronic valvular lesions; to record certain cases of spontaneous valvular disease in the dog which have come under our observation, and finally to comment on the possibilities of future surgical measures in man directed toward the alleviation particularly of the lesion characterizing mitral stenosis." Thus, interest at Johns Hopkins in cardiovascular surgery goes back further than most realize. Cushing could scarcely foresee in December 1907 the attainment of this goal (an operation for mitral stenosis) which was to eventuate some forty years later.

As one looks at the investigations carried out in the laboratory, several distinctive features emerge: first, the same excellence of performance demanded by Dr. Halsted in the operating room was required of the workers in the laboratory. Every detail of his meticulous surgical technique was applied to the operations on animals; second, the majority of the problems studied were basic in nature; and third, a true spirit of thoughtful inquiry and creative scholarship pervaded the laboratory. Experience in this laboratory had an immeasurable influence on students, fellows and visitors from this country and abroad.

Cushing recorded his reminiscences about the laboratory in 1920 in response to a letter from Jay McLean, who was at that time in charge of the Hunterian: "Not long after my return in 1901 I was given a position on the surgical staff as an assistant. The delightful feature of the Johns Hopkins Hospital organization in those days was the absence of any obvious departmental machinery and I hope it may always stay so. The professor's junior associates practically agreed among themselves as to what they would teach, and they were allowed to go about it in their own way. Dr. Finney had for many years given a course in operative surgery on the cadaver and this he relinquished in order to give me something to do. Though untrained in laboratory methods except for my short period abroad in the physiological laboratories of Kronecker and Sherrington, I had been introduced to some experimental work on animals by Dr. Halsted, through an investigation we started together on parathyroid extirpations. The third year students occasionally attended these experiments as onlookers, but I always felt that they did not profit much thereby. The experience . . . suf-

ficed to make me think that something might be done with a course on animals at which the students should do their own operations, and such a course in operative surgery was started in the year 1901–02. There was, of course, nothing particularly new in this; the only novel features lay in the attempt to liken the exercise so far as possible to the actual performance of surgery as conducted on a patient in the hospital. . . The course was offered as an optional exercise for third year students and during the first year I took only two groups with two tables of five men each—only twenty men in all. R.T. Miller, Jr. and M.T. Hutchins of the class of 1903 were the first volunteer prosectors.

"The first paper, which appeared in the *Johns Hopkins Bulletin* in May 1905 while the laboratory was in course of erection, was a collection of papers by third year students: Faris, Thacker, Ortschild and Beall of the class of 1906 describing a number of pathological conditions in animals which we had encountered.

"The laboratory was ready for occupancy in the summer of 1905, and Philip K. Gilman, a graduate of that year became the first surgical assistant there. He was succeeded a year later by J.F. Ortschild, 1906, and there followed in the same position, Lewis Reford of Montreal, 1907, S.J. Crowe, 1908, Emil Goetsch, 1909, W.E. Dandy, 1910, and Conrad Jacobson, 1911.

"We finally came to depend greatly on the offices of a cadaverous little man called Jimmie, to whom a monument should be erected, for how he managed to survive the buffets from the many departments of the School that wanted animals of the right size, sex and disposition at the right moment; how he managed with hose, mop and carbolic to keep the place tolerable under the rays of a hot Baltimore sun, how he managed to keep up the supply of animals in competition with the local society that collected and electrocuted them—all this is beyond me. I can see him now, tripping down Monument Street with his buckets of garbage from the hospital kitchen, and had it not been for his extraordinary moral control over the occupants of our kennels in his charge, their vociferousness would have driven the neighbors distracted. . .

"The second 'Comparative Surgery' series was published from the Hunterian Laboratory by members of the class of 1907: F.W. Bancroft, E.S. Cross, G.W. Henry, W.D. Gatch, J.G. Hopkins, A.R. Dochez, W. von Gerber and G.J. Heuer, which appeared in the *Bulletin* for December, 1906. A year later a third series in which J.T. Geraghty, J.W. Churchman, S.J. Crowe, F.F. Gundrum, C.W. Mills, R.D. McClure, H.F. Derge, C.H. Bryant, H.M. Evans, and A.G. Brenizer, Jr. of the class of 1908 participated. This was the last of the collected comparative surgery reports, for we had begun to get more interested in experimental work as our equipment was perfected. In 1908 a paper by J.R.B. Branch, later of the Hunan-Yale Hospital, and in 1909 papers by James Bordley, Jr., by S.J. Crowe, by Lewis L. Reford, B.M. Bernheim, R.D. McClure, P.W. Harrison, and S. Griffith Davis were published together in the April *Bulletin*. Reford's paper was the first of the studies on the pituitary body which came to engross us during the next few years when Crowe, Goetsch, Dandy, and Jacobson were successively the assistants in the laboratory.... All told, it has been a useful line of investigation and has served at least to put the pituitary body on the map..." It was here that Cushing began his work with Weed on the cerebrospinal fluid which was later finished after he went to Boston. Cushing states that more credit should have been given to the Hunterian than the reprint records.

"I had hoped to keep up the traditions of the old place in the surgical laboratory here at Harvard which has been successively under the direction of Dr. John Homans and William C. Quinby, both of whom have worked in Baltimore in the old Hunterian. The Arthur Tracy Cabot fellowship here has been assigned to the assistant in charge of the laboratory and the post has been held successively by Lewis H. Weed, 1912–13, Gilbert Horrax, 1914, Samuel C. Harvey, 1915, William S. McCann, 1916 and George B. Wislocki, 1917–19; and though to my everlasting regret, I am unable to be in the laboratory as much as I used to be in Baltimore, I feel that these men are first cousins to those of you who have succeeded Gilman, Ortschild and the others in the Hunterian.

"I have said little of MacCallum's and Whipple's department, undoubtedly much more productive than our half of the house.... There were many workers from time to time, Bernheim, Stone, and Staige Davis having worked more or less continually during my last few years, as I presume they have continued to do; and Dr. Halsted always had a problem on foot and came to the laboratory frequently during its early days.

"The most gratifying tribute the laboratory received was in 1912 when Abraham Flexner, at the time the Rockefeller funds were about to be turned over to the University, recommended that $100,000 be utilized for the enlargement of the Hunterian Laboratory."

NEUROSURGERY

Interest in surgery of the brain had its origin from two directions: one proceeding from the problem presented by head injuries, particularly blood clots and fractures, and the other proceeding from the problem of brain tumors and their surgical removal. The first report of successful removal of a brain tumor was that of Francesco Durante of Rome who took out an olfactory groove tumor in May 1884.

Fulton has traced Cushing's interest in brain surgery as it developed during his period of training. In 1890 he removed a dog's brain for Professor Ladd at Yale and also dissected the cranial nerves of a frog. His lecture notes at Harvard showed a deep interest in the physiology of the nervous system, with drawings of the motor area, the nerve pathways from the eye and the decussation of the fibers of the optic chiasma. At the Massachusetts General Hospital, "Jack" Elliott (John Wheelock Elliott) first turned Cushing's attention to surgery of the brain. Elliott had met Horsley in England in 1889 and upon his return to Boston in 1890 he solicited his colleagues to refer cases of brain tumor to him. Elliott's first successful operation on an intracranial tumor was in 1895 and during that summer Cushing assisted him at two operations for brain tumors. Cushing was impressed by how often the neurologic signs made it possible to accurately localize the tumor prior to operation.

Cushing had operated on an occasional neurologic case between 1897 and 1899, but in 1900 he began to devote himself more completely to disorders of the central nervous system, writing a careful history on each case he saw. He particularly concerned himself with the surgical relief of trigeminal neuralgia, an operative procedure suggested originally by W.G. Spiller, the Philadelphia neurologist. Cushing, at the invitation of W.W. Keen, published a paper on this subject on April 28, 1900 in the *Journal of the American Medical Association* entitled "A method of extirpation of the gasserian ganglion for trigeminal neuralgia by a route through the temporal fossa and beneath the middle meningeal artery." This paper, an important landmark in the history of neurosurgery, was illustrated by Cushing's own drawings.

As a result of his interest in the gasserian ganglion, Cushing studied the sensory distribution not only of the trigeminal nerve but also those supplying the skin in other parts of the body. His analysis of the skin areas supplied by the various branches of the trigeminal nerve is a classical neuroanatomical study. Following each fifth nerve operation, Cushing plotted the sensory deficit on the face. He demonstrated that the posterior limit of skin anesthesia involved the anterior margin of the ear, including the "auricular vagus" and the anterior wall of the external ear canal. These findings he regarded as predictable from knowledge of the embryological development of the ear in relation to the other cranial nerves. He also described the disturbances in taste, recording the relation of the gasserian ganglion to the taste buds of the tongue. Cushing studied sensory distribution in patients with herpes zoster and published several papers on problems of peripheral nerve regeneration. As a result, he was asked to contribute several chapters and diagrams to the 1905 edition of Osler's *Principles and Practice of Medicine*.

In November 1904 he gave his first report on the special field of neurological surgery in an address before the Academy of Medicine at Cleveland. "I shall attempt," he said, "to formulate some personal views concerning a branch of surgery which, in this country at least, largely owing to the allurement of other and more promising fields of operative endeavor, has hardly received the attention it deserves.... Through the generosity of Dr. Halsted, his junior associates have been given in a measure the privilege of directing the work in some of the subdivisions of his large surgical clinic, in order that they may concentrate their efforts toward advancement along particular lines. It has thus fallen my lot temporarily and under his guidance, to control the group of cases which present features chiefly of neurological interest; and it is upon the present possibilities and limitations, as well as upon the future outlook for this Department of Surgery, that I shall briefly dwell tonight..." He described the physiological work of Sherrington on the motor area and stated that reports of removal of such tumors in the motor area were becoming more frequent. In a footnote, Cushing added prophetically: "It is not impossible that a diseased pituitary body may someday be successfully attacked."

Although he had attempted brain tumor removals at that time, he did not have a successful case to report and his paper was largely concerned with the technique of "palliative trepanation" (cerebral decompression). He also discussed surgery of the spinal cord and the physiological problems involved in the management of cases of spinal injury, as well as the surgery of peripheral nerves and the problem of peripheral regeneration. His family was very much amused by a local Cleveland newspaper reporting that: "Dr. Harvey W. Cushing of Baltimore addressed the Academy of Music on Nemological Surgery."

During 1906 and 1907 Cushing devoted a major effort to the preparation of a section on "Surgery of the Head" for Keen's five-volume *Surgery*. His elaborate manuscript was eventually compressed into a monograph of 276 pages and 154 illustrations which appeared in 1908. As a result of this book, neurological surgery was recognized im-

mediately as a definitive field of surgery (Figs. 7 and 8).

At first Cushing's mortality rates from operations were so high that he was often deeply discouraged. His chief contributions during the first six years were mainly technical. In addition to the use of blood pressure recordings during operations, he had developed a number of ingenious ways of diminishing hemorrhage, including a special cranial tourniquet. He improved the burrs and saws for opening the skull and devised electrodes for applying stimuli to the exposed surface of the brain. A major contribution was the groundwork he laid for gaining information on the natural history of brain tumors. He early realized that certain tumors were much more favorable for surgery than others in that they grew slowly and tended not to recur.

THE PITUITARY BODY

From 1908 to 1912 Cushing was at the peak of his active career—a period during which he devoted his efforts to the study of the normal functions and clinical disorders of the pituitary gland and the surgical treatment of its tumors. After his return to Baltimore from Sherrington's laboratory (where he had met Alfred Fröhlich), Cushing operated on a girl who entered his clinic in December 1901 complain-

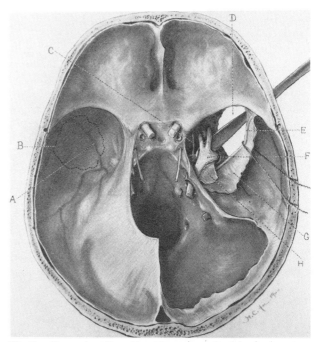

Fig 7.   Gasserian Ganglion Operation. Cushing's drawing showing the position of the Gasserian Ganglion at the base of the skull and its relationships to other structures.
From Fulton JF: Harvey Cushing, A Biography. Springfield, Ill.: Charles C Thomas, 1946.

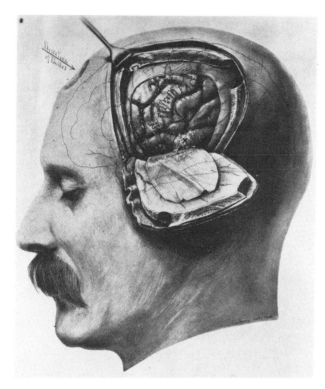

Fig 8. Motor area of the brain. Drawn by Cushing in 1906 and first printed in Keen's *Surgery*, 1908. Note that the face is that of his hero, William Osler.

From Fulton JF: Harvey Cushing. A Biography. Springfield, Ill.: Charles C Thomas, 1946.

ing of headaches and failure of vision: ". . .The patient was fat and although fourteen years of age, she had failed to mature sexually." His diagnosis was incorrect and he decompressed the brain first on one side and then on the other. The headache improved but vision continued to deteriorate. Cushing then concluded that she had a tumor in the occipital area and made a cerebellar exposure after which the patient died. At autopsy there was a large pituitary cyst which was undoubtedly a Rathke's pouch defect. Soon after this, Cushing received a reprint from Fröhlich in which he described a similar patient seen in October 1901. This was the first description of Fröhlich's syndrome. Cushing's pride was hurt by his erroneous diagnosis and from then on the pituitary became an obsessive interest. Cushing did not describe his case until November 1906 when he reported it along with a similar case under the title "Sexual infantilism with optic atrophy in cases of tumor affecting the hypophysis cerebri" (J Nerv Ment Dis 33: 704, 1906). A real dividend for neurosurgical science came from the fact that the importance of the first case was not appreciated at the time of autopsy. Several years

later Cushing requested the tissue from the Department of Pathology and found that it had disappeared. From then on he insisted that he be responsible for the pathological study of all intracranial specimens removed at surgery. Fortunately he had understanding friends such as William H. Welch and W.G. MacCallum. Later when he went to Harvard he encountered similar difficulties. His unyielding demand for the material resulted in the foundation of the Cushing Tumor Registry in which are preserved specimens of over 2,000 brain tumors that he saw during the next 30 years.

Another key event occurred in 1908 when Schaefer, in his Herter lectures, described his work on the physiology of the pituitary gland, including the discovery of the active principle of the posterior pituitary in 1898. The four lectures were entitled: "The Ductless Secreting Glands and the Doctrine of Internal Secretion"; "The Structure and Development of the Pituitary Body"; "The Physiology of the Pituitary Bodies"; and "The Pituitary Body in Disease: Its Relation to Diabetes and Acromegaly." Cushing's experimental studies on the pituitary at the old Hunterian "went into high gear" shortly after this occasion. Cushing's important advantage over Schaefer was his command of the surgical techniques essential for approaching the pituitary gland of higher animals.

In 1907 Paulesco devised a new surgical approach to the canine pituitary which permitted complete removal. His animals invariably succumbed in a state of cachexia. Later in that year Cushing and Reford repeated these experiments and reached the same conclusions. Occasionally, however, their animals merely became fat and did not die. In September 1908 John Homans, the son of Cushing's teacher at Harvard, joined in the pituitary study. In describing their work, Homan stated: ". . .He set Crowe and the rest of us to making hypophysectomized animals. It soon appeared that many of these died within a few days in a state of what was called "cachexia hypophysiopriva," of which many photographs were taken showing dogs in extraordinary attitudes. Some animals survived for many months. These animals were carefully looked after, but, on the whole, were passed by for the time being as freaks in which something had marred the completeness of the hypophysetomy. Finally, I remembered that one of these animals died; an extraordinarily fat, logy sexless creature. I made the autopsy merely noting the fact of the asexual adiposity which made no impression upon me whatever. One day Cushing caught sight of another of these animals while it was still alive, I'm quite certain, and said at once 'Here is Fröhlich's asexual adiposity.' From the fact that the animal was nearly or perhaps entirely without hypophysis, he judged that this represented a state due to hypophyseal deficiency, as opposed to acromegaly which must represent an overfunction of the gland. This latter condition was beginning to be recognized as such, but the asexual adiposity had been very confusing because this also seemed to be due to an enlargement of the hypophysis. Thus, it was Cushing's quickness and insight in connecting the hypophyseal adiposity of the dog with the Fröhlich syndrome which straightened out the confusion and made Cushing the leader in this field."

In 1909 Cushing wrote to his father as follows: "We have been working hard over the pituitary body question in the Hunterian Laboratory and have made some progress. It seems to be an important gland and one which is surgically accessible. I have had one clinical case—an acromegaly patient. It is quite extraordinary how he has improved . . .Charles Mayo sent him down to me from Rochester and the chap walked in the clinic on his sixth day after operation when our surgical club was here—as much to my astonishment as to theirs. I think it is the first case in this country though there have been a few in London by Horsley. . . ."

As a result of the work done in 1909 with Drs. Samuel J. Crowe and John Homans, an important monograph was published entitled "Experimental hypophysectomy" (Johns Hopkins Hosp Bull 21: 127, 1910). It was demonstrated that the pituitary of animals normally exerts an important influence on metabolic processes of the body. The disturbances which follow partial and complete removal of the gland were described and correlated with the symptoms of pituitary disease in man. In a paper presented to the American Medical Association in June 1909, Cushing introduced the terms hypo- and hyperpituitarism. ("The hypophysis cerebri—clinical aspects of hyperpituitarism and of hypopituitarism," JAMA 53: 249, 1909). At the time, Cushing was unaware that Marburg had used the terms hypo- and hyperpituitarism the previous year. But Marburg had made his deduction from clinical material without experimental verification. Cushing's paper was an important milestone. The summary was as follows: "Two conditions, one due to a pathologically increased activity of the pars anterior of the hypophysis (hyperpituitarism), the other to a diminished activity of the same epithelial structure (hypopituitarism), seem capable of clinical differentiation. The former expresses itself chiefly as an excessive, often a rapid, deposition of fat with persistence of infantile sexual characteristics when the process dates from youth and a tendency toward a loss of the acquired signs of adolescence when it appears in adult life.

"Experimental observations show not only

that the anterior lobe of the hypophysis is a structure of such importance that a condition of apituitarism is incompatible with the long maintenance of life, but also that its partial removal leads to symptoms comparable to those which we regard as characteristic of lessened secretion (hypopituitarism) in man. A tumor of the gland itself, or one arising in its neighbor and implicating the gland by pressure, is naturally the lesion to which one or the other of these conditions has heretofore been attributed, though it is probable that oversecretion from simple hypertrophy, or undersecretion from atrophy, will be found to occur irrespective of tumor growth when examination of the pituitary body becomes a routine measure in the postmortem examination of all cases in which the condition suggests one or the other of the symptom-complexes described. When due to tumor, surgery is the treatment that these conditions demand, and at present there are reasonably satisfactory ways of approaching the gland; but clinicians and surgeons must clearly distinguish between the local manifestations of the neoplasm due to the involvement of structures in its neighborhood other than hypophysis, and those of a general character from disturbances of metabolism due to alterations of the hypophysis itself.

"When the anterior lobe of the pituitary exhibits increased activity and enlargements in adults, the bones of the extremities become heavy, as do the viscera, since after adolescence the long bones cannot increase in length, the growing points at the ends of the bones having become fixed and incapable of further growth (acromegaly).

"If, however, cells in the anterior pituitary become excessively active before the long bones have stopped growing then they become longer and longer and a human giant may be the result. Gigantism then is a condition akin to acromegaly, but the onset occurs earlier in life."

Cushing clearly recognized that the anterior pituitary cells elaborate a secretion that influences growth, especially growth of the skeleton. Herbert M. Evans, who had been one of his students and colleagues at Johns Hopkins, later isolated and purified the growth hormone, thus reinforcing Cushing's early deductions based upon experimental studies on dogs and clinical observations in man. In Cushing's monograph on the pituitary he described several cases of gigantism. Cushing was as much interested in dwarfs as in giants, and during the summer of 1929 when his family was on summer vacation he filled the house with dwarfs in order to test the effect of the growth hormone which had been purified by Evans.

Fulton emphasized that as an investigator, Cushing had faults as well as virtues. He was wedded to the idea that posterior pituitary secretion found its way into the spinal fluid and Conrad Jacobson worked hard to find proof for this. In spite of good evidence to the contrary, Cushing never really admitted that his theory was incorrect. A succession of junior associates wasted valuable time trying to confirm Cushing's concept. Jacobson wrote as follows: "As a research man he was of the deductive type of mind. Some investigators gathered their data and tried to draw their conclusions from them. He was inclined to have a theory and then use all of his efforts and ingenuity to prove the validity of it. One of the last papers he published while he was at Hopkins was on the blood pressure-raising effect of spinal fluid. He always had the idea that pituitary gland secretion found its way into the spinal fluid. For several years every spinal fluid that was taken in his clinic or operating room in any amount was sent to me for kymograph tracings and many a Saturday afternoon was spent in the laboratory with Dr. Cushing on this problem looking intently for something to bear out his theory. He would be quite elated when with a little added force in injecting the fluid, there would be an increased blood pressure effect and rather crestfallen when the identical result would be obtained by the artificial spinal fluid . . . .Cushing's interpretation of certain facts which were produced experimentally under his direction undoubtedly has been rather too enthusiastic and has been and will be questioned. When he was reminded of these facts by some of his contemporaries, he usually remarked, 'I never expected to settle these things; I have set others thinking about them and this is the main purpose after all.' . . .One feels that Cushing's greatness in the research line is due more to his interpretation of clinical findings from his operative cases than to the experimental work on animals."

By 1911 the neurosurgical service had become extremely busy and Cushing's assistant had to work hard to keep up with him. Conrad Jacobson has described this period: "While Dr. Cushing was in charge of Neurosurgery at the Johns Hopkins Hospital the service was conducted by himself and an assistant known throughout the hospital as 'Cushing's man.' This individual was selected from the graduating class. While several men were considered for the position, it was given to the one who possessed what was spoken of as 'Geist.' This expression was a favorite one of the 'Chief.' Such an individual was supposed to have some tendency toward research work, some special ability to work alone and to possess the usual qualifications of a good medical student. The choice was not one limited to scholarship but rather to personal fitness. This man had charge of the Hunterian Laboratory of Surgical

Research for a year. During this year he was a free lance devoting himself mainly to research work and occasionally brought into contact with the hospital, if his research work was in any way related to the clinical aspects of the patients. It was understood, however, that the research work undertaken should be along neurological lines, both he and Dr. Cushing collaborating in the articles published. After spending a year in the Hunterian Laboratory, he was given the hospital year on Cushing's service. The hospital year was a particularly hard one. At this time, every little detail regarding the patient, concerning the various special examinations and pertaining to new and exacting operations was a personal affair with Dr. Cushing. He was an extremely hard taskmaster and drove his men incessantly, almost to the point of exhaustion. He was an indefatigable worker and expected the same of his assistant. 'Cushing's man' was looked upon by the rest of the hospital staff with considerable sympathy for what was ahead of him, as well as respect for the honor associated with this position . . .Cushing's selections of the first few assistants were, on the whole, harmonious. It soon became evident that 'Geist' not only concerned the innate ability of the assistant for work but also concerned a temperament which could meet or put up with the demands of a most exacting taskmaster."

Walter Dandy was selected from the class of 1910 to be Cushing's assistant (Fig 9). While in the Hunterian, he became interested in the problem of absorption from the pleural cavity. This was not a neurological problem so it led to a conflict of personalities and may have contributed to the beginning of the antagonism which existed between the two men. Fox has published the most extensive analysis of this famous controversy. Dandy recalled (1945) that he and Cushing first battled over some experiments on the relation of the sympathetic nervous system to glycosuria. Dandy had obtained results contrary to those that were expected and those about to be reported by Cushing with Weed and Jacobson (Johns Hopkins Hosp Bull 24: 50, 1913). He told Cushing that in stimulating the central end of the sympathetics, a "tremendous glycosuria" had resulted. Cushing was elated and rushed out to relay the news to Emil Goetsch who had been Cushing's appointee the preceding year. Dandy then felt compelled to add that when he stimulated the central end of the cut sympathetics, he obtained the same results. Cushing replied in an irritated manner, "Dandy, nobody could think of such a thing as that but you. . ." "I told him," said Dandy, "I was only trying to check the results." At the end of that year when Cushing was preparing to leave for Boston, another incident arose which served further to fire the flames of antagonism. Dandy relates that Cushing came to the Hunterian Laboratory to see his (Dandy's) results in his experiments on hydrocephalus. "I showed them to him," Dandy said in a letter to John Fulton, "and he put them in his box of materials from the Hunterian. I took them out and told him they were going to stay there as they were mine and he had nothing to do with them. He flared up, quickly calmed down and said he guessed they did not amount to anything anyhow." By this time Cushing had told Dandy that he was not taking him to Boston. This was a deep disappointment to Dandy according to Sam Crowe, not because Cushing had changed his mind, but because the lateness of his change had deprived Dandy of his position on Halsted's staff. Halsted subsequently found him a place on his surgical staff having meanwhile been greatly impressed with the importance of the work that Dandy and Blackfan, the resident in pediatrics, had done on hydrocephalus.

In view of the antagonism between the two men, many felt that it was not surprising that Cushing was reluctant to adopt ventriculography for many years. In a letter written to Dandy in the spring of 1922 Cushing remarked: "I was glad that you brought up the ventriculography (sic) matter before the neurological association, and hope that you

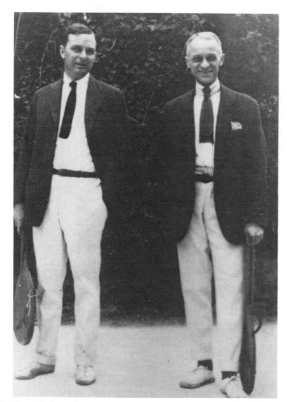

Fig 9. Walter Dandy and Harvey Cushing.
From the Archives Office, Johns Hopkins Medical Institutions.

don't feel that we were too critical. It has been an important contribution, but you must be very careful not to overdo it, lest you make people expect too much of it, for under these circumstances, it is likely to get a black eye." Others have observed that Cushing, although conservative, should have at once visualized the possibilities of this new diagnostic aid, but as they point out, it was introduced by his old assistant at the Hunterian, Walter E. Dandy, which likely had something to do with Cushing's reluctance to adopt this new technique immediately. One of the "reasons beneath the surface," it has been suggested, was the older man's jealously of his younger trainee's superb accomplishment.

Fox describes how in September 1922 the final episode of the Cushing–Dandy controversy took place. Dandy had recently published in the *Johns Hopkins Hospital Bulletin* a note entitled "An operation for the total extirpation of tumors of the acoustic nerve." This apparently irritated Cushing immensely, who apparently believed that Dandy desired the credit for an operative approach which the older neurosurgeon had described previously. Cushing sat down and wrote a letter to Dr. Winford H. Smith, the director of the Johns Hopkins Hospital at that time, which he later decided to send directly to Dandy instead. This letter read as follows:

"My dear Smithie:
I assume that you are editor of the *Bulletin*, but if not, you will know to whom this letter should be referred. I have been very much disturbed by seeing an article by Dandy in the last issue which, in the shape of a preliminary report, consists of nothing more than a promise, so far as I can see, that he is going to describe in the future an operation for a certain kind of brain tumor. It is exceedingly bad for me, inasmuch as many people know that I had something to do with Dr. Dandy's training; it is equally bad for Dr. Dandy himself, inasmuch as general professional esteem is concerned; but what affects all of us still more is that it is very bad for the Hopkins to have the *Bulletin* accept and permit the title of such an incomplete and promissory article to get into the literature. . . ."

Cushing then sent this letter directly to Dandy with the following additional note written in long hand enclosed:

"Dear Dandy,
I have cogitated over this letter a good deal. I think I will send it to you instead of to Dr. Smith. Perhaps you will wish to show it to him and get his advice. After all, it is as important to you as it is for me that you stand in a high plane of professional ethics.
I think you are doing yourself a great deal of

harm by the tone of some of your publications. You are an independent thinker and worker, and that is not a bad thing. But you must not forget your manners, and this last note of yours is in extremely bad taste.

Always your friend,
Harvey Cushing"

As Fox points out, Dandy was greatly offended by this attack, believing that he was completely justified in making his preliminary report on the total extirpation of acoustic tumors using the Cushing approach, and that it was not required of him to cite the literature which would be done when the final and definitive paper was published. Dandy submitted Cushing's letter to the Board of Editors of the *Bulletin* and in an accompanying note said that he was "absolutely at a loss to discover the point for such a letter other than personal animus." He went on to say that the only reason he submitted the preliminary note was "to establish priority for a procedure which is directed toward the total enucleation of these tumors." Dandy pointed out that neither Cushing nor others had published up until that time any procedure for the safe total extirpation of acoustic tumors.

Subsequently a penned letter to Dandy written by Cushing was found in the Cushing papers in the Yale Library of Medicine—a letter which was never mailed. In it, he said: "Everyone knows that you were once a pupil of mine, and though most of them know that you have far surpassed your teacher, there are at the same time certain amenities which most of us try to observe."

Dandy apparently never forgave Cushing for these various episodes, although the two men in the many years that followed maintained outwardly a gentlemanly attitude toward each other. Dandy, in a note written to Fulton (Cushing's biographer) on November 26, 1945 concerning his relationships with his mentor, said the following of Cushing: "I think he realized his unfairness in later life and in some slight way tried to make amends, to which I did not at all reciprocate. You can use your own judgment about publishing this. You have my permission to do so, but I do not think anything would be gained and I think it would be better left out. Cushing certainly was not a big man; he was a selfish one and certainly not the type who wished his pupils to excel, and I have never felt that his scientific contributions were trustworthy." However, in an earlier paragraph in this same letter, Dandy expressed his debt to Cushing: "He gave me my start in neurosurgery and I, of course, owe a great debt to him for that. He certainly was far and away above all others in neurosurgery at that time and it was par-

ticularly fortunate for me to be associated with the master." Fox contends that Cushing was obviously the antagonist in this difficult controversy. He concludes that Cushing had an insatiable ambition to be tops in his field and that perhaps he unconsciously felt threatened by one with Dandy's ability. On the other hand, he notes that Dandy, like Cushing, was also a perfectionist and was equally demanding.

Cushing's sixteen years in Baltimore ended with the publication of his classical monograph entitled "The Pituitary Body and Its Disorders," which bore the subtitle, "Clinical States Produced by Disorders of the Hypophysis Cerebri." This monograph is a landmark in the history of endocrinology, for it introduced a clinical concept of endocrine function which served to synthesize the growing body of knowledge. In cases of acromegaly, it revealed a preponderance of cells that stained with eosin, leading him to conclude that these cells produced the growth hormone and that the basophilic cells probably elaborate some other essential secretion. This prediction illustrates his extraordinary clinical acumen. He had to wait 20 years before his ideas crystallized sufficiently to allow him to recognize the syndrome that now bears his name.

CUSHING'S SYNDROME

Perhaps Cushing's most original contribution to clinical research came in his 63rd year when he was about ready to retire—his description of an entirely new disease entity. Among the patients seen by Cushing over the years there was a small group with a condition which had been vaguely referred to as "polyglandular syndrome." Patients in this group rarely came to operation since they did not show visual impairment or signs of increased intracranial pressure. As he had not had the opportunity to examine any of these patients at autopsy, his suspicions as to the nature of this disease could not be clearly established. Cushing tells how his interest in this subject was crystallized, leading to the description of this syndrome: "The next came in a report made from Professor Biedl's clinic in Prague in 1924 by Dr. William Raab on the general topic of hypophysial and cerebral adiposity, or what is commonly called adiposo-genital dystrophy. The subject was approached largely from its roentgenological aspects, and it was a mere chance that in 1930 when preparing for my Lister lecture I happened to hit upon the fact in reading this paper that in one of the patients (Case 2) a basophil adenoma had been disclosed at autopsy. The photographs of the patient were so striking and bore such a close resemblance to the appearance of a patient at the time under observation in my own wards that I felt little doubt that they had been afflicted in all certainty with the same disorder." Cushing described his case in detail, and as the patient responded favorably to x ray, he returned home without operation. He was examined frequently and died in 1935 several years after Cushing's paper on the new disease was published. Cushing did not learn of his death until three days after the funeral but he persuaded the family to have the body exhumed, and a well-circumscribed basophilic adenoma was found.

Following the clue provided by the Raab case, Cushing was further stimulated by H.M. Teel's report of a basophilic tumor in 1931 entitled "Basophilic adenoma of the hypophysis with associated pluriglandular syndrome (Arch Neurol Psych 26: 593, 1931) and his enthusiasm became unrestrained. As indicated at the time of Cushing's original paper on basophilism, none of his own cases had come to autopsy. However, soon three patients were autopsied and all had basophilic adenomas. Cushing first reported the syndrome associated with the basophil tumors before the New York Neurological Society on January 5, 1932. He presented the same material at the Harvard Medical School Society on January 20, and then as an Alpha Omega Alpha lecture at Yale on February 24. These first three accounts of basophilism were preliminary talks for his official presentation given before the Johns Hopkins Medical Society on February 29. The full text appeared in the March issue of the *Johns Hopkins Hopkins Bulletin*: "The basophil adenomas of the pituitary body and their clinical manifestations (pituitary basophilism)." It is remarkable that Cushing from clinical observations alone was able to deduce a whole new concept in endocrinology, i.e., that of a master gland, the pituitary, which influenced the level of function of other endocrine glands such as the thyroid, the gonads, and the adrenals.

While a second year student in medicine, I attended that meeting of the Johns Hopkins Medical Society and heard Dr. Cushing present the description of his new syndrome. He did this in beautiful fashion but pronounced the word syndrome incorrectly. After his presentation was finished, Dr. William H. Welch, who had sat listening intently in the first row, took the podium. Welch then proceeded for the next forty minutes to trace the derivation of the word syndrome and to politely inform Dr. Cushing that the accent should be on the first syllable. Dr. Welch did this in such a fascinating manner that I could not recall the major manifestations of Cushing's syndrome after that evening, although I could remember all of Dr. Welch's delightful remarks. I had to wait for the *Bulletin* the following month to learn the manifestations of Cushing's syndrome. The day after his lecture I saw Dr. Cushing walking down the hall with Dean Lewis, who was then the Professor of Surgery. I noticed that they would walk only a few steps and then Dr. Cushing would stop and look out the large windows along the corridors of the hospital into the courtyard. He would continue to talk and after one to two minutes of standing proceed down the hall only to stop shortly at another window. When I reached my course entitled "Introduction to Clinical Medicine" later in the year, I was able to make the diagnosis—severe intermittent claudication (Fig 10).

In 1926 Cushing, in memory of his old love the Hunterian Laboratory, made an anonymous gift of $25,000 to establish a fellowship for surgical research in that laboratory. He announced this in a letter of March 27 to President Goodnow: "As our contribution to the Johns Hopkins Endowment Fund, Mrs. Cushing and I wish to give the University the sum of $25,000, the income of which we would like to have used to provide a salary for the fellow in charge of the Hunterian Laboratory at the medical school. The reasons for wishing to establish this fellowship are purely sentimental ones. I feel under great obligation to the University for having permitted me, some 20 and more years ago together with Dr. W.G. MacCallum, to organize the original Hunterian Laboratory in which I subsequently passed some most happy and profitable years. During that period, I was permitted to appoint each year a recent graduate into whose hands the general supervision of the laboratory was put. . . . It is my desire that the selection of the incumbent for this proposed Hunterian Fellowship should be in the hands of the Professor of Surgery at the Johns Hopkins, or of the senior Professor of Surgery, should the department ever grow to be of such a size that it comes to be under two heads . . . May I request further that the names of the donors not be made public, at least until I shall have retired from my present academic post." Dr. Lewis H. Weed wrote in reply: "Under Dean Lewis and Ferdinand Lee the Hunterian is coming back into its own. There is tremendous activity in the old building and it calls to my mind the type of work carried out when I was there with you. I miss, however, in that laboratory only one thing: there is no longer the group of happy people around Joe seated at a microtome."

A most revealing analysis of Cushing is that made by a surgeon who worked under him as a student and surgeon-in-training. These were remarks made by Dr. P.W. Harrison in a letter to his son, written after reading Fulton's "Life of Cushing": "There are things to be learned and imitated and there are things in it to be learned so they can be avoided. He was a very remarkable man, I imagine the greatest surgeon America's likely to produce for a

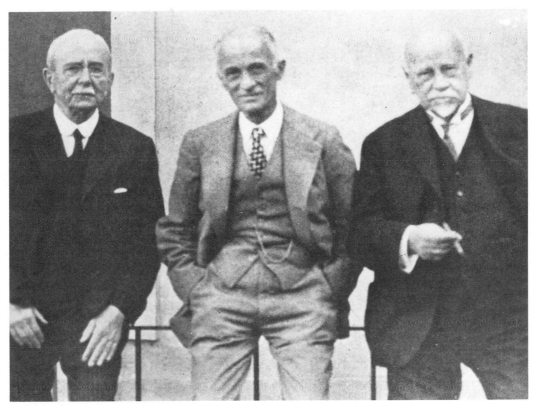

Fig 10.   Sir Charles Sherrington, Harvey Cushing and William H. Welch, 1931.
From Fulton JF: Harvey Cushing, A Biography. Springfield, Ill.: Charles C Thomas, 1946.

long time. He was three things, and three not often combined in one person. He was a genuine scientist, with a real love for truth in and of itself. Not many doctors in actual practice are that. I think that the greatest thrill that he got in his life or nearly the greatest at least, was the fact that he had discovered a new little piece of truth. In the second place he was a technician of the grade that not a half a dozen men in a generation could equal, taking the world as your field of search. But he was far more than a mere technician; in that he was an unusual artist which is not the same thing. The pure beauty of an operative procedure or result meant a great deal to him. Cushing was not a first-string scientist, but his technical equipment was so incredible that with it he was able to carry out investigations that were unreachable by the first-stringers nearly always as they are, third-grade technicians. And finally as developed in his life later he was a really first-class writer. His life of Osler I think is a permanent piece of work. . .

"In the field of human relations he did not do well. His patients he treated very well, indeed, and there was no difference between the rich and poor, but he left no community behind him to mourn his passing as some of the other giants of those days, e.g.,

Finney. His professional colleagues meant very little to him. You will wonder as you read his life how he could have been such a worshipper of Osler and not try to follow that great teacher along this line. About the community as a whole, he knew little and as the phrase of my own childhood put it, cared less. His assistants though, those who stayed with him for any length of time, came to be great admirers of his and to think very much of him. I was one of them, and am still. He had lots of charm, and ability and could be fascinating when he was in the mood."

"The devotion that he brought to this ideal of neurological surgery, 20% scientific, 75% artistry, 5% community benefit burned like a high-pressure blowtorch till he lay down and died, at the age of 70. The devotion of an artist has to be a self-centered thing, I guess, and every assistant that comes along is sucked into this vortex. Cushing's critics, even in my day, called him utterly selfish, and in one sense he was. But his assistants got a lot of valuable training from being his assistants and most of them went out with his blessing, but he was pretty anxious to stay at the top; and when Dandy rather took that place away from him, his appreciation of Dandy evaporated.

"Late in life as he got older, Cushing developed a taste for applause, especially the applause of foreign audiences; that was a very great surprise to me, who knew him only in his very early days. His weakness for foreign praise with its aristocratic trappings, scientific and political both, came strongly to the front, and doubtless was the price he paid for getting old. . .

"But I think that the reason that the less desirable aspects of Cushing's life tend to be emphasized more as he grew older was that he seems to have been a complete stranger to religion. We all of us start with a lot of selfishness in our souls, but if we give God a steady chance at our hearts, we grow to put at least our families ahead of our selfishness, and eventually some of our companions, and assistants, and to take a genuine interest in the community. I do not know whether or not you ever heard of Dr. J.M.T. Finney referred to in Baltimore. There was a man who worked all of his life to develop the personal and community side of surgery as Cushing did to develop its scientific and technical side. I think perhaps that in adjusting surgery to the world that we are entering now J.M.T. made just as great a contribution as Cushing did . . . Well, that will do as a review of Harvey Cushing. He will stand for a long time as a sort of tremendous example of what can be done, and perhaps of the dangers of that way of doing it."

In commenting on Cushing's character and personality, Dr. Franklin S. Newell, who had served under Cushing at the Massachusetts General Hospital and later became professor of obstetrics at Harvard Medical School, stated: He was recognized as perhaps the ablest man in his class at the medical school and was an extremely hard worker. As house officer I was his junior and suffered severely in that position for a year. He was an extremely hard man to work with, whether one was over him or under him, as his tremendous ambition for success made it impossible for him to allow anyone else to get any credit for work done. As you know, when he wanted to be, he was one of the most charming people in the world, but working with him, I found that he couldn't tolerate anyone else in the limelight."

Ted Scarff has contributed a story which shows another side of Cushing's character: "This story was told to me by Dr. William MacCallum, the great and beloved Professor of Pathology at Johns Hopkins, and one of Dr. Cushing's close friends, at a small dinner for Dr. MacCallum in New York. When Dr. Cushing and Dr. MacCallum were young medical men they had enjoyed a good holiday together in Paris and talked over their plans and hopes for the future. At that time they said: 'Let's meet in Paris ten years from now and talk things over.' And they agreed that they should meet on the 4th of July at high noon on the top of the Eiffel Tower. For ten years neither man ever mentioned the pact. But on the appointed day, Dr. MacCallum happened to be in Paris and thought it would be great fun to pay a quick visit to the Eiffel Tower and then, on his return to the states, to gently reproach his old friend for having failed to keep their ten-year engagement. So he went to the Eiffel Tower a little before noon and took the elevator as high as it would go, to the top station where there was an observation deck and promenade. He spent 15 or 20 minutes there walking around and looking out over Paris and enjoying the exhilarating sight. Then feeling he had made his point and would have some fun chiding Dr. Cushing when he next saw him, he started to leave. Some deep instinct, however, compelled him at this point to ask the guard if this was 'the top' of the Tower. The guard said 'Well, yes, for all practical purposes; there is a rickety iron staircase that goes up about a hundred steps to a small lookout but visitors rarely go up there.' Dr. MacCallum's instinct stayed strong, and he decided to go on up to the top. Just as he got his head above the floor he heard a familiar voice say, 'Well, Willy, I had almost despaired of your getting here.' It was, of course, Dr. Cushing."

ACKNOWLEDGEMENTS

I am indebted to Carol Bocchini for her editorial assistance.

REFERENCES

1. Bancroft FW et al.: Comparative Surgery. Second series of reports. Johns Hopkins Hosp Bull 17: 369, 1906

2. Brown HA: The Harvey Cushing Society: Past, present and future. J Neurosurg 15: 587, 1958

3. Bucher HK: The first anesthesia records (Codman, Cushing). Surg Gynec Obstet 71: 689, 1940

4. Crile G: Blood Pressure in Surgery. Philadelphia: Lippincott, 1903

5. Cushing H: Haematomyelia from gunshot wounds of the spine. A report of two cases, with recovery following symptoms of hemilesion of the cord. Amer J Med Sci 15: 654, 1898

6. Cushing H: Cocaine anesthesia in the treatment of certain cases of hernia and in operations for thyroid tumors. Johns Hopkins Hosp Bull 9: 192, 1898

7. Cushing H: Laparectomy for intestinal perforation in typhoid fever. A report of four cases with a discussion of the diagnostic signs of perforation. Johns Hopkins Hosp Bull 9: 257, 1898

8. Cushing H: A method of extirpation of the gasserian ganglion for trigeminal neuralgia by a route through the temporal fossa and beneath the middle meningeal artery. JAMA 34: 1035, 1900

9. Cushing H: Concerning the poisonous effect of pure sodium chloride solutions on the nerve-muscle preparations. Amer J Physiol 6: 77, 1901

10. Cushing H: On the avoidance of shock in major

amputations by cocainization of larynx nerve trunks preliminary to their division with observations on blood pressure changes in surgical cases. Ann Surg 36: 321, 1902

11. Cushing H: On routine determinations of arterial tension in operating room and clinic. Bost Med Surg J 148: 250, 1903

12. Cushing H: The sensory distribution of the fifth nerve. Johns Hopkins Hosp Bull 15: 213, 1904

13. Cushing H: The special field of neurological surgery. Cleveland Med J 4: 1, 1905

14. Cushing H: Comparative surgery with illustrative cases. Johns Hopkins Hosp Bull 16: 179, 1905

15. Cushing H: Instruction in operative medicine, with the description of a course in the Hunterian Laboratory of Experimental Medicine. Johns Hopkins Hosp Bull 17: 124, 1906

16. Cushing H: Sexual infantilism with optic atrophy in cases of tumor affecting the hypophysis cerebri. J Nerv Mental Dis 33: 704, 1906

17. Cushing H: The hypophysis cerebri: Clinical aspects of hyperpituitarism and hypopituitarism. JAMA 53: 249, 1909

18. Cushing H: Partial hypophysectomy for acromegaly with remarks on the function of the hypophysis. Ann Surg 50: 1002, 1909

19. Cushing H: The basophil adenomas of the pituitary body and their clinical manifestations (pituitary basophilism). Johns Hopkins Hosp Bull 50: 137, 1932

20. Cushing H and Branch JRB: Experimental and clinical notes on chronic valvular lesions in the dog and their possible relation to a future surgery of the cardiac valve. J Med Research 17: 471, 1908

21. Cushing H and Goetsch E: Concerning the secretion of the infundibular lobe of the pituitary body and its presence in the cerebrospinal fluid. Amer J Physiol 27: 60, 1910

22. Cushing H, Crowe SJ, and Homans J: Experimental hypophysectomy. Johns Hopkins Hosp Bull 21: 127, 1910

23. Cushing H and Eisenhardt L: Notes on the first reasonably successful removal of an intracranial tumor. Bull LA Neurol Society 3: 95, 1938

24. Fox WL: The Cushing–Dandy controversy. Surg Neurol 3: 61, 1975

25. Fulton JF: Harvey Cushing, A Biography. Springfield, Ill.; Charles C Thomas, 1946. (Extensive use has been made of this excellent biography in the preparation of this essay.)

26. Harrison PW: Letter written to his son, the late Dr. Clinton Harrison, after reading Fulton's biography of Cushing.

27. Heyl HL (Ed.): A selection of Harvey Cushing anecdotes. J Neurosurg 30: 365, 1969

28. Holman E: Sir William Osler, William Stewart Halsted, Harvey Cushing: Some personal reminiscences. Surgery 57: 589, 1965

29. Moore FD: Harvey Cushing, general surgeon, biologist, professor. J Neurosurg 31: 262, 1969

30. Osler W: The Principles and Practice of Medicine (Ed. VI) New York and London: D. Appleton and Company, 1905. Section X: Diseases of the Nervous System. (H. C. did some of the illustrations).

31. Reford LL and Cushing H: Is the pituitary gland essential to the maintenance of life? Johns Hopkins Hosp Bull 20: 105, 1909

32. Viets HA: Notes on the Formative Period of a Neurological Surgeon. Harvey Cushing's Seventieth Birthday Party, Springfield, Ill.: Charles C Thomas, p. 118, 1939

7.

Halsted's Innovative Ventures in the Surgical Specialties: Samuel J. Crowe and the Development of Otolaryngology at Johns Hopkins

THE EARLY PERIOD (1889–1912)

The Outpatient Department of the Johns Hopkins Hospital was organized in 1889 with William S. Halsted as chief of the dispensary. Its divisions were: (1) Department of General Medicine, William Osler; (2) Department of Diseases of Children, William Osler and W. D. Booker; (3) Department of Nervous Diseases, William Osler and H. M. Thomas; (4) Department of General Surgery, W. S. Halsted, assisted by J. M. T. Finney; (5) Department of Genitourinary Diseases, W. S. Halsted and James Brown; (6) Department of Gynecology, H. A. Kelly, assisted by Hunter Robb; (7) Department of Ophthalmology and Otology, S. Theobald and R. L. Randolph; (8) Department of Laryngology, John N. Mackenzie; (9) Department of Dermatology, R. B. Morison.

From the outset, the hospital relied heavily upon a group of private practitioners in Baltimore for the conduct of the outpatient department. Many of these men had obtained their special training abroad, as was the custom in those days. Dr. Samuel Theobald, who was initially in charge of the Outpatient Department of Ophthalmology and Otology, was born in Baltimore on November 12, 1846. He received his M.D. degree from the University of Maryland in 1867 and subsequently studied in Vienna and London in preparation for the practice of his specialty. He was appointed clinical professor of ophthalmology and otology in the Johns Hopkins University in 1896 and remained in charge of ophthalmology, which was organized as a sub-department of surgery, until 1925, when he retired. He was a founder of the Baltimore Eye, Ear and Throat Charity Hospital and served as ophthalmic and aural surgeon to that institution. He died September 20, 1930.

Reprinted from the *Johns Hopkins Medical Journal* **140:** 101, 1977.

Dr. Robert L. Randolph, Theobald's associate in the Department of Ophthalmology and Otology, was born in Baltimore on December 1, 1861. He was also a graduate of the University of Maryland (M.D., 1884). He had taken the preliminary medical course in the Johns Hopkins University in 1881–82 as a non-matriculated student, and later took courses in pathology under Dr. Welch. After medical school graduation, he went to Vienna (1886) to study ophthalmology and was for a time assistant in ophthalmology in the polyclinic in that city. He was appointed associate in ophthalmology and otology at Johns Hopkins University in 1896, and at the time of his death, December 11, 1919, was associate professor of clinical ophthalmology and otology. He carried a heavy share of the instruction in ophthalmology during his connection with the university and hospital and was a very effective teacher.

Dr. John N. Mackenzie, who had charge of the Outpatient Department of Laryngology, was born in Baltimore on October 20, 1853. He received his M.D. at the University of Virginia in 1876. He also studied at the Universities of Vienna and Munich and later was chief of clinic under Dr. Morell Mackenzie at the Hospital for Diseases of the Throat and Chest in Golden Square, London. He was clinical professor of diseases of the throat and nose at the University of Maryland from 1888 to 1897 and was president of the American Laryngological Association in 1889. In 1896 he was appointed clinical professor of laryngology at the Johns Hopkins University and remained at that post until 1912. He died on May 21, 1925.

According to the first announcement issued by the hospital regarding postgraduate education, courses were to be offered in the following subjects: pathology (Drs. Welch and Councilman) ... laryngology (Dr. Mackenzie) ... ophthalmology and otology (Drs. Theobald and Randolph). All of these courses consisted of lectures, demonstrations and practical work. They were repeated for several years and were well attended. Later on, when the school of medicine was opened and the wards had to be made available to the undergraduate students, it was necessary to curtail and finally to abandon for a time this type of instruction, which had proved so successful in the first years of the hospital's existence.

This arrangement for the practice and teaching of otology and laryngology, which continued until 1912, was unsatisfactory to the doctors, to the patients and to the students as well. The quarters were overcrowded and poorly equipped. No public ward beds were assigned to these departments. Many of the patients were operated on in the chair or in the room in which they were examined. Some of these operations were performed under local anesthesia, but many patients were given ether and then sent home. All nose, throat, ear and larynx cases admitted to the hospital were operated on by Dr. Finney, Dr. Bloodgood or the resident surgeon. Thus, the men Halsted invited to take charge of the ear, nose and throat clinics in 1889 served for 23 years without being permitted to operate on the patients they sent into the hospital, or receiving a salary or compensation of any kind.

SAMUEL J. CROWE ASSUMES COMMAND

A rare blending of learning and humanity, incisiveness of intellect and sensitiveness of spirit which occasionally come together in an individual who chooses the calling of medicine—and then we have the great physician (or surgeon).

Hans Zinsser (1930)

In 1912 Halsted asked Samuel J. Crowe (Fig. 1) to remain in Baltimore and to organize a university department of laryngology and otology, rather than go to Boston with Harvey Cushing as he had planned. Crowe protested that he knew nothing about this specialty, that he had never seen a tonsillectomy or a mastoid operation and that his ambition was to become a good neurosurgeon. Halsted replied that surgery of the upper air passages and lungs could be combined in one department and felt that such a plan could be successfully launched at Johns Hopkins. Crowe departed in a "bewildered state." The next day he received a note from Dr. Welch asking him to come to his office that afternoon. When Crowe arrived, Welch was very cordial and said that Halsted had asked him to talk to him about the proposed appointment; he strongly advised Crowe to accept it. Welch said nothing about the specialty which was the subject of discussion but stressed that Halsted considered every appointment with great care, and an invitation to become a member of his surgical staff should not be lightly refused. Crowe left Welch's office "a potential otolaryngologist." Who was

Samuel James Crowe in whom Halsted had so much confidence?

Crowe's father was born on a farm in Washington County, Virginia. He received his medical education at the College of Physicians and Surgeons in New York and interned at Bellevue where he attended Welch's lectures. Although he never knew Welch or Halsted, he was greatly impressed with the "new medicine" that these men had brought from Europe and were teaching in New York. The elder Crowe returned to Virginia and for a time did country practice on horseback. After his wife's death he moved to Atlanta in 1884. The South was impoverished at that time and he had to work very hard. Crowe remembered his father as "always tired, pale and thin," and he never knew him to take a vacation. As a result, medicine, to young Crowe, seemed the most undesirable profession. Crowe attended the University of Georgia where the professor of physics encouraged him to pursue a career in electrical engineering. However, his father's one idea was that he should study medicine, return to Atlanta and gradually take over his practice. Although Crowe never discussed his distaste for this idea with his father, he did take the courses that would enable him to enter a technical school and only the biology and premedical work required for a B.A. degree. Shortly after graduation, his father told him of the new Johns Hopkins School of Medicine and urged him to go to Baltimore where he would come under the influence of Welch, Osler and Halsted. He could not refuse, and entered the Johns Hopkins School of

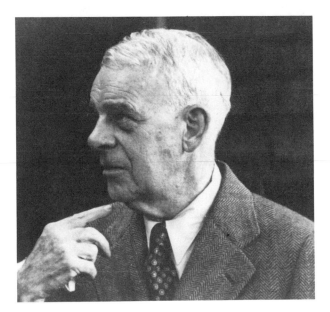

Fig 1.   Samuel J. Crowe

Medicine in 1904 much against his will and with no real interest in medicine.

During the summer after his first year of medical school, he and two of his friends took a camping trip in the North Carolina mountains. After an unusually cold and rainy night one of the horses was found with head hanging, legs far apart and stiff in every joint. Crowe did not know what to do about his dilemma and set off to find help. After an hour or more of walking, he came to a side road and saw a cabin in the distance. He found an elderly man sitting on the porch smoking a corncob pipe who told him after much questioning (he was most likely suspected of being a revenue agent on a hunt for illicit stills) about a friendly "Doc Halsted" who lived only two miles up the road, who also came from Baltimore, and whose barn was the only one in those mountains large enough for a horse of the size that Crowe had with him. Crowe's knock on the door of Halsted's home was answered by a maid in a white uniform and cap. Crowe was quite embarrassed as he looked at that point more like a tramp than a medical student. About an hour later Halsted appeared in spotless white flannels, a silk shirt, and patent leather pumps. Instead of sending his stable man with Crowe he had his buggy brought around and drove down to see the sick horse. He could not have been more polite and helpful to this medical student in dire distress. In spite of the muddy road, Halsted got out of the buggy and for fully twenty minutes palpated every joint and muscle of the horse. After this close examination, Halsted, who had become intensely interested in the problem, finally said that he thought the horse had muscular rheumatism and not hip disease. The horse was hitched to the back of the buggy, and they slowly returned to Halsted's barn. There the advised method of treatment with Sloan's liniment followed by bandaging the horse from head to foot with oil cloth was carried out. Within a few days, the horse fully recovered and Crowe went on his way. However, he stayed at High Hampton during the week of the horse's convalescence, struck up a friendship with Halsted, and discussed his career in medicine with him. Crowe soon learned of Halsted's philosophy that medicine is a living, growing, constantly changing and rewarding profession. The doctor, Halsted said, must know how to diagnose and treat the sick. He must also try to find, by laboratory work and research, new ways to reduce the number of cripples from disease who constantly flow into the hospital. That chance meeting in the mountains with Halsted changed Crowe's entire life. He acquired a new concept of medicine and returned to school a few weeks later with great enthusiasm.

During his second year in medical school,

Crowe spent the evenings and holidays working in the anatomical laboratory with a classmate, Herbert Evans. They injected dyes of various kinds into the ear veins of rabbits and later made frozen sections of the various organs in an effort to learn something of the physiological activities of the ductless glands. In the third year, while listening to Dr. Barker's discourse on the etiology of gallstones, it occurred to Crowe that it might be beneficial for acute as well as for chronic biliary tract infections to determine whether or not hexamethylenamine (urotropin) was excreted in the bile. While working in Dr. Hugh Young's urological dispensary, Crowe had seen this drug used as an antiseptic for the genitourinary tract. Two days later Crowe presented the problem to Professor Abel in the Department of Pharmacology. They searched the literature and found that no report had ever been published on the excretion of the drug in the bile, pancreatic juice or cerebrospinal fluid. This led to a series of experiments in which it was found that the drug is excreted in the bile and cerebrospinal fluid; the drug was later used in the hospital to "prevent" meningeal infections in patients with compound fractures of the skull. This work in the pharmacology laboratory led to a close friendship between Crowe and that inspiring scientist, Professor John Jacob Abel.

Also in his third year, Crowe came to know another stimulating investigator, Harvey Cushing, with whom he worked for the next five years. In 1907 he took Cushing's course in operative surgery in the Hunterian Laboratory. At the conclusion of the course, Crowe, Roy D. McClure, Herbert M. Evans, and five other classmates were asked by Cushing to undertake a special investigation during their free time for the remainder of the year. Cushing assigned a topic to each of them; Crowe's assignment was to study the parasites of Baltimore dogs. All of the students invited by Cushing to participate in this third series of studies from the Hunterian Laboratory of Experimental Surgery and Medicine distinguished themselves by their originality, enthusiasm and willingness to do work not required in the curriculum of the medical school. Cushing, like Halsted, was always on the lookout for such men.

During 1908–09 Crowe worked on experimental hypophysectomy (Fig. 2) with Dr. John Homans. This work, under the supervision of Dr. Cushing, led to the production in the dog of a syndrome similar to Fröhlich's asexual adiposity. In the following year Crowe assisted Cushing in operations on acromegalics; a preliminary tracheostomy was done in order to provide adequate breathing space for the smooth administration of ether. The tongues of these patients were enormous, necessitating the tracheostomy which Cushing vainly looked for some means to avoid. In early 1910 Crowe chanced to see in the catalog of a Chicago instrument maker the cut of a mouth gag with a tongue depressor attached. He sent for one of these instruments, and Cushing's anesthetist, Griffith Davis, modified it for this special purpose by making the framework and tongue depressor heavier and stronger and by attaching a metal tube to the tongue blade through which ether vapor was given. Many years later this gag was used in the operation Crowe devised for removing tonsils.

During this period, Cushing was the only neurosurgeon on the hospital staff and Crowe his only assistant. In the private and public wards combined, Cushing usually had about 40 patients at all times. It was the assistant's duty to write in a legible manner the patient's history and to make and record a physical and neurological examination, as well as a perimetric examination of the visual fields. He was also responsible for assisting in long and tedious intracranial or spinal cord operations, making dressings on the wards, and answering all night calls.

HALSTED'S PLAN FOR THE SURGICAL SPECIALTIES

William Stewart Halsted had an unusual approach to the development of the Department of Surgery. At an early stage Halsted suggested to his fourth resident surgeon, Joseph C. Bloodgood, that he should undertake in a more systematic manner than had hitherto been done the study of all tumors and other tissues removed at operation. Thus, surgical pathology was the first specialty established in the surgical department and Bloodgood was the first of a group of young men invited by Halsted to develop one of the surgical specialties. Later in his apparently casual way, Halsted steered Baetjer into roentgenology; Cushing and then Dandy into neurosurgery; Young into urology; Baer into orthopedics; and Crowe into otolaryngology.

There is evidence that suggests that this apparent casualness on Halsted's part was actually a well-designed plan for the development of clinical

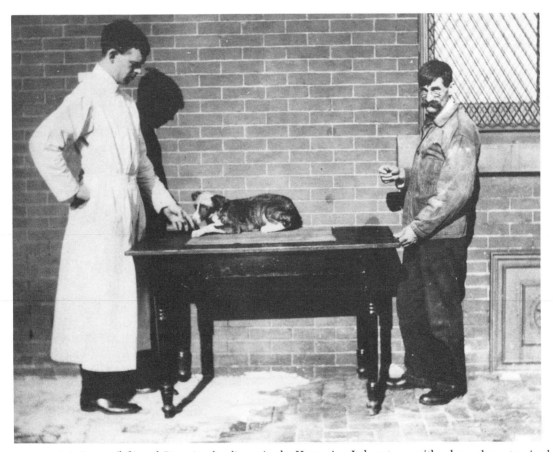

Fig 2.   Samuel J. Crowe *(left)* and Jimmie, the diener in the Hunterian Laboratory, with a hypophysectomized dog, 1910.

investigation in surgery. The idea may well have been inspired by Franklin Paine Mall, just as Mall had inspired Lewellys Barker to begin full-time research divisions in the fields of bacteriology, chemistry and physiology in the department of medicine.

Franklin Mall, during his period in the laboratory of Carl Ludwig in Leipzig, witnessed the application of the methods of science to the study of disease in man in the institute for clinical investigation set up by Hugo von Ziemssen. In these laboratory facilities physicians were engaged in the study of disease without the necessity of supporting themselves in private practice. Mall later advanced the idea that such a step would logically follow the placing of the preclinical departments on a full-time basis. Mall understood disease as the price of ignorance and worked continually behind the scenes after his return to Baltimore to introduce the methods and the trained investigators who would make the clinics more scientific. It is well known that in his early years in Baltimore Mall discussed this goal with his colleagues and his students. Lewellys Barker, who was responsible for the course in neuroanatomy, was one of Mall's articulate spokesmen for this basic idea that for medicine to advance clinical investigation had to become a recognized, important responsibility in a clinical department.

Halsted and Mall became close friends while collaborating on a number of investigations. In 1887 they worked in Welch's laboratory on intestinal anastomosis and no doubt Mall's studies on the structure of the intestinal wall contributed largely to their finding that inclusion of the submucosa or fibrous layer in the suture is essential for a successful result. Other joint investigations included the circular suture of the intestine, isolation of an intestinal loop and reversal of the intestines—all experimental studies on dogs. Councilman noted that: "the entry of Mall into the laboratory marked a period of brilliant activity. Mall's first work here was on the structure of the intestinal canal, and in the course of this he demonstrated the peculiar character of the submucosa. The two men were very congenial and they worked together in the large south room of the laboratory, each receiving from and giving to the other. Halsted made full use of the work of Mall in the development of his method of intestinal suture. I remember very well the experimental work in intestinal anastomosis and the huge distended circles which were produced by sewing together the ends of a severed, reversed loop of small intestine." Halsted was already an ardent experimentalist in the laboratory and he had this drive reinforced by association with Mall. As noted by Florence Sabin in her biography of Franklin Paine Mall: "The companionship of these two men was very close and

only after Mall's death did I realize how closely they had followed each other's work; for then Dr. Halsted used to come over to the anatomical department and talk to me about his research, just as he said he had always done with Mall. To me this was a rare experience to hear his plans for all the work he was undertaking. Thus Halsted and Mall formed a friendship rich in enjoyment and Dr. Welch told me that after Mall left Baltimore there was never a vacancy in any department of the university whatsoever for which Halsted did not urge Mall's appointment." It seems reasonable to assume that Mall and Halsted must have talked frequently about the development of the department of surgery and for the need to identify promising young surgeons who had the curiosity and originality to apply the methods of science to the study of the problems of surgery in man.

CROWE'S EARLY STRUGGLES

In view of the fact that Randolph and Mackenzie had worked in the dispensary for 23 years with no compensation or any opportunity to operate on their patients in the hospital, it is easy to understand their indignation when it was announced that a young man, four years out of medical school and with no training whatever in their specialty, had been appointed to supersede them. They immediately ceased to attend the dispensary and Crowe in February 1912 suddenly found himself faced with the responsibility of trying to examine 25 to 30 patients each afternoon.

Dr. Winford Smith, who was at that time superintendent of the Johns Hopkins Hospital, told an amusing story about the Medical Board Meeting in 1912 at which Halsted proposed to combine laryngology and otology in one department, and to place Crowe in charge of it. Halsted explained that Crowe had been on his staff for four years and that although he had had no training in either of the specialties involved, he would go abroad from time to time for study. Halsted also proposed a small salary for Crowe which, Smith noted, was unusual at that time. Howard A. Kelly interrupted Halsted and asked if this reorganization had been discussed with Mackenzie, Theobald and Randolph and the other men now doing the work. Halsted replied that he had not spoken to these men, that he was a little embarrassed about it, but thought everything would work out all right. Kelly pounded on the table and said, "Halsted, I am opposed to this. Everything we do here must be open and above board." Halsted flushed but promptly replied: "Kelly, you are absolutely right. How could I have perpetrated such an offense? It was an awful thing for me to do. I am ashamed, and I apologize for bringing such a recommendation before this dignified board—" and on and on, but never did he offer to withdraw the recommendation. Finally Kelly interrupted again to say, "Halsted, stop it. I'll vote for it."

Crowe found that writing the many histories and examination notes on such a large number of patients was a laborious process so he purchased a typewriter and employed a stenographer. Because of Crowe's inexperience, his records from the medical point of view might not have been too helpful to the other departments who sent patients for consultation, but they were legible, and it was not long before typists were employed throughout the dispensary.

During this difficult break-in period, and for many years thereafter, Crowe was ably assisted by Harry R. Slack, Jr. (Fig. 3). Slack graduated from the Johns Hopkins School of Medicine in June 1912, and from February to June of that year he helped Crowe in the dispensary almost every afternoon. They were a remarkable combination, since neither of them knew much about otolaryngology. Slack continued to work with Crowe and to assist in operations and in the care of the patients on the wards until June 1913

when both of them went to Germany to work in the clinic of Professor Killian at the University of Freiburg in Breisgau, and in Vienna under Alexander. When they returned to Baltimore in September 1913, Slack became the first resident in otolaryngology at the Johns Hopkins Hospital. When World War I broke out about a year later, Slack enlisted in the American Red Cross and spent a year in France. There he had a severe attack of influenza and returned to Baltimore in the summer of 1915 to recuperate. In October of that year he resumed his position as resident in otolaryngology and served in that capacity until October 1916 when he opened an office in Baltimore and began to practice his specialty.

Halsted, upon the inauguration of this new department, assigned a certain number of beds on the public wards to ear, nose and throat cases. These beds, however, were never in one ward or in one building but were mixed in with the general surgical beds. In Crowe's opinion this was a wise arrangement for the training of young men, because house officers in otolaryngology were then in contact with general surgeons on the wards and absorbed much

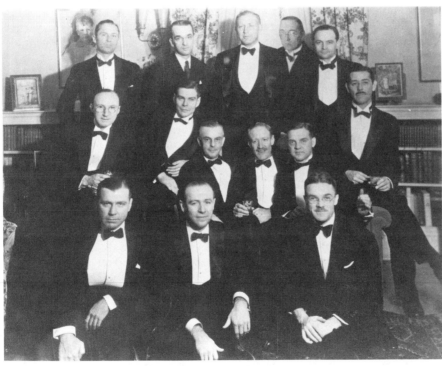

Fig 3. Some faculty members of the Zend-Avesta Medical Dinner Club, early 1930s. Harry Slack, Jr. and Edwin Broyles were members.
Bottom row, from left: W. F. Rienhoff, W. S. Tillett, E. Hanrahan
Middle row, from left: E. N. Broyles, J. T. King, S. R. Miller, H. M. Thomas, J. C. Colston, Ben Tappan
Back row, from left: D. C. Wharton Smith, John Dorsey, Robert Johnson, Walter Hughson, Harry R. Slack, Jr.

knowledge from them that was essential to their development as good technical surgeons in their chosen specialty.

As Edwards A. Park pointed out, Halsted recognized in 1912 that the time had come to raise the department of otolaryngology to a major division of the surgical service because he realized that the man for whom he had been waiting had at last emerged on the scene. The selection of Sam Crowe to head the service was the signal, and, as time proved, was the only step necessary to that end. The promotion of Crowe, only 29 years old at the time, to head a division of surgery in a field in which he had had no experience whatsoever, was, to say the least, a daring move on Halsted's part. It provides a wonderful illustration of Halsted's prescience in the perception of worth and also of his complete faith in the power of native ability to surmount obstacles, including that of complete inexperience. Halsted must have believed also that only a general surgeon was capable of developing otolaryngology on a sufficiently broad basis and he undoubtedly realized that Crowe's experience in neurosurgery and his demonstrated investigative abilities were essential assets. Crowe found himself plunged by his appointment into an extremely difficult situation. The practical problem presented by the mass exodus of the existing staff must have been balanced, however, by the opportunity which it afforded Crowe to reorganize his department in complete freedom. To add to his difficulties there was a lack of financial resources for the department while the demand for patient service was tremendous. Considering all of this, the only course open to him was to work along as well as he could, supporting himself from private practice and to hope to develop his own men. As indicated, he and Harry Slack fought the good fight shoulder to shoulder. Park points out that Crowe felt the strain keenly for he began to suffer from severe headaches and repeatedly spent his entire weekends in bed. However, hard-earned knowledge of the subject soon took root and as time went on everyone was impressed by his mastery of the field. Step by step, he explored and standardized each method and procedure, not so much by copying from others in the field as by shaping them according to his own ideas and in harmony with the principles and techniques of general surgery as worked out by Halsted. This development of the new department must have been exactly what Halsted had desired and envisioned when he selected Crowe. Crowe advanced the department in an orderly way, gradually building up a solid foundation. As assistants trained in his ideas and methods accumulated and lent their aid, his department grew to become the first great clinic of otolaryngology in this country, organized with a unique breadth and

soundness. Once the security of the routine responsibilities had been tended to, Crowe increasingly turned his attention from clinical development to the great problem in the field, notably the physiology and pathology of hearing.

Most men in medicine reach their peak and then remain stationary or decline. Crowe's career both from the clinical and scientific points of view was a steady upward progression and the work of the last years was perhaps the best of all.

THE "NEW" OTOLARYNGOLOGY

In 1912 tonsillectomy was the most frequently performed operation. Many patients were referred from the medical or pediatric wards with rheumatic fever, acute nephritis or some other systemic disorder aggravated by infected tonsils and lymphoid tissue in the upper air passages.

In most clinics at that time postoperative lung abscesses in patients undergoing tonsillectomy were a serious problem. Cutler and his associates, as well as Holman and others, ascribed these abscesses to the liberation of infected emboli. Tonsillectomies were done with the patient in the upright position. Crowe, however, placed the patient with the head at least 15 inches below the feet. Anesthesia was given at a level to keep the patient quiet but never to the point of abolition of the swallowing reflex. Suction was employed to keep the pharynx absolutely free of mucus and blood, and all bleeding points were ligated promptly. Over 3500 patients had their tonsils removed in this manner without the occurrence of a single lung abscess. In 1924 Crowe and his collaborators began the study of experimentally produced lung abscesses. After two years of diligent effort they were able to produce abscesses limited to a single lobe by introducing through a bronchoscope a small piece of cotton saturated with fresh scrapings from pyorrhea cavities in patients. Such scrapings were swarming with spirochetes and other bacteria. In several animals they inserted the material into a frontal sinus and a localized abscess resulted indicating that pus from the frontal sinus flowed into the trachea during sleep and produced the localized pulmonary lesions.

To perform a tonsillectomy satisfactorily, it was imperative that the general anesthesia be given by an experienced person. During the first 25 or 30 years of the operation's existence, only ether was used. Halsted had come to Baltimore with the conviction that the administration of ether in the operating room was an essential part of the training of a young surgeon. As given by the intern, however, ether was a hazard and Dr. Cushing had been permitted to have a professional anesthetist. When

Cushing left for Boston and Crowe began to remove tonsils, he longed to hire Cushing's anesthetist (Griffith Davis) but could not afford to pay the fee. Ether, as administered by the surgical interns, resulted in so much gagging and vomiting that Crowe purchased a water suction pump to keep the pharynx clear of mucus. Thus otolaryngology was the first department to use suction in the operating rooms of the Johns Hopkins Hospital.

Hugh Young and Sam Crowe eventually teamed up to hire Miss Margaret Boise, a graduate nurse who had been giving anesthetics in the New York Hospital for several years, to take over this responsibility for them. This was in opposition to the wishes of Dr. Halsted, who said: "My interest is in someone who will advance our knowledge of anesthesia." Miss Boise succeeded so well, however, that Halsted soon offered her the position of anesthetist-in-chief for general surgery. He asked her to supervise every anesthesia given by an intern and also to instruct third year medical students in anesthesia during their course in operative surgery. In addition, he permitted her to train graduate nurses; thus was started a school, which, under the direction of her pupil, Miss Olive Berger, continued for many years to supply nurse anesthetists to hospitals throughout the country.

Another of Crowe's particular interests at the time was the frequency with which tuberculous lesions were found unexpectedly in the sections of tonsils removed at operation. In 1917 with Watkins and Rothholz he reported a careful study of 46 cases with histopathological confirmation. Seven years later, while he was working in the department of pathology, he published a further study on the subject with Paul MacCready of his resident staff in which he discussed the manner in which the bacilli reached the tonsils and the significance of the lesions in relation to the subsequent development of clinical tuberculosis. A follow-up study of these same patients fifteen years later by John Baylor, of Crowe's staff, and James Bordley, III, of the department of medicine, supported the law of Marfan, which stated that persons who had recovered from cervical tuberculosis rarely developed pulmonary tuberculosis afterwards.

There was a very good reason for Crowe's deep and continuing interest in this problem. He himself had tuberculosis of the pharynx and had a dramatic experience with a rather harrowing method of treatment. Dr. Halsted simply burned away the lesions with a red-hot soldering iron. Crowe had severe burns of the pharynx, larynx and trachea and was "in torture" for days afterwards. For a much longer time he feared that he would have a permanent impairment of his voice. Halsted was equally concerned and apparently never attempted that maneuver again.

PURSUING THE CAUSE AND TREATMENT OF DEAFNESS: THE OTOLOGICAL RESEARCH LABORATORY

One of the major examples of Crowe's power of intuition was his recognition of the role that the audiometer would play in his specialty. In most clinics at that time there was very little interest in the causes of impaired hearing. Although there was some understanding of the pathology of hearing loss from tumors and infections, there were still large numbers of patients with hearing impairment in whom no obvious cause could be identified. With only such tools as tuning forks and whistles, supplemented by the whisper and the spoken word, no reliable measurement could be made of the acuity for the various tones in the speech range. All of this, as Crowe clearly recognized, would be changed by the development of an accurate method for permanent recording of levels of hearing acuity.

Important events in medicine often come about by the chance association of two apparently unrelated events. Crowe's recognition of the importance of the audiometer coincided with the admission to the hospital late in 1923 of Dr. Wallace Buttrick, chairman of the General Education Board of the Rockefeller Foundation. Buttrick had come to see Halsted about an epithelioma on his face, and Halsted had asked Crowe to examine Buttrick's upper air passages and ears. During the course of their conversation, Buttrick asked Crowe what research efforts he had in progress. Crowe told him about his interest in the ear and of his many trips abroad in search of information about the cause, the location and the histologic appearance of lesions in various types of impaired hearing. It was not the impairment caused by infection or tumor in the temporal bone that interested Crowe, but the more common variety that occurred both in children and adults and about which little or nothing was known at the time. Crowe related to Buttrick the story of an instrument, called an audiometer, which had been developed in the Bell laboratory of the American Telephone and Telegraph Company, that could be used to determine the hearing acuity of a cross-section of people of all ages. With this apparatus it was possible for the first time to measure and record accurately the acuity of hearing, which opened the way for the study of the nature and causes of impaired hearing. Crowe reasoned that to learn anything about the causes of impaired hearing the functional performance of the ear would have to be correlated with the pathology seen in histologic sections of the middle and inner ear. This, he knew, was the method by which much of the knowledge of clinical medicine had been acquired up to that time: clinical-pathological correlation. If he had an audiometer and permission from the various hospitals of Baltimore to examine the ears and test the hearing of all patients in their wards who had a potentially fatal disease, he would soon have some basic material to work with. When these patients died, the temporal bones could be removed at necropsy, sectioned serially, and the histologic findings correlated with the functional test. It did not matter whether the patients tested with the audiometer had normal or impaired hearing. The important objective was to correlate functional tests with the histologic appearance of the various components of the hearing apparatus in the temporal bone. From this brilliant idea, the Otological Research Laboratory evolved.

At Buttrick's suggestion, Crowe wrote the following proposal to be presented to Mr. Rockefeller:

"My proposal is that we collect for microscopical study the temporal bones of individuals upon whom we have previously made a functional test of the auditory and vestibular apparatus. The object is to try and coordinate the pathological changes as seen in the microscopical sections of the inner and middle ear with the clinical symptoms, if any, that were observed during life.

"In order to obtain material it will be necessary to make a clinical examination of the ear and vestibular apparatus on large numbers of patients in the hospitals of Baltimore; and, subsequently, to follow these patients so closely that in the event of their death we may be able to obtain their temporal bones for microscopical study. In this way we may gradually collect material that will be invaluable for determining the cause, and will probably point the way to the prevention of deafness.

"This plan would require: (1) the whole time service of a man trained to make accurate functional tests of the auditory and vestibular nerves. A new man should be assigned to this position each year. Such a position would afford a man ample opportunity to acquaint himself with all the literature, the clinical and the pathological aspects of the ear. He should have a salary equal to that of an instructor in other departments of the university, (2) the services of an expert technician are required. His salary should be adequate to obtain the services of a man already trained in technical methods, otherwise much valuable material will be spoiled, (3) a well-equipped laboratory. Suitable quarters have been provided and equipped through the courtesy of Dr. MacCallum."

Buttrick, in replying on January 29, 1924, commented that the brevity and clarity of the proposal had impressed Mr. Rockefeller and he had approved it.

The next step was to gather a group capable of carrying such a project to successful conclusion. Dr.

Stacy R. Guild (Fig. 4) was the first of this group to be recruited. Guild was an anatomist at the University of Michigan who was interested in the finer structure of the middle and inner ear of animals. He had produced excellent histologic sections of the ear in animals, but soon found that the technique he had employed for animals did not produce good histologic sections of human temporal bones. Another member of the group, Leroy Polvogt, was a Johns Hopkins Medical School graduate (1921) who had served as a resident in otolaryngology from 1922 to 1925. Polvogt was sent to Europe, where he spent the better part of a year studying with Wittmack, Alexander and Nager, in whose laboratories sectioning of human temporal bones was being carried out. He returned with voluminous notes, which were carefully reviewed and revised. The new techniques were installed in the laboratory, and the first successful temporal bone sections produced.

An audiometric survey that was carried out by Guild and Bunch soon revealed that with progressive aging, there was no loss of hearing for low tones, but for high tones the loss increased in each successive decade. It became evident that the degree of impairment for the higher frequencies varied from patient to patient, in much the same way that changes in the vision or in the skin with aging varied among individuals. Thus clinicians learned that in interpreting the audiogram of a patient with a systemic, central nervous system, or local ear disease, it is essential to take into consideration the age of the patient as well as the history and findings on examination.

Another important contribution from the new laboratory was proof that hearing is not impaired in

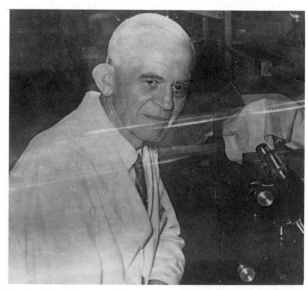

Fig 4.   Stacy R. Guild

either ear after removal of the right cerebral hemisphere. In 1927–1928, Walter Dandy removed the entire right hemisphere in five patients with brain tumors. After operation, three of these patients answered questions just as accurately and promptly as they did before the operation; they had no evident mental impairment or loss of memory. Careful tests were made on one patient who, one month after the operation, could repeat words whispered into both the right and left ear. An audiogram made three months after the operation revealed her hearing for all tones to be equally good in both ears. This indicated that total deafness in one or both ears is always a result of a lesion of the inner ear or in that part of the auditory nerve that lies between the cochlea and the brain stem but never in the middle ear alone or in the central auditory pathways.

A paper entitled "Observations on the pathology of high tone deafness," published in 1934 by Crowe, Guild and Polvogt, was the first large-scale report on the program Crowe had outlined for the Rockefeller Foundation in 1922. It was a giant step forward to be able to interpret an audiogram in terms of the location and the type of lesion that caused the hearing impairment.

EUSTACHIAN TUBE BLOCKAGE AND THE USE OF RADON

During the first 14 years after the audiometer was introduced, hearing tests were made on approximately 15,000 patients at Johns Hopkins. It became apparent that impaired hearing for high tones was not uncommon in children. This led Crowe's group to doubt the accepted theory that impaired hearing for high tones with good hearing for low tones was always caused by an inner ear or nerve lesion. Use of an electrically lighted otoscope and a nasopharyngoscope for every examination of the ear and nasopharynx of children disclosed that some adenoid tissue often remains even after careful surgical removal, or recurs in or around the pharyngeal orifice of the Eustachian tubes following an upper respiratory infection. The Eustachian tube equalizes atmospheric pressure on both sides of the tympanic membrane. Therefore, even a partial occlusion upsets this balance, causing congestion of the blood vessels in the middle ear, edema of the mucous membrane, and an outpouring of serum in the middle ear to offset the partial vacuum. It is a well-known complication of flying, when it is referred to as aerotitis. Abundant evidence indicates that it is a condition similar to that seen in children.

In searching for a safe and effective therapy for this condition, it was found that Heineke in 1903 had observed that lymphocytes are more sensitive to irradiation than the adjacent epithelium, muscle, bone or cartilage. This suggested to Crowe that hearing might be restored by reducing with radium the amount of lymphoid tissue causing tubal obstruction. In 1927, with the advice of Dr. Curtis F. Burnam, Crowe and his colleagues began to treat the hypertrophied lymphoid tissue around the Eustachian tubes with roentgen rays through portals near the angle of the jaw and with radium in an applicator small enough to pass along the floor of the nose. The radium was placed in a brass tube, the wall of which was 1 mm thick, allowing the passage of gamma rays but filtering out most of the beta rays. They used from 2 to 2.5 gram minutes of radiation on each side of the nasopharynx. These early studies were the subject of a preliminary report by Crowe and Guild in 1938. In a later paper entitled "The prevention of deafness," Crowe and Baylor described a series of cases in more detail. Extracts from the summary of that paper are as follows:

A long continued partial obstruction of the Eustachian tubes in children causes retraction of the tympanic membranes, impaired hearing for high tones with relatively good hearing for low tones, and sometimes a total loss of hearing by bone conduction. This revolutionary statement is based on detailed observation of 60 children in some cases for 10 years. . . . The most satisfactory method of treatment is irradiation with radium or roentgen rays. After the hyperplastic lymphoid tissue has been reduced . . . the hearing for high tones and for bone-conducted sounds often returns to the normal level and it remains there so long as the Eustachian tubes are clear . . . We feel that if school children in the primary grades were examined with a nasopharyngoscope at least once a year and those with hyperplastic lymphoid tissue in and around the orifice of the Eustachian tubes were treated with radiation as often as necessary to ensure normal functioning of the tubes, the number of deaf adults in the next generation could be reduced by 50 percent.

Starting in 1939 large scale examinations were done on randomly selected school children with the object of finding how many had a type of hearing impairment that could be arrested or restored with nasopharyngeal irradiation treatments, sometimes supplemented with antibiotics or surgical removal of tonsils and adenoids.

In 1941 Crowe and Burnam published another paper on the subject, "The recognition, treatment and prevention of hearing impairment in children." They substantiated the previous findings and noted that lymphoid tissue is so sensitive to radiation that the dosage employed in the treatment of the nasopharynx is far below the amount that could cause any irritation or injury to the mucous membranes or surrounding structures.

Early in 1942 W. R. Willard, who was then health officer of the Washington County Maryland Health Department, became interested in the problem of the prevention of deafness. He conferred with the otolaryngologic staff of the Johns Hopkins Hospital; Dr. Curtis Burnam, who developed the radon applicator for treating adenoid tissues; representatives of the Maryland League for the Hard of Hearing; representatives of the State Department of Health; the United States Children's Bureau; State and County Departments of Education; the County Medical Society, and with other interested persons and agencies. Eventually an Advisory Committee was established in which these various interests were represented. It was decided to organize a program to identify as high a percentage as possible of the children in Washington County who were suffering from early impairment of hearing or with aural infection or disease of the nose and throat predisposing to such difficulties. Early treatment would thus be possible. Dr. Donald Proctor, at that time an instructor in laryngology and otology at Johns Hopkins, was placed in charge of the examinations to be conducted at a clinic in Hagerstown, Maryland. The program, which got underway in 1943, was an immediate success. In a report of the program in 1946, Proctor and Willard stressed that (1) an adequate, interested and cooperative health department was absolutely necessary for such a program, and (2) no amount of planning could make up for the lack of a health officer and an otolaryngologist who were capable of meeting the specific problems peculiar to the community involved. This clinic in Hagerstown became the model for a statewide program which was organized through the State Health Department of Maryland over the next few years. Many members of the Hopkins and Maryland communities participated in the implementation of this program, including Edward Davens, Jean Stifler, and John Whitridge.

The original applicator used by Crowe when these studies began changed very little in seventeen years. The handle of the instrument was 13 centimeters long and the tube into which the handle screwed was 2 centimeters long. The small glass tube containing radon was 1½ cm long. The thickness of the brass tube wall was 1 millimeter. Fifty milligrams of pure anhydrous radium sulphate could be put into the tube. When radon was used, they could introduce any amount up to the equivalent of a gram or more of radium. With this applicator a dose of 2 gram minutes could be given to either side of the nasopharynx and repeated at intervals of four weeks or longer without causing disagreeable symptoms of any kind. The mixture of rays emitted from the applicator was 95.5 percent gamma and 4.5 percent beta rays. At that time it was thought that beta rays were harmful and the shielding was constructed to eliminate these rays to the greatest extent possible. The 1 millimeter of brass filtration removed all alpha rays and a large portion of the beta rays.

In 1944 Burnam and Crowe published the description of a new type of applicator in a paper entitled "The monel metal radium applicator designed for maximum use of hard beta rays in the treatment of nasopharyngeal hyperplastic lymphoid tissue" (Fig. 5). The active part of this new applicator was a monel metal or a stainless steel tubular chamber 15 millimeters in length with an inside diameter of 1.7 millimeters and a wall thickness of 0.3 millimeters. Its chamber contained 50 milligrams of radium sulphate. Practically all of the beta rays emitted by the applicator were absorbed by the tissues of the nasopharynx, seventy-five percent of the beta rays being absorbed in the first 3 millimeters of tissue. After 1943 this type of applicator was used by Proctor in the Hagerstown clinic. This provided a practical form of therapy, which could be used in localities where radon was not easily available. The use of 0.3 mm of monel metal as a filter provided a large percentage of beta rays and reduced the time factor for treatment.

Another study was started in 1948 with the additional object of determining what changes in hearing occurred in treated and untreated children between the ages of 7 and 14 years during a five-year period of observation. One hundred and ninety-three children treated with radon and 192 children who had received treatment with blank applicators were followed. The record showed that the adenoids of children who had been treated with radon greatly decreased in size or disappeared entirely during the first three years. The adenoids in the untreated group also decreased in size, but this change did not occur until the fourth or fifth years of observation. These studies were reported by John E. Bordley and W. G. Hardy in 1955.

There has been no evidence subsequently in these patients of any untoward effect on distant organs, such as the thyroid, by the use of this type of nasopharyngeal irradiation.

THE PHYSIOLOGY OF HEARING

In February 1930 Wever and Bray, working in the psychological laboratory of Princeton University, discovered that when a tone was sounded in the ear of an animal, the frequency of the action current set up in the auditory nerve was the same as that of the stimulating tone. After amplification, the action current became audible, and the tone was found to be identical with the original stimulus. In short, the ear

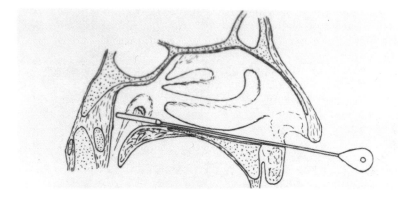

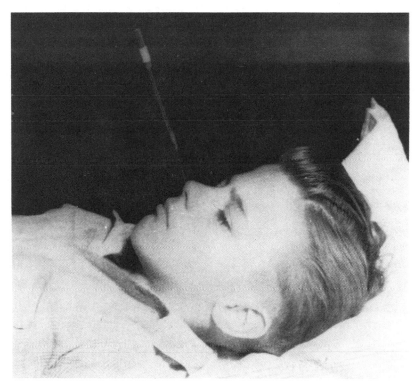

Fig 5. *Top*, Cross section to show position of monel metal radium applicator in nasopharynx. *Bottom*, Photograph of child during treatment with applicator in position.

From: Proctor, D. F., Polvogt, L. M. and Crowe, S. J.: Irradiation of lymphoid tissue in diseases of the upper respiratory tract. Bull. Johns Hopkins Hosp., 83: 383, 1948.

could be used as a telephone and the auditory nerve as a telephone wire from which impulses could be recorded and, when amplified, proved to be the same sounds that were transmitted to the ear. Using this technique, a series of investigations were carried out in Crowe's department by Walter Hughson, Stacy Guild, John E. Bordley and Edward Walzl. One of their publications in 1934 on the localization of tones along the length of the cochlea of man stimulated physiological studies to determine whether a similar arrangement of the hearing apparatus could be demonstrated in animals.

Crowe and Guild realized that they could learn a great deal by dismantling the ear part by part while recording the changes in the cochlear potentials. They set up a laboratory for this study and shortly after the work was begun, they persuaded Walter Hughson, a full-time assistant professor who had been doing research in general surgery, to take over the direction of the laboratory.

Dr. John E. Bordley, a second-year resident in otology, was permitted to drop out of the residency training program for six months to work in this laboratory with Guild and Hughson. Bordley's evenings were spent in the Temporal Bone Laboratory studying sections and dissecting the temporal bones under Guild's direction. This experience greatly influenced Bordley's future career. When he completed his residency training in October 1933 he received an appointment as instructor. He entered private practice in Baltimore but continued to work part-time with Hughson. In 1932 when Hughson left to take charge of a laboratory in Philadelphia, Bordley assumed charge of the Baltimore laboratory, working there two days a week. With Mary Hardy, he studied the effect of various lesions on the tympanic membrane in animals. After each incision was made in the membrane, audiograms, employing the Wever–Bray technique, were taken. Two years later, they published the first paper on this subject, entitled "Effect of lesions of the tympanic membrane on the hearing acuity. Observations on experimental animals and on man."

In 1937 Dr. Edward McColgan Walzl (Fig. 6) joined the laboratory. Walzl proved to be one of the most ingenious investigators in Crowe's group of outstanding otolaryngologists. Born on January 22, 1910, Walzl had suffered a damaging attack of poliomyelitis during his childhood, which left him severely incapacitated. The prolonged hospitalization interfered with any formal schooling, but with great persistence he accomplished the high school work that would admit him to Mount St. Mary's College, where he spent the years 1929 to 1931. He then entered the Johns Hopkins University and received his Ph.D. in zoology at the age of 25. His graduate thesis dealt with the actions of electrolytes on the oyster heart—actions which proved to be the opposite of the effects of these same electrolytes on vertebrate hearts. In 1936 he became an assistant to Professor E. K. Marshall, Jr., in the department of pharmacology, and co-authored with Marshall papers on sulfanilamide cyanosis and on picrotoxin as a respiratory stimulant in barbiturate poisoning.

When he joined the Otological Research Laboratory, he adapted to the cochlea the perfusion techniques that he had used in the oyster heart and studied the effects on cochlear microphonics of crystals of NaCl and KCl applied to the exposed endosteum of either the scali tympani or the scala vestibuli of the basal turn. Response to high tones was first impaired when the salts were applied at the

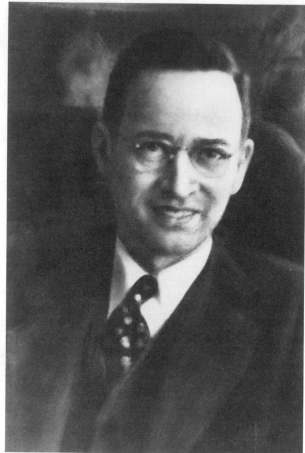

Fig 6.   Edward McColgan Walzl

basal end of the cochlea and to low tones when applied to the apex. The next step was to test the effects of small lesions of the organ of Corti on cochlear potentials, experiments that were carried out in collaboration with John E. Bordley. They developed a method for thinning out the otic capsule and crushing small lengths of the organ of Corti. These studies confirmed that there was a pattern of tonal localization along the organ of Corti.

During the period when Walzl and Bordley were carrying out these experiments, Clinton N. Woolsey, who was a research fellow in orthopedic surgery, was developing an electrophysiological setup in the laboratory adjacent to Walzl's. When he saw the exquisite way in which the organ of Corti was approached through the otic capsule, Woolsey proposed that he and Walzl attempt to stimulate the cochlea electrically by employing the same technique and explore the auditory cortex for localized responses. At first the experiments were unsuccessful. It was then decided to remove the fluids from the cochlea, which Walzl believed could be done most easily by opening the cochlea widely and applying electrical stimuli to the cochlear nerve fibers as they entered the osseous spiral lamina. This method was at once successful. In these experiments they produced evidence for a two-fold representation of the cochlea in each cerebral hemisphere. They next decided to investigate the effects of cochlear lesions, which produced selective impairments of cochlear microphonics for high or low tones, on cortical activation by click stimuli in animals in which the ipsilateral cochlea had first been destroyed. When the cortex was explored for responses to the clicks, after destruction of the apical turn, only those parts of the cortex found responsive to basal coil stimulation in other experiments were activated; the apical areas of the cortex remained silent, suggesting that there must be frequency representation in the cortex. Walzl and Woolsey extended these studies to the monkey in 1943.

While these experiments were being carried out, Walzl was also enrolled as a medical student at Johns Hopkins. After receiving his M.D. in 1942, Walzl spent three years in the residency training program of the department of otolaryngology. During this time he participated in clinical research with Dr. Crowe, studying the effects of irradiation of hyperplastic lymphoid tissue in the nasopharynx.

After completion of residency training he took the course in fenestration surgery with Lempert in New York in 1946. The surgical skill which he had used to such effect in the laboratory was applied with great success in the clinic, where he soon was doing many of the total laryngectomies performed at Johns Hopkins for cancer of the larynx. In 1948 with Broyles he reported on the postoperative course of 27 patients who had received subperichondral total laryngectomies.

In spite of his clinical activities, and, indeed, stimulated by them, as Woolsey pointed out, Walzl continued his interests in laboratory research. In 1949 he studied the effect of streptomycin on the hearing mechanism. He produced damage in cats with the drug and determined the site of the lesion using a technique similar to that used in the studies of tone localization in the cochlea and in the cerebral cortex. These experiments showed that the dizziness from streptomycin toxicity is a symptom of central nervous system damage. No evidence of a lesion was found in the peripheral end organ.

The last experimental study reported by Walzl was carried out with Vernon Mountcastle in the department of physiology on the projection of the vestibular nerve to the cerebral cortex of the cat. An initial attempt to look for a cortical vestibular area in 1944 did not succeed, but Walzl then made the necessary dissections to reach as many of the ves-

tibular receptor areas for electrical stimulation as could be exposed surgically. Some preliminary results on the vestibular nuclei were obtained by recording from the dorsal surface of the medulla. In the experiments with Mountcastle, peripheral excitation was accomplished either by brief mechanical stimulation of the vestibular end organ through minute fenestrations or by electrical stimulation of the vestibular nerve. These experiments constituted the first clear demonstration of a projection of the vestibular nerve to the cerebral cortex.

In 1949 Walzl had the great misfortune to develop a second major neurological disorder, myasthenia gravis. The sequelae of his previous poliomyelitis with the added problem of myasthenia could not be overcome, and he died on August 10, 1950 at the peak of a brilliant research career.

BROYLES AND THE BRONCHOSCOPIC CLINIC

Halsted had told Crowe that he believed the department of otolaryngology should also include diseases of the thorax. At the time, bronchoscopy was performed at the Johns Hopkins Hospital on rare occasions for the removal of foreign bodies or for the diagnosis of esophageal obstruction; diagnostic bronchoscopy was seldom done. One of Crowe's residents, Edwin N. Broyles (Fig. 3), took a particular interest in this field. He recalled that he frequently assisted Crowe at the Hunterian Laboratory while Crowe was working on methods of occlusion of the primary bronchi.

After completing his residency training in 1922, Broyles worked for a time with Hasslinger of the Hajack Clinic in Vienna. When he returned to Baltimore, Slack recommended that he be given the responsibility of endoscopic examinations in the Johns Hopkins Hospital. Broyles assumed this duty after spending several months in Philadelphia with Dr. Chevalier Jackson and his assistants, Drs. Gabriel Tucker and Louis Clerf. Under Broyles's direction, a special endoscopic clinic was started at Johns Hopkins in 1923. It was at first situated in a side room on the fourth floor of the old surgical building, but when the Dispensary, or Carnegie Building, was completed in 1927, the clinic was moved to a room at the east end of this building on the fourth floor. It was not long before the surgical, medical and pediatric departments were sending patients to the endoscopic clinic for examination.

One of Broyles's great contributions to endoscopy was the development of a bronchoscope with a series of telescopes that could be inserted into its lumen. These telescopes brightly illuminated and magnified the structures in the field of vision. A telescope with a right-angled lens afforded a clear view of the upper lobe bronchi.

From the time the endoscopy clinic opened, Broyles was never content merely to report what he saw in patients, but exhibited a personal interest in the patients and a concern with finding a way to cure their basic problems. This trait came to the fore one day when Dr. Park referred a girl to Dr. Crowe for examination because of a large shadow by x-ray and an absence of breath sounds in the left chest. Crowe sent the patient to Broyles for a bronchoscopic examination, which disclosed a smooth tumor filling the left main bronchus and protruding into the trachea. Attempts to remove the tumor through the bronchoscope were unsuccessful, and in July 1933 Broyles sought the aid of Dr. William F. Rienhoff. Rienhoff removed the entire left lung with no postoperative complications. This was the first total pneumonectomy at the Johns Hopkins Hospital. At first it was believed to have been the first in the United States, but it was later learned that in April 1933 Dr. Evarts Graham at Washington University had performed the first one-stage pneumonectomy for cancer of the lung with a cure. Graham advocated a thoracoplasty when pneumonectomy was performed because he feared that overdistention of the only good lung would produce emphysema and that the shift of the mediastinum to the operated side would kink the large blood vessels. Rienhoff disagreed, however, on the basis of observations made on animals by Heuer and Dunn in 1920 in the Hunterian Laboratory, which showed that the space left after extirpation of one lung was soon filled by a shift of the mediastinum, elevation of the diaphragm and distention of the remaining lung.

After these dramatic cases, the days on which the bronchoscopic clinic met had to be doubled and then tripled because of the rapidly increasing number of cases referred there. The number soon reached 2000 annually. Thoracic surgery blossomed in the hospital, and many patients with lung tumors were admitted.

Crowe stimulated Broyles's interest not only in lung conditions but in laryngeal and esophageal lesions as well. In 1938 Broyles, in collaboration with Crowe, devised an operation for the cure of selected cases of carcinoma of the larynx. It was designed to cure patients with laryngeal cancer that was too far advanced for a localized surgical procedure, but that had not yet spread to the lymph nodes in the neck. The operation entailed removal of the entire larynx, a permanent tracheostomy and loss of the normal speaking voice. These patients now learn esophageal speech and get along very well.

In patients with the common type of malig-

nant tumor in the larynx—squamous cell carcinoma—Broyles noted, as had others, that cancer had a tendency to invade and destroy a local area of the thyroid cartilage just under the skin and midline of the neck. It rarely invaded cartilage in other parts of the larynx. Broyles and Guild developed methods to serially section the whole larynx. Broyles found that the tendon of the vocal cords and its associated thyroarytenoideus muscles penetrate the thyroid cartilage anteriorly. Many tumors spread along this tendon and destroy the anterior part of the thyroid cartilage. This was a valuable clinical contribution. When examination of the patient shows a malignant growth in the anterior part of the larynx, the possibility is always present that cancer cells may have already invaded the thyroid cartilage by way of this tendon. In such a case laryngectomy, rather than local removal of the growth, should be considered.

THE HEARING AND SPEECH CLINIC

The advances made in the Otological Research Laboratory opened up opportunities for the rehabilitation of the deaf. The idea for a special hearing and speech clinic, in which the new knowledge could be applied, originated with John E. Bordley (Fig. 7). After his discharge from military service in World War II, he made a tour of the rehabilitation services of the Armed Forces and studied a number of their audiology centers in which otologists, speech specialists and audiologists worked together on the problem of deafness. He eagerly proposed the development of a hearing and speech unit to Crowe, but was met with a complete rebuff. He was surprised the next morning when Mrs. Bordley told him that Sam Crowe was on the telephone. Bordley had been so discouraged by the previous day's discussion that he really did not want to talk further about the proposal. Mrs. Bordley pointed out that "Dr. Crowe's voice sounded very pleasant." When he took up the receiver, Crowe told him that upon reconsideration he found Bordley's idea an excellent one. Once Crowe had made this decision, he immediately looked for funds to support the project. He took a train to Wilmington and persuaded Mr. Copeland, a member of the Du Pont family, to donate $75,000 to establish the clinic. Bordley then went to Philadelphia and recruited William G. Hardy, who was chief of the rehabilitation service at the Naval Hospital there. Under Bordley and Hardy's brilliant direction, the hearing and speech unit was set up as a division of the department of otolaryngology in the Johns Hopkins School of Medicine. It was the first such unit to be connected with a medical school. Following its organization, the unit was also made a division of the department of environmental medicine within the School of Hygiene and Public Health. Since the medical school provided only for the M.D. degree, this arrangement allowed students in the unit to earn a masters or a doctorate.

Shortly after the new Division of Hearing and Speech was organized, research began on methods for the early identification of hearing loss in children and infants. Modern electronic equipment, speech training and the hearing aid made it possible for the severely deaf child to go to public schools and grow up with normal-hearing children. Training, however, had to begin at the age of two or three years, and it was essential to know how much, if any, hearing defect a child had. The test for hearing had to be accurate and show which tones in the sound spectrum were heard and which were most impaired.

It was known that sensory or emotional stimuli changed the resistance of the skin to the passage of an electric current. In 1928 Curt Richter developed a technique for recording graphically the change in skin-resistance that follows a mild electric shock. The electric shock stimulates the sympathetic nerves in the skin, which in turn increases the activity of the sweat glands and lessens the resistance of the skin in the sweating area to the passage of a minute electric current. Bordley and Hardy, after consultating with Richter, devised a method using the conditional reflex of Pavlov to test the hearing of children and the observations of Richter to measure and record this response. They conditioned the child to a tone by first introducing the tone and then following the tone with a mild electrical shock. Following the shock, a drop in skin resistance could be recorded. After the child was conditioned, the skin resistance would drop on hearing the tone without the electrical shock. If the child failed to hear the tone, there would be no change in skin resistance. Using this method for recording the audiogram in very young children, Bordley and Hardy began a long-term study of hearing loss in children; the study was carried on for over ten years and included more than 6000 children. This technique could distinguish between severe congenital deafness and mental deficiency, and the whole course of a child's life might depend on an accurate diagnosis. This test was also used later in the detection of malingering in adults.

John E. Bordley was born on November 8, 1902 in Baltimore, Maryland. He was educated at the Gilman School in Baltimore and graduated with a Ph.D. from Yale in 1925. He received his M.D. from Johns Hopkins in 1929. His family background led him into the field of medicine. In 1896 his father joined the faculty of the Johns Hopkins University School of Medicine as an assistant in ophthalmology. He soon met Harvey Cushing and they studied the various ophthalmologic changes which develop in tumors of the brain. Discussions about ophthalmology and otology were frequent in the Bordley family circle, and young John Bordley developed an early interest in the field of otolaryngology. In his senior year at medical school, he talked with Dr. Crowe about this interest and was advised to take a year's internship in surgery before entering specialty training. In 1930 Bordley was a surgical intern at the Union Memorial Hospital in Baltimore at which time Dr. J. M. T. Finney and Dr. W. A. Fisher, who was later to become Bordley's father-in-law, were the leading surgeons. At the end of his internship in surgery, Bordley married Ellen Bruce Fisher. Becoming a married resident trainee in those days was a complicated procedure. Bordley first had to get permission to marry from Crowe, who in turn had to get approval from the director of the hospital to bring a married resident trainee on his service. When approved, the married trainee had to live within five

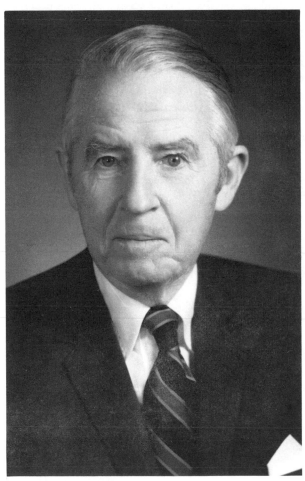

Fig 7.   John E. Bordley

minutes of the emergency room. The accident room in those days was watched over by Miss Kitty Brady, who took a great interest in all of the young house officers and their wives. She provided in a back room, a number of chairs and small tables and bought games that could be played in the evening by the wives of the resident trainees whose husbands were on duty. The social life in the accident room was probably never more interesting in the history of Hopkins than under Miss Kitty's guidance and supervision.

The residency years were influenced by two individuals in the department: Dr. Stacy Guild and Dr. Crowe himself. Guild conducted regular meetings for the staff during which he showed the new sections on temporal bones. Crowe gave a great deal of time to his second and third year house officers. They were invited to help him examine his patients, he made rounds with them and spent hours with them on Saturday afternoons or Sundays reviewing slides, reviewing the research that was being done in the temporal bone laboratory, and describing the research problems in otolaryngology.

Bordley's early work in the otology laboratory was interrupted by the advent of World War II. He became a member of the Johns Hopkins 118th General Hospital, serving in Australia, New Guinea and the Philippines. He played an important role in making radium applicators available for the treatment of aerotitis media, which was an important problem for the pilots in that combat area.

In 1950 Bordley was invited to join a group headed by Dr. A. McGehee Harvey, the Professor of Medicine, to study the effect of ACTH and cortisone in allergy and hypersensitivity. Bordley's assignment was to observe the effect of these substances on the allergic nose, particularly when polyps were present. The polyps decreased rapidly in size in patients receiving these hormones. These studies resulted in the first publication of the beneficial effect of ACTH and cortisone in allergic conditions.

Upon the retirement of Dr. Crowe, Bordley became the first full-time chairman of the Department of Otolaryngology in June 1952.

CROWE'S CONTRIBUTIONS TO THE U.S. AIR FORCE

Samuel Crowe was a responsible and effective consultant for the U.S. Air Force at home and abroad. In World War II it became apparent that Air Force pilots were developing a pattern of symptoms comparable to those of the children with blockade of the Eustachian tubes. While training in altitude chambers, and in actual flight, some pilots suffered ear pain in descent, as well as other symptoms of aerotitis. Crowe organized a course at Johns Hopkins to train medical officers in the use of the nasopharyngoscope and in his technique of radon therapy. In addition, during World War II, Crowe went to many air bases to advise officers and treat patients. When the same symptoms as those in flyers were reported by the Navy in men being trained for submarine work during practice of methods of escape from great depths, Dr. Crowe undertook to develop the same services for the Navy.

In 1951 Crowe, who disliked the hot Baltimore summers, gladly accepted an invitation to work with the Air Force at Wiesbaden, Germany, where he had regular office hours, saw patients, taught and counseled young doctors. In recognition of Crowe's service the Secretary of the Air Force in January 1952 presented to him, in a Pentagon ceremony, the Air Force Scroll of Appreciation. The citation read in part: "Dr. Samuel J. Crowe distinguished himself by rendering meritorious service to the department of the Air Force. Realizing the critical need existing in the European theatre for a consultant with his training and experience, Crowe volunteered his services to the Wiesbaden Military Post Hospital, Germany. He gave unstintingly of his time and energy to treat numerous complicated cases, to conduct lectures in the field of his specialty, and to instruct medical personnel. As a result of Dr. Crowe's efforts, the professional services provided for military and civilian members of the United States Occupation Forces were improved. Dr. Crowe's contributions and accomplishments reflect the highest credit upon himself and the medical profession."

CROWE AND HALSTED

Pasteur once stated that had he been steeped in the traditions and disciplined in the classic school of medicine, he would have had little chance to develop his original ideas. Perhaps the same can be said of Samuel Crowe. He entered otolaryngology superbly trained to observe, to experiment and to think along the broad planes of the physiological, pathological and surgical approaches which were being developed in his environment, yet he was untrammeled by the archaic and rigid blinds which had gradually been drawn in otolaryngology at that time.

E. A. Park

Crowe learned a great deal from Halsted. They not only worked together closely, but they lived just around the corner from each other, and Crowe was a frequent visitor at Halsted's home. Of all of Halsted's assistants, Park felt that Crowe was the closest to the Professor spiritually, occupying the position nearest, perhaps, to a son. Halsted's feelings toward Crowe, he thought, were a combination of pride and deep affection. Although quite different in many ways, Halsted and Crowe were alike in others. Both were thinkers in the field of their work and spent much time at it; both were perfectionists and intolerant of slack ways and loose thinking; they despised pretense and abhorred intellectual dishonesty; each exerted his influence, not by interference, but by example. Both put thoroughness and care in their surgical work first and were contemptuous of speed as an end in itself. At a time when tonsils were being taken out all over the country with guillotine and snare, Crowe insisted on dissecting them out with the same meticulous care which Halsted used in amputation of the breast. Both thought only in terms of the ultimate welfare of the patient. Neither looked on money as an end in itself; Halsted forgot fees and Crowe's bills were moderate. Crowe, of course, worshipped Halsted, and some might ascribe these qualities in Crowe to Halsted's influence. However, Park felt, knowing them both, that the qualities were inherent—the two men were kindred spirits.

CROWE AS A SURGEON AND INVESTIGATOR

As Park witnessed Crowe's development, both as a surgeon and investigator, he was continually made conscious of the great advantage which Crowe derived from his training in general surgery, particularly in brain surgery. Crowe was never confined by the geographical boundaries of his specialty and was as much a master outside them as inside. In summarizing Crowe as an investigator, Park stated that Crowe's initial studies in his specialty were really steps in his own education. As his knowledge of the specialty grew, his studies assumed a more fundamental character, increasingly aimed at physiological knowledge or interpretation. Taken as a whole, his thinking was on a large scale. His studies revealed a remarkable combination of intelligence and imagination, which enabled him to seize new methods as they were developed in the fundamental science laboratory and to apply them to his own purposes. Illustrative of this was his immediate recognition of the potential value of the audiometer and also of the Wever–Bray method for studying sound transmission along the auditory tract. The introduction of the audiometer into clinical otology was a noteworthy achievement, for it placed the testing of hearing at once on an exact scientific basis. The employment of the audiometer, serial reconstruction of the temporal bone and the Wever–Bray method formed the basis for a series of investigations on hearing by Crowe and Guild and later by Hughson, Bordley, Walzl, Woolsey and Mountcastle, which remain classics. These pioneer investigations on hearing rank among the most important contributions to knowledge ever produced at Johns Hopkins. Crowe's projects were daring in their magnitude. One need only consider the boldness of his attempt to correlate specific defects of hearing in living human beings with the corresponding defects or injuries in the cochlea, or his development of the use of radon for the treatment or prevention of deafness due to the growth of lymphoid tissue in and around the orifices of the Eustachian tubes.

One of Crowe's most striking traits was his ability to get things done. When under the pervading influence of an idea, all else was excluded from his mind and he followed it up with a burning enthusiasm like one possessed, but always by a carefully organized methodical process. This directness of approach to the essential issue and the thoroughness with which he proceeded were as characteristic of Crowe in the operating room as in other activities. When Crowe had finished anything to his satisfaction, he never returned to it but turned to something new instead.

It is doubtful that any head of a department at Johns Hopkins has ever commanded more loyalty than that accorded Crowe by the members of his staff. John Bordley, in describing Crowe as head of his department, indicates the secret of this devotion to Crowe:

> Dr. Crowe expected loyalty from his staff. On the other hand, he was always extremely loyal to his staff, and was perfectly willing to fight for them whenever they were criticized or if he felt that anything unfair had been said about them. The loyalty of his staff, I think, was really born during the residency training which all the staff underwent. During this period Crowe was a stern disciplinarian and on several occasions dismissed house officers whom he felt were not doing the type of work that he expected. He was ever critical of the notes the house officers wrote and was a stern task master in the operating room. However, he more than made up for this by calling his residents into his office when he was seeing patients following surgery, and explaining to the patient that his good results were the result of excellent work of the house officer in question.

Crowe created a large, closely knit organization, whose members not only practiced his methods and extended his ideas but kept on making important contributions of their own. The development of a successful department of clinical medicine or surgery requires a certain bigness on the part of its head, quite apart from other prerequisites for leadership. The "chief" must be able to trust his subordinates and at the same time be willing to subordinate himself for them. He must have the vision to realize that collectively the department will diversify and be of much greater usefulness, and accomplish far more than if contained in himself. Moreover, he must be prepared to be surpassed and he must be so constituted as to feel the same pride in the successes of those working under him that he would experience if the triumphs had been his own.

Crowe's beliefs on this subject are illustrated by a conversation which he had with John Bordley. Shortly after his retirement Crowe came to Bordley and asked what he was going to do in the summer. Bordley told him that he felt he had too many irons in the fire to go away very far or for very long. Crowe then told him that he had always gone away for two or three months each summer because he could not stand the Baltimore heat; that he had been able to do this because he had developed an organization that could run itself and he trusted the man to whom he turned it over each summer; that if Bordley expected to run a department he had better start picking young individuals in whom he had faith and plan to give them the experience and responsibility of handling the department in his absence; and that he should plan to take two months off every summer.

Perhaps no better summary of Samuel J. Crowe as a person and as a scientist could be constructed than the citation when he was awarded the degree of doctor of science by the Johns Hopkins University on February 22, 1955:

> "Samuel James Crowe, Virginian, son of a physician, graduate of the University of Georgia, bent on becoming an engineer but persuaded by his father to study medicine; faltering in allegiance to medicine during his first year at Johns Hopkins until by accident encountering Professor William S. Halsted in a peculiarly personal way; then overnight falling under the spell of that great man and transformed into his ardent disciple. Intern, assistant resident, research student for five years, ushered into investigation through the doorway of surgery under that dynamic perfectionist in technique, Harvey Cushing; planning on a career in brain surgery with him at Harvard, but in a dramatic moment suddenly invited by Dr. Halsted to alter the course of his life by accepting the directorship of the newly planned division of otolaryngology, a subject about which he knew nothing. Bewildered but accepting, he began his independent career at the age of 29.
>
> "Among his far flung accomplishments which have extended even to studies on the physiology of the adrenal gland and hypophysis, these:—the creation of the first great clinic of otolaryngology in this country, conceived in the grand perspective of general surgery, pervaded by the spirit and example of its head, an oasis in a desert of medical practice; the first penetration into the terra incognita of deafness in the human being, coincident with the founding of the otological research laboratory, accomplished through painstaking correlations between specific

defects in hearing and the corresponding anatomical defects in the organ of Corti of the inner ear; the first to recognize as a major cause of deafness in children lymphoid ingrowths about the Eustachian tubes, the development by him of a method for prevention and treatment through radium, now widely adopted and organized throughout this country and in Europe which has safeguarded the hearing of countless persons.

> "Taciturn, shy, with heart of gold, unconscious of himself in his consecration to ideals, skilled surgeon, foremost explorer and acknowledged intellectual leader in his subject, teacher of teachers, in his inner demand for perfection in the mold of his great master, the life and light of his department, a constant joy to his friends, bulwark to his colleagues and a pride to the medical school as one of its great sons, in honoring whom the university is but doing homage to itself."

ACKNOWLEDGMENTS

I wish to thank the following for their help in the preparation of this essay: Carol Bocchini, John E. Bordley, Donald F. Proctor, George T. Nager, Clinton N. Woolsey, and Martin W. Donner.

REFERENCES

1. Bordley JE and Hardy M: Effect of lesions of the tympanic membrane on the hearing acuity. Observations on experimental animals and on man. Arch Otolaryngol 26: 649, 1937

2. Bordley JE, Hardy WG and Richter CP: Audiometry with the use of galvanic skin-resistance response. Bull Johns Hopkins Hosp 82: 569, 1948

3. Bordley JE and Hardy WG: A study in objective audiometry with the use of a psychogalvanometric response. Ann Otol Rhinol Laryngol 58: 751, 1949

4. Bordley JE and Hardy WG: The efficacy of nasopharyngeal irradiation for the prevention of deafness in children. Acta Otolaryngol (Stockh) Suppl 120, 1955

5. Broyles EN; Optical and visual aids in bronchoesophagology. Ann Otol Rhinol Laryngol 58: 1165, 1949

6. Broyles EN and Rienhoff WF: Local resection of carcinoma of the right main bronchus. The Laryngoscope 59: 666, 1949

7. Bunch CC: Auditory acuity after removal of the entire right cerebral hemisphere. JAMA 90: 2102, 1928

8. Burnam CF and Crowe SJ: The monel metal radium applicator designed for maximum use of hard beta rays in the treatment of nasopharyngeal hyperplastic lymphoid tissue. Miss Valley Med J 1945, p. 2

9. Crowe SJ: A new method for the study of the physiology and pathology of the ear. Milwaukee Proc Interstate Postgrad Med Assn North Am 1931, p. 185

10. Crowe SJ and Baylor JW: The prevention of deafness. JAMA 112: 585, 1939

11. Crowe SJ and Broyles EN: Carcinoma of the larynx and total laryngectomy. Ann Otol Rhinol Laryngol 47: 875, 1938

12. Crowe SJ and Burnam CF: Recognition, treatment and prevention of hearing impairment in children. Ann Otol Rhinol Laryngol 50: 15, 1941

13. Crowe SJ and Guild SR: Impaired hearing for high tones. Acta Otolaryngol 26: 138, 1938

14. Crowe SJ and Scarff JE: Experimental production of lung abscess in the dog. Int Surg Dig 3: 323, 1927

15. Crowe SJ and Walzl EM: Irradiation of hyperplastic lymphoid tissue in the nasopharynx. JAMA 134: 124, 1947

16. Guild SR: Nasopharyngeal irradiation and hearing acuity—A follow-up study of children. The Laryngoscope 60: 55, 1950

17. Guild SR: Edward McColgan Walzl, 1910–1950. Anat Rec 109: 554, 1951

18. Guild SR, Crowe SJ, Bunch CC and Polvogt LM: Correlations of differences in the density of innervation of the organ of Corti with differences in the acuity of hearing, including evidence as to the location in the human cochlea of the receptors for certain tones. Acta Otolaryngol 15: 269, 1931

19. Heuer GJ and Dunn JR: Experimental pneumonectomy. Bull Johns Hopkins Hosp 31: 32, 1920

20. Hughson W and Crowe SJ: Experimental investigation of the physiology of the ear. Acta Otolaryngol 18: 291, 1933

21. MacCready PB and Crowe SJ: Tuberculosis of the tonsils and adenoids. Am J Dis Child 27: 113, 1924

22. Marshall EK Jr. and Walzl EM: On the cyanosis from sulfanilamide. Bull Johns Hopkins Hosp 61: 140, 1937

23. Park EA: Dr. Crowe, the man. Memorial Program for Samuel James Crowe, 1883–1955. On the occasion of the biennial meeting, The Johns Hopkins Medical and Surgical Association, March 1, 1957

24. Polvogt LM: Histologic variations in the middle and inner ears of patients with normal hearing. Arch Otolaryngol 23: 48, 1936

25. Proctor DF: Irradiation for the elimination of nasopharyngeal lymphoid tissue. Arch Otolaryngol 43: 473, 1946

26. Proctor DF and Willard WR: Washington County (Maryland) Program for the prevention of deafness in children. Arch Otolaryngol 43: 462, 1946

27. Proctor DF, Polvogt LM, and Crowe SJ: Irradiation of the lymphoid tissue in diseases of the upper respiratory tract. Bull Johns Hopkins Hosp 83: 383, 1948

28. Richter CP: Electrical skin resistance. Arch Neurol Psychiatr 19: 488, 1928

29. Rienhoff WE and Broyles EN: The surgical treatment of carcinoma of the lung. JAMA 103: 1121, 1934

30. Walzl EM: Effect of chemicals on cochlear potentials. Am J Physiol 125: 688, 1939

31. Walzl EM: Representation of the cochlea in the cerebral cortex. The Laryngoscope 57: 778, 1947

32. Walzl EM and Bordley JE: Effect of small lesions of the organ of Corti on cochlear potentials. Am J Physiol 135: 351, 1942

33. Walzl EM and Woolsey CN: Cortical auditory areas of the monkey as determined by electrical excitation of nerve fibers in the osseous spiral lamina and by click stimulation. Fed Proc 2: 52, 1943

34. Walzl EM and Woolsey CN: Effects of cochlear lesions on click responses in the auditory cortex of the cat. Bull Johns Hopkins Hosp 79: 309, 1946

35. Walzl EM and Broyles EN: Report of postoperative course of subperichondral total laryngectomies. Ann Otol 57: 686, 1948

36. Walzl EM and Mountcastle V: Projection of vestibular nerve to cerebral cortex of the cat. Am J Physiol 159: 595, 1949

37. Willard WR and Proctor DF: Results and problems after four years of a conservation of hearing program. Am J Public Health 38: 1424, 1948

38. Woolsey CN: Dedication of the workshop to the memory of Edwin McColgan Walzl. *In* Physiology of the Auditory System, Sachs MB, Ed. Baltimore: National Educational Consultants, 1971

39. Woolsey CN and Walzl EM: Topical projection of nerve fibers from local regions of the cochlea to the cerebral cortex of the cat. Bull Johns Hopkins Hosp 71: 315, 1942

8.

The Department of Physiological Chemistry: Its Historical Evolution

The original plan for the "Medical Department" of the Johns Hopkins University included the teaching of chemistry to medical students under the auspices of the Department of Chemistry. The first University announcement listed the head of that department, Ira Remsen, as Professor of Chemistry in the roster of the medical faculty. With the opening of the medical school in 1893, however, this original plan of teaching the preclinical subjects was modified, and the teaching of physiological chemistry was entrusted to the professional school (Medical Department).

As William Mansfield Clark pointed out, physiological chemistry was given a unique position in this new school. The reasons for this were adequately stated by William H. Welch in 1894: "Physiological chemistry means much more than what is usually taught in our medical schools as medicinal chemistry, which includes little more than the chemical analysis of certain fluids of the body for diagnostic purposes." He expressed full approval of Hoppe-Seyler's statement: "I cannot understand how in this present day a physician can recognize, follow in their course, and suitably treat diseases of the stomach and alimentary tract, of the blood, liver, kidneys and urinary passages, and the different forms of poisoning; how he can suitably regulate the diet in these and in constitutional diseases, without knowledge of the methods of physiological chemistry. . . ." Welch further remarked: "When studying chemistry, it should be done with the object of learning the general principles." Thus, in general, the effort was made to keep the Medical Department more than just nominally a part of the University. ". . . Ideals of the University," Welch said, "must inspire the whole life and activities of the medical department." These ideals were to permeate the clinical department where

Reprinted from the *Johns Hopkins Medical Journal* **139**: 257, 1976.

medicine would be treated as "one of the natural sciences."

These thoughts were the basis of the guiding principles set down in the medical school's catalog in the early phase: "The medical art should rest upon a suitable preliminary education and upon a thorough training in the underlying medical sciences." Chemistry was made an important member of the "underlying medical sciences" by imposing an unusual entrance requirement and by making physiological chemistry a prerequisite to the study of clinical subjects.

The instruction in physiological chemistry was placed "under the charge of Dr. John J. Abel, Professor of Pharmacology, with the aid of an assistant." Its placement in the Department of Pharmacology broke an historical tradition that had made the subject the foster child of physiology. It is particularly important that the Hopkins arrangement entrusted the teaching to John J. Abel. Abel had been under the influence of a number of German investigators, who, although trained in the general field of medicine, had acquired an expertise in chemistry and were devoted to fundamental work in that subject. This influence, and Abel's own appreciation of the role of chemistry in the development of the scientific basis of medicine, led him to give this science its full measure of importance. He wanted to avoid the limitation of the purely "analytic school" and the subordinate place of chemistry suggested by the term "chemical physiology." Abel's attitude is undoubtedly reflected in Walter Jones' advertisement for an assistant that he was seeking in 1925, some 35 years later: "We want a man who has a Ph.D. degree, who has teaching ability as well as research ability and who is well grounded in the fundamentals of chemistry. Of course, it is desirable that he should also have had a training in physiological chemistry and the biological sciences but he must be a chemist primarily."

Since pharmacology had been designated a second-year subject in the curriculum when the school opened in 1893, Abel, with his first assistant, Dr. Thomas B. Aldrich, was able to handle the introductory course in chemistry. When the first course in pharmacology was given the following year, Abel turned over the instruction in chemistry to Aldrich. In addition there was a spatial separation of the work; chemistry being left for a time in the old Pathological Building, and pharmacology going with anatomy to the newly built (1894) Women's Fund Memorial Building until chemistry and pharmacology were reassembled in the "Old" Physiology Building in 1898.

The order of arrival of those who assisted Professor Abel and were designated as Assistants in Physiological Chemistry were: Thomas B. Aldrich (1893–1899), Edwin S. Faust (1895–1896), Walter Jones (1896–1908), and Arthur S. Loevenhart (1905–1908).

WALTER JONES—THE FIRST PROFESSOR OF PHYSIOLOGICAL CHEMISTRY

When Walter Jones came to assist in the teaching of physiological chemistry in 1896, there was, as mentioned, no separate department for that subject, although it was taught as a distinct discipline. The list of Jones' successive titles at Johns Hopkins is worth recording: 1896–1898, Assistant in Physiological Chemistry; 1898–1899, Assistant in Physiological Chemistry and Toxicology; 1899–1902, Associate in Physiological Chemistry and Toxicology; 1902–1908, Associate Professor of Physiological Chemistry and Toxicology; (1908, Department of Physiological Chemistry established), 1908–1923, Professor of Physiological Chemistry; 1923–1927, De Lamar Professor of Physiological Chemistry. Thus, when Jones was made full Professor in 1908 the Department of Physiological Chemistry was created. (Clark points out that the choice of Professorship of Physiological Chemistry, which later received the benefactor Captain De Lamar's name as one of several means of commemoration, gave recognition to De Lamar's acquaintance with one branch of chemistry and to the specific part of his will that referred to his interest in nutrition.)

Jones' assistants in the teaching of physiological chemistry were: Arthur H. Koelker (1908–1911), Eli Kennerly Marshall, Jr. (1911–1914), D. Wright Wilson (1914–1922), Annabella E. Richards (substituting for Wilson, 1918–1919, during his leave on military service), Mary Van Rensselaer Buell (1921–1930), Marie E. Perkins (1921–1927), Lawrence Wesson (1922–1925), William Hoffman (1922–1927) and Herbert O. Calvery (1925–1927).

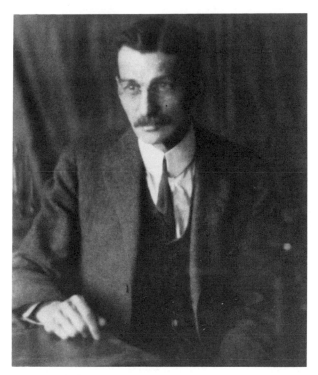

Fig 1.   Walter Jones

EARLY LIFE

Walter Jones was a native of Baltimore. He was born on April 28, 1865, two weeks after the death of President Lincoln. This was a sad period for Baltimore as described by Gerald Johnson of the *Baltimore Sun*: "Driven by internal dissension, drawn by affection in one direction and by interest in another, suspected and reviled by both sides, exposed to all the horrors of war without enjoying its fierce exultation, sharing the dangers, the losses, and the woe of both North and South, but never with any part in the triumphs of either, Maryland was trampled under the feet of both contestants and emerged beaten and broken." Perhaps after his exposure to this unfortunate period, Jones grew up into a man who felt the world to be "out of joint."

Jones' forebears were Marylanders through several generations, his paternal ancestors having been dwellers on the Eastern shore of the Chesapeake Bay and his maternal ancestors on the Western shore. His family took pride in having descended from Welsh ancestry and from early settlers of Maryland and Virginia, but it was characteristic of Walter Jones that he was quite indifferent to his ancestral history. The most famous of his collateral ancestors was Colonel John Jones who fought in the War of Independence. Levin Jones, Walter's father, left the Eastern shore and settled in Baltimore where he became a successful ship chandler.

The following quotation is from William Mansfield Clark's excellent biographical sketch of Walter Jones:

"Those who knew Walter Jones used thread of gold for the warp of the tapestry that they weave on the loom of memory. They float the golden warp for the figures of the eloquent teacher, the keen investigator and the kind friend. Because the unique personality made extraordinary impressions, every weaver uses highly colored, homespun yarn for the wefts of his tapestry."

The only things left as records of the career of this unusual man were an incomplete set of reprints, a list thereof, and three diplomas. It was his habit to tear up a letter while he still mused upon its contents. He wrote very few extensive letters and when after many years he had a secretary he was known to go to the typist of another department in order to be certain that the carbon copy would not be filed. It seems quite probable that much of the mischief that he indulged in so gayly each day was his own peculiar way of telling people not to take too seriously the depth of his feeling about many things that he felt obliged to take quite seriously.

As Clark points out, the tradition of the family seems to have established that the youngest member had the inalienable right to be mischievous. As the 13th child, Walter was clearly then in a favorable position to claim this right. No occasion during his career was so oppressed with dignity as to suppress his sense of humor; no personage so high that he would not dare to banter. His greatest opportunity for mischief arose from his ability to articulate. He was a brilliant conversationalist and yet so forthright that he said of himself, "When I talk the loudest, I know the least." He could be frank to the verge of offense and yet he had a student say of him, "One always knew where one stood with Walter Jones and that was a great comfort."

Jones had talent in many areas. He was active in sports, a good tennis player, and "one of the best fancy ice skaters in Baltimore, the envy of the younger ones as he performed in Sumalt's ice pond." He was an ardent lacrosse fan and a vigorous critic of the players not only in their contests but also in their routine practice. He played the piano well enough to afford entertainment and collected records of classical music which he knew well. Baltimore in those days offered many opportunities in this direction that Jones always took advantage of. On one occasion he addressed a class as follows: "The usual recitation is scheduled at 4 o'clock tomorrow. Those of you who are uncivilized do not know that the Boston Symphony Orchestra is to give a special concert at that hour and so you will report here promptly. I

shall not be here!"

Jones' early education was obtained partly in small, neighborhood private schools and partly in public schools. His sister Anne, who followed his studies keenly, once said that she had attained a college education through Walter's eyes. During his brilliant career as a student, Walter's image of a lesson was always clear as attested to by college classmates who heard him recite. When he became a mature professor he expected the same of his pupils. They could laugh at his extravagance while feeling the significance of his exclamation to a forgetful student: "Even the Baltimore streetcar conductors know the amino acids!"

Jones entered the City College of Baltimore in 1879 and completed the five-year course in the spring of 1884. The following autumn, he entered the Johns Hopkins University and took the courses then known as Group 4 with chemistry and physics predominating in the last two years. He received his B.A. in 1888 and won a university scholarship for the year 1888–1889. Work for his dissertation was done under Professor Ira Remsen and he was granted his Ph.D. in June 1891.

On September 1, 1891, Walter Jennings Jones and Grace Crary Clarke were married in Ocean Grove, New Jersey. A short time later they settled in Springfield, Ohio where Jones was Acting Professor of Natural Science in Wittenberg College. This was only a temporary assignment and after a year the young couple returned to Baltimore where on August 13, 1892 their only child, Marion Eleanor, was born. In September 1892 Jones went to Purdue University as Professor of Analytical Chemistry. He was apparently not happy there and after a few years returned to Baltimore without a job, taking up work under Remsen as a "fellow by courtesy" for the year 1895–1896, after which followed in March 1896, his appointment as Assistant in Physiological Chemistry.

PIONEER IN THE STUDY OF NUCLEIC ACIDS

After Jones had been at Hopkins for a few years, Abel advised him to study under Albrecht Kossel in Germany. Jones was receptive to the idea, but financial difficulty stood in the way. Appreciating this, Abel had an inspiration one day when a sheriff appeared with the organs of a woman suspected of having been poisoned. While Abel was loathe to have his laboratory burdened with such cases, he arranged to have Jones take this one. When Jones had identified strychnine, he went to the distant town with his evidence, eventually testified, and used his fee for his passage to Europe.

Jones' visit to Germany was a short one lasting only from June to December, 1899, but during that short time he accumulated the data for two papers and became so inspired by Kossel that he devoted himself exclusively thereafter to Kossel's interest, the study of the nucleic acids. In Germany he was welcomed by Dr. P. A. Levene, later of the Rockefeller Institute. Levene, himself a pioneer in nucleic acid chemistry, recalled: "My memory pictures the arrival one day of a lean, tallish American of rather indefinite age somewhat forlorn in a foreign land which he was visiting for the first time . . . I am certain Jones was not a man to permit a day to pass without leaving some impression on it . . . I remember clearly that as soon as Jones discovered that English was the dominating tongue . . . he dropped his shyness and was ready for argument, great enthusiasm and force of expression revealed themselves soon and, before long, I became a victim of them . . . So the friendship of Jones and myself began with an argument and continued in the same way for many years for we were warm friends regardless of our temporary scientific disagreements." It was in the year of Jones' migration to Marburg that the long series of papers on nucleic acid chemistry that constitute the greater part of his contribution to science began.

Investigation of the nucleic acids started with the classic work of Friederich Miescher. While a student under the anatomist His, Miescher became interested in foraging beyond the range of the microscope in search of a chemical description of the cell nucleus and selected Hoppe–Seyler's laboratory for his work. He began by digesting the more easily attacked parts of pus cells in order to isolate the nuclear material; by this and other methods, he obtained a powdered substance which was rich in nuclear material and which had chemical properties quite unlike anything that had previously been described. Miescher called the characteristic constituent of this material nuclein. In 1869 he submitted a paper on this material to the *Zeitschrift für Physiologische Chemie* of which Hoppe–Seyler was the editor. Hoppe–Seyler held up publication until his students had confirmed Miescher's observations by separating nucleins from various sources. Shortly thereafter, Miescher transferred his activities to Basel where he recognized the opportunity presented by the Rhine salmon. During their ascent up the river these salmon developed their reproductive organs enormously and the males were a huge source of material, since their spermatic fluid consisted largely of a suspension of spermatozoa, the "heads" of which are largely nuclei. Miescher, of course, was working with what later proved to be deoxyribonucleic acid (DNA).

Jones' mentor, Albrecht Kossel, was one of the numerous investigators who entered the field following Miescher's pioneering work. In the period 1879 to 1886 Kossel was the first to identify purines among the products of the hydrolysis of nuclein and to recognize their source in the part later to be called nucleic acid rather than in the protamine moiety. He was also the first to recognize a pyrimidine in the hydrolysate. With the identification of purines and pyrimidines in the hydrolysates of nuclein, the story of the nucleic acids became linked with that of uric acid which had been more than a century in the making.

In order to put Jones' work in proper perspective, it should be emphasized that he found a literature full of discrepancies. The material he had to work with was a very complex mixture of macromolecules; it was difficult to prepare nucleic acids sufficiently pure for refined analysis. The hydrolysates did not lend themselves well to the usual physicochemical tests of homogeneity and molecular composition. P. H. Levene later said of this field of chemical study: "It is singular that in the history of the chemistry of nucleic acids each new conclusion was reached by a path of disagreements, controversies, and errors, and that error often led to progress."

Jones' first contribution came in 1899 when he prepared a bromine derivative of thymine and confirmed Kossel's opinion that thymine was distinct from 4-methyl uracil. These early studies revealed the presence of oxypurines as well as aminopurines in tissue hydrolysates. Four were found of basic importance: guanine, adenine, xanthine and hypoxanthine. The obvious problem was the relation of these four purines to true nucleic acids.

One of the first to work with Jones at Johns Hopkins on the nucleic acids was George H. Whipple, who later received the Nobel Prize for his work on the nutritional aspects of blood regeneration. As their basic materials Jones and Whipple studied residues of the adrenal gland which Abel was using in his studies of epinephrine. From their work (1902) they drew the conclusion that the nucleins of the suprarenal glands of sheep and beef are similar to those of the pancreas and that each yields adenine and guanine but no demonstrable amounts of other purines. Later Jones surmised that the presence of xanthine and hypoxanthine arose from deamination of the aminopurines. In 1904 Jones found that while guanine, adenine and thymine could be identified among the products of hydrolysis of thymus nucleic acid if acid hydrolysis was used, autolysis or self-digestion of the gland resulted in the formation of xanthine and hypoxanthine. The tissues were then examined for deaminating enzymes—guanase was found by Jones and Partridge in 1904, and adenase by Jones and Winternitz in 1905. This work on the deaminating enzymes was summarized by Jones in the following diagram:

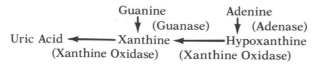

If a solid arrow represents the indicated enzymatic activity and a dotted arrow represents its absence, the distribution of these enzymes may be shown as follows:

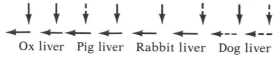

Much of this work was done in collaboration with Dr. Charles Austrian. That these enzymes were formed during embryonic growth was shown by Jones and Austrian in 1907 and by Jones and deAngula in 1908.

Levene and Jacobs then demonstrated (1909) the order of linkage in inosinic acid to be: hypoxanthine-pentose-phosphoric acid. By acid hydrolysis they obtained a nucleoside, discovering its pentose to be the hitherto unknown d-ribose (Levene and Jacobs, 1909–1912). They extended these methods to yeast nucleic acids and obtained the four nucleosides: guanosine, adenosine, cytidine and uridine. Thus the evidence at that stage indicated that yeast nucleic acid was composed of the residues of four nucleotides in which the orders of linkage were:

guanine-ribose-phosphoric acid
adenine-ribose-phosphoric acid } Purine nucleotides

cytosine-ribose-phosphoric acid
uracil-ribose-phosphoric acid } Pyrimidine nucleotides

Jones continued work in this area, and in his lectures he often emphasized that an enzymatic action upon a specific group might depend upon the mode of linkage of the group carrier with some other residue. He anticipated in some measure what was to be shown subsequently regarding phosphorylated metabolites in general. Thus, Levene and Jones were to a large degree responsible for working out the scheme of enzymatic degradation of nucleic acids.

The sequence of enzymatic activities leading from nucleic acids to uric acid (in man) clearly has a bearing upon the problem of gout. Jones recognized that the clarification of the enzymatic processes in man was an important goal. The few articles in which Jones touched upon this subject are characteristically confined to items that could be discussed with available experimental data. This is a true mark of the man, because few other subjects had received more speculative treatment in medical circles. Osler of course was cautious as usual, and it was not until the 8th edition (1912) of his *Principles and Practice of Medicine* that the discussion of the etiology of gout included what chemical data were available up to that time.

In an article entitled "On the Threefold Physiological Origin of Uric Acid" Jones reviewed the enzymatic studies up to 1910 with particular reference to the subject of gout. He indicated that uric acid might arise from the degradation of ingested nucleic acid, from the hypoxanthine (or its precursor) of the muscle, or through a *de novo* synthesis of the purine ring. However, Jones, although an enthusiast on the subject of purine metabolism, continued to show restraint in his occasional writings on gout, a subject that for many years remained completely obscure. Later Jones' work was directed more specifically to the constitution of the nucleic acids and the polynucleotide structure comprising them. It is not possible here to detail the further chemical ventures of Jones and his co-workers in the nucleic acid field. However, his work was outstanding and laid solid groundwork for what was to follow in the meteoric rise in importance of the nucleic acids in biology. It is difficult to imagine what would have come to pass from Walter Jones' work if his illness had not cut short his own work and altered the staff in the department. He came close to touching grounds of research that had previously not been encountered—catalysis of phosphorylation and of oxidation-reduction, vitamins of the B group, and the structure of chromosomes.

Jones' monograph entitled *Nucleic Acids*, the first edition of which was published in 1914 and the second in 1920, remained for years the only comprehensive review of the subject in the English language. It provided a brief historical background and then discussed the chemistry of the known components of nucleic acids and their structures. Much attention was given to their enzymatic transformations, a field largely developed by Jones and his group.

JONES AS A TEACHER

Evidence indicates that Walter Jones was not only a student of medical education but also an inspiring teacher. He was not a propagandist for the evolving science of physiological chemistry, but he was a creator of one main area of the field. His department offered advanced courses which were intended for physicians in training, but it seems clear that very few enrolled in these courses. Only on very rare occasions was a graduate student accepted. Replying to an inquiry from Homewood of what he was doing for graduate students, Jones wrote in 1922: "Physiological chemistry . . . is treated exclusively as a medical subject and the entire resources of the department are devoted to medicine. No attempt is made to train men for philosophical degrees."

Jones was obviously an eloquent lecturer, as Robert P. Kennedy wrote: "Walter Jones' lectures both in classrooms and in private conversation were virile and impressive. No matter what sort of tirade his dissertation may have sounded like, his thoughts were logical, his expressions extremely accurate and if the listener was inclined to argue he was always worsted by a better piece of argumentative effort."

Jones was a stimulating teacher but not a soft one. For example, a student who poured the materials of his experiment down the sink with the explanation, "It didn't work the way the book said," would probably never forget the explosive remarks of the Professor: "My God, man, if you threw a brick out of the window and it went up instead of the way the books say, wouldn't you stick your head out?"

Jones had entered Hopkins as an organic chemist with no particular interest in medical affairs, without specific training in the evolving science of physiological chemistry, without recorded training even in biology, and he was valued initially and throughout his career primarily as an investigator. He nevertheless felt at home in the medical school not only because his teaching fit the declared scheme, but also because of one of the outstanding characteristics of university life in that period. Jones was distinctly a specialist and was honored as such. Americans at that period had been converted to an enthusiasm for research so intense that it swept aside didactic teaching and "book learning" in favor of direct demonstration and observation in the laboratory.

Knowledge in biochemistry was expanding so rapidly that many American teachers in the field were beginning to demand longer introductory courses. Jones would not be drawn into this controversy. Not only did he accept the plan for the shortened courses in all departments agreed upon at Johns Hopkins shortly before his retirement, but he also wrote as follows: "I should say that the time devoted in the medical curriculum to physiological chemistry depends to a considerable extent upon what portion of this subject is taken up in other departments on the borderline. I think the tendency is to teach clinical medicine in departments of physiological chemistry and this greatly lengthens the time allotted to the subject."

As one looks at the list of co-authors in Jones'

bibliography, it includes a number of members of the clinical departments. In the early years of the school the preclinical laboratories were centers of a good deal of research by members of the clinical staff. Later the introduction of the full-time system in clinical departments was accompanied by a more systematic organization of research in those departments, and the participation of clinicians in the types of investigations that were influenced by the points of view in the basic sciences measurably declined. The greater part of Jones' co-author list is made up of medical students, and their subsequent careers show him to have been a good judge of character. Of the 14 medical students and 4 graduate students who published with Jones, 9 obtained academic distinction by professorial rank; 1 later won the Nobel Prize. Thus, Jones selected wisely and contributed importantly to the training of those who later made this remarkable record.

In the autumn of 1923 Jones wrote of "a remarkable weariness in my left leg after walking a few blocks." It soon became evident that he was suffering from atherosclerosis with intermittent claudication. By January he was unable to meet his classes after the first lecture and appeared at the laboratory only to discuss general matters. He soon abandoned work entirely and retired in 1927.

In 1921 tentative plans had been made for a "new building for physiological chemistry." The necessity arose from the expanding work in the departments of physiology, pharmacology and physiological chemistry and the offices of the medical school administration, all housed in the old Physiology Building. Chemistry was confined to the attic. The hood available for students was so inadequately ventilated that adjustments of Kjeldahl digestions had to be made by rushing into the fume-filled room and out again for gasps of air. Every inch of space, including that under the eaves, was in use. Jones accepted the chairmanship of a committee on plans for the new building. However, nothing concrete was accomplished until after he retired.

The new Physiology Building opened in 1929 and Jones appeared, after an absence of years, to lunch with the new staff. As in the past, he led the course of the conversation and after lunch was taken to the laboratory that had been reserved for him. There he became for a moment his old self, sending the faithful Andy, the Department's diener, on trips for glassware and reagents. One day he disappeared, never to return to the laboratory. It was later learned that he had been overcome by a discouraging sense of ground lost and lack of energy. He died in Baltimore on February 28, 1935.

Jones had been elected to membership in the

National Academy of Sciences in 1918. He was President of the American Society of Biological Chemists in 1915 and 1916.

WILLIAM MANSFIELD CLARK

When Walter Jones retired in 1927, he was succeeded by William Mansfield Clark. Clark had previously received offers of appointment to a university chair, but he had always declined because "I had had no formal training in any of the subjects I was supposed to 'profess.'" He was notified of his appointment as director of the Department of Physiological Chemistry at Johns Hopkins without any preliminary consultation. A short time after his nomination to the Johns Hopkins faculty, he remarked to Abel that he "did not know, for example, the difference between the thymus and the thyroid glands and knew less of their function." Abel's reply was, "My dear boy, that is why we want you." Thus Clark accepted the appointment in spite of the fact that: "I had had no formal training in biochemistry, had an inadequate appreciation of the needs of medical students, and I inherited laboratory equipment and space totally deficient for my research and student instruction. I needed support desperately. It was given effectively. Funds were provided for equipment needed immediately. I was allowed to modify plans for a new building, and then everyone left me completely alone as a token of confidence." Clark was a scientist who, once he accepted a responsibility, tenaciously carried it out—a conclusion supported by his enrolling, shortly after his arrival in Baltimore, in the gross anatomy class and dissecting a cadaver along with the students to whom he would soon be teaching physiological chemistry.

During the 25 years that Clark served as head of the department, physiological chemistry developed into a major branch of chemistry. He was constantly faced with the problem, as were all teachers of biochemistry in medical schools, of what aspects of the subject to include in his course. He made a decision that would be expected of a sound and talented scientist: "To provide a basis on which the students could build, we should pick up the threads of thought in basic chemistry before weaving them into biochemistry . . . In the 1930's it was estimated that about half of the entering students had had inadequate instruction in those more elementary parts of physical chemistry that are involved in almost all parts of the science, and that are essential in a first approach to an understanding of matters of clinical importance." Clark was essentially a physical chemist so that he was ideally equipped to carry out this approach.

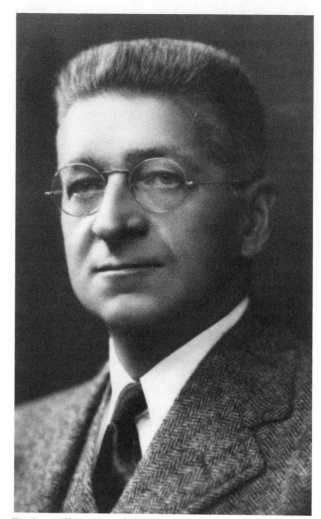

Fig 2.   William Mansfield Clark

Mansfield Clark became an excellent teacher, always insisting that the student must acquire a sound knowledge of fundamental principles. As commented on by Philip Bard in a Minute prepared for the Advisory Board of the School of Medicine at the time of Clark's retirement: "To some students he appeared at times stern, one who demanded precision and definition, for his approach was necessarily a quantitative one. Many students with an insufficient background in chemistry, especially quantitative chemistry, had a hard time in his course. But he was as fair to such individuals as he was encouraging to the good students. He liked the students and they, conscious of his high scientific repute and integrity, admired and respected him . . . There can be no doubt that he was a great force for good teaching in this medical school."

THE EARLY YEARS

What was the background of this brilliant and conscientious man? He was the son of James Starr Clark, an 1850 graduate of King's College (now Columbia University) and an Episcopal clergyman who established and administered a succession of boys' schools. His son received his elementary education at one of these, Trinity School in Privoli, New York, founded in 1867 and conducted on military principles. William Mansfield Clark ultimately obtained a scholarship at the Hotchkiss School in Connecticut, where he excelled in English, was a member of the debating team, and became an expert in gymnastics. It was during his period at Williams College that he became interested in chemistry when his teacher, Professor Leverette Mears, suggested that he read Remsen's textbook in preference to a more elementary text used by the others in the class. He received an M.A. in 1908 and was accepted as a graduate student at the Johns Hopkins University by Professor Harmon Morse. In the Department of Chemistry, Clark worked on the osmotic pressure of cane sugar solutions and received his Ph.D. in 1910. His period at Hopkins at this time, however, was not particularly happy as Remsen's lectures had lost much of their earlier stimulation and Morse, while an excellent experimenter interested in the study of osmotic pressure, was a very dull lecturer.

During his college years Clark spent the summers working in laboratories of the U. S. Bureau of Fisheries at Woods Hole. When a chemical research laboratory was set up there, Clark was employed as an assistant. Carl Alsberg, a physiological chemist from Harvard in charge of the laboratory, was the one who first turned Clark's attention to biochemistry. In 1909 D. D. Van Slyke became head of the laboratory and an incident occurred which had an important influence on Mansfield Clark's later career. At the start of the summer session Van Slyke became ill. Clark, knowing that his chief would need accurate standard dye solutions on his return to the laboratory, prepared a solution of redistilled ammonia and titrated it with standard acid. To make certain of the titer, he tried the equivalence point with every indicator dye available, as well as with a number of histological stains, and discovered to his bewilderment that no two dyes yielded the same result. Another puzzle which was to provide an important stimulus to his future research interests was a question regarding the behavior of phenolphthalein that was asked him during his oral examination for his Ph.D. at Hopkins. The question gave rise to a disagreement between two of his examiners, which, to his delight, took up a large portion of the examination period.

GOVERNMENT SERVICE

After obtaining his Ph.D., Clark's first appointment was in the research laboratories of the dairy division of the U. S. Department of Agriculture. When he reported for work in 1910, he independently began a study of the composition of gases in the characteristic "eyes" of cheese. Clark became an expert in the design and construction of special apparatus for the manipulation and analysis of the gases produced by bacterial fermentation, and his techniques were valuable to his chief, who was investigating the bacteria found in milk. One of the special tests used in the examination of the culture solutions was a titration with alkali. It was while he was concerned with the problems of acid development in cultures and in milk products that he remembered the work done by a fellow graduate student at Hopkins with the hydrogen electrode. He had never discussed the problem with the student and knew only what he had read in a text of physical chemistry. Undertaking a literature search, he came across the basic papers of Sørensen, immediately understood the importance of this area, and began his own systematic studies.

Clark's first publication in this field came in 1915 in the *Journal of Medical Research*. It concerned the procedure of adding alkali to cow's milk for infant feeding with the alleged purpose of "correcting the high acidity of cow's milk." The technique was based on the fact that more alkali was needed to titrate cow's milk to neutrality to phenolphthalein than was needed by human milk. Clark showed that the hydrogen ion concentration of the two kinds of milk was essentially the same, the difference being attributable to the high salt and protein content of cow's milk. It was in this paper that Clark used for the first time the term "buffer" and the symbol "pH." His conclusion was that the practice of adding alkali to cow's milk was based upon incorrect principles.

About this time Clark began his collaboration with H. A. Lubs, an excellent organic chemist. Their studies showed that the organisms of the coli-aerogenes group, which had been differentiated by the ratio of carbon dioxide to hydrogen in the gas produced, could be more easily separated by measurements of the hydrogen ion concentration of the culture medium with the electrode, or by means of an indicator. For many years the "Clark and Lubs methyl-red test" was used in the investigation of the organisms of this group.

Clark and Lubs then set out to study all of the indicators that they could find. Clark obtained samples of phenolsulphonphthalein and several of the derivatives which had been studied by Professor

Acree at Johns Hopkins. Lubs prepared additional homologues. They ultimately selected some 13 dyes useful as indicators which covered essentially the whole range of pH and also were quite reliable in the presence of salts or of proteins. The description of these indicators was published in 1915 as was the description of the widely known Clark hydrogen electrode vessel. This very productive team then began the study of buffer mixtures and in a paper published in 1916 they described the phthalate, phosphate and borate mixtures which became standard. The next year a comprehensive paper appeared on the colorimetric determination of hydrogen ion concentration and its application in bacteriology. This 106-page paper was soon in wide demand. It was suggested first that the publisher reprint the paper, but ultimately Clark brought together the broader aspects of the field. What emerged was the first edition in 1920 of his famous book, *The Determination of Hydrogen Ions*. The original paper had only 160 references, while the first edition of the book had over 1200 titles in the bibliography. The second edition, which appeared in 1923, contained almost 2000. Clark's modesty in view of the success of the book was typical; he indicated that anyone who took the trouble to search the literature could have found what was in the book.

Vickery, in his memoir of William Mansfield Clark for the National Academy of Sciences, states that Clark's interest in the measurement of oxidation-reduction potentials was aroused first during a chance conversation in 1915 with L. J. Gillespie. According to Vickery, Gillespie had set up a calomel half-cell against an electrode of mercury overlaid by a culture of bacteria and had found that the mercury electrode became progressively more negative as the culture grew. He recognized that he was observing a reduction potential. Clark saw immediately that this technique offered great promise in the study of the differential reduction of dyes which was often seen in cultures of bacteria. As he stated a number of years later, "... There was hope that a method had been revealed whereby it might be possible to accumulate *quantitative* data and, step by step, build up exact evidence upon one of the manifold aspects of the general problem." Clark encountered considerable difficulty with the bacteria in these studies and the work with biological systems was stopped so that a comprehensive study could be done of the oxidation-reduction potential of various dyes in equilibrium with their reduction products. Clark had a great advantage over other workers in the field because he was familiar with the use of buffer systems. All of his experiments were carried out at constant pH. This resulted in stable and reproducible potentials and the observations "lined up beautifully on a diagram like nothing seen before. I was elated. I recall saying to myself: 'This general subject will keep me busy for years.' It did." The preliminary results of these studies were published in 1920 in a short paper concerned with indigo sulfonate and methylene blue. In the introduction to this paper, Clark wrote, "So far as the writer is aware such indicators have not been regarded in their possible relation to oxidation-reduced potentials in a manner analogous to the well-systematized relation of hydrogen ion indicators to hydrogen–electrode potentials. That such a relationship if established will aid in the interpretation of various biochemical phenomena will be evident, but the significance of such data is of broader scope, because the efforts that have previously been made to bring organic compounds within the range of potential measurements have yielded few data of value." Thus Clark was well on the path of his life work.

Clark became chief of the Division of Chemistry of the Hygienic Laboratory of the U. S. Public Health Service in 1920. At this time he conducted his systematic study of the oxidation–reduction potentials of dye systems. He published a remarkable series of papers in the *Public Health Reports* between 1923 and 1926. There was no restriction on space so that Clark was able to present a comprehensive and detailed description of the theory of oxidation–reduction potentials. In a review paper which he published in 1925, Clark commented on the significance of these observations as follows: "With a convenient method of formulating the somewhat complex relations . . . we shall not only gain a better understanding of how it is that accurate data on organic systems are now being obtained, but we shall also see that the potentiometric methods are furnishing precise data on free energy relations, opening new methods of analyses, broadening the methods of determining hydrogen ion concentration, aiding in the solutions of problems in structural chemistry, furnishing valuable data on the effects of substitution, and suggesting new approaches to fundamental problems of biological oxidation–reduction." It was on the basis of this outstanding work that Clark was invited to Johns Hopkins.

RESEARCH AT JOHNS HOPKINS

During his period at Hopkins, Clark devoted the major portion of his time to the study of the metalloporphyrins—compounds concerned with respiration (cytochrome), with the transport of oxygen, and with many enzyme processes in the living cell. He believed each system must be characterized by a certain electron-escaping tendency. Clark outlined the problem in a lecture given in 1952: "What modification of the electron escaping tendency exhibited by the prosthetic system follows the incorporation of oxidant and reductant in complexes? . . . Suppose the complexes form reversibly so that in the same solution there will be uncombined prosthetic compound in both oxidized and reduced states, uncombined ligand, and both oxidized and reduced complexes. Suppose also that these components can serve as a proton donor or as a proton acceptor in one or another region of pH. How shall we formulate the equilibrium states of so complex a system in such a way as to make them subject to experimental evaluation?'' Clark recognized that more stable substances would be required for the experimental studies although in the living cell a specific protein frequently plays the role of coordinating substance with the metalloporphyrin. He thus chose to examine the coordination compounds of a number of available metalloporphyrins with such bases as pyridine, nicotine, cyanide and various imidazoles. He had no practical application in mind and was entirely concerned with elucidating the general principles which control the interactions among such components. This is why it was necessary in his view to use stable reproducible model systems. As Vickery points out, Clark's mastery of the mathematical complexities involved in the theory of the subject was clearly shown in his paper published in the *Journal of Biological Chemistry* in 1940. "Here the theoretical relations were described in detail in the form of a series of 16 propositions dealing with the 5 types of reactions which can occur. He derived a general equation for the potentials which contained five logarithmetic terms. In addition he derived an equation for the use of spectrophotometric data in determining various constants. Following this, he outlined the simplification that could be made so that graphical methods could be used in analyzing the data. The depth of his intellectual capacity and knowledge of his subject was evident, and the experimental difficulties which he encountered were formidable enough to have thoroughly discouraged any less qualified individual. However, he was able by manipulation of the necessary equations to devise a mathematical or graphical test which led to a judgment. Clark went on to develop a concept that underlies all of his works, the idea, based upon the smooth behavior of the electrode even in complex systems, of what he called a chemical continuum.'' Proton donors and their conjugate acceptors form an acid-base continuum. A more complex system that contains potential oxidants and reductants constitutes an oxidation-reduction acid base continuum involving electron and proton transfers, and sometimes the incorporation of oxygen. Further there are cases where the oxidant, the reductant, or both enter into the processes of coordination. Where such still more complex systems occur in nature, there is an at least four dimensional continuum. The experimentalist works on this continuum by a series of zigs and zags since he must control all parameters save the one under investigation. Nature is under no such restriction. As Clark put it when considering the degrees of freedom opened to the metabolism of the amoeba,

> I once met a lively young cell
> Whom I then proceeded to tell
> Of pH, electrons,
> P wiggles and protons;
> To which he replied:
> "Go to ____."

(Clark was class poet at the Hotchkiss School.)

WAR SERVICE

Mansfield Clark made valuable contributions to the national defense in both world wars. In 1917 he was faced with the problem of how to make casein for the glues which were essential in assembling the plywood used in the wings and other parts of the aircraft of that period. Vickery describes his work on this subject as follows: "Most of the casein was imported from Argentina, American-made casein being rejected by the glue manufacturers on grounds of lack of uniformity. At the time, Clark was fresh from his studies of the papers of Sørensen and knew that proteins passed through a minimum of solubility at their iso-electric points. Accordingly, when supervising the precipitation of casein from the skim-milk in a huge vat, he insisted that the addition of acid should be continued until the pH of the whey reached the iso-electric point of casein in spite of the fact that all of the casein appeared to have separated long before this point was reached. As a result the casein aggregated into large firm granular curds which could be easily washed free from the whey and secured in a reproducible form. This material was entirely satisfactory for glue manufacturers." Thus, he provided a simple solution to a difficult problem to which at the time few if any young chemists in America could have found the answer so readily.

His participation in World War II was much more on the administrative side. He was a member of the Executive Committee of the National Academy of Sciences and from 1941 to 1946 was chairman of the Division of Chemistry and Chemical Technology of the National Research Council. Their investigations dealt with the physiological action of toxic agents which were a matter of great concern during the early part of the war. Later they were called upon to examine the purity of atabrine of domestic origin, since at that time toxicity was thought to be due to impurities. The importance of research on malaria led to the formation under the Division of an office of information known as the Survey of Antimalarial Drugs. An important function was the screening for antimalarial use of the enormous numbers of drugs submitted by manufacturers, as well as the organization of new synthetic work on drugs. Clark was also for a period chairman of the Academy committee on biological warfare.

William Mansfield Clark retired in 1952, becoming De Lamar Emeritus Professor and Research Professor of Chemistry. He moved to the Remsen laboratory on the Homewood campus and during the next several years finished the writing of his last book entitled *Oxidation–Reduction Potentials of Organic Systems* which appeared in 1960.

During his distinguished career Clark received many honors. He was President of the Society of American Bacteriologists in 1933 and of the American Chemical Society in 1933 and 1934. He was elected to the National Academy of Sciences in 1928 and to the American Philosophical Society in 1939. He received numerous honorary degrees and was awarded the Nichols Medal of the New York Section of the American Society in 1936, the Borden Award in 1944, and the Passano Award in 1957.

Bill Clark had a wonderful sense of humor and was a delightful companion. In 1910 he married Rose Willard Goddard and two daughters were born while they were living in Washington. He was an ardent golfer and a gardener. It is a measure of the man that a scientist who had phenomenal knowledge in a very complex field of chemistry still listed his two holes-in-one as among the important highlights of his life. He was interested in unusual varieties of flowers and shrubs and, of course, used only their scientific names.

Clark always had a keen sense of history. In his final book he began his account of oxidation with a discussion of Lavoisier, Priestley and Scheele; he defined ion, anode, cathode, electrolyte, and correlative terms by quoting Faraday, who had invented the words. His delightful sense of humor came out in a footnote which stated that he had heard that "one librarian classified the author's book on hydrogen ions under Greek mythology." His books were always embellished with quotations chosen from many sources. One chapter on techniques carried the following Turkish proverb: "Don't descend into the well with a rotten rope." Bill Clark never did. He came close "to the ideal of what a professor in an American university should be." Modest and unassuming though he was, his strength of character, his total mastery of his subject and enthusiasm for it, his independence of thought, and his personal mag-

netism impressed themselves on all who came into contact with him.

In the words of Philip Bard, "He was worthy to walk with the great founders of the medical school, Welch, Howell, Abel and Halsted."

ALBERT LESTER LEHNINGER

No less distinguished than his two predecessors is the third De Lamar Professor of Physiological Chemistry, Albert Lester Lehninger. Born in Connecticut, he received his undergraduate education at Wesleyan University. He had entered with the plan to become an English major, devoting himself to the writing of stories and poetry, but soon became more interested in chemistry. In the late 1930's he first heard from his teacher, Ross Fortner, Jr., about the fascinating developments in the new field of biochemistry. Otto Warburg was then unfolding his monumental work on the "Wasserstoffübertragende Fermente" in Berlin, and Hans Krebs was doing equally exciting work on the tricarboxylic acid cycle in Sheffield. Lehninger was intrigued by these developments, and in his senior year decided to embark upon a combined career of medicine and biochemistry. He chose as the ideal institution for his graduate work the University of Wisconsin, where some of the most important discoveries in the field of nutrition and biochemistry were then being made. He completed his Ph.D. dissertation in 1942 under Edgar Witzemann on ketone body oxidation, but the discovery of oxidative phosphorylation, which occurred in the late 1930s, seized his imagination and from then on the whole field of capture and transduction in cells was never far from his interests. Soon, however, because of the exigencies of World War II, he became involved full-time in the Plasma Fractionation Program at the University of Wisconsin, which was being masterminded in Boston by E. J. Cohn and his associates. Lehninger's assignment in this program was to modify plasma globulins to be useful as plasma extenders. This work came to a halt when it was discovered that the globulins themselves had valuable therapeutic properties as sources of antibodies.

In 1945 Lehninger, then an Instructor in Physiological Chemistry at the University of Wisconsin, moved to the University of Chicago where he was appointed Assistant Professor of Biochemistry in the Department of Surgery. He was closely associated with the laboratory of Dr. Charles Huggins (which was later to be known as the Ben May Laboratory for Cancer Research). It is clear that Huggins, who later became a Nobel Laureate, profoundly influenced Lehninger's scientific career. It was on the basis of Lehninger's extraordinarily imaginative work on the

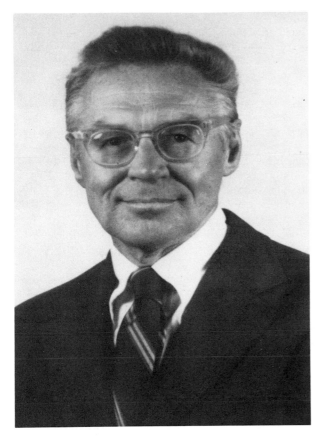

Fig 3. Albert Lester Lehninger

enzymatic aspects of fatty acid oxidation and oxidative phosphorylation in the years 1945 to 1951 that he received the invitation to succeed William Mansfield Clark. Lehninger became De Lamar Professor of Physiological Chemistry and director of the Department of Physiological Chemistry at the Johns Hopkins University School of Medicine in 1952 at the age of 35.

SCIENTIFIC CONTRIBUTIONS

Lehninger's most important scientific contributions center around three themes: (1) discovery of some of the main features of oxidative phosphorylation and other energy-coupling mechanisms associated with the electron transport chain; (2) discovery of the major role of the mitochondrion in respiration and in the compartmentation of metabolism in the cell; and (3) the role of mitochondria in regulating Ca^{2+} distribution in cells and tissues and in biological calcification. These advances had origins in his very early work begun soon after completing his Ph.D. dissertation. At that time he had established that the capacity for the oxidation of

fatty acids and of pyruvate via the tricarboxylic acid cycle resided in a particulate fraction of rat liver homogenates, an observation later confirmed by others. This was also the period in which attempts to refine the differential centrifugation method earlier developed by Albert Claude were taking place.

Lehninger made several early attempts to determine whether the organized oxidation of fatty acids and pyruvate in cell particles took place in one or another cell organelle isolated by centrifugation. However, it was not until 1948, when Hogeboom, Schneider and Palade first described the sucrose procedure for centrifugal recovery of cell organelles, that success was achieved. He and his graduate student E. P. Kennedy (now Hamilton Kuhn Professor of Biological Chemistry at Harvard Medical School) were able to find, only weeks after the sucrose method was described, that the mitochondrial fraction of liver contained virtually all the organized oxidative activity of the cell. Until that time it had been known that the succinoxidase and cytochrome oxidase systems were present in the mitochondria. But with the new work it became clear that the entire enzymatic apparatus for the fatty acid oxidation cycle, the tricarboxylic acid cycle, and oxidative phosphorylation were organized into the structure of the mitochondria. This basic discovery in Lehninger's laboratory started a new direction in biochemistry—an awareness and appreciation of the metabolic role of intracellular structure and of highly organized enzyme complexes, at a time when the conventional goal of most enzymologists was to discard cell "debris" and to solubilize and purify enzymes as chemical entities. These observations of Kennedy and Lehninger were made when there was intense interest in oxidative phosphorylation and its enzymatic mechanism. From 1948 on, mitochondrial compartmentation of metabolism and the mechanism of oxidative phosphorylation represented Lehninger's dual interests. An extensive series of important investigations followed.

In the period 1949–1951 Lehninger became the first to show that oxidative phosphorylation of ADP is coupled to the flow of electrons along the respiratory chain from NADH to oxygen. Although thermodynamic analysis had predicted this to be the case as early as 1939, it was not until 1951 that this was proved experimentally. Success came with Lehninger's recognition that oxidative phosphorylation takes place *within* the mitochondria and that the membrane presents a permeability barrier to the entry of NADH and other reduced coenzymes.

Shortly after his move to Johns Hopkins, Lehninger, together with his student, Sigurd Òlaf Nielsen, demonstrated that one of the three respiratory-chain phosphorylations occurs on electron transport from cytochrome c to oxygen. With another colleague, Bengt Borgstrom, he showed that two phosphorylations occur between NADH and cytochrome c.

Lehninger's discovery in 1951 that NADH cannot pass through the membrane of intact mitochondria was a crucial element in his demonstration that oxidative phosphorylation occurs during electron transport. But he also foresaw that this fact had very fundamental significance in the compartmentation of oxidation-reduction reactions in the cell. Lehninger pointed out that the failure of NADH to pass through the membrane effectively compartments the nicotinamide adenine dinucleotide of the cell into cytosolic and mitochondrial pools. Moreover, he showed that NADH formed by glycolysis could not directly enter the mitochondria and indicated that some other pathway was required, one that would necessarily be of crucial importance in the integration and regulation of glycolysis and respiration. This paper began a new era in the understanding of cell metabolism and later led to the recognition that many other metabolites, such as tricarboxylic acid cycle intermediates, and coenzymes, such as ATP and CoA, are compartmented into separate pools.

In a series of papers which appeared in 1955–1956, Lehninger, with his students Cecil Cooper and Thomas Devlin, first reported the preparation and properties of submitochondrial particulate systems capable of catalyzing electron transport and oxidative phosphorylation. These membrane preparations, later found to be vesicles, were shown to promote the partial reactions of oxidative phosphorylation and to be lacking in organized tricarboxylic acid cycle activity.

Lehninger was among the earliest investigators of respiratory energy coupling to give serious consideration to ion transport as an important means of energy conservation by mitochondria. Early work in his laboratory with James Gamble on K^+ transport revealed a very rapid incorporation of K^+ into respiring mitochondria and submitochondrial vesicles. Later, following the observations by his associate Frank Vasington that calcium ions are rapidly accumulated by respiring mitochondria, Lehninger and his colleague, C. S. Rossi, carried out a classical study of the stoichiometric relationship between the number of Ca^{2+} ions transported into the mitochondrial matrix and the number of electrons flowing from substrate to oxygen. Their first paper, published in the Warburg Festschrift of 1963, was the first to report stoichiometric coupling of ion transport to electron flow in mitochondria. They found that two Ca^{2+} ions were transported inward as a pair of electrons passed each of the three energy-

conserving sites of the respiratory chain. Similarly, they showed that ATP hydrolysis led to Ca^{2+} uptake. Soon they also found that phosphate is accumulated together with the Ca^{2+} and defined the quantitative relationship between the uptake of Ca^{2+}, the uptake of phosphate, electron flow, and respiratory activation by Ca^{2+}. Subsequently, Lehninger and his students, Rossi, Carafoli, Bielawski, Greenawalt, and others, filled in much detail on Ca^{2+} transport by mitochondria, which they summarized in an important review in 1967. The capacity for stoichiometric coupling between electron transport and ion transport so demonstrated gave much impetus to the chemiosmotic coupling hypothesis of Mitchell. This hypothesis was proposed in 1961 but was not given much serious consideration until the mid-1960s, when ion transport activities became widely accepted as an important mitochondrial activity.

In 1963 Lehninger, with his colleagues Rossi and Greenawalt, had observed that accumulation of calcium and phosphate by isolated mitochondria leads to formation of electron-dense insoluble deposits in the mitochondrial matrix, and that these could be visualized by electron microscopy. These deposits of calcium phosphate, which were found to be amorphous by x-ray diffraction, were suggested by Lehninger (*The Mitochondrion*, 1964) to be involved in biological calcification processes. Later in 1970 he assembled this and other evidence into a general hypothesis of biological calcification, which has received strong support and acceptance within the past five years. Lehninger postulated that the mitochondria are responsible for generating amorphous tricalcium phosphate deposits after concentration of both Ca^{2+} and phosphate in the intramitochondrial compartment at the expense of respiratory energy. He postulated that such "micropackets" of calcium phosphate, stabilized by naturally occurring inhibitors, passed through the mitochondrial membrane(s), through the cytosol, thence through the plasma membrane toward the extracellular collagen nidus where the micropackets are inserted and converted into hydroxyapatite. The mitochondrial stage in this process was postulated to be essential because only in the mitochondria can the solubility product of amorphous calcium phosphate, the obligatory precursor of hydroxyapatite, be exceeded, at the expense of energy generated by electron transport and subsequent inward active transport of Ca^{2+} ions and phosphate.

Recent experiments reported by Lehninger and his colleagues, Chen and Becker, on calcium phosphate segregation in mitochondria of the crab hepatopancreas and on the formation of extramitochondrial calcium phosphate granules, found to contain nearly 8% ATP which stabilized the granules in amorphous form, have provided important supporting evidence for this calcification hypothesis.

With his colleagues Brand and Reynafarje, Lehninger has reported new evidence on the H^+/site coupling ratio for H^+ ejection associated with mitochondrial electron transport. Early experiments of Mitchell in England appeared to show that one H^+ ion was ejected per pair of electrons per site during mitochondrial electron transport; in his later oxygen pulse measurements he concluded the true value was 2.0. His stoichiometry is central to Mitchell's chemiosmotic coupling hypothesis for oxidative and photosynthetic phosphorylation.

Lehninger and his colleagues have reasoned that the H^+/site ratio of 2.0 may not be correct, since it is incompatible with the now well-established fact that 2 Ca^{2+} ions are transported per 2 electrons per site, a total of 4 positive electrical charges. Moreover, workers in other laboratories have indicated that the H^+/site ratio of 210 is inadequate to account for the energetics of ATP formation.

Lehninger and his associates have recently found that Mitchell's oxygen pulse experiments of the H^+/site ratio were compromised by a systematic error occasioned by transmembrane movements of endogenous phosphate. They found that the true value, when phosphate movements are eliminated, is at least 3.0, and may be as high as 4.0. They have also developed two other methods for evaluation of the H^+/site ratio, namely, the "Ca^{2+} pulse" and "reductant pulse" methods, which yielded values of the H^+/site ratio of 3.5 to 4.0. From these recent experiments by Lehninger's group, it has become necessary to modify the chemiosmotic hypothesis significantly in order to account for these higher stoichiometric ratios. Lehninger thus has been a leader in the long-standing and intensive research in many laboratories to elucidate the molecular mechanism and pathway of energy conservation in oxidative phosphorylation, one of the major unsolved problems in biochemistry today.

LEHNINGER AS A TEACHER

The medical students who have passed through Johns Hopkins during the past 83 years have benefited from exposure to three of the greatest American teachers of physiological chemistry. Lehninger's ability as a lecturer capable of developing in a comprehensive yet simple and understandable style the important principles of physiological chemistry and their relationship to medicine has been outstanding. His talent as a teacher and the value of his research has resulted in his being chosen to give such important lectures as the Harvey Lec-

ture of the New York Academy of Medicine, the Herter Lecture of the New York University College of Medicine, the Prather Lecture at Harvard, the Bloor Lecture at the University of Rochester and many others.

Although graduate education was recognized and approved in some of the basic science departments at Johns Hopkins before Albert Lehninger joined the faculty, no significant number of graduate students were trained until his influence became felt in the Department of Physiological Chemistry. Within a few years of his arrival Lehninger set as a specific goal the training of graduate students. In 1958 the first NIH training grant specifically designated for graduate study was awarded at the Johns Hopkins School of Medicine to Albert Lehninger as the Program Director. The graduate program in physiological chemistry has continued to be quantitatively the most important graduate training program of the School of Medicine. In recent years it has been combined with training programs in biophysics, molecular biology and cellular biology, so that a unified training program in Biochemistry, Molecular and Cellular Biology is operated from the base in the Department of Physiological Chemistry.

Lehninger's perception of the important issues that are essential in the proper conduct of a high quality medical school have enabled him to play a leading role in the academic affairs of the Johns Hopkins School of Medicine. Because of his effectiveness in administration, he has been called upon to participate in many important decision-making bodies at the national and international level. For the National Academy of Sciences, he has been chairman of the Panel on Metabolism and Nutrition of the Committee on Growth, National Research Council, and a member of the Committee on Science and Public Policy. He was recently elected a member of the Council of the National Academy of Sciences and also a member of the Council of the Institute of Medicine. He was appointed in 1975 by President Ford to the President's Panel on Biomedical Research mandated by act of Congress. He served as president of the American Society of Biological Chemists in 1972–1973 and is a member of the Scientific Advisory Committee of the Massachusetts General Hospital. In 1975 he was elected vice president of the American Philosophical Society. He has also been a member of the Editorial Board of many important journals, including the *Journal of Biological Chemistry, Physiological Reviews, Journal of Biophysical and Biochemical Cytology, Biochemistry*, and the *Journal of Membrane Biology*.

Among Lehninger's best-known accomplishments is the writing of a comprehensive biochemistry text, which was first published in 1970. The second edition appeared in 1975. This book, a unique achievement, is generally recognized as the outstanding textbook in biochemistry on a worldwide basis. It may well represent the last time that a single author can successfully write a comprehensive account of general biochemistry suitable for undergraduates, medical students and graduate students. Lehninger is the author of two other excellent monographs of major importance: *The Mitochondrion* (1964) and *Bioenergetics* (1965; 1971). All of these books have been translated into many foreign languages.

Thus Lehninger has added lustre to the accomplishments of his two predecessors in the directorship of the Department of Physiological Chemistry. He exemplifies well the requirements in Walter Jones' advertisement for an assistant. But Johns Hopkins received much more than "a man who has a Ph.D. degree, who has teaching ability as well as research ability and who is well grounded in the fundamentals of chemistry." When Albert Lehninger came to Baltimore, Johns Hopkins also acquired an outstanding medical statesman who has contributed immensely to the progress of medicine not only at Johns Hopkins but throughout the world.

ACKNOWLEDGMENTS

The account of Dr. Albert Lehninger was prepared in collaboration with Dr. Paul Talalay. I wish to thank Dr. Kenneth Blanchard for valuable suggestions and Ms. Carol Bocchini for her editorial assistance.

REFERENCES

1. Becker GL et al.: Calcium phosphate granules in the hepatopancreas of the blue crab (*Callinectes sapidus*). J Cell Biol 61: 316, 1974

2. Betts F et al.: The atomic structure of intracellular amorphous calcium phosphate deposits. Proc Natl Acad Sci 72: 2088, 1975

3. Brand MD and Lehninger AL: Superstoichiometric Ca^{2+} uptake supported by hydrolysis of endogenous ATP in rat liver mitochondria. J Biol Chem 250: 7958, 1975

4. Brand MD, Chen C-H, and Lehninger AL: The stoichiometry of H^+ ejection during respiration-dependent accumulation of Ca^{2+} by rat liver mitochondria. J Biol Chem 251: 968, 1976

5. Brand MD, Reynafarje B, and Lehninger AL: The stoichiometric relationship between energy-dependent proton ejection and electron transport in mitochondria. Proc Natl Acad Sci 73: 473, 1976

6. Brand MD, Reynafarje B, and Lehninger AL: Reevaluation of the H^+/site ratio of mitochondrial electron transport in oxygen pulse technique. J Biol Chem 251: 5670, 1976

7. Carafoli E and Lehninger AL: Binding of Adenine nucleotides by mitochondria during active uptake of Ca^{++}. Biochem Biophys Res Comm 16: 66, 1964

8. Chen C-H and Lehninger AL: Respiration and phosphorylation by mitochondria from the hepatopancreas of the blue crab (*Callinectes sapidus*). Arch Biochem Biophys 154: 449, 1973

9. Chen C-H, Greenawalt JW, and Lehninger AL: Biochemical and ultrastructural aspects of Ca^{2+} transport by mitochondria of the hepatopancreas of the blue crab (*Callinectes sapidus*). J Cell Biol 61: 301, 1974

10. Clark WM: A contribution to the investigation of the temperature coefficient of osmotic pressure: A redetermination of the osmotic pressures of cane sugar solutions at 20°. Ph.D. Dissertation, Johns Hopkins University, 1910

11. Clark WM and Lubs HA: The colorimetric determination of hydrogen-ion concentration and its applications in bacteriology. J Bacteriol 2: 1, 109, 191, 1917

12. Clark WM: On the formation of "eyes" in Emmental cheese. J Dairy Science 1: 91, 1917

13. Clark WM: The determination of Hydrogen Ions. Baltimore: Williams and Wilkins Co., 1920

14. Clark WM: Studies on oxidation-reduction. I. Introduction. Public Health Rept 38: 443, 1923 (Reprint 823)

15. Clark WM: Recent studies on reversible oxidation-reduction in organic systems. Chem Rev 2: 127, 1925

16. Clark WM: The potential energies of oxidation-reduction systems and their biochemical significance. Harvey Lectures, 1933–1934, p. 67; Medicine 13: 207, 1934

17. Clark WM: Walter Jones. Science 81: 307, 1935

18. Clark WM: Walter (Jennings) Jones: 1865–1935. Biog Mem Natl Acad Sci 20: 79, 1938

19. Clark WM: Potentiometric and spectrophotometric studies of metalloporphyrins in coordination with nitrogenous bases. Cold Spring Harbor Symp Quant Biol 7: 18, 1939

20. Clark WM et al.: Metalloporphyrins. I. Coordination with nitrogenous bases. Theoretical relations. J Biol Chem 135: 543, 1940

21. Clark WM: Topics in Physical Chemistry. Baltimore: Williams and Wilkins Co., 1948

22. Clark WM: Oxidation-Reduction Potentials of Organic Systems. Baltimore: Williams and Wilkins Co., 1960

23. Cooper C and Lehninger AL: Oxidative phosphorylation by an enzyme complex from extracts of mitochondria. IV. Adenosine-triphosphatase activity. J Biol Chem 224: 547, 1957

24. Cooper C and Lehninger AL: Oxidative phosphorylation by an enzyme complex from extracts of mitochondria. V. The adenosine triphosphate exchange reaction. J Biol Chem 224: 561, 1957

25. Friedkin M and Lehninger AL: Esterification of inorganic phosphate coupled to electron transport between dihydrodiphosphopyridine nucleotide and oxygen. I. J Biol Chem 178: 611, 1949

26. Greenawalt JW, Rossi CS, and Lehninger AL: Effect of active accumulation of calcium and phosphate ions on structure of rat liver mitochondria. J Cell Biol 23: 21, 1964

27. Jones W and Whipple GH: The nucleoproteid of the suprarenal gland. Amer J Physiol 7: 423, 1902

28. Jones W and Winternitz MC: Uber die Adenase. Ztschr Physiol Chem 44: 1, 1905

29. Jones W and Austrian CR: Uber die Verteilung der Fermente des Nucleinstoffwechself. Ztschr Physiol Chem 48: 110, 1906

30. Jones W and Austrian CR: On thymus nucleic acid. J Biol Chem 3: 1, 1907

31. Jones W and Austrian CR: On the nuclein ferments of embryos. J Biol Chem 3: 227, 1907

32. Jones W and Austrian CR: The occurrence of ferments in embryos. J Biol Chem 3: Proc. XXVIII, 1907

33. Jones W and Rowntree LG: On the guanylic acid of the spleen. J Biol Chem 4: 289, 1908

34. Jones W and Perkins ME: The preparation of nucleotides from yeast nucleic acid. Johns Hopkins Hosp Bull 34: 63, 1923

35. Kennedy EP and Lehninger AL: Intracellular structures and fatty acid oxidation. J Biol Chem 172: 847, 1948

36. Kennedy EP and Lehninger AL: Oxidation of fatty acids and tricarboxylic acid cycle intermediates by isolated rat liver mitochondria. J Biol Chem 179: 957, 1949

37. Kennedy EP and Lehninger AL: Activation of fatty acid oxidation by dihydrodiphosphopyridine nucleotide. J Biol Chem 190: 361, 1951

38. Lehninger AL: The relationship of adenosine polyphosphates to fatty acid oxidation in homogenized liver preparations. J Biol Chem 154: 309, 1944

39. Lehninger AL: Fatty acid oxidation and the Krebs tricarboxylic acid cycle. J Biol Chem 161: 413, 1945

40. Lehninger AL: A quantitative study of the products of fatty acid oxidation in liver suspensions. J Biol Chem 164: 291, 1946

41. Lehninger AL: The fatty acid oxidase system of liver. Josiah Macy, Jr. Foundation Conference on Biological Antioxidants, New York, October, 1947

42. Lehninger AL and Kennedy EP: The requirements of the fatty acid oxidase system of rat liver. J Biol Chem 173: 753, 1948

43. Lehninger AL: Esterification of inorganic phosphate coupled to electron transport between dihydrodiphosphopyridine nucleotide and oxygen. II. J Biol Chem 178: 625, 1949

44. Lehninger AL: The organized respiratory activity of isolated rat liver mitochondria. In Enzymes and Enzyme Systems. Cambridge: Harvard University Press, 1951

45. Lehninger AL: Phosphorylation coupled to oxidation of dihydrodiphosphopyridine nucleotide. J Biol Chem 190: 345, 1951

46. Lehninger AL: Oxidative phosphorylation in diphosphopyridine nucleotide-linked systems. In Phosphorus Metabolism. Vol. I. Baltimore: The Johns Hopkins Press, 1951

47. Lehninger AL: Oxidative phosphorylation. The Harvey Lectures, Series XIL. New York: Academic Press, Inc., 1955

48. Lehninger AL: Physiology of mitochondria. In Enzymes: Units of Biological Structure and Function, Henry Ford Hospital International Symposium, Detroit. New York: Academic Press, Inc., 1956

49. Lehninger AL: Oxidation of fatty acid. In The Chemistry of Lipids Related to Atherosclerosis. Page I, Ed. Springfield, Ill.: Charles C Thomas, 1958

50. Lehninger AL: Relation of oxidation, phosphorylation and active transport to the structure of mitochondria. In A Symposium on Molecular Biology. Zirkle RE, Ed. Chicago: University of Chicago Press, 1959

51. Lehninger AL: Respiratory energy transformation. Rev Modern Phys 31: 136, 1959

52. Lehninger AL: The enzymatic and morphological organization of mitochondria. In The Cell: A Symposium. IX International Congress of Paediatrics, Montreal, 1959, Paediatrics 26: 3, 1960

53. Lehninger AL: Energy transformations in the cell. Sci Amer 202: 102, 1960

54. Lehninger AL: Oxidative phosphorylation in submitochondrial systems. Symposium Issue, Fed Proc 19: 952, 1960

55. Lehninger AL: How cells transform energy. Sci Amer, September, 1961

56. Lehninger AL: Components of the energy-coupling mechanism and mitochondrial structure. Proc of the First IUB/IUBS International Symposium held in Stockholm. In Biological Structure and Function. Vol. II. Goodwin TW and Lindberg O, Eds. New York: Academic Press, p. 31, 1961

57. Lehninger AL and Wadkins CL: Oxidative phosphorylation. Ann Rev Biochem 31: 47, 1962

58. Lehninger AL, Rossi CS, and Greenawalt JW: Respiration-dependent accumulation of inorganic phosphate and Ca++ by rat liver mitochondria. Biochem Biophys Res Comm 10: 444, 1963

59. Lehninger AL: Mitochondrial ion and water transport. Symposium Proceedings, VI Int Cong Biochem, New York City, VIII SII, 623, 1964

60. Lehninger AL, Carafoli E, and Rossi CS: Energy-linked ion accumulation in mitochondrial systems. Adv Enzymol 29: 259, 1967

61. Lehninger AL: The neuronal membrane. Proc Natl Acad Sci 60: 1069, 1968

62. Lehninger AL: Mitochondria and the physiology of Ca²⁺. The Gordon Wilson Lecture, October, 1971, Hot Springs, Virginia. Trans Amer Clin Climatol Ass 83: 83, 1971

63. Lehninger AL: Role of phosphate and other proton-donating anions in respiration-coupled transport of Ca²⁺ by mitochondria. Proc Natl Acad Sci 71: 1520, 1974

64. Lehninger AL and Brand MD: Pathways and stoichiometry of H⁺ and Ca²⁺ transport coupled to electron transport, IUB-IUPAB Symposium, Tehran, Iran, May, 1975. In The Structural Basis of Membrane Function. Hatefi Y, Ed. New York: Academic Press, pp. 329–334, 1975

65. Lehninger AL, Brand MD, and Reynafarje B: Pathways and stoichiometry of H⁺ and Ca²⁺ transport coupled to mitochondrial electron transport. International Symposium, Bari, Italy, September, 1975. In Electron-Transfer Chains and Oxidative Phosphorylation. Quagliariello E et al., Eds. Amsterdam: North-Holland Publishing Co., 1975

66. Nielsen SO and Lehninger AL: Oxidative phosphorylation in the cytochrome system of mitochondria. J Amer Chem Soc 76: 3860, 1954

67. Nielsen SO and Lehninger AL: Phosphorylation coupled to the oxidation of ferrocytochrome c. J Biol Chem 215: 555, 1955

68. Reynafarje B and Lehninger AL: Ca²⁺ transport by mitochondria from L1210 mouse ascites tumor cells. Proc Natl Acad Sci 70: 1744, 1973

69. Reynafarje B and Lehninger AL: Super-stoichiometry of H⁺ ejection on addition of Ca²⁺ pulses to mitochondria. *In* Dynamics of Energy-Transducing Membranes, BBA Library 13. Ernster L, Estabrook RW, and Slater EC, Eds. Amsterdam: Elsevier, pp. 447–454, 1974

70. Rossi CS and Lehninger AL: Stoichiometric relationships between mitochondrial ion accumulation and oxidative phosphorylation. Biochem Biophys Res Comm 11: 441, 1963

71. Rosse CS et al.: The stoichiometry and the dynamics of energy-linked accumulation of Ca²⁺ stoichiometry and the dynamics of energy-linked accumulation of Ca²⁺ by mitochondria. *In* Regulation of Metabolic Processes in Mitochondria. Vol. 7 Tager JM et al., Eds. Amsterdam: Elsevier Publishing Co., p. 317, 1966

72. Rossi CS, Carafoli E, and Lehninger AL: Active ion transport by mitochondria. Symposium on Biophysics and Physiology of Biological Transport. Frascati, Italy, Springer, Protoplasma, 63: 90, 1967

73. Talalay P: Personal communication

74. Vickery HB: William Mansfield Clark (1884–1964). Biog Mem Natl Acad Sci 39: 1, 1967

75. Wadkins CL and Lehninger AL: The role of the ATP-ADP exchange reaction in oxidative phosphorylation. Symposium Issue, Fed Proc, Vol. 22, 1963

9.
Johns Hopkins's Pioneer Venture into International Medicine: The Commission to the Philippine Islands

INTRODUCTION

The Johns Hopkins University's first involvement overseas was an outgrowth of the Spanish–American War. That war left the United States government with the Philippine Islands on its hands and, as an aftermath, an insurrection of Filipinos under the leadership of Emilio Aguinaldo.[1] American interest in this newly acquired overseas responsibility was great at the time and the enthusiasm spread to two members of the staff of The Johns Hopkins University School of Medicine who conceived the idea of forming a group to go to the Philippines to study the diseases which were prevalent there. Lewellys Franklin Barker, in his autobiography, describes the background as follows: "Flexner and I were close companions at this time [Fig 1].[2] In several conver-

sations we discussed the importance of the study of tropical diseases in America's new possession in the Orient. European governments had during the preceding 15 years been sending specially trained medical investigators into tropical regions. Thus Koch and Gaffky had gone to Egypt and India to study Asiatic cholera with the result that the cause of the disease, the 'comma bacillus,' was discovered and at Hong Kong, Yersin had in 1894 isolated the bacillus that is the cause of bubonic plague."

THE IDEA TAKES FORM

On March 8, 1899 Simon Flexner wrote the following in his diary:[3]

Early . . . January . . . Rupert Norton paid Barker and me a visit in Baltimore. Barker invited us to dine with him at the country club [Fig 2]. The dinner was a pleasant one and after it we retired into the general room where we sat before the great open log fire and talked over past experiences, present occupations and future prospects. . . . The sense of well-being and contentment which follows a good dinner and a moderate quantity of good wine was never in my experience greater than that night. In the course of the conversation I developed a scheme to pay a visit to the Philippines in the summer in order to study the tropical diseases prevailing in the Islands. The plan was to enlist the interest of the Surgeon-General who, it was thought, might be willing to send a Commission for this purpose. The idea was vigorously pursued for the remainder of the evening, and on bidding Norton good-bye at the station about midnight, it was decided to carry the proposal into effect. The request was to be made by me of the Surgeon-General. Barker and I were to go and we were to endeavor to secure Norton's transference from Santiago.[4]

. . . Finally on Saturday, February 18 . . . I called upon General Sternberg. The Surgeon-General failed to

---

[1] In the course of the Spanish–American War, Commodore George Dewey vanquished the Spanish fleet of Admiral Montojo in the Battle of Manila Bay in the spring of 1898, and occupied Cavité. Dewey permitted the insurrectionist Emilio Aguinaldo, who had been banished to Hong Kong in 1897, to return to Cavité and allowed him to be supplied with arms. Aguinaldo fought the Spanish and gained control of most of the island of Luzon, except Manila and the immediate environs. Spain, on making peace at the end of 1898, ceded the Islands to the United States. Unfortunately, the Filipinos, led by Aguinaldo, who with his troops had been refused permission to enter Manila when General Merritt captured the city, felt deep resentment against the Americans and in February 1899, revolt erupted. Although the American army under General Otis was successful in early encounters with the Filipinos, reinforcements from the United States were necessary to complete their conquest and the war continued until Aguinaldo was captured.

[2] In 1894 it was decided by the Trustees, after a thorough consideration of the subject by the Medical Board, to organize Pathology as a department of the hospital and to give it equal standing in the medical staff by appointing a resident pathologist and an assistant resident pathologist. In consequence of this action, Dr. Simon Flexner, associate in pathology in the medical school, was appointed resident pathologist and Dr. L. F. Barker, the associate in anatomy, was appointed assistant resident pathologist. This was the first instance in which similar officers were appointed with staff standing in connection with any hospital in the United States.

Reprinted from the *Johns Hopkins Medical Journal* **147**: 13, 1980.

[3] Flexner's diary was made available by the Library of the American Philosophical Society.

[4] Rupert Norton took his M.D. from Harvard in 1893. He came to The Johns Hopkins Hospital in the spring of 1893, but according to some misunderstanding, was not actually given the formal appointment of assistant resident physician until a year later, at which time it was officially back-dated to March 1, 1893. During all that time, however, he served as a member of the resident staff of the hospital. When the Spanish–American

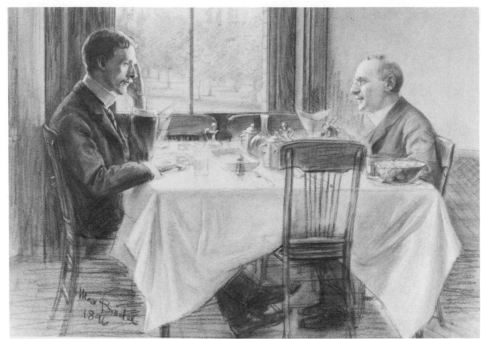

Fig 1.   Lewellys F. Barker (left) and Simon Flexner (Drawn in 1896 by Max Brödel).

show a special enthusiasm. However, he was interested and he proposed to send me under contract to Manila for one year in the capacity of assistant surgeon.

This is not at all what was envisioned, but instead that a Commission might be appointed in order to have better facilities for work. After leaving the General, Flexner noticed that there was a matineé at the National Theater which he went to with Walter Reed. During the afternoon, he unfolded to Reed the plan of going to the Philippines. Reed was very enthusiastic and promised to lend his aid. He advised enlisting the interest of Drs. Welch and Osler, and President Gilman. On his return to Baltimore, Flexner consulted Barker and they decided to put the matter before President Gilman first; if he discouraged it, their intention was to go no further. However, if he approved, they would then talk to Welch and Osler. They made arrangements to see Gilman on Friday morning, February 24, after carefully working out a plan of presentation. They reviewed the Commissions which had, in recent years, been sent by England, Germany, France, Japan and Austria to investigate certain tropical diseases. It was decided to bring out these data in the course of the conversation with Gilman. At that time, Barker was giving lectures to the graduating class of the university on the physiology and anatomy of the brain. These were delivered in one of the rooms at McCoy Col-

lege. When he and Flexner met at luncheon to discuss the matter further, Barker indicated that he hoped Flexner was in earnest about the proposition, because he had called upon President Gilman after his lecture and "Mr. Gilman had caught fire" at the idea. Barker then developed to Flexner the plan as he had unfolded it and: "I could readily understand from his account delivered so modestly that he himself did not appreciate the force of the presentation and the quiet eloquence of the arguments." Flexner commented that it was, indeed, necessary to be in earnest, for a meeting was projected at Mr. Gilman's home that evening. Flexner was to see Welch and briefly present the subject to him, and Barker was to do the same with Dr. Osler, all the parties coming together at half past eight to have a general conference.

Welch, of course, was taken by surprise and in a jocular mood said, "Why, the Filipinos would certainly capture you and if you escape them you must certainly succumb to the climate or even if you escape both these dangers you would surely be destroyed by earthquakes."

Welch was late for the evening meeting, and while waiting for him the subject was opened. The enthusiasm of Gilman and Osler broke out and soon swelled to "an uncontrollable volume." In the middle of this conversation Welch arrived, but the matter was now out of the control of Barker and Flexner. The president unfolded his views and gave his impressions, bringing forward many cogent reasons in support of the undertaking, but also dwelling on the dangers to be found. When the question of time of departure arose, the president was for immediate action, even wishing that they might leave on the hospital ship *Relief* scheduled to sail for Manila via Suez in a few days. He proposed calling the Surgeon-General by phone in order to confer upon the possibility of this

---

War broke out in 1898, Norton entered the U.S. Army as acting assistant surgeon and served in one of the army camps in the south, doing pathologic work for the most part. He had been on a leave of absence in Boston and was in the process of going to his next assignment in Santiago when he visited Barker and Flexner in Baltimore.

plan. Finally, reason prevailed, as the start of such a Commission could hardly be made so quickly. Since both Barker and Flexner had teaching responsibilities, further discussion led to the selection of April 1 as the departure date. In terms of defraying the expenses, it was proposed to raise a sum of 5,000 dollars by appealing to a few friends of the university. From that point on matters proceeded very quickly.

Welch and Osler visited Surgeon-General Sternberg and his counterpart in the Navy, who offered all the aid in their power. In addition to the opportunity of visiting hospitals, it was arranged that free transportation for the party was to be supplied by the government. Two thousand dollars in subscriptions for the cost of the expedition were soon in hand and this was considered enough to proceed with preparations. Further investigation made it clear that it would take too long to go by government transport. Flexner found that the Empress of India was sailing from Vancouver, British Columbia on March 27, so that plans were made to catch this vessel.[5] They began acquiring complete laboratory equipment for bacteriological, pathological and clinical studies. The next question was the necessity of having some assistants in the party, but this posed difficulty as there were no funds available for this purpose. The idea surfaced that some of the medical students who were financially able to pay their expenses would be willing to come on these terms. Mr. F. P. Gay and Mr. Joseph M. Flint quickly volunteered to go (Figs 3 and 4). Mr. John W. Garrett, a friend of Mr. Flint and of Dr. Barker, also proposed joining the party. The start was to be made from Chicago on

[5]   "TO CIRCLE THE GLOBE
First Time Such Trip Tickets Have Been Sold
At the Starting Point
THE JOHNS HOPKINS PARTY
Will Leave Chicago Tomorrow for Manila

After Studying Diseases Prevalent In The Philippines They Will Proceed On A Trip Around The World—Stops Will Be Made At A Number Of Interesting Places.

Members of the Expedition which will go to Manila for the Johns Hopkins University will meet in Chicago tomorrow and start on their long journey. As has already been announced, the purpose of the expedition is to study diseases prevalent in the tropics by modern methods, clinical as well as pathological.

From Chicago the party will go to St. Paul and there take the Canadian Pacific Railway. From St. Paul they will go to Vancouver and take the steamer Empress of India, which sails from Vancouver March 27. Yokohama and Kobe, in China, will be points where stops will be made in the journey. From Hong Kong the party will go to Manila, and after making their investigations, will return to take up the rest of the globe-circling route of the Canadian Pacific Railway . . .

There will be five in the party, and through tickets for the trip are furnished them on starting. In ticketing such a trip the marvelous organization in which the transportation interests are concerned appears. The arrangements for the party were made by Mr. C. G. Osburn, Baltimore agent of the Canadian Pacific Railway, and this is said to be the first time that a party of five bought trip tickets around the world . . ." (Baltimore Sun—March 21, 1899)

Wednesday evening, March 22 at 6:25 p.m. on the Wisconsin Central Railroad.

Letters were given to the Commission by the Secretary of the Navy, the Surgeon-Generals of the Army and Navy and influential government officials, as well as by private persons which it was believed would open up all the avenues for work and also for social recreation that they might desire.

Flexner had recently accepted an invitation to become professor of pathology at the University of Pennsylvania. Coming to Baltimore from Louisville, Kentucky in 1890, at the age of 27, only one year after graduation from medical school, he had the good fortune to be accepted as a graduate student in Welch's laboratory at a time when Welch was still active in the daily work of the department. His talents were quickly recognized and he became Welch's close associate and first assistant when Councilman left in 1892 to become Shattuck Professor of Pathology at Harvard. From that time until his departure, Flexner carried the main burden of the routine work of the department, including a major share of the teaching load. Although Flexner left the Hopkins environment in March 1899, never to again serve as a member of the staff, he continued throughout his life his interest in the institutions and on February 23, 1937 accepted an appointment as Trustee of the University, serving until October 1942. While director of the Rockefeller Institute for Medical Research, he played an important role in fostering the close relationship between Johns Hopkins and that Institute. In 1898 Flexner was given the title "professor of pathological anatomy." A short while before he had received a call to the chair of pathology in the Medical College of Cornell University. He paid a visit to the institution and later discussed the opportunity with Mall. Mall immediately wrote to Welch about this matter, urging that Flexner should be kept in Baltimore if possible. In his first letter in reply, Welch suggested that if a moderate increase in Flexner's salary would keep him here he thought that this should be done. Welch stated in his letter: "I do not want him to go where the scientific atmosphere is dispiriting, and I think that this is what he fears most if he goes to New York. After all, if one has enough to subsist, the environment is everything for a scientific man; and environment is our strong point, stronger than the means of subsistence." In a second letter dated July 3, 1898, just four days after the first note to Mall, he continued: "Of course we cannot compete with New York in the matter of salary. I should suppose that $2500 would be as high as we could think of going . . ." In the final letter of the series, written on August 1, Welch wrote as follows: "Dr. Hurd has just been in and tells me that you think that if Flexner was given the title of professor he might be influenced to stay. I'm quite willing to favor this. I think that probably it would be better to give him the title of professor of pathological anatomy than that of professor of pathology." This was the first time more than one individual in a single department held the rank of full professor. Flexner elected to stay in Baltimore, but as we have seen, he remained for only one year more and then left for good.

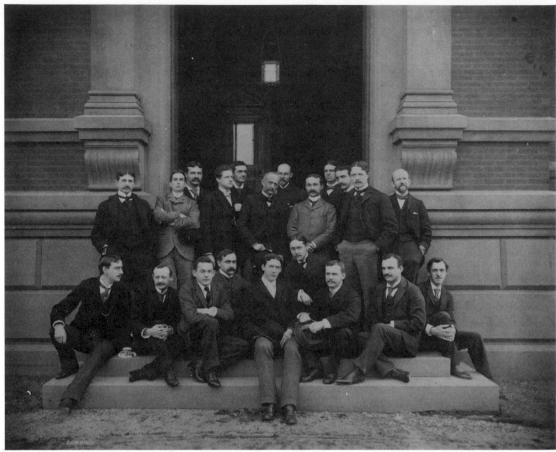

Fig 2.   Johns Hopkins Hospital House Staff, 1892. Bottom row (seated) second from left, Simon Flexner; fifth from left, L. F. Barker; far right, Rupert Norton.

VISIT TO JAPAN EN ROUTE

The party reached Yokohama on Tuesday, April 11. Since the diseases of the Philippines had much in common with those of Japan, it was decided to spend a week there as modern hospitals could be visited and advantage taken of the results of the study of tropical diseases by eminent Japanese physicians. The day of their arrival they were invited to a reception by the Mikado, which required top hats and morning coats. There was no choice but to have these made by a tailor especially for the purpose.

In Tokyo, Flexner visited the Institute for Infectious Disease, presided over by Kitasato and the Second Hospital where Aogama was in charge. The Institute was modeled on that of Koch's in Berlin, although smaller. Shiga, Kitasato's assistant, had recently isolated a bacillus from epidemic dysentery which he believed to be the specific causative organism.

Flexner wrote: "Aogama showed us the hospital and pointed out a number of interesting cases. Most important was several cases of beri-beri, the first we had seen . . . He demonstrated cultures of a streptothrix obtained from the lung of a patient. The organism injected into guinea pigs produces pseudotubercles. No publication had yet been made."

In Kyoto they saw lacquer in preparation. The chief workman, who was making a box in lacquer to be exhibited at the Paris Exposition, showed them how the work was done. Flexner wrote: "He is regarded as one of the cleverest workmen in this line. The box on which he is at work will have taken two years to complete. Garrett bought a considerable number of pieces of lacquer from Ikeda."

HONG KONG

The party reached Hong Kong on Wednesday, April 27 aboard the Rosetta. They found many things of medical interest. Thus, their study of plague began at that time and was extended when several months later Barker and Flint returned to Hong Kong en route to America. At that time a considerable increase in incidence of the disease had taken place and within a week or ten days, they saw scores of cases and performed many autopsies. The various forms of infection—inguinal, axillary, tonsillar, cervical and pulmonary—were encountered. Flexner wrote:

Through the courtesy of Dr. J. A. Lawson, we saw, for the first time, bubonic plague, the famous "black death" that destroyed one quarter of the population of Europe in the 14th century. Lawson had

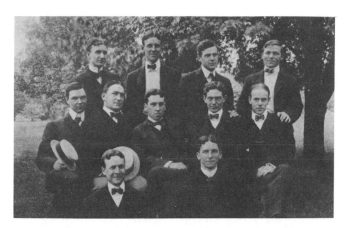

Fig 3. Pithotomy Club, Senior members, 1900. Middle row, second from left, Joseph M. Flint. Others: top row, left to right: Henry C. Evans, Mortimer Warren, Warren H. Lewis and Albion W. Hewlett. Middle Row, left to right: Herbert W. Allen, Flint, J. B. MacCallum (brother of W. G. MacCallum), W. F. M. Sowers, Henry A. Christian. Bottom row: Arthur L. Fisher, Preston Keyes.

studied the great outbreak of the disease in Hong Kong in 1894, and epidemics had also occurred there in 1896, 1898 and in the year of our visit 1899. Kitasato and Yersin had studied the causative agent, *Bacillus pestis*, in 1894. We were permitted to examine plague patients in the wards of the isolation hospital and to see the pathological findings in the autopsy room. It was the Chinese inhabitants who were most often attacked. Cases among whites were rare. One member of our group commented upon the curious psychological reactions we manifested on encountering this much dreaded disease. On our first visit to the morgue, containing bodies of patients that had died of plague, we were all careful not to come into personal contact with the cadavers and even avoided drafts of air leading from their vicinity. On the second day we began cautiously to palpate the swellings (buboes) due to enlargement of the lymph glands (in the groins, armpits, or neck), and on the third day we found ourselves making postmortem examinations of the internal organs.

It had not yet become generally known that infection is most often due to the bites of fleas that have bitten infected rats (a fact not established until 1907). Direct infection of one patient by another occurs only rarely, except in cases of pneumonic plague.

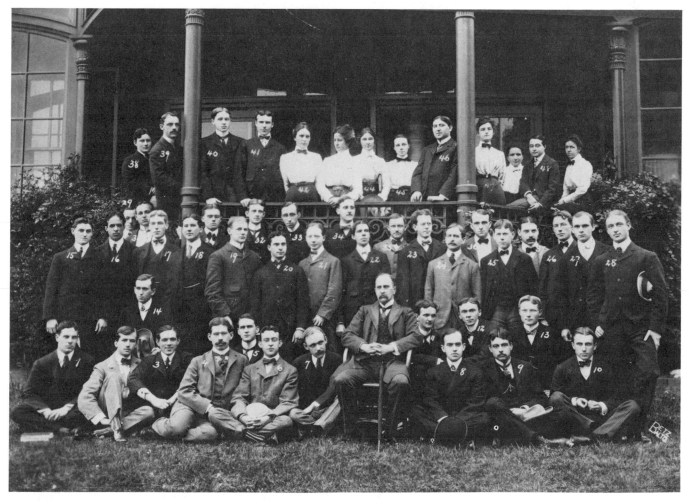

Fig 4. Class of 1901. Johns Hopkins University School of Medicine. Seated, center: William Osler. Seated to his right: F. P. Gay. Back row, third from right: Gertrude Stein (who did not graduate).

ARRIVAL IN MANILA

The Commission arrived in Manila, some 600 miles southeast of Hong Kong, on May 4, 1899, and established quarters at the Hotel de Oriente. They stayed there for only a short time, as accommodations were insufficient owing to the sudden descent on the hotel of families of army and navy officers. Having been forewarned of the living conditions in Manila, the group took the precaution of bringing with them from Hong Kong a group of Chinese servants, intending to set up housekeeping.

The group lived at Calle Malacanan, Number 1, which was formerly the palace of the governor; thus life was reasonably enjoyable for them during their stay. Jacob Gould Schurman, who had been president of Cornell University, was in Manila in 1899. As the first president of the United States Philippine Commission, he extended every courtesy to the group.

Since the members of the Johns Hopkins Commission were all young and healthy they were able to withstand the continuous heat, the high degree of humidity and the increased discomfort due to the rains which began in July. The Americans who had lived in Manila gave them good advice as how to conduct themselves— careful selection of foods, avoidance of iced drinks and of any excesses (physical or mental), tropical clothing, tepid baths rather than cold baths, staying indoors during the hottest part of the day and sleeping under mosquito netting. They found the water in Manila safe to drink without boiling, but recognized the importance of drinking only boiled water outside the city.

Within a few hours of their arrival, credentials and private letters were presented to Colonel Woodhull, Surgeon-in-Chief to the 8th Army Corps, and to General Otis. They were afforded the opportunity to pursue their work in the military hospitals. Although they had no special introduction, they quickly met Dr. Bournes, chief health officer of Manila, who opened to them the hospitals under his charge. The civilian facilities consisted of a large hospital within the walled city, San Juán de Dios, with a capacity of 250 to 300 beds, accommodating both natives and Europeans. San Lázaro, a leper hospital in the outskirts of Manila, usually had 80 to 100 patients, most of whom had come from Luzon—mainly from Manila and its immediate surroundings. One wing of the building having a private entrance was devoted to native prostitutes who applied regularly for examination and were incarcerated there and treated medically when found to be suffering from venereal disease.

In addition to the regimental hospitals which were virtually detention camps, the army had three Reserve Hospitals, the First, Second and Third; a convalescent hospital on Corregidor; and the hospital ship *Relief* which was anchored in the bay. The First Reserve under the command of Major Crosby had been originally the Spanish Military Hospital. By the erection of tents over platforms, it was raised a foot or two from the ground and increased in capacity to 1200 or more beds. The Second Reserve, under Major Keefer, was a transformed

modern school building with a capacity of 250 beds. There were high ceilings and wide corridors, making it a model hospital. The Third Reserve, of more recent origin, was smaller and intended as a convalescent hospital, as was the hospital at Corregidor. The *Relief* was used as a hospital for acute cases. After an outbreak of beri-beri at Cavité, a hospital under military control was established at San Roque in the remains of the Spanish Marine Hospital which had been wrecked by the insurgents. A small hospital for sick seamen and marines was established at Cavité. Through the courtesy of Dr. Pearson this was open to them for clinical studies.

Through the kindness of Colonel Woodhull and Major Crosby, a small Filipino house situated on the banks of the Pasig was provided as a laboratory (Figs 5 and 6). The expense of putting up working tables was borne by the Medical Corps of the Army. Laboratory equipment was soon set up and within a few days work was begun. The members of the Commission were able to visit the wards and were assisted in their clinical and pathological work by the medical staff of the various hospitals. They were particularly grateful for the assistance of Lieutenant Richard P. Strong, a graduate in the first class of The Johns Hopkins University School of Medicine.[6] It was found necessary to establish laboratories in the other hospitals since all were connected with the First Reserve by the Signal Corps telegraphic system which they were free to use, and all the dead were carried to the morgue connected with the First Reserve Hospital. Commission members went frequently to other hospitals to make clinical and bacteriological examinations.

Flexner's diary for May 6 recorded immediate activity:

> At 6 a.m. the following morning, an orderly from the First Reserve Hospital arrived with a note from Strong saying there were three bodies awaiting autopsy. One supposed to have mucous colitis, the second suspected to have typhoid fever and the third, gunshot wounds. We arrived about 9 o'clock and autopsied a case of amebic dysentery with typical and extensive intestinal ulceration extending into the cecum . . . In the sigmoid flexure there was a perforating ulcer and general peritonitis was found, although there was no liver abscess . . . In the afternoon, we again called on Colonel Woodhull. He received us with a smile, saying that we were regarded as dangerous characters and not proper persons to be given passes permitting us to remain out later than 7 p.m. This pleasantry was the result of a request to General Otis, through his aide, for passes for our party, which request was declined . . . Colonel Woodhull proposed to appoint Barker and me assistant surgeons, admitting us to the rank of First Lieutenant, which rank would secure for us the privileges we desired. The Colonel also spoke of an out-

[6] Strong was in charge of the laboratory in the First Reserve Hospital. He had established the Army Pathological Laboratory and was appointed by the Secretary of War in 1899 as the president of a board for the investigation of tropical diseases in the Philippine Islands.

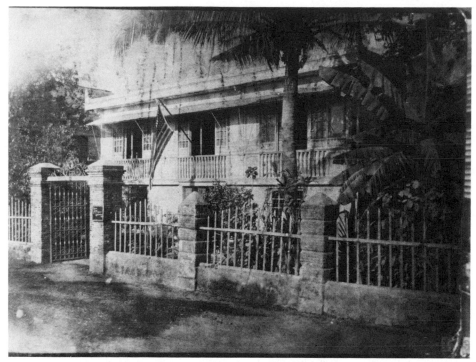

Fig 5.   Laboratory building of the Johns Hopkins Commission in Manila, Philippine Islands.

break of beri-beri reported from the Filipino prison at Cavité. He desired us to visit the prison and see the cases. . . . After tiffin, Mr. Woods' launch, the Victory, was waiting. We were carried to the boat by Filipinos and cruised about, visiting the hospital ship "Relief" anchored in the bay. The "Relief" was comfortably and beautifully fitted up as a hospital ship . . . The Misses Irvine and Fulkerson of The Johns Hopkins Hospital were on board as nurses. They were in charge of the operating room and the methods of the Hopkins were seen at every turn. The operating room was by far the best we had seen in the east, far surpassing the one in the Civil Hospital in Hong Kong.

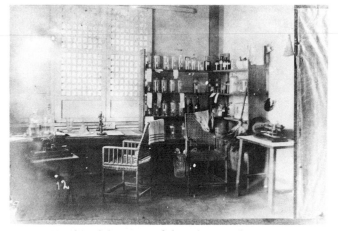

Fig 6.   Histology laboratory of the Johns Hopkins Commission, Manila, Philippine Islands.

A VISIT TO THE COMBAT AREA

The group wanted to visit the combat zone before settling down and departed at 7:30 a.m. by train the next day (May 8): "The train carried provisions and water from the city and other freight as well as soldiers and officers. The train ran very slowly over a track much the worse for wear and the insurgents, and was more or less open to obstruction from the latter . . . Their trenches were easily visible on both sides of the road from the train . . . They were of earth, enclosed in bamboo and often covered with a shed of bamboo; 'bomb proofs, so-called. We were destined to see them at close quarters later, but the general statement of officers was that they were well and skillfully made. That the Filipinos should not have held them longer was the greatest wonder." The heat of the sun about noon was intense. They camped just beside a detachment of the Third Artillery, acting as infantry and commanded by Captain Randolph. Transportation never arrived and it was decided to push forward on foot, leaving Garrett with the luggage to go forward by Strong's bullock cart, while he was to come on Strong's mount.[7] The distance they had to travel was about 10 miles. They passed through a small village stretching for miles along the road, with rows of parallel native houses covered with straw, some of which were very pretty. The village had not been burned but the

[7] From the railroad on the Bag Bag River they walked several miles to San Fernando, but before the end of the trip they found themselves, contrary to all advice, drinking any water that was available, some of it certainly far from pure.

haste with which it had been abandoned was shown in the household articles which were strewn about. There were a few natives searching in the ruins and an American soldier in pursuit of a chicken for dinner. The Commission reached Santo Tomás, about 4–5 miles distance, which was the seat of considerable resistance by the insurgents. Trenches crossed, flanked, or ran parallel with the road. A couple of dead oxen were passed and a few abandoned and upturned carriages. Bullet marks on the shrubs and trees could be made out and empty shells were found along the road. Sentries were passed more frequently now. By this time the party was hot, tired, hungry and thirsty and in a few instances, the sentries were distinctly agitated by their approach. They finally reached San Fernando after dark and immediately went to headquarters. They were escorted to the General Hospital which had been established in two abandoned residences. The mosquitoes were bad, and after vainly trying to get to sleep by covering his face with a handkerchief, Flexner removed his undershirt and in its place put on his khaki coat and drew the shirt over his head. Garrett finally arrived, having gotten a ride on the bullock cart with the luggage. The next night the members of the party were given mosquito netting, a supply of which had just arrived on the wagon trains. The following morning they made an excursion to the front line where a Filipino outpost could be seen in the distance across the railroad track. With the glasses sentries could be seen. Flint and Lieutenant Archer, who acted as his guide, went much closer. The city had been largely burned. It was a sad and desolate sight. Many of the natives left in the neighborhood were quite friendly, but it was difficult to distinguish whether they were "amigos" or were insurgents who were roaming about hiding their arms whenever a party appeared, but quickly recovering them when they left. There were many unexplained disappearances and murders. On their return, the members of the Commission found their new house in good order and their Chinese staff provided an excellent meal.

Life was gay in Manila. On May 21 Flexner went to the laboratory for a short time to examine cultures from dysentery cases made the day before. Then he attended a lunch party aboard the *Victoria* given by Wood and Jones:

> Also attending were Strong, Mrs. Beveridge (the wife of Senator Beveridge of Indiana), Flint, Gay and myself. The "Victoria" welcomed each boatload with music from a native orchestra. After boarding, cocktails were passed around. The "Victoria" steamed for Cavité and in going, we passed the sunken Spanish vessels in the harbor. When we landed, a carpet was spread under a tree, full table service at hand and delightful "tiffin" of 6 or 7 courses was served. Each course was brought warm and served admirably. Several kinds of wine were at hand including sherry, claret, champagne and finally Old Port for the toast—"Old Folks at Home," which seems never to be omitted in the east on Sundays. We then went aboard the "Victoria" and steamed to old Cavité where we walked around, saw the town, visited the naval hospital and naval yard, the Filipino prison and saw the church. The next day we went to the San Juan de Dios Hospital to

autopsy a case of beri-beri. The sister in charge of the dispensary showed us around and then served sherry, muscatel and cognac. The next day we did an autopsy on a case of acute malaria with mitral stenosis. The following day, autopsies on two cases of leprosy at San Lazaro were done.

Flexner's diary for May 25 noted that: "The laboratory is running smoothly and . . . in time should yield results. The work on dysenteric stools goes on . . . although thus far the cases . . . have been of rather long-standing and under treatment for a long time. Barker . . . is looking for malaria, typhoid fever, etc. Gay is endeavoring to assist both Barker and me. He does Widal tests and odd things as they come up. Thus far he wants in independence and initiative. Flint does well; active, alert and independent."

On June 3 Flexner learned that a move was to be made from the southern lines after the insurgents and he and the others decided to proceed to the water pumping station from which it was said they might watch the movement. Flexner left early but Flint and Garrett stayed and saw a rather sharp engagement from their position on the bluff, one in which the gunboats in Lagoona Bay also participated. The bursting of the shells could be watched and they saw the village burned. The enemy made practically no resistance and the American troops occupied the town.

"On June 10 went down with Garrett to fort to take photographs of the interior, showing the destructive effects of bombardment and in the hope of seeing something of the movement in Paranaque and Panoi begun that morning. The number of wounded on the American side was considerable." They came under fire with the whirl of bullets frequently quite close to them. Thus, their daily life consisted of visits to the laboratory to take care of their work there, visits to the hospital for observation of patients and for autopsies, and efforts to see the war first-hand.

The work was carried on under rather difficult conditions. On July 1 they went to the Cavité hospital where there were two Filipino doctors. They immediately set to work, made blood cultures from 15 patients with beri-beri and two patients who had died during the morning. They established themselves in the corridor outside the main ward, in which there were some cots and some patients on mats on the floor.

> We employed only selected cases; the most recent ones. At first there was some resistance; that is, the patients were reluctant. In a little while, those who could walk lined up and others, the paralyzed and very weak ones, clamored to be used. While we were engaged in this work, Barker drawing the blood and Gay mixing, keeping syringes sterilized and pouring the cultures, an officer, minus coat but with two bars on his shirt collar walked into the corridor in which we were working with much excitement. He proved to be the army surgeon of the First California Volunteers who had succeeded Major Nef. He began by abusing the place for being dirty and neglected and then asked rather gruffly who we were. Barker told him in a word. He then asked by whose authority we were working; this was explained. He careened around for some

minutes utterly dissatisfied with the state of the hospital, a proper enough attitude. But he got into a rage and finally a fever, much to his discomfort and disadvantage. There was, however, no little provocation, for besides the inadequacy of the hospital and its neglected condition, there were few cots and very little attention, either medical or hygienic, could be given the patients. It appeared that for two days no commissary supplies had been obtained and the sick had only a little rice and fish caught under the pier in the bay. We saw natives unable to walk and women fishing on the pier. The fish caught were a little larger than minnows and these were being relied upon for animal food. It appears that the Captain had asked for an allowance for food—$1500 was voted and at once the commissary supplies cut off. Whether the money was or was not delivered in time to obtain supplies in the interim I do not know, but the fact remains that these poor people were left barely with food to keep them from starvation for this period. The floor was dirty, the prisoners crowded in the room, the mats upon which they lay were filthy, all the sick were infested with vermin, especially with scabies, which in some had led to deep ulcers from scratching.

DISEASES STUDIED

The Commission studied many febrile diseases including typhoid fever, malaria, tuberculosis, dengue, smallpox and dysentery. They examined cases of beriberi and also became interested in the skin diseases prevalent among the natives and the American soldiers as well, many of whom were attacked by what was called "dhobi itch" or "washerman's itch" which appeared to be a type of eczematous ringworm due to invasion of the skin by a vegetable fungus. One of the most important observations was the isolation by Flexner from the dejecta of patients suffering from acute epidemic dysentery of a pathogenic bacillus.

The group had no difficulty in isolating the malarial parasites from the blood of patients with both tertian and aestivo-autumnal types. They were well prepared to make such blood studies since they had observed many cases in The Johns Hopkins Hospital where Thayer and Hewetson had made their classic studies on the disease just four years earlier (1895). They were interested to learn of a statement in the records of the Jesuits in Mindanao that the natives of that island had recognized more than two centuries before a relation between the malarial intermittent fevers and the prevalence of mosquitoes.

At Cavité the Commission had an excellent opportunity to study the clinical and pathological aspects of beri-beri, as some 200 cases had occurred among Filipino prisoners who lived mainly on polished rice. All varieties of the disease (neuritic or "dry form," cardiovascular or "wet form," etc.) were observed. Historically, the Philippine Archipelago has the unenviable record of being the country in which beri-beri has been most frequent. Ten thousand deaths due to beri-beri had occurred there in a single year among the population of about 12 million people, with some 58% of these deaths being in suckling infants. This relative frequency exceeded that of Japan where there were some 20,000 deaths yearly among the population of about 80 million people. At the time the Commission was in the Philippines the true cause of beri-beri had not yet been discovered. It was not until 1916 that the Dutch investigator, Eijkmann, working in Java, proved that pigeons fed on polished rice developed paralysis (polyneuritis gallinarum), due to deficiency of vitamin B1 in the diet.

While the Commission was in Cavité a large epidemic of dengue fever occurred. Eight years afterwards, this disease was carefully studied in the same locale by Asburn and Craig of the Army Medical Research Board for the Investigation of Tropical Diseases who showed that it was due to infection with a filterable virus transmitted by a mosquito (*Culex fatigans*).

Another disease that the group had not previously seen was leprosy. They examined patients with the nodular (or tuberous) form, some with the neural (or anesthetic) form, and some patients who had mixtures of the two.

Smallpox, which had previously been prevalent in Manila and had claimed many victims among the American soldiers at the beginning of the occupation, had been largely eliminated, although there were still a few cases in the city. The rapid control of the disease was due to the energetic activity of Major Bournes, who made vaccination compulsory and re-established a carabao (water buffalo) form of the vaccine.

When the time came to pack up their belongings in July, including a large amount of pathological material to be studied later in Baltimore, the Commission members were all sorry to see their venture come to an end. They had developed a fondness for the Malay people (Tagalogs) and the mestizos. They had learned the art of boiling rice so that each individual grain stands out separately, as they were to demonstrate to their friends many times on return to the United States. On the return trip, the party divided. John W. Garrett went to Java to become acquainted with the affairs of the Dutch East Indies, gaining knowledge that doubtless was helpful to him in his distinguished career as a diplomat. He became Secretary to the American Legation at The Hague in 1901, was made Envoy Extraordinary and Minister Plenipotentiary to the Netherlands and Luxembourg during the first world war, and in 1929 Ambassador to Italy.[8] Flexner and Gay returned by way of Ceylon and the Suez Canal, while Flint and Barker came back by way of British India, spending three weeks in that country.

[8] Garrett's return was reported in the Herald on October 14, 1899.

"FROM THE FAR EAST
Mr. John W. Garrett Returns From A World's Tour
HIS IMPRESSIONS OF MANILA

Commends The Results Thus Far Of American Occupation of Philippines—A Field For The South.
Mr. John W. Garrett returned Thursday night to his country place, the Evergreens, after a trip around the world, which included a stay in Manila for a study of social and economic questions in the Philippines . . .

STUDIES ON DYSENTERY

The history of dysentery is obscured by the confusion which existed between the bacillary and amebic types before the recognition of the causal agents. Various observers noted, however, that the types of dysentery seen in the tropics were often associated with liver abscess, whereas such a lesion was conspicuously absent in the dysenteries of temperate climates. However, one is not certain, with many of the early articles, whether the writer was dealing with amebic or bacillary dysentery. It is difficult to believe today what a major problem this was in the last half of the 19th century and at the time Flexner began his studies in the Philippines. During the Civil War, it was known as the "camp disease." Woodward contributed a monumental volume on the *Alvine Fluxes* to the "Medical and Surgical History of the War of the Rebellion (1861–65), Part II. Vol. I, being the second medical volume." This tremendous folio of nearly nine hundred pages deals in intimate detail with every phase of the subject—statistical, clinical, pathological, and epidemiological. "These disorders occurred with more frequency and produced more sickness and mortality than any other form of disease. . . . Soon no army could move without leaving behind it a host of victims. They crowded the ambulance trains, the railroad cars, the steamboats. In the general hospitals they were often more numerous than the sick from all other diseases, and rivalled the wounded in multitude." There was a total of 1,739,135 cases of dysentery during the Civil War, with 44,558 deaths.

In the latter part of the nineteenth century, the dysentery problem was a very serious one in Japan, where there were 90,000 cases with 20,000 deaths in 6 months. This impelled Kiyoshi Shiga to look for the causal agent. Since animals were resistant to the production of dysentery, Shiga sought an organism in the dejecta of patients which would be agglutinated by their blood serum in a manner similar to that of the Widal test in typhoid fever. He found this reaction with an organism recovered from 36 patients with dysentery. He laid great stress on the specific agglutination test. As in the history of so many infectious diseases, the worker who first isolated the correct causal organism "skimmed the cream" and left relatively little for his successors to prove. However, the contributions of Flexner and Strong were significant ones.

Flexner, while the Commission was in Manila, directed his attention to a study of the dysentery prevailing in and around that city. The Report of the Surgeon General of the Army for 1899 contained a tabulation of diseases observed among the American troops during the first four months of the American occupation of Manila. In it the dysenteries were included with the diarrheal diseases. The total number of cases reported was 445, with a death rate of 0.48%. This compilation, however, failed to present an adequate reflection of the extent, severity and mortality from dysentery in Manila. Although he could not obtain exact figures, Flexner was convinced from nearly three months' residence in Manila, that the enteric diseases, of which dysentery was the most frequent and important, were the principal causes of disability and mortality among the land forces of the American army.

The disease occurred in two main forms: acute and chronic. Flexner scrutinized the stools and intestinal contents for amebae. These organisms were either absent or extremely difficult to find in the acute cases. In the chronic forms of the disease, in which ulcers were present, the amebae were variable as to actual occurrence and number. Large hepatic abscesses, usually single, were encountered in the number of cases. Thus, the morbid anatomy of the chronic disease, as Flexner saw it, agreed with that of so-called amebic dysentery. The pathological changes in the acute disease differed greatly from those of the chronic cases.

In his study of the bacterial flora of the disease, both acute and chronic cases were utilized. Two distinct types of organisms could be distinguished, especially in acute cases. Results of the agglutination tests varied. With the host there was frequently a reaction in low dilutions; with another person the reaction was rarely obtained. Neither organism could be isolated in the healthy dejecta from normal persons, including army personnel, natives and patients with beri-beri. The organism was also absent from cases of chronic dysentery. Flexner also demonstrated that the bacillus was pathogenic for laboratory animals. The organism proved to be closely related to, but not identical with, that isolated by Shiga in Japan and has since been known as the Flexner bacillus.

R. P. Strong and W. E. Musgrave made important studies on dysentery in the American forces in the Philippines simultaneously with those of Flexner. They found *Bacillus dysenteriae* in the acute stage of the dis-

---

From his observations in Manila and the surrounding territory of the island of Luzon, which was occupied by the American troops, Mr. Garrett says that he was struck with the adaptability of the country surrounding Manila for the establishment of 'hill stations,' as they are called in tropical settlements, or stations where the Europeans and Americans may retire to the hills at night in order to retain their health.

'Much good has already been accomplished in Manila in improving the sanitation of the city. I am afraid many persons do not realize what a city Manila is. Leaving out China and one or two places in Japan, it is the largest city in the far East. The houses there are especially well built, many of them being constructed of stone. Probably the best result has been secured in the stamping out of smallpox. Formerly the average death rate from this disease in Manila was 22 persons a month. At the present time the rate has been reduced to about two fatal cases a month, some months being without deaths.

Benefits To The South

'Looking at the question from a standpoint of dollars and cents alone, the great commercial development of the future will be on the shores of the Pacific. With the completion of the Nicaragua Canal, the South will benefit probably more than any other section of the United States in this trade. At that time I look to the far East as the market for the cotton crop of the South, which is now held back by the long railroad haul to the Pacific Coast . . .' "

eases, both in the discharges and in the superficial necrotic layer of the intestinal mucosa. They described in detail the reactions of the bacillus which they isolated and which they regarded as similar to, if not identical with, that isolated by Shiga in Japan.

Richard Pierson Strong was born in Fortress Monroe, Virginia on March 18, 1872 and died in Boston, Massachusetts in July 1948, at which time he was professor of tropical medicine emeritus in the faculty of the Harvard School of Public Health. Strong, who graduated from Yale in 1893, was a member of the first class to receive the M.D. from Johns Hopkins (1897) (Fig 7). Following postgraduate training at Johns Hopkins, he was commissioned in the United States Army as a first lieutenant during the Spanish–American War. After the war he was assigned to the Philippine Islands as the first president of the Army's Medical Research Board for the Investigation of Tropical Diseases. Strong resigned from the Army in 1902, and after a period of research and study in Germany, was made director of the biological laboratories of the government of the Philippine Islands located in the Bureau of Science, Manila. During this period he was chief of medicine in the Philippine General Hospital and a professor of tropical medicine at the medical school of the University of the Philippines. His investigations of plague, cholera, bacillary dysentery, balantidial dysentery and other diseases gained for him an international reputation as a leader in the field of tropical medicine.

In 1911, when the Manchurian Plague Commission was formed to combat a widespread epidemic of pneumonic plague, Strong was appointed as a member representing the United States government. He and his associate, Oscar Teague, performed heroic service during this dangerous epidemic.

In 1913 Strong was called to Harvard University, where he became the first professor of tropical medicine and organized postgraduate teaching in this subject. He had hoped also to build a school of tropical medicine, the first of its kind in America, which would compare favorably with the leading schools of England and Europe. The project was initiated and well financed for a time; however, shrinkage of available funds subsequently led to the reduction of the school to the status of a department. (In 1922 when the Harvard School of Public Health was organized, the department of tropical medicine was transferred to that school.) Strong was recognized throughout the world as a leader in tropical medicine. He conducted important research in the laboratories of the department and on various field expeditions made to many parts of the world. The more important of these were to Peru, 1913; the Amazon Basin, 1925; Liberia and the Belgian Congo, 1926–27; Guatemala, 1931–1932; and again to the Belgian Congo, 1934.

In 1915 Strong went to Serbia as head of a Red Cross unit to combat the typhus epidemic of that year. He and his associates demonstrated the transmission of trench fever by the louse.

After his retirement at Harvard, Strong, at the request of Admiral Stitt, rewrote Stitt's *Textbook of Tropical Diseases*, which was published in two volumes. This

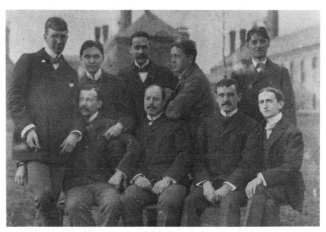

Fig 7. Members of the Pithotomy Club, Class of 1897 (first class), The Johns Hopkins University School of Medicine. Left to right, standing: Thomas R. Brown, Eugene L. Opie, James F. Mitchell, William G. MacCallum, Charles R. Bardeen. Seated, left to right: Joseph L. Nichols, Richard P. Strong, L. W. Day (did not graduate), Louis P. Hamburger.

work was the best current reference on tropical medicine and was of great service to the armed forces during the second World War.

Shortly after the United States entered World War II, the Preventive Medicine Section of the Surgeon General's Office recommended that Strong organize and direct a series of intensive courses in tropical medicine at the Army Medical School. The training of these men was of enormous importance to the Army in meeting the conditions faced by American troops in the tropical regions in which they had to operate.

VISIT TO INDIA WITH INSPECTION OF THE PLAGUE DISTRICTS

After leaving Hong Kong on the journey home, Barker and Flint took a steamer which called at Singapore and then went northwest across the Bay of Bengal, up the Hugli River to Calcutta. School memories of English history were revived for them as they visited the site of the "black hole" of Calcutta. But they remained in the city just long enough to visit the medical school, look at the monuments and principal buildings and drive in the Maidan Park, along the Red Road, and up and down the Chowringhee, on which the principal hotels, clubs and shops were located.

In Bombay and Poona, Flint and Barker studied as fully as they could the measures adopted by the English officers for combating bubonic plague. In Bombay they were taken through the hospitals, bazaars, and native quarters by Colonel Weir, the chief health officer of the city; he was a man who had a profound knowledge of the character of the people of India and leavened his duty as plague official with such a degree of respect for Indian traditions that he was greatly admired by the natives.

Three years before their visit there had been a serious outbreak of plague in the city and island of Bombay. The disease was still very prevalent there during their visit—more than 50,000 persons dying of plague in the city of Bombay alone in 1899. The outlook for controlling it seemed to the plague authorities indefinite and not very hopeful. The problem would have been difficult even if medical officers had met with intelligent appreciation of their efforts on the part of the people, but in Bombay they encountered, at first, nothing but prejudice, bigotry and resistance. Weir, in his 1897 report, had said: "So bitter was the opposition to the capture of rats that monstrous stories were invented of our officers throwing live rats on the fires, as if to give pleasure to men tired and weary, and knowing the danger of handling rats, doing what they need not do, even if a sense of humanity did not forbid them." Thus the plague authorities had to deal with people who were more careful of the lives of animals than of their own. The measures necessary in fighting plague clashed with the interests, the customs, and the deepest feeling of the inhabitants. On one occasion the picking up of a few sick pigeons had caused great excitement, nearly leading to a riot. Peaceful traders threatened to raze the city for the sake of ten sick pigeons. Actual plague riots had occurred, causing the death of several soldiers and policemen. The natives believed that human sacrifice was necessary to palliate the gods who controlled the plague, so they killed some of the Sahibs. The sanitary measures at first adopted interfered with the strict castes of the Hindus, and house-to-house inspection violated the seclusion in which the Musselmen guard their women. Haffkine vaccine for prophylactic inoculation was made from meat broth, and the high caste Hindus would have none of it. Haffkine tried to prepare it by using a substrate of gluten or other substances free from meat extracts. All efforts of the plague authorities were misinterpreted. It was even said openly that the doctors were killing the patients by subcutaneous injections in order to stop further ravages of the plague. Fantastic stories were invented, including a statement that patients were purposely killed and their hearts removed in order that the latter might be sent to Her Majesty, the Queen Empress, to appease her wrath on account of the disfigurement of her statue in Calcutta, which had occurred early in the epidemic.

The high point of their observations of plague in India was reached when they visited Poona, where the disease was more prevalent than elsewhere. Poona had suffered a severe drought in the preceding year and the general resistance of the population was low. When Barker and Flint alighted from the train they were astonished at what they saw. The population was in flight. One-third of the people had already left the city or had died from the disease. Panic prevailed among the people, all desiring to escape. Hundreds of natives rushed into the third-class compartments of the trains until they were entirely filled; those who could not get in fell asleep on the station platform waiting for the next train. The town was preternaturally quiet and dismal; it suggested the atmosphere of a gigantic sickroom. Barker and Flint passed a Mohammedan funeral headed by chanting Mullahs bearing clanking cymbals in their hands. The body of the deceased, borne on a litter, was partially covered with a white muslin cloth, but they could see the emaciated face with its open staring eyes directly blankly upward toward the sky. Their guide led them into the court of an old Hindu temple where on the floor of a little room at one side of the yard lay a girl of 16, unconscious, with a plague bubo in her right armpit. A naked yogi, leering at them, stood before the shrine of the court, his body littered with ashes and his face painted as he bowed. On the road leading to the general hospital they passed bullock carts laden with plague patients. At the hospital 100 plague patients were being admitted daily and 80 patients died each day. Major Windle, who was in charge, had great difficulty in keeping servants, ward boys or grave diggers, for despite the offer of larger wages than usual the fear of the pest made them refuse to accept jobs. The mortuary at the hospital consisted of four corrugated iron shanties—one for Mohammedans, one for high-caste Hindus, a third for low-caste Hindus, and the fourth for Christians and Parsees. Mohammedans were being buried in long rows of shallow graves, whereas the dead Hindus were placed upon funeral pyres built of dry cakes of cow dung, each pyre being fired from the top so that the body was slowly cremated. Hindu relatives watched the burning; some left when the skull of the deceased exploded; others remained until the incineration was complete. Some, who were of frugal inclination, sold the ashes to speculators who scratched away in the ruins of the pyre searching for melted jewelry.

Leaving Poona, Flint and Barker clearly recognized that they had witnessed plague devastation as dire as anything observed in modern times. What they saw in Poona left them with an indelible impression of a dreadful nightmare. The words "stricken, pest-ridden, and pestilence" have their full meaning only to those who have looked upon such scenes. For the first time they realized what the horrors of the "black death" of Europe in earlier centuries must have been like. It provided an enormous stimulus to their devotion to medical research with the confident expectation that ultimately great epidemics of infectious disease would be abolished.

PLAGUE IN SAN FRANCISCO

Barker could not have known at the time that within two years his experience with plague would lead to his contact with the disease in his own country. Early in 1901 his work as professor of anatomy at Chicago was temporarily interrupted by his appointment to a federal commission on the plague in the United States. Bubonic plague had been reported as occurring in San Francisco, but its existence had been strenuously denied by the local politicians. It was admitted that some Chinese had died with "swollen lymph glands," but physicians who had been in practice for long periods in the city maintained that the glandular swellings had been occurring among the Asiatic inhabitants of the city for at least 30 years and no epidemic of plague had occurred. It was quite natural for the politicians of the city and state to hope that this explanation was correct.

However, from reports that he had received from the Marine Hospital Service and the Treasury Department in Washington, Dr. Walter Wyman, Surgeon-General of the U.S. Public Health Service, was convinced that it was not safe to accept such statements as evidence that no plague existed in San Francisco, and at his request, President McKinley appointed on January 19, 1901 a commission "for the purpose of ascertaining the existence or nonexistence of bubonic plague in the city of San Francisco, California under instructions that the members of the commission would receive from Dr. Wyman." The Commission was composed of Professor Simon Flexner of the University of Pennsylvania, as chairman; Professor L. F. Barker of the University of Chicago, as recorder; and Professor F. G. Novy of the University of Michigan, a skillful bacteriologist who had worked in Koch's laboratory in Berlin and in the Pasteur Institute in Paris.

The Commission was told by Wyman that their "investigation should be entirely unprejudiced and independent"; the findings were not to be revealed until authorized by the Bureau. Barker arrived in San Francisco on January 25, 1901 and Flexner and Novy reached the city two days later. The City Board of Health supplied them with a map of Chinatown on which were charted the location of the patients that the Board had examined and had reported as having plague. They interviewed a number of physicians whose opinions were divided, some being confident that plague had occurred, others being just as certain that it had not. These preliminary steps proved of value, for through them the commissioners learned how to gain access to the sick and dead Chinese and how to proceed without exciting the opposition or suspicion of those among whom they had to work. A room at City Hall was placed at their disposal; this was converted into a laboratory. The attorney of the so-called Chinese six companies advised the Chinese to cooperate with the Commission, and proclamations were issued ordering the Chinese to report all cases of sickness and death no matter what the cause. Because of his clinical experience, visits of inspection were delegated to Barker, whereas Flexner was to do the pathological work and Novy, the bacteriological.

Beginning on February 6, Mr. Wong Chung took Barker to visit the rooms of all patients reported as sick. Many turned out to have advanced tuberculosis or other chronic diseases and needed only one visit. In any doubtful case, subsequent visits were made and the progress of the illness watched closely. Barker also inspected daily every dead body in the undertaking establishments in Chinatown, and those persons suspected of having died of plague were studied pathologically and bacteriologically, both by the City Board of Health and by Flexner and Novy. In the eight days from February 6 to February 13 they saw three patients with bubonic plague while they were still alive; in two of them, the clinical diagnosis of plague was made before death. In addition, the pathologic and bacteriologic diagnoses of plague were made in three dead Chinese. Of the 13 deaths that came to their attention, 6 were found to be due to infection

with plague. When they telegraphed their conclusions to Surgeon–General Wyman, orders were sent from Washington that immediate steps should be taken to admit the existence of plague and to institute promptly the measures necessary to exterminate the disease. The public was not alarmed earlier because there had been no large epidemic, but the progress of the plague in California had been characteristic of the disease elsewhere before a large outbreak, the same kind of "sneaking" progress that was observed in Hong Kong, Calcutta and Bombay for months before large numbers of people were attacked.

The Commission found that before their visit to San Francisco at least 25 deaths due to plague had been discovered during the 11 months from March 1900 to January 1901. These cases had been reported by Drs. Kellogg and Kinyoun, and these physicians, together with Dr. John M. Williamson, president of the San Francisco Board of Health, affirmed that bubonic plague existed and should be vigorously combated. If the California people, and especially those in authority, had been willing to accept the findings of these competent observers, it would not have been necessary for the federal government to appoint a special commission. Unfortunately, the physicians, who announced the existence of the plague, were subjected to a vicious and unjust vilification. After the Commission made its report, city and state authorities adopted measures for stamping out the disease. Chinatown was cleaned up and only an occasional sporadic case of plague was reported between 1901 and 1904.

THE REPORT

After the return of those on the expedition to the Philippines, there was a frequent exchange of letters between Barker and Flexner while the report was being written and the expenses of the trip straightened out. In a letter to Barker on September 13, 1900 Flexner said the following:

You will be interested in learning that I worked out the vaccine in Paris at the Pasteur. By cultivating the virulent bacilli upon a wide thin surface of agar in special flasks and then making a suspension, which was killed by heat (60°) and afterwards preserved with lysol, I got a definite product. The method is capable of yielding any quantity of vaccine. I shall, on getting settled in Philadelphia, prepare a large quantity which I shall turn over to the Surgeon–General ... In England I also had a pleasant time. In London through the Chief (Osler) I met a number of the best men ... I went to the BMA [British Medical Association] at Ipswich and talked on "Cirrhosis of the Liver" and "Dysentery." For the latter I had the advantage of Manson's discussion. He was, apparently, both interested in and impressed with, the bacillus; he expressed himself as regarding the amebae as epi-phenomena. You will see my position if you ever read the Middleton–Goldsmith Lecture.

In a later letter: "The Bulletin account I considered very good. I suspected it was the manuscript prepared for Harper's, who seem not to know 'pearls.'"

In a further letter on August 10, Flexner wrote as follows: "Thanks for the congratulations. I think that the observations [on an outbreak of dysentery] on the 'kids' will be of help to us. There seems little doubt of its correctness. We have worked with 40–50 positive cases at the Wilson Sanitarium [Mt. Wilson Tuberculosis Sanitarium near Baltimore]. The blood is positive in 90 percent of the cases. We have failed completely to obtain the organism from healthy children and from 10 to 12 cases of gastric disturbances clinically differentiated from the summer diarrheas . . . We are trying to carry out a tentative experiment with the serum. It is very difficult to get at fresh cases, partly because they do not get into the hospitals and partly because the season is rather advanced and rather cool." Thus Flexner's interest in the work on bacillary dysentery continued.

In a letter to Barker on July 26, 1902 written by William H. Welch, the following paragraph appears: "Flexner is here today out at the Wilson Sanitarium. They have found there the Shiga bacillus in nearly every case of summer diarrhea in infants and children. A really exciting discovery. Flexner will be here for several days. I have not yet seen him, but expect him and Gay at dinner."

The report was addressed to "President Gilman, Drs. Welch and Osler, Philippine Committee of The Johns Hopkins University Medical School" and was published in President Gilman's official report as president of the University for the year 1899 and in other publications. A short account of the expedition was published by Barker in the *Bulletin* of the hospital.

A letter to Barker provides evidence of Walter Reed's interest in their venture (October 16, 1899): "Well, my Dear Doctor, I am delighted to know that you are back once more, sound and well, and that you were kindly treated by the Med. Dept. in Manila. I saw dear old Flexner and had a long talk with him. That *Bacillus dysenteriae*, of which you speak, is a most important finding. What will Councilman say? Shall we have an antitoxic serum for this disease? What a God-send it would be to the poor sick devils in the Philippines!

"It begins to look as if I would go to Manila, sometime in December. I want to go, and shall certainly come over and have a long talk with you, before I start on my journey."

THE SUBSEQUENT CAREER OF FLINT AND GAY—THE MEDICAL STUDENTS

Both of the medical students who accompanied Flexner and Barker on the expedition to the Philippines later had distinguished careers. John Marshall Flint received the B.S. degree from Chicago in 1895, and entered The Johns Hopkins University School of Medicine in 1896. Anatomy with Mall remained throughout his stay in Baltimore the inspirational and, to a considerable degree, his working locus.

In 1900 Flint went to Leipzig, as so many of Mall's pupils did. He then went with Barker to Chicago where he was associate in anatomy for the year 1900–1901. His stay was short, for he was offered the professorship of anatomy at the University of California, which he held from 1901 to 1907. He organized the anatomical laboratory there and published 12 papers, of which 10 concerned the histogenesis and organization of the structure of the adrenal, submaxillary, thyroid, parathyroid glands, lung and esophagus. He later took a prolonged sabbatical year in Germany where he completed his anatomical work on the lungs and esophagus. While surveying most of the university clinics in surgery, he centered his activities with von Eiselberg, a pupil of Billroth. Obviously Flint was preparing himself to enter the field of surgery, having, as Mall had been advised, first perfected himself in a preclinical discipline.

His opportunity came for this transition from anatomy to surgery when he was offered the professorship at Yale in 1907. Flint accepted on condition that laboratories, classrooms and offices be provided in close contiguity with the hospital and dispensary and that adequate technical assistants be provided for these. All the essential and basic conditions of a university department on "whole time" were introduced, although it was not as yet an established policy at Yale.

Out of his war experiences (1913–1916), Flint accumulated material for several papers on military medicine which provided valuable information before our own entrance into the war. From the Greco–Bulgarian experience came the "Balkan frame" and knowledge of the suspension methods for treating fractures. Another valuable contribution was a method for the precise location of foreign bodies by roentgenography.

Following naturally upon his anatomical studies of the lung and esophagus, Flint was interested in surgery of the thorax. First he developed an apparatus for the administration of ether vapor within the pharynx, collaborating with Herbert Thoms, a student. This was also employed intratracheally by the technique of Meltzer, and finally, a modification was made by which positive pressures could be maintained, thus making it possible to carry on operations within the open thorax. Sauerbruch and Willy Meyer were working with massive chambers for this purpose, but Flint's approach was the forerunner of the present day methods employed in thoracic surgery.

A large number of lobectomies and pneumonectomies were successfully done upon dogs and such physiological observations made as were possible at the time. The capacity of the remaining lung to expand and fill out the thorax was demonstrated. Flint remained as professor of surgery at Yale until 1920.

Frederick Parker Gay received his education at Harvard College and then at the Johns Hopkins medical school. On graduation, one year later than Flint, he received one of the first fellowships from the Rockefeller Institute and started as assistant demonstrator in pathology at the University of Pennsylvania under Simon Flexner. Perhaps the most important influence in his life was Jules Bordet of Brussels, with whom he studied for three years. Returning to this country, he occupied various posts until in 1910 he was called to the University of

California, where he remained for 13 years. In 1923 he moved to the College of Physicians and Surgeons, Columbia University, and remained in charge of the department of bacteriology until his death in 1939. Gay devoted himself chiefly to studies on cellular immunity, using particularly the streptococcus as a pathogenic agent. In 1935 he compiled an extensive work entitled "Agents of Disease and Host Resistance," written almost entirely by men who had worked in his laboratory in New York. The year before his death he was elected to the National Academy of Sciences.

EPILOGUE

Johns Hopkins's first international venture was a success from many points of view. The University demonstrated an interest in world medicine, which it has maintained and which over the years has greatly expanded its educational and scientific contributions. For the members of the faculty, it was an experience which enlarged their appreciation of medicine in its broader, worldwide context. It prepared Barker for his subsequent role in the San Francisco plague episode and gave Flexner additional background which undoubtedly stood him well in his future role as scientific director of the Rockefeller Institute for Medical Research. For the students, it must have been an unforgettable introduction to the real world of medicine as a major problem not only in the United States but also in the less well-developed countries. It is reasonable to assume that Gay's career interest in microbiology stemmed from this experience. Another important benefit was the realization that American medicine has a unique opportunity and a responsibility to help solve the health problems abroad as well as at home. Medicine has no national boundaries. In spite of the current lack of tropical diseases in the United States, World War II demonstrated the need for medical personnel experienced in those problems. Lastly, in spite of the limited time that the group was in Manila, definitive scientific contributions resulted, in particular the work which Flexner accomplished on dysentery—a study which he continued after his return. Among the remaining disease problems, some of the most common and important are those in tropical areas. The time has come to see that the new basic advances in biochemistry and

pharmacology are appropriately applied to the solution of those problems.

ACKNOWLEDGMENTS

I wish to thank Dr. Thomas B. Turner and Patricia King for help in the preparation of the manuscript and to Susan Tripp for providing the newspaper clippings from the Homewood Archives.

REFERENCES

1. Barker LF: Medical commission to the Philippines. Bull Johns Hopkins Hosp 11: 26, 1900 (Also see 11: 37, 1900)

2. Barker LF: Time and the Physician. New York: G. P. Putnam's Sons, 1942

3. Barker–Reed Letter: Barker papers. Alan M. Chesney Archives, Johns Hopkins University School of Medicine

4. Barker LF and Flint JM: A visit to the plague districts in India. NY State Med J 71: 145, 1900

5. Bloomfield AL: A Bibliography of Internal Medicine; Communicable Diseases. Chicago: University of Chicago Press, pp 33–41, 1958

6. Diary of Simon Flexner: Kindly made available by the Library of the American Philosophical Society, Philadelphia

7. DuBois EF: Frederick Parker Gay (1874–1939). Trans Assoc Am Physicians 55:15, 1940

8. Flexner S: Etiology of dysentery. JAMA 36: 6, 1901

9. Flexner S and Barker LF: The prevalent diseases in the Philippines. Science 11: 521, 1900

10. Flexner–Barker Letters: Barker papers. Alan M. Chesney Archives, Johns Hopkins University School of Medicine

11. Harvey SC: Joseph Marshall Flint. Yale J Biol Med 17: 503, 1945

12. Johns Hopkins University Circulars, Johns Hopkins Press, 1900. Volume XIX, Number 143, pp 13–16. (Gilman's Annual Report for 1899 which contains report of the Commission to the Philippines)

13. Opie EL: Simon Flexner, M.D., 1863–1946. Arch Pathol 42: 234, 1946

14. Shiga K: Ueber den erreger der dysenterie in Japan. Centralbl f Bakt 23: 599, 1898

15. Shiga K: Ueber der dysenterie bacillus (Bacillus dysenteriae). Centralbl f Bakt 24: 817, 870, 913, 1898

16. Simmons JS: Richard Pierson Strong, 1872–1948. Trans Assoc Am Physicians 62: 20, 1949

17. Strong RP and Musgrave WE: The bacillus of Philippine dysentery. JAMA 35: 498, 1900

10.
Arthur D. Hirschfelder—Johns Hopkins's First Full-Time Cardiologist

Arthur D. Hirschfelder was born in San Francisco, California, on September 29, 1879. He was the only son of Dr. Joseph Oakland Hirschfelder, the first child born in Oakland, California. Joseph Hirschfelder had graduated in the first class at the University of California (Berkeley) and then studied medicine in Leipzig under such masters as Carl Ludwig, the celebrated German physiologist, and Franz Hoffman. Upon returning to California, he became professor of medicine in the Cooper Medical College (now Leland Stanford University). He is reputed to have been an excellent teacher of clinical medicine from whom the students and interns learned more about history taking than from any other member of the faculty. His clinics were given at the bedside in the medical wards of the City and County Hospital, the students and interns sitting in a semicircle around the bed of the patient used as a text. His discussions at daily rounds were founded on long experience and extensive study of the literature, especially of English and German medical journals. George Dock recalled a remark Hirschfelder made to an intern who spelled syphilis with two "ll's": "My God, doctor, syphilis with one 'l' is bad enough." In 1873 he translated from the German an interesting small book entitled *A Pocket Manual of Percussion and Auscultation for Physicians and Students*.

Joseph Hirschfelder was also an investigator working experimentally for years to find a cure for tuberculosis (Fig 1). In 1896, in the November issue of the *Occidental Medical Times*, Hirschfelder first described his method of treatment. His theory was conceived in early October 1895 and the treatment of patients was cautiously begun on October 22, 1895.

In 1864 Spencer Wells had performed a laparotomy in consequence of an erroneous diagnosis upon a case of tuberculous peritonitis. Contrary to all expectations, the patient recovered. Similar cases were soon reported. It was Hirschfelder's hypothesis that the entry of air into the peritoneal cavity brought about oxidation of the tuberculin present in the effusion and that it was oxytuberculin which brought about the cure. It seemed plausible to him that by oxidation the toxin was changed into an antitoxin. Acting on this hypothesis, he prepared tuberculin and then subjected it to oxidation with hydrogen peroxide, thus making the oxytuberculin

Reprinted from the *Johns Hopkins Medical Journal* **143**: 129, 1978.

that he used. His description of the results was rather dramatic: "Within a few days (of beginning treatment) the cough and expectoration diminish and the most striking effect is the rapid improvement in the appearance of the patient. His eyes become bright and his color changes from the gray hue of tuberculosis to one more nearly resembling that of health. The appetite rapidly returns and with it a feeling of vigor. . ."

It was a crowded meeting of the Medical Society of the State of California at which he demonstrated his patients as well as his culture tubes showing inhibition of growth of the tubercle bacillus by oxytuberculin. Dr. Levi C. Lane closed the extensive discussion of Hirschfelder's report as follows:

As we have been occupied here for a long time, I will say but little. I have followed the work of Dr. Hirschfelder from the time he began it, and in the beginning was very skeptical. I did not believe that he had made a discovery. There was a committee selected by him of members from two medical schools here, of which I was one of the members, to examine into his claims for his discovery. We were partially but not wholly convinced; we believed in going very slowly and told him so, though he was fully convinced a year ago that he had made the discovery. Time has gone on and he has done a great deal more work. He has brought here to-night specimens in the test-tubes showing demonstrably, certainly, that this oxytuberculin will control the bacillus and the spores of bacillus tuberculosis. He has worked that out of the test-tube. He has brought here to-night forty consumptives, some of whom were in the last stages of the disease, and would certainly have been in their graves. They here appear as persons well, and I have carefully listened during the last three hours, and not one of them has coughed. I will say nothing further.

In 1901 J. O. Hirschfelder was the physician to President McKinley's wife during a visit of the President to San Francisco.[1] In a letter to his son, Hirschfelder

[1] An extensive trip around the country was planned at the beginning of McKinley's second term in office. He was to leave Washington at the end of April for six weeks. The highlight of his visit to San Francisco was to be the launching of one of the new battleships, the *Ohio*.

Mrs. McKinley was in her usual poor state of health, but her maid was on hand to take care of her, and her physician, Dr. Rixey, was in the party. The second week of May, during their stay in Los Angeles, a bone felon on her forefinger had become so inflamed that Dr. Rixey had lanced it. However, this procedure failed to bring relief—she was febrile and had developed diarrhea. On the way to San Francisco the train was stopped for

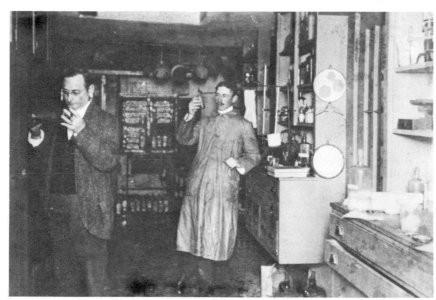

Fig 1.   Joseph O. Hirschfelder (foreground) and Arthur D. Hirschfelder. This photograph was taken in 1904 in the laboratory on the top floor of J. O. Hirschfelder's home at 1392 Geary Street in San Francisco.

Courtesy of Joseph O. Hirschfelder, director, Theoretical Chemistry Institute, University of Wisconsin

mentions this and then discusses his efforts to make available to the public his treatment for tuberculosis:

My dear Arthur,   May 25, 1901

As you have already learned through the daily press my task has been well finished. I have just received a telegram from Wells, Nev. stating that Mrs. McKinley passed a very comfortable night and is standing the trip well. She has therefore passed safely out of the state of Cal. and I may consider that my duty has been done. As you can easily imagine I experience a great feeling of relief for I was in great dread that she would die on my hands. Her condition as I told the President was very precarious and I am certain that only the salt hypodermoclysis saved her. However, all is over and I can return to

my ordinary duties again. Your mother has kept you informed of all details and I need not refer to them. But far above the prestige that I have derived from my connection with the case I have reaped a reward that is far dearer to me. I have found a way of putting your brother "oxy" (the child of my brain) upon the road to success. For a long time past I have been looking around for ways and means of giving "oxy" the trial that is absolutely necessary to establishing its value. Some months ago I spoke first with the members of the family and then with Drs. Lane and Rixford of a plan that I had. It has been my dream to found a sort of Pasteur Institute for the investigation and treatment of disease, especially tuberculosis. An institute in which experiments upon cultures and animals could be performed and in which patients could be treated gratuitously. It was and is my purpose that unlimited quantities of "oxy" should be made and distributed gratuitously to rich and poor both here and abroad. Such an institute could be built for about $100,000 and would take at least $10,000 a year to run. My second plan was more modest. I wanted about $5,000 to equip a clinic with x-ray, blood apparatus, chemical and bact. labs and to treat the poor gratis with "oxy" having a sufficient number of assistants to run easily. This would take about $5,000 a year. Neither plan would cause me very much additional work. Dr. Lane thought most favorably of the plan, but Dr. Rixford advised waiting a few years—for what reason was not perfectly clear except that he thought my evidence should first be far more conclusive than it yet is. After very careful deliberation and discussion with Rixford (whom I had selected as I thought he would be on the other side and I wanted to hear what objections could be made to my plan), I concluded that it was wise and proper to start my clinic if I could. The main objection that R. made was that I would get worn out again as I had been before and that the strain upon me would be too great. I did not and do not agree with him for the two things that disturbed me before were (1) the

nearly an hour while Dr. Rixey again lanced Mrs. McKinley's finger. On Sunday, May 12, she was so ill that the President made an exception to his strict rule against travel on Sunday, and took her quickly to San Francisco. Mr. H. T. Scott, the head of the Union Iron Works which had built the battleship *Ohio*, placed his house at the President's disposal, and trained nurses were obtained.

During the next three days, Mrs. McKinley became more critically ill. Local physicians called in consultation made the diagnosis, later confirmed, of a blood-stream infection. On May 13 McKinley gave up all thought of continuing his tour. When she sank into a stupor before morning, a medical consultation (Hirschfelder) was called, and heart stimulants were administered. As her heart responded to the stimulants, the "new treatment" of injections of salt were tried with good results. On Saturday, May 16, the President attended the launching ceremony and clearly expressed his relief as he opened his address as follows: "I am inexpressibly thankful to the Ruler of us all for His goodness and His mercy, which have made it possible for me to be with you here today." (This account of Mrs. McKinley's illness was abstracted from Leech M: In the Days of McKinley. New York: Harper and Row, 1959.)

loss of faith in my own results which were due, I am certain, to deterioration of my "oxy" on account of my germ having become a laboratory germ and to too long oxidation (130 hours) of my "oxy" which was made with tuberculin 1/10 N acid. I have now and can always have a fresh germ raised from the pig on our own farm. I also oxidize my tuberculin (1/10 N acid) only 108 hours and have better results than ever both in my lupus and in my tubercular patients.[2] My x-ray photographs show the improvement objectively as you will see when you come out. (2) I was upset by the worries caused by selling the "oxy." This shall never again occur for although I will give "oxy" away I shall never again sell a drop.

I consequently paid one respect to what Rixford said but decided that my plan was wise for with all the evidence I could possibly collect in the ordinary way I would not be much nearer the proof in 10 years than I am now.

My first plan was to enlist the interest of Tom Williams but he was so much taken up with a fight over his race track and with his marriage immediately after followed by a trip to the McCloud River where he now is that I could not see him. I next gently brought the subject to Mr. McNear, the father of the young lady whom I had cured of tuberculosis. He seemed interested and said the rich ought to pay for the remedy but the matter stopped there. He did not volunteer any contributions and I did not ask for any.

After I had consulted several times with Dr. Rixey he asked me for anything I had written and so I gave him my "oxy" pamphlet. He was much interested and we had several conversations on the subject. He read some passages to the President who said to him: "That reads well." I showed and gave him some of my x-ray photographs and also took him through my lab. I then thought that I might speak to Scott for the first time on the subject, believing that he had made a good deal of money and would jump at the chance to give me my chance. I spoke but he did not jump. The next day he came to my office and said that the President had opened up the subject to him and had asked him what he knew of my treatment. Scott told him I had spent $20,000 to $40,000 on the thing and that he believed I was correct. Scott told me that when he was through with the President, the strike and his daughter's marriage he would write to Carnegie and see what could be done. When Mr. Hay was at my office with Mrs. Hay I took the opportunity while Mrs. Hay was lying on the x-ray table under Hubbel's supervision to show Mrs. Hay my photographs and to speak of my treatment and plans. She said that it ought to be easy to raise the money and mentioned Mr. Carnegie's name. I said I did not know him whereupon she answered that my friends did. Then he said Morgan was coming to S. F. in October and that he might do something. I asked her to take the matter under her

protection. She seemed very friendly and spoke of a friend whom she would induce to come to be treated.

After matters had reached this stage I thought it wise to have a talk with the President. I did not want to take advantage of my official position and bring up the subject while we were smoking and chatting together nor did I care to call upon him without special permission as Dr. Rixey suggested but preferred to send him a note asking for the privilege of a few minutes conversation with him on my treatment of tuberculosis if his time and inclination permitted. He set a time and on entering the room said that he had heard of my treatment and was favorably impressed therewith, that he had watched me for two weeks in the sick room and believed in me. I told him of my plans and desires and that I wanted nothing for myself. He said: "That is not right. You should be rewarded for your discovery." I answered that it was a holy subject with me and that commercial gain was repulsive to me. He said: "Your larger project is modest and your present demand is very small," that it ought to be very easy to raise the small sum from the rich men of S. F. I told him that Mrs. Scott had said that it was very hard to raise money here and that I did not like to ask anything of anyone, etc. "Well," he said, "it will be a very easy thing for me to get you the money. You should have $5,000 to establish your experimental station, if I may call it so, and a fund of about $20,000 to run it. Of course as President I cannot take the initiative, but if Mrs. Scott will speak to me I will have no difficulty in getting the sum: Hay will give a thousand and so will Moore and Hanna. Why, I will get half the amount on the train." I thanked him most heartily as you can well imagine and immediately told Scott of what had occurred. Scott did not promise to speak but said "That is all right, old man." Scott went on to Ogden with the party and will be back in a few days. Unless some very unforeseen accident occurs, I will have what I wish. Still it has been my fate so often to have the cup dashed from my lips that if that occurs this time I shall merely wipe my lips instead of smacking them and shall not be disheartened. For me the main thing is to have faith in myself and I have it.

Dr. Rixey asked that you should call upon him in Washington and I would like you to do so when you can. I may want you to give him a special message. I would also like you to call on the President, as Mrs. McK. especially asked for you. Dr. Rixey can take you there. Telegraph me the date of your departure from Baltimore a few days before you leave for I may want to telegraph to you to call on Dr. Rixey and the President with a message from me. At any rate even if I do not telegraph, I wish you to present my greetings to both of them.

As I am very tired we will go to Monterey on Wednesday or Thursday for a good rest. Your mother will write other news.

Much love from your
Father

I told the President that Scott had said he would write to Carnegie whereupon the Lord of the Land exclaimed: I would not let Carnegie do all that.

---

[2] At the tenth International Medical Congress at Berlin in 1890, Koch announced that he had found a remedy for tuberculosis. The introduction of tuberculin, his one mistake, was hailed all over the world as an event of the greatest importance. Although he had limited his claims to the possible cure of early cases, great hopes were widely entertained which, of course, did not materialize. Hirschfelder appears to have thought his particular method of preparation could surmount any difficulties. In 1897 he published a paper entitled "The Cure of Tuberculosis by Oxy-tuberculine with experiments on patients, animals and cultures" (Trans Med Soc Calif, San Francisco, 1897, p. 250).

With such a heritage, it was natural for Arthur Hirschfelder to elect a career in medicine. He attended a small private school where his performance put him in the child genius class. He memorized all of the books and passages which interested him, including many of Shakespeare's and Sir Walter Scott's books; all of Cicero

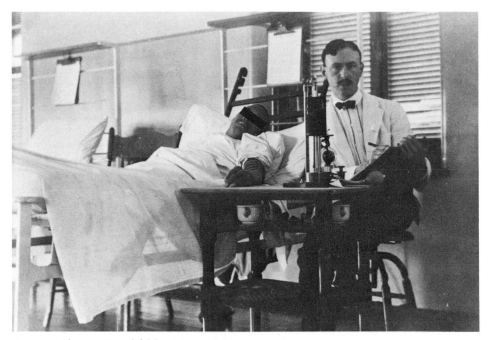

Fig 2.   Arthur D. Hirschfelder (about 1905)
From the Alan M. Chesney Medical Archives, The Johns Hopkins Medical Institutions

and Caesar, etc., in Latin. After obtaining his B.S. degree from the University of California in 1897 as the school's youngest graduate, he began the study of medicine in Europe. In Heidelberg, where he was a classmate of Herbert Freundlich, he studied physical chemistry under Lommel, protozoology under Butschli, physiology under Kühne, and physiological chemistry under Otto Cohnheim. He then entered The Johns Hopkins University School of Medicine, receiving the M.D. degree in 1903. The next year was spent as an intern under William Osler and the following year as a resident in medicine under his father at the San Francisco General Hospital. During that year he was also an assistant in medicine in the Cooper Medical College.

THE FIRST CARDIOVASCULAR RESEARCH DIVISION

In 1905 when Lewellys Barker succeeded William Osler as professor of medicine at Johns Hopkins he established three full-time clinical research divisions—the first of their kind in the United States—in physiology, in biology and in chemistry. Arthur D. Hirschfelder assumed the position of director of the physiological laboratory of the medical clinic (Fig 2). This laboratory began official operation in October 1905 to study diseases from the standpoint of disturbance in function.[3] The facilities consisted of one laboratory in the new Surgical Building of the hospital which was for the clinical study of patients by the special methods in use at the time, particularly the graphic methods. A second facility was available in the Hunterian Laboratory where dis-

[3] Barker LF: The Laboratories of the Medical Clinic. Johns Hopkins Hosp Bull 18: 193, 1907

eases seen in the medical wards could be reproduced in animals and studied by physiological methods. It was the aim in these laboratories "to bring the studies upon the patient as closely as possible into relation with the findings upon animals and mechanical models and to turn these results to practical use."

Hirschfelder had been attracted to a career in medical investigation as a result of stimuli from three sources: one, the influence of his father for whom he had the greatest admiration; two, the frequent contacts which he had with Jacques Loeb when Loeb was at the University of California; and three, his friendship with his Johns Hopkins classmate Arthur Loevenhart, who later became professor of pharmacology at the University of Wisconsin.

Hirschfelder's early research was carried out on problems relating to the circulation. He made some of the early determinations of blood pressure in man using the wide cuff. Under the guidance of his father he began a study of the venous pulse and an analysis of cardiac arrhythmias. Upon his return to Johns Hopkins in 1905 he studied experimental heart block in dogs with Joseph Erlanger. Erlanger spoke of this work in his "Reminiscences of a Physiologist": "During the 1905 summer vacation, a medical student, Arthur D. Hirschfelder, collaborated with me in some experiments designed to ascertain the relative action of the cardiac nerves, the inhibitors and the accelerators, during complete heart block when these two parts of the heart are functioning independently of each other." (Erlanger erred in his memories of this early period. Hirschfelder had graduated in 1903 and was head of the cardiovascular research division in the department of medicine in 1905!) The results of this work appeared in two publications. The first article, entitled "Eine vorläufige Mitteilung über weitere studien in

Bezug auf an Herzblock in Saügetieren," was published in the *Zentralblatt für Physiologie, Leipzig und Wien*, and the second, entitled "Further Studies on the Physiology of Heart Block in Mammals," was published in the *American Journal of Physiology*.[4] During 1906 Hirschfelder published three papers: "Graphic Methods in the Study of Heart Diseases," "Observations on a Case of Palpitation of the Heart" and "Observations Upon Paroxysmal Tachycardia." In the following year, in collaboration with J.A.E. Eyster, a study was reported on extrasystoles in the mammalian heart.

In 1907 the *Johns Hopkins Hospital Bulletin* published a series of papers which emanated from the research laboratories organized by Barker. Three of these papers came from the physiological division of the medical laboratory and were presented by its director, Arthur D. Hirschfelder.

In Hirschfelder's first paper, entitled "Some Observations Upon Blood Pressure and Pulse Form," he discussed the Strasburger method for the determination of minimal blood pressure and pointed out its inaccuracies. In this method the pressure in the cuff upon the upper arm was gradually increased while the observer palpated the pulse at the wrist and determined the point at which the volume of the pulse was maximal. On careful estimation Hirschfelder found the error to be only 5 to 8 millimeters. The method had been put into use in The Johns Hopkins Hospital during the preceding year for routine blood pressures taken by medical students. For them it proved quite unsatisfactory, the discrepancy lying mainly in the lack of uniformity of pressure exerted by the palpating finger upon the radial artery. Hirschfelder also made observations on the dicrotic pulse in typhoid fever, concluding that it was the result of the coincidence of a very marked peripheral dilatation with somewhat increased heart action.

In the next paper Hirschfelder discussed "Some Variations in the Form of the Venous Pulse." He encountered a slight variation of form occurring in the diastolic portion of the cardiac cycle, which might well be confused with disturbances in conduction or with atrial extrasystoles. He presented evidence that this wave was to be regarded as an event in the normal diastole, more pronounced in some hearts than in others.

The third paper was entitled "The Rapid Formation of Endocarditic Vegetations." Hirschfelder, in collaboration with Harold A. Stewart, a recent graduate of The Johns Hopkins Medical School who later worked with Alfred Cohn at the Hospital of the Rockefeller Institute and then as a cardiologist at Cornell Medical School, showed that in some cases the cauliflower-like form of the vegetations of verrucose endocarditis may be determined by the thrombotic deposit which collects upon the valve immediately after the production of the lesion. They produced lesions in dogs by means of a blunt

button-pointed probe introduced into the left carotid artery and thrust through the aortic valve. These papers illustrate what primitive techniques were available for application to the study of clinical problems by physiological methods at the turn of the century.

In 1908 Hirschfelder published papers on "Recent Studies on the Circulation and Their Importance to the Practice of Medicine"; "The Volume Curve of the Ventricles in Experimental Mitral Stenosis and its Relation to Physical Signs"; and a description of his contributions to the study of auricular fibrillation, paroxysmal tachycardia and the so-called auriculo-(atrio)ventricular extrasystoles.

In the following year Hirschfelder and his chief L. F. Barker related "The Effects of Cutting the Branch of His Bundle Going to the Left Ventricle."

In 1910 Hirschfelder expressed his interest in other areas in papers entitled "Another Point of Resemblance Between Anaphylactic Intoxication and Poisoning with Witte's Peptone" and "Cutaneous Tests with Corn Extracts in Pellagrins." There were also in that year articles in the cardiovascular field, including one entitled "The Functional Disturbances in Paroxysmal Tachycardia," and another, "Functional Tests of Cardiac Efficiency."

As described in another of these essays,[5] 1910 saw the early use of the electrocardiograph machine in America at Johns Hopkins. Hirschfelder participated in this work, which was carried out largely by George M. Bond at the instigation of Lewellys F. Barker, who had ordered the Edelmann string galvanometer while on a trip to Europe the preceding summer. The three published their first paper on this subject, "Personal Experience in Electrocardiographic Work with the Use of the Edelmann String Galvanometer (smaller model)," in the *Transactions of the Association of American Physicians*; a second paper, entitled "The Electrocardiogram in Clinical Diagnosis," appeared in the *Journal of the American Medical Association*.

THE FIRST AMERICAN MONOGRAPH ON CARDIOLOGY

The first edition of Hirschfelder's treatise entitled *Diseases of the Heart and Aorta* (Fig 3) was published in 1910. Although other books relating to the cardiovascular system had been published earlier,[6] Hirschfelder's was the first comprehensive monograph on the subject published in the United States.

---

[4] Some years later, when Hirschfelder had become professor of pharmacology at Minnesota, he sent Erlanger a copy of his newly published, massive *Textbook of Pharmacology*. To it was attached a card reading: "The harvest of the seed you planted in the summer of 1905."

[5] Harvey, A McG: Creators of clinical medicine's scientific base: Franklin Paine Mall, Lewellys F. Barker and Rufus Cole. *In* Adventures in Medical Research: A Century of Discovery at Johns Hopkins. Baltimore: Johns Hopkins University Press, p. 124, 1976.

[6] In 1884 Alonzo Clark, professor of medicine at the College of Physicians and Surgeons of Columbia University, published his lectures on "Diseases of the Heart." Even earlier (1852) Austin Flint wrote a book entitled *A Practical Treatise on the Diagnosis, Pathology and Treatment of Diseases of the Heart*. There was a second edition of this book published in 1870. In 1887 John M. Keating published his book entitled *Diseases of the Heart in In-*

DISEASES
of the
HEART AND AORTA

BY

ARTHUR DOUGLASS HIRSCHFELDER, M.D.
ASSOCIATE IN MEDICINE, JOHNS HOPKINS UNIVERSITY

WITH AN INTRODUCTORY NOTE
BY
LEWELLYS F. BARKER, M.D., LL.D.
PROFESSOR OF MEDICINE, JOHNS HOPKINS UNIVERSITY

329 ILLUSTRATIONS BY THE AUTHOR

PHILADELPHIA & LONDON
J. B. LIPPINCOTT COMPANY

Fig 3. Title page of the first edition of Hirschfelder's monograph.

The investigations in the broad field of internal medicine had so multiplied in the decade before 1910 that it became desirable to have from time to time, in addition to the summaries of progress which were contained in the general textbooks on medical practice, monographs which pictured more completely the status of knowledge in the special divisions of the subject. During the first decade of the twentieth century new methods introduced for the study of diseases of the circulatory system led to the discovery of an enormous array of information, and the field had attracted a large body of investigators. Beginning in 1905, Hirschfelder had occupied himself exclusively with such studies in the medical clinic at the Johns Hopkins Hospital. His monograph attempted to epitomize the actual condition of the subject at the time as viewed from the standpoint of an active investigator with extensive first-hand experience who also had a wide acquaintance with the literature of the physiology and pathology of the circulatory apparatus. It was no easy task to combine adequately the most recent results of anatomical, physiological,

---

fancy and Adolescence, while Robert Babcock published a monograph entitled *Diseases of the Heart and Arterial System* in 1903. The following year Theodore C. Janeway's "The Clinical Study of Blood Pressure" appeared. Five years after the publication of Hirschfelder's book, Carl J. Wiggers brought out his "Circulation in Health and Disease" and in 1926 Richard Cabot's "Facts on the Heart," which was pathologically oriented, was published.

pathological and clinical studies in a form which would satisfy the critical demands of the scientific investigator and at the same time be useful as a guide to the everyday practitioner. Special attention was paid in the volume to the practical facts involved in the diagnosis and treatment of circulatory disease; in the theoretical portions there was evidence of careful, critical sifting of the information and an appreciation of the distinction between what was essential and what nonessential for the more general reader. There were ample bibliographic references at the end of each chapter giving those who desired to do so the opportunity to consult the most important and especially the most recent treatises, monographs and original articles on that particular area of circulatory function.

In the preface Hirschfelder stated that his goal was to present side-by-side the phenomena observed at the bedside and the facts learned in the laboratory in order to show how each supplements the other in teaching the physician how to observe the patient and to direct the treatment. He pointed out that many of the laboratory results had not yet attained practical importance because they had been scattered throughout the literature and had not reached the eye of the clinician. However, he emphasized that wherever clinicians have looked to the laboratory or laboratory workers have looked to the clinic for verification or application of their theories, the great pillars of progress have been raised. Based on this idea, the clinical presentation in each chapter was preceded by an introductory section dealing with the experimental pathology and more fundamental principles of the subject, which were frequently referred to in the clinical discussion.

Hirschfelder described how the trend of clinical observation during the past two decades had been toward more accurate study of disturbances of function and toward the introduction of mechanical methods for their observation; methods of precision which tended to supplement or supplant the older and simpler methods of physical diagnosis. Chief among these were the study of blood pressure, the graphic studies upon alterations in cardiac rhythm by means of the venous pulse, the outlining of the heart and vessels by use of the x-ray, and a phonographic recording of the heart sounds. Hirschfelder reviewed each of these subjects with special reference to the general principles upon which the method was based, in order to point out its applicability, its limitations, the character of information which it yielded in clinical conditions, the conditions under which the same information might be gained by simpler methods, the conditions under which its employment was essential and those under which it was superfluous.

The fatigue of the heart was traced through its various stages, from the simple fatigue of the normal heart in exercise, through the stage of "primary overstrain," to that of broken compensation, special attention being given to the states of broken pulmonary compensation arising from failure of the left ventricle and of broken systemic compensation from failure of the right ventricle. The pathogenesis of cardiac symptoms was fully discussed, with their pathological physiology, occurrence and the symptomatic treatment for their relief.

The general methods of treatment in cardiac diseases—dietetic, pharmacological, gymnastic, hydrotherapeutic and electrical—were considered, both as empirical procedures and as experimental methods to correct definite disturbances in the physiology of the circulation, especially changes in cardiac force, cardiac tonicity and peripheral resistance.

In the chapters on the individual organic lesions, discussions were included of pathological anatomy, pathogenesis, pathological physiology, and of symptomatology, course, notes of typical cases, diagnosis, treatment and prognosis. Hirschfelder paid particular attention to functional disturbances such as valvular deficiencies which might bring about conditions similar to those resulting from organic changes or which might accompany the latter. It was his conclusion that the Adams–Stokes syndrome was so definitely associated with lesions of the auriculoventricular muscle bundles as to justify its classification among those conditions resulting from organic lesions. The congenital heart lesions were viewed as disturbances in embryologic development in which primary malformations or states in fetal life had diverted the blood current, modifying the further course of development and producing concomitant secondary malformations. The effects of these lesions upon the adult circulation and their relation to "overstrain" in producing the syndrome of the "morbus coeruleus" were discussed, as well as the various signs, the diagnosis, the prognosis and the treatment.

Hirschfelder devoted short chapters to the subjects of pregnancy in heart disease and the effects of trauma and wounds of the heart. Considerable space was given to the purely functional disturbances of cardiac action, especially to the physiological mechanisms by which many of them result from disturbances in distant organs as well as to the improvements resulting when these disturbances are corrected. This was an area in which Hirschfelder's own research interest was centered.

There were certain interesting omissions. For example, in the first chapter dealing with physiological considerations, although he stated that even the mammalian heart could be readily revived and kept beating outside the body if perfused with a solution containing the essential ions together with sodium bicarbonate and saturated with oxygen, he simply gave a reference to Howell and made no mention of the pioneer studies of Henry Newell Martin. He must have discussed this chapter with Howell and it seems unusual that Howell,[7] who worked in Martin's laboratory, did not point out to Hirschfelder the importance of Martin's contributions.

Hirschfelder described fully the work of Ringer and Howell concerning the role of the various salts in the function of the heart, and in his discussion of the mode of

action of the cardiac nerves he mentioned the "brilliant series of researches" by Howell and Duke who showed that potassium is given off from the heart muscle and can be found in increased quantity in the perfusion liquid after the vagus has been stimulated, noting that it would therefore appear that vagus inhibition is a true potassium effect.

Hirschfelder pointed out in Chapter 2 on blood pressure and blood viscosity that the most accurate and satisfactory, if somewhat bulky, sphygmomanometer was that of Erlanger with which graphic records of both maximal and minimal pressures might be obtained. Hirschfelder devised a polygraph attachment for this apparatus which is shown in Fig 4. He also described the modification of the method for determination of the venous pressure in man (V. Basch) and the modification introduced by Eyster and Hooker while working in the department of physiology at Johns Hopkins (Fig. 5).

Of course, Hirschfelder's monograph appeared just before Herrick's classical description of coronary thrombosis and myocardial infarction with survival and also just at the beginning of the era in which the electrocardiograph was extensively applied in the clinical study of heart disease. There is an extensive discussion of angina pectoris, including a reproduction of Heberden's original description and an interesting discussion of the

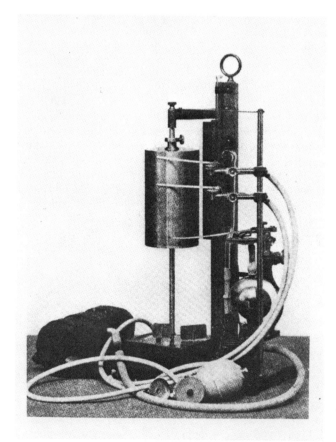

Fig 4.   Erlanger's blood-pressure apparatus with Hirschfelder's polygraph attachment.
Fig. 22, p. 21, in first edition of Hirschfelder's monograph, Diseases of the Heart and Aorta. Philadelphia: J. B. Lippincott, 1910

---

[7] See Harvey, A. Mc.G.: Fountainhead of American physiology: H. Newell Martin and his pupil William Henry Howell. *In* Adventures in Medical Research: A Century of Discovery at Johns Hopkins. Baltimore: The Johns Hopkins Press, p. 84, 1976.

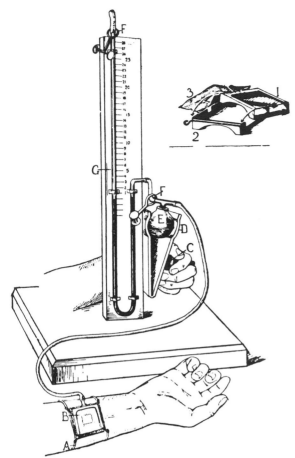

Fig 5. Hooker and Eyster's modification of von Reckling-hausen's method of determining the venous pressure in man.
Fig. 31, p. 33, in Diseases of the Heart and Aorta. Philadelphia: J. B. Lippincott, 1910

theories of the cause of anginal pain. Treatment at that time did include the use of amyl nitrite which had been introduced as early as 1867 by Lauder-Brunton. He also quoted the old treatment of Heberden: quiet, warmth, and hot drinks even if spiritous, also "opium," best in the form of morphine hypodermically or by mouth, during the attack, and repeated if necessary. As Heberden stated, it is well to bring on perspiration (and hence vasodilatation) in any way possible. Hirschfelder discussed the use of caffeine and of diet as well as local treatment of the chest wall by vigorous counterirritation, by blistering and so forth. He stated that in five cases his father had obtained striking relief of the symptoms by treatment with the galvanic current, applying the anode to the neck over the course of the vagus, and the cathode to the precordium and passing a current of 20 milliamperes for five minutes to each side of the neck.

It is interesting that in Hirschfelder's book he did all of the line drawings which helped greatly to clarify the various aspects of circulatory function.

PROFESSOR OF PHARMACOLOGY

Hirschfelder was studying, with Milton C. Winternitz of the department of pathology, experimental pneumonia in rabbits when he was called to the College

of Medicine at the University of Minnesota as professor and chairman of the new department of pharmacology.

At the time the College of Medicine was initiated at Minnesota (1883), pharmacology was not an independent department in American medical schools. The only mention of drugs had to do with courses in materia medica and therapeutics. Pharmacology as a medical school discipline had only come into being some 50 years earlier in Germany. However, in 1907 the University of Minnesota organized a department of physiology and pharmacology. Edgar D. Brown from Torald Sollmann's department of pharmacology at Western Reserve was brought to Minnesota to initiate this new discipline. He was given a modest amount of space, allotted curriculum time for teaching and encouraged to develop a research program. Having little or no funds, he had to outfit the laboratory himself which he did by constructing essentially all of the laboratory equipment. Fortunately, he was an expert glassblower and a skilled worker in wood and metal.

In 1912 Millard Hall was built and the Institute of Anatomy (Jackson Hall) was also constructed. At the same time a reorganization of the medical school took place. Dean Wesbrook resigned and was succeeded by a physiologist, Elias P. Lyon, who took office in the fall of 1913. A search committee was formed to recommend a professor for a new and independent department of pharmacology. Charles Lyman Green of St. Paul, an internist, was chairman of the search committee. In the spring of 1913 the American Medical Association held its meeting in Minneapolis. At this meeting Arthur D. Hirschfelder presented a paper entitled "Diuretics in Cardiac Disease." Hirschfelder was at that time head of the cardiovascular research division in the department of medicine at Johns Hopkins. In this paper Hirschfelder considered the advisability of resorting to diuretic measures in five forms of circulatory disease: (1) infective endocarditis; (2) arteriosclerosis with periodic attacks of the various disturbances associated with localized arteriosclerosis, vertigo, headaches, transitory cardiac asthma or pulmonary edema, angina pectoris, and vasomotor crises; (3) chronic or paroxysmal hypertension without edema; (4) acute cardiac overstrain; and (5) broken systemic compensation with chronic passive congestion, and edema with or without general anasarca, ascites, hydrothorax or hydropericardium, arising from myocardial weakness, valvular insufficiency or adherent pericardium. His concluding statement read as follows: "In general, we should aim first to know the exact state of the kidneys; second, to improve the circulation with digitalis or to spare it with the Karell diet; and, thirdly, to resort to theocin or the saline diuretics to relieve edema if the renal epithelium is not severely injured." His paper greatly impressed Dr. Green, who wished to have a clinician teaching pharmacology. After this meeting Green read Hirschfelder's recently published book, Diseases of the Heart and Aorta, and shortly thereafter the committee recommended Hirschfelder's appointment as professor and head of the new department of pharmacology. On July 7, 1913 the following letter was sent to Hirschfelder:

My dear Dr. Hirschfelder:

At a meeting of the Administrative Board of the medical school you were nominated to the president and Board of Regents for the position of professor of pharmacology and director of the department of pharmacology. The nomination will go to the Board of Regents at its next meeting, after which you will undoubtedly receive an official communication from the president.

This is a matter of personal information, merely, so that you may be prepared to act upon the appointment when you receive regular notice of it.

I am looking forward to much pleasure and profit in our future association.

With very kind regards, I am,
Sincerely yours,
R. O. Beard

Less than 10 days later George E. Vincent, president of the University, wrote to Hirschfelder. The tone of this letter sent some 65 years ago would hardly be appropriate today. It read as follows:

My dear Dr. Hirschfelder:

I am glad to learn that you have accepted our invitation to join our staff. I extend to you a hearty welcome. I am sure that your coming will add to the strength of our medical staff and will be a stimulus to the research spirit which we feel is growing steadily in the university.

I am, Sincerely yours,
George E. Vincent

In accepting this position Hirschfelder had as his goal the application of chemistry to pharmacology and chemotherapy.

When he arrived in Minnesota, Hirschfelder did some work in basic pharmacology (Fig 6). During Hirschfelder's early years there, an organic chemist, Merrill C. Hart, was a member of his department. Hart synthesized a series of organic compounds that were studied for their antiseptic and local anesthetic actions. Hirschfelder had a tremendous admiration for Paul Ehrlich and believed that specific bacterial chemotherapy was possible. He had not only a deep interest in this field but a remarkable store of ideas. It

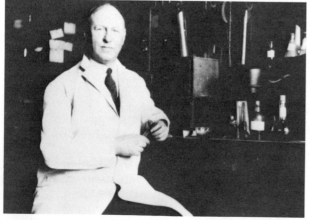

Fig 6. A. D. Hirschfelder in his laboratory, Department of Pharmacology, University of Minnesota School of Medicine.
Courtesy of R. N. Bieter

seems likely that if funds for this type of research had been abundantly available in his time, he would have made some outstanding contributions.

One of the major achievements of Hirschfelder and Hart was the synthesis and discovery of the local anesthetic action of saligenin. This local anesthetic—the least toxic of all local anesthetics up to that time—proved effective on injection and on local application to mucous membranes. Its only drawback was that the anesthesia was of too short a duration for clinical use. Hirschfelder himself directed the clinical pharmacological studies on this drug. In this endeavor and in his approach to teaching in which he made great use of his clinical training, he ranks clearly as one of the early proponents of clinical pharmacology.

His shift to research in basic pharmacology and his withdrawal from clinical medicine were to a significant degree due to his inability to obtain a license to practice medicine in Minnesota. Minnesota had established a Medical Practice Act in 1887 which, it was said: " . . . except for South Carolina, was a model for all the Medical Practice Acts for most of the states. It was a challenge to the efficacy of the medical diploma as a test of the fitness of a candidate to practice and did more to elevate the standards of medical education than any other single factor." When Hirschfelder was a medical student, there was no formal course given in physical diagnosis at Johns Hopkins. The Minnesota Medical Practice Act required a course in this subject. Consequently, the Board of Medical Examiners would not give him a license to practice either by reciprocity or on the basis of taking their examinations.

During his first decade as professor at Minnesota Hirschfelder had very few graduate students; however, there were very few in any department. Hirschfelder encouraged medical students to take electives and to do pharmacological research with him. The elective system had been introduced in Minnesota at about the time of his arrival and he made good use of it in the conduct of his research.

During World War I Hirschfelder helped organize and teach in a school for pharmacist mates of the U.S. Navy at the University of Minnesota. Through a National Research Council project he synthesized a number of brominated and chlorinated cresols. When cloth impregnated with these compounds was worn next to the skin, louse killing vapors were given off for about 13 days whereas ordinary cresol and naphthol lost this capability after about 24 hours. In the latter part of 1918 he was called to serve as pharmacologist to the Johns Hopkins Research Unit of the chemical warfare service. From 1922 to 1925 he was a member of the Board of Consultants of the Chemical Warfare Service at Edgewood Arsenal.

Hirschfelder died on October 11, 1942 as a result of the complications of coronary sclerosis. He had his first difficulty in 1929 and from that time on he was forced to take life a little easier. In his career as a pharmacologist he always strove to apply chemistry to the action of drugs and to stimulate this same scientific interest in all problems relating to clinical medicine. This did not prevent him from utilizing his practical knowledge of drugs used in the treatment of disease in an effective way in his teaching of undergraduates. It was his belief that both of these viewpoints were essential to the development of a creative department of pharmacology.

ACKNOWLEDGMENTS

I am grateful to Dr. Joseph O. Hirschfelder for information about his father and grandfather and for permission to publish figure 1; to R. N. Bieter for information and the use of figure 6; to Carol Bocchini for editorial assistance; and to Patricia King for typing the manuscript.

REFERENCES

1. Barker LF and Hirschfelder AD: The effects of cutting the branch of the His bundle going to the left ventricle. Trans Assoc Am Physicians 24: 313, 1909; Arch Intern Med 4: 193, 1909

2. Barker LF, Hirschfelder AD and Bond GM: Personal experience in electrocardiographic work with the use of the Edelmann string galvanometer (smaller model). Trans Assoc Am Physicians 25: 648, 1910

3. Bieter RN: Department of Pharmacology at the University of Minnesota, unpublished manuscript, 1962

4. Bieter RN and Hirschfelder AD: The effect of sodium benzoate and sodium hippurate and other drugs upon the glomerular circulation in the frog. Proc Soc Exp Biol Med 19: 352, 1922

5. Erlanger J and Hirschfelder AD: Further studies on the physiology of heart block in mammals. Am J Physiol 15: 153, 1905

6. Erlanger J and Hirschfelder AD: Eine vorlaufige Mitteilung uber weitere studien in Bezug auf an Herzblock in Saugetieren. Zentralblatt fur Physiologie, Leipzig und Wien 19: 270, 1905

7. Grey EG and Hirschfelder AD: A clinical investigation of the carbonic acid in alveolar air. Arch Intern Med 11: 551, 1913

8. Hirschfelder AD: Graphic methods in the study of cardiac diseases. Am J Med Sci 132: 378, 1906

9. Hirschfelder AD: Observations on a case of palpitation of the heart. Johns Hopkins Hosp Bull 17: 299, 1906

10. Hirschfelder AD: Observations upon paroxysmal tachycardia. Johns Hopkins Hosp Bull 17: 337, 1906

11. Hirschfelder AD: Some observations upon blood pressure and pulse form. Johns Hopkins Hosp Bull 18: 262, 1907

12. Hirschfelder AD: Some variations in the form of the venous pulse. Johns Hopkins Hosp Bull 18: 265, 1907

13. Hirschfelder AD: The rapid formation of endocarditis vegetations. Bull Johns Hopkins Hosp 18: 267, 1907

14. Hirschfelder AD: Inspection of the jugular vein; its value and its limitations in functional diagnosis (heart block): A criticism by Dr. Hirschfelder and a reply by Dr. McCaskey, a criticism. JAMA 48: 1105, 1907

15. Hirschfelder AD: Recent studies on the circulation and their importance to the practice of medicine. JAMA 51: 437, 1908

16. Hirschfelder AD: The volume curve of the ventricles in experimental mitral stenosis and its relation to physical signs. Johns Hopkins Hosp Bull 19: 319, 1908

17. Hirschfelder AD: Contributions to the study of auricular fibrillation, paroxysmal tachycardia and the so-called auriculo-(atrio)ventricular extrasystoles. Johns Hopkins Hosp Bull 19: 322, 1908

18. Hirschfelder AD: The functional disturbances in paroxysmal tachycardia. Arch Intern Med 6: 380, 1910

19. Hirschfelder AD: Cutaneous tests with corn extracts in pellagrins. Arch Intern Med 6: 614, 1910

20. Hirschfelder AD: Functional tests of cardiac efficiency. Int Clinic, 20th series, 6: 39, 1910

21. Hirschfelder AD: Another point of resemblance between anaphylactic intoxication and poisoning with Witte's peptone. J Exp Med 12: 586, 1910

22. Hirschfelder AD: Diseases of the Heart and Aorta. Philadelphia: J. B. Lippincott, 1910

23. Hirschfelder AD: Recent studies upon the electrocardiogram and upon the changes in the volume of the heart. Interstate Med J 18: 557, 1911

24. Hirschfelder AD: Gibt es besondere fluoreszierende Substanzen im Serum bei Pellagra? Centralbl f Bakteriol (etc.) 1 Abt Jena 66: 537, 1912

25. Hirschfelder AD: Are specific fluorescent substances present in the blood serum of pellagrins? Trans Natl Assoc Study Pellagra 2: 275, 1912

26. Hirschfelder AD: An experiment for training students in the technique of intravenous and intraspinal injections. Am J Physiol 45: 568, 1913

27. Hirschfelder AD: Diuretics in cardiac disease: A general review. JAMA 61: 340, 1913

28. Hirschfelder AD: Methods of diagnosis in circulatory troubles. Trans Int Cong Med Sect 6, Med Pt 2: 271, 1913

29. Hirschfelder AD: Simple methods in cardiac diagnosis. Va Med Semi-month 18: 573, 1913–14

30. Hirschfelder AD: The relation of pharmacology to the practice of medicine. St Paul Med J 16: 16, 1914

31. Hirschfelder AD: Gehirnlipoid als Hämostaticum. Berl klin Wchnschr 52: 976, 1915

32. Hirschfelder AD: Effect of digitalis in experimental auricular fibrillation. J Pharmacol Exp Ther 6: 597, 1915

33. Hirschfelder AD: Effect of drugs upon the vessels of the pia mater and retina. J Pharmacol Exp Ther 6: 597, 1915

34. Hirschfelder AD: The clinical use of digitalis. St Paul Med J 17: 255, 1915

35. Hirschfelder AD: Brain lipoid as a haemostatic. Lancet 2: 542, 1915; Science 44: 251, 1916

36. Hirschfelder AD: Applications of saligenin and other aromatic alcohols and their derivatives to the problems of therapeutics. Trans Assoc Am Physicians 36: 387, 1921

37. Hirschfelder AD: Some newer tendencies in therapeutics. Northwest Med 21: 39, 1922

38. Hirschfelder AD: The direct applications of chemistry in the study and practice of medicine. Chem Educ 2: 431, 1925

39. Hirschfelder AD: Antagonization of the narcotic action of magnesium salts by potassium sodium and other monovalent cations, with a contribution to the theory of narcosis and analgesia. J Pharmacol Exp Ther 37: 399, 1929

40. Hirschfelder AD (with the technical assistance of Victor G. Haury): Clinical manifestations of high and low plasma magnesium: Dangers of epsom salt purgation in nephritis. JAMA 102: 1138, 1934

41. Hirschfelder AD (with the technical assistance of Victor G. Haury): Effect of renal insufficiency upon plasma magnesium and magnesium excretion after ingestion of magnesium sulfate. J Biol Chem 104: 647, 1934

42. Hirschfelder AD and Eyster JAE: Extrasystoles in the mammalian heart. Am J Physiol 18: 222, 1907

43. Hirschfelder AD, Barker LF, and Bond GM: The electrocardiogram in clinical diagnosis. JAMA 55: 1350, 1910

44. Hirschfelder AD and Schlutz FH: Clinical and experimental studies in chemotherapy with ethyl-hydrocuprein in

measles, scarlet fever and other infections. Proc Soc Exp Biol Med 12: 208, 1914–15

45. Hirschfelder AD and Hart MC: Some derivatives of saligenin. J Am Chem Soc 18: 1688, 1921

46. Hirschfelder AD and Hart MC: A simple pressure bottle for laboratory use. J Med Eng Chem 14: 623, 1922

47. Hirschfelder AD, Wethall AG and Thomas GJ: Saligenin as a local anaesthetic for cystoscopy in men. J Urol 7: 329, 1922

48. Hirschfelder AD and Bieter RN: The effect of phenolsulphonephthalein upon the glomerular circulation in the frog. Proc Soc Exp Biol Med 19: 415, 1922

49. Hirschfelder AD and Serles ER: A physico-chemical study of the antagonistic action of magnesium and calcium salts and the mode of action of some analgesic drugs. J Pharmacol Exp Ther 29: 441, 1926

50. Hirschfelder AD and Wright HN: Studies on the colloid chemistry of antisepsis and chemotherapy I. The mode of combination of antiseptic dyes with proteins. J Pharmacol Exp Ther 38: 411, 1930

51. Hirschfelder AD and Wright HN: Studies on the colloid chemistry of antisepsis and chemotherapy III. The ultramicroscopic examination of neoarsphenamine and of certain antiseptics and their effects upon protein solutions. J Pharmacol Exp Ther 39: 13, 1930

52. Hirschfelder AD and Serles ER (with the technical assistance of Victor G. Haury): A simple adaptation of Kolthoff's colorimetric method for the determination of magnesium in biological fluids. J Biol Chem 104: 635, 1934

53. Hirschfelder AD and Haury VG: Variations in magnesium and potassium associated with essential epilepsy. Arch Neurol Psychiatr 40: 66, 1938

54. Winternitz MC and Hirschfelder AD: Studies upon experimental pneumonia in rabbits. Parts I–III. J Exp Med 17: 657, 1913

55. Wright HN and Hirschfelder AD: Studies on the colloid chemistry of antisepsis and chemotherapy II. Does the fraction of an antiseptic which has been adsorbed on protein still exert an antiseptic action? J Pharmacol Exp Ther 38: 433, 1930

56. Wright HN and Hirschfelder AD: Studies on the colloid chemistry of antisepsis and chemotherapy IV. The duplication in vitro of the "Interference phenomenon" in combination chemotherapy. J Pharmacol Exp Ther 39: 39, 1930

11.
Pioneer American Virologist—Charles E. Simon

Charles E. Simon, a professor of filterable viruses in the School of Hygiene and Public Health of The Johns Hopkins University, was one of the first scientists to recognize the importance of these organisms for medicine (Fig. 1). Of him, William H. Howell, dean of the school in the 1920s, said: "The development of the subject of filterable viruses as a separate branch of study was entirely due to his initiative. His own investigations and those of his students, his writings and the character of his courses of instruction, have been responsible for developing a general interest in this subject throughout the country and have added greatly to the reputation and influence of this school as a center of research in preventive medicine." Simon organized the first formal course in filterable viruses, and under his direction the first doctorate degrees in filterable viruses were awarded. Indeed, he was the first to establish the subject clearly as a separate discipline in a school of medicine or public health. As a result of his efforts, the development of virology as an independent area of medical research received a major impetus.

VIROLOGY BEFORE SIMON

The term virus is derived from the Latin and means poison or slime. It was applied to the noxious stench emanating from swamps that was thought to be the cause of a variety of diseases before the establishment of a specific relation between microbes and illness in man. It was almost a hundred years after the discovery by Jenner of the effectiveness of cowpox vaccine as a prophylactic measure against smallpox that the relationship of a true virus to a disease was established. Of importance was the observation that causal agents could not always be detected microscopically in infectious material. In 1885 Pasteur made the remarkable discovery in his research on rabies that a vaccine could be prepared without prior identification of the infectious agent. Although filtration as a procedure in chemistry dates from antiquity, only in the latter half of the 19th century was it used for the separation of microorganisms from the fluids in which they are contained. Casimir Davaine, in his investigation of anthrax in the 1860s, used the placenta of a living guinea pig and also a "porous partition" to separate the bacilli from blood in an attempt to prove that they, rather than a bacterial toxin, were the cause of the disease. In 1871, Ernst Tiegel, a Swiss physiologist, improved the process of bacterial filtration by connecting unglazed clay cells to a Bunson air pump. By this technique, he succeeded in isolating anthrax bacilli from blood. A filter which came to be widely employed was the Berkefeld filter of "Kieselguhr" or diatomaceous earth which was introduced by Nordtmeyer in 1891 and named for the owner of the mine in which the filtering properties of the earth were first noted.

The first representative of the filterable viruses was discovered in 1892 by Iwanowski, a graduate student in botany at the University of St. Petersburg, in the course of his investigations into the etiology of mosaic disease of tobacco. He was able to produce the disease in healthy plants by inoculating them with the filtered juice obtained from diseased leaves. In 1898, Martinus Beijerinck, unaware of Iwanowski's work, published the results of his

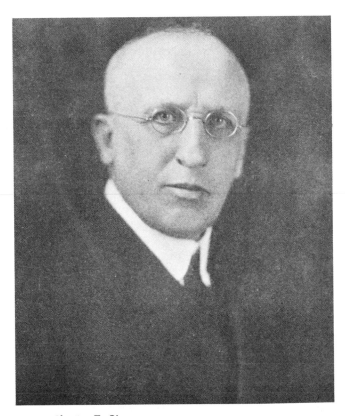

Fig 1. Charles E. Simon

Reprinted from the *Johns Hopkins Medical Journal* **142:** 161, 1978.

observations on the etiology of the same disease, describing the virus as a "contagium vivum fluidum." In the same year there also appeared Loeffler and Frosch's epoch-making studies on the etiology of hoof and mouth disease. These investigators found that they could produce the disease in question by inoculating animals with Berkefeld filtrates of the contents of the specific vesicles, and that the disease could thus be transmitted in passage ad infinitum. They fully realized the basic importance of their results and suggested that other infectious diseases of hitherto unknown etiology, such as variola, vaccinia, scarlatina, and measles, might be due to organisms of this order. The virus of yellow fever, discovered by Reed and Carrel, was the first viral agent proved to be the cause of a human illness. The first human disease shown to be related to a virus, then, was also the first demonstrated to be transmitted to humans by the bite of an insect. Thus, older observers were on the right track with their concept of miasmas and vapors from swamps as the cause of disease since such areas were the sites in which mosquitoes bred and multiplied.

Research in the early decades of the 20th century focused primarily on viral diseases rather than on the precise nature of viruses which could not be visualized or grown in vitro. The spectrum of animals susceptible to viral diseases of man was relatively small. An important event was the recognition of viral inclusions and elementary bodies. Cellular inclusions had long been observed in association with certain infectious diseases and they became the focus of considerable debate toward the end of the first decade of the 20th century. They were thought to be visible evidence of the presence of viruses but it was not clear whether or not they were the actual pathogens. Prowazek, a Bohemian microscopist, suggested that the inclusions were of dual composition. He believed that they were filterable microorganisms which developed intracellularly and were enveloped in a mantle of cellular reaction material. He was unsure of their classification but thought that they were more closely related to the protozoa than to bacteria. In 1909 Lipschütz placed the microscopically visible and filterable agents into a separate group which he called Strongyloplasma. He described them as round, darkly staining bodies which were usually obligate parasites of the host cell. These bodies, as is now known, were microscopically visible viruses. By 1913 Lipschütz had listed 41 diseases thought to be caused by filterable infectious agents of which 16 were microscopically visible as inclusion or elementary bodies. The presence of these bodies and their varied forms continued to provoke questions about their identity. These questions were resolved in 1929 when C. E. Woodruff and E. W. Goodpasture showed that the inclusion bodies of fowl pox contained elementary bodies which were actually the virus.

In 1908 Ellermann and Bang discovered that leukemia of hens could be transmitted by cell free filtrates and three years later Rous demonstrated that a sarcoma of fowls could be transmitted in the same manner. The fact that the pathogen was filterable suggested to many that it might be a virus.

In 1913 Steinhardt, Israeli and Lambert demonstrated that the vaccinia virus could be grown in tissue cultures of rabbit or guinea pig cornea. In the same year Levaditi used in vitro cultures of spinal ganglia to grow polio virus. Tissue culture simplified research since before its introduction isolation of a virus depended on the use of the intact animal. However, because of the problems involved in maintaining aseptic conditions, the technique was not widely used in virus research until the 1950s.

In 1915 the British bacteriologist Frederick William Twort published a short paper entitled "An Investigation on the Nature of the Ultramicroscopic Viruses." This study marked the beginning of a new phase of virus research. Twort described a filterable principle which caused lysis of bacterial colonies, a condition which could be transmitted to fresh cultures for an indefinite number of generations. This was the first demonstration that bacteria, as well as plants and animals, are susceptible to disease. Two years later, d'Herelle rediscovered Twort's lytic principle. He observed that filtrates from lysed cultures of the dysentery bacillus produced further lysis when transferred to fresh cultures. He concluded that the lysis was caused by "an invisible microbe endowed with antagonistic properties against the Shiga dysentery bacillus."

SIMON'S EARLY CAREER

Charles Edmund Simon was born in Baltimore on September 23, 1866, the son of Charles Simon, Jr., a well-known merchant of the city. His primary and secondary education was obtained in Germany, where he lived from his sixth to his eighteenth years, at Baden-Baden and later at the Gymnasium at Hanover. The imprint of this German training remained with him throughout his life, exhibiting itself in occasional German modes of expression and coloring his ideals of scientific work.

When Simon returned to Baltimore, he enrolled in The Johns Hopkins University, taking the Chemical-Biological course in the group system of studies devised by President Gilman and the early members of the faculty. This course provided preparation for the study of medicine. After receiving his bachelor of arts in 1888, Simon studied at the University of Pennsylvania and then transferred to the University of Maryland, from which he received the degree of doctor of medicine in 1890. At that time the course in medicine in most American schools was a two-year program.

Simon received an appointment as assistant resident physician on the medical service under William Osler in the newly opened Johns Hopkins Hospital (1889), serving from May 1890 to April 1891. During this year, under the influence of Osler's magnetic personality, Simon became and remained one of his most devoted admirers. His contemporaries on the resident staff were William Sydney Thayer, who was an assistant resident from November 1890 to September 1891; August Hoch, who later became a prominent professor of psychiatry in New York State; and John Hewetson, who wrote the monograph "Studies of Malarial Fever" with Thayer.

It was at Osler's suggestion, and with anticipation of a future position at The Johns Hopkins Hospital, that Simon spent the year 1891–1892 in Paris doing special work with Gautier in physiological chemistry. He then studied for three months in Basel, working with Bunge. This choice was not entirely dependent on the great reputation of Bunge as a physiological chemist—it was perhaps more important that Miss Lina Stumm, who was to become his wife, lived in that city. They were married in the spring of 1892, and returned to Baltimore later that year.

When the position at the hospital, which had been promised to him by Osler, did not materialize, Simon was allowed the use of a room under one of the wards as a laboratory with the opportunity of offering a special course to the postgraduate students. With the assistance of Dr. Salzer,[1] a prominent physician in Baltimore, Simon opened a private practice specializing in gastro-intestinal diseases. He became widely known for his work in this field and was one of the founding members of the American Gastroenterological Association in 1897. (He resigned from the Association in 1901.) Simon also became busily engaged in preparing his *Manual of Clinical Diagnosis*, which was published in 1896 and which went through some 10 editions, becoming one of the standard textbooks on the subject in this country.

As a result of the intensity with which Simon approached these various activities after his return to Baltimore, he suffered a serious breakdown in his health just after finishing the textbook. For the succeeding 10 years he had emotional difficulties which made it virtually impossible for him to continue the active life of a practitioner of medicine. Osler, who was his personal physician, suggested a way out. "There is a stable," he said, "in the rear of your house. Get the landlord to fix it up and start a diagnostic laboratory." This Simon did. It was the first laboratory of its kind in Baltimore and probably one of the first in the country. It was heavily patronized by the local physicians and its reputation soon spread far beyond the confines of Baltimore. In addition, many physicians came to Simon to study the new laboratory methods of diagnosis. This group continued to enlarge so that soon his laboratory was a training ground from which many physician students went out to establish similar laboratories in other cities or to engage in practice on the basis of the excellent instruction they received. To the extent that his physical and emotional problems permitted, Simon also engaged in scientific investigations. He made numerous contributions to scientific journals which established his reputation as an investigator and which won for him membership in some of the leading scientific societies. He was

one of the charter members of the American Society for Clinical Investigation.

SIMON'S RESEARCH GRANTS FROM THE ROCKEFELLER INSTITUTE[2]

As Simon increased the amount of time he spent in research during his period of ill health, he had great difficulty financing his work. His correspondence with various members of the Scientific Advisory Board of the Rockefeller Institute reveals not only these financial difficulties but also Simon's drive to gain a reputation for his scientific accomplishments (24). His work at this time included the development of a method for testing the opsonic content of blood and other tissues and studies to determine the relationship of this reaction to the stimulation of phagocytosis and immunity in infection. For four years he secured a small sum of money from the Rockefeller Institute. It is clear that while the scientific directors of the Institute exhibited interest and some confidence in his work, they were not overwhelmed by its importance.

Simon first applied for a grant to William Henry Welch, chairman of the Board of Scientific Directors, in 1904. He inquired about his eligibility for a fellowship to carry out experimental work into the chemical mechanism involved in the peculiar tendency of eosinophilic leucocytes to disappear from the circulation in certain infections. He outlined the approach he had used thus far in this work and then indicated that his laboratory would require little new apparatus for the study. The chief expense would be for animals. He stated that the

---

[1] Henry Salzer, born in Germany in 1841, received his M.D. degree from Giessen in 1866. He settled in Baltimore in 1872, specializing in gastric diseases. He was lecturer on diseases of the stomach at the Baltimore Medical College. He died in 1896.

[2] The first duty of the Board of Directors of the Rockefeller Institute was to begin using the money put at its disposal. They decided not to centralize work at once in a single place but to create a number of scholarships and fellowships to be used in existing laboratories throughout the country. In the first fiscal period ending June 30, 1902, $13,200 was allotted in 23 grants of $250 to $1,500 each. Recipients of the grants were classified, according to age, as "research students," "research scholars," and "fellows of the Institute." For the second year, 1902–1903, there were 25 similar grants, the total amount voted for that year being $14,450. Welch took care of practically all the correspondence. Writing in longhand, he approved the expense accounts and sent them to Herter, treasurer of the Board, for payment.

This program diminished in significance after 1903 when the Institute's own laboratories were opened. At the dedication of the new buildings in May 1906, Holt referred to the grants recently made and said it was not intended that the program be discontinued altogether. In 1907, grants totalling more than $11,000 were allocated. In 1914, the Board voted to curtail such grants and made only two or three more in the next three years, discontinuing them altogether in 1917.

Various accounts have treated these grants as scarcely more than a stopgap measure but as Corner pointed out it was a pioneering experiment with a way of promoting research which a few decades later was to become a major factor in American scientific effort in medical research. (Corner, G.W.: A History of the Rockefeller Institute, 1901–1953: Origins and Growth. The Rockefeller Institute Press: New York, 1964, pp. 43–46.)

little he had been able to accomplish in the preceding two years was done altogether from his own limited private resources which depended on royalties from his books. In the closing paragraph, he wrote: "I hope you will understand my sentiments which prompt me to write you on this matter. Through my ill health in the past years, I have been practically forced out of practice. I must confess that I am much happier doing research—still I have the feeling that unless I attempt some little research work in my leisure hours that there is something lacking in my life. Ergo, if I am not entirely out of order I should be grateful if I could obtain some little financial aid for my work. Contrariwise, as I have said, please pardon me for troubling you." Simon was given no encouragement for a grant in the current year, but on April 22, 1905 he again wrote to Welch:

> I have tried to formulate the theme anew, and have embodied a number of points which suggested themselves to me after our conversation. If you think it sufficiently detailed I shall be very much indebted indeed to you, if you will submit it to the Board...
>
> As it has been demonstrated that phagocytic activity on the part of leucocytes is dependent in part on the presence of certain substances in the blood plasma, and serum, which Wright and Douglas have termed opsonins, and as the existence of such substances appears of signal importance in connection with problems of immunity, it would seem of interest to investigate (1) the existence of such substances in the various organs of the animal body (lymph glands, bone marrow, spleen, liver, muscle, brain, etc.); (2) to determine the possibility of the formation of opsonins during the autolysis of the various organs; (3) to isolate such products chemically as may prove practical.
>
> As there is evidence further to show that in certain bacterial infections the opsonin content of the blood may be diminished, it would also seem important to determine the extent to which autolytic products of bacterial origin may be of moment in diminishing (1) the opsonin content of the blood; (2) the opsonin producing power of the various organs; and (3) to separate such products chemically, so far as may prove practical.
>
> In conclusion, experiments would be indicated to determine the possibility of increasing the opsonic power of the blood by active and passive immunization.

Welch could not attend the meeting at which this grant application was to be discussed, but turned the correspondence and the application over to L. Emmett Holt, another member of the Board. In a letter written to Holt on April 4, 1905, Welch indicated that Simon was well qualified to undertake work along the lines indicated. Simon had not asked for a specific sum of money, but Welch suggested to Holt that, if Simon's application was considered favorably, $350 would be appropriate. The grant was approved.

The next year Simon wrote to Simon Flexner, the director of the Institute, stating that his first year under the grant had to be spent largely on the gaps in the information concerning opsonins before he could really proceed with the question concerning immunity. He indicated that much of this had been accomplished but that there was more material to be worked up before he

(Simon) would be justified in discussing certain phases of the subject. He wanted to spend the remainder of the winter creating a firm basis for the next year's work and inquired if Flexner thought that the results were worthy of another grant. He pointed out:

> You know, of course, that I have given up the practice of medicine some years ago and I devote my entire time to laboratory work. Hitherto, I had been severely handicapped for the reason that I have had no financial support and I am profoundly grateful for the grant. I am most anxious to continue the work but must, of course, also think of the question of bread and butter. Do you suppose a larger grant could be obtained which would make matters a little easier for me? This also sounds like I am begging but my position is a little anomalous. I depend on my work in the laboratory to a great extent for my livelihood, and I would like nothing better than to devote my entire time or most of it to the work.

Again, Simon was awarded a grant.

In a letter to Holt written on April 28, 1907, Simon stated that the work performed under his two grants had shown that Wright's opsonic index could not be utilized as a measure of the degree of immunity which had been acquired as the result of the effects produced by bacterial vaccination, and that bacterial vaccination could not be used to advantage without an index to dosage and time of inoculation. Research in this direction, he felt, was no longer warranted. Under a new grant his objective would be to ascertain whether or not the principle of complement deviation could be advantageously employed to the same end. He said that the experiments of Wasserman and his co-workers in this area seemed to offer some hope of success. His personal research led him to the conclusion that the technique could be conveniently modified so as to become a practical method. With this method, he proposed to study the degree of immunity which could be produced by bacterial vaccination both in the human being and in experiments on animals. He pointed out that it was incidentally his purpose to determine by the aid of Wasserman's method whether, with suitable antigenic material, evidence of the production of immune bodies could be obtained in cases of malignant disease. He indicated that should it be possible to demonstrate the formation of immune bodies in such cases, attempts at vaccination with carcinomatous vaccine would not be out of place.

Flexner wrote to Simon on June 14, 1907 requesting the completed paper on the opsonins in acute infection so that he could publish it immediately. He also gave Simon the news of a new grant awarded to him and offered to supply his laboratory with tumor mice if Simon decided to pursue that line of study.

With the help of the mouse cancer material sent to him by Flexner, Simon continued his work on malignant disease. On February 18, 1908, he wrote to Flexner:

> Tomorrow is the meeting of the Society of Experimental Biology and I had hoped to attend this meeting. I find, however, that it is impossible for me to get off. If you think it desirable, would you be so kind as to make a brief

statement in my name that I have succeeded in obtaining a serum reaction along the principle of complement fixation which seems to be specific for carcinoma. I have been able to make the diagnosis of carcinoma by the aid of this reaction without having seen the patients, the diagnosis being confirmed at operation. By taking the cases as they come, some before operation, some a number of weeks after operation, our percentage of positive results with the method . . . has been over sixty. By improvements in technique, we hope to increase this still further.

I am of course anxious to secure priority rights but desire very much also to keep the field undisturbed for myself, for a while at least. What would you recommend? If you think it well to make this brief announcement, please do so.

There is no indication in the correspondence as to whether or not the statement was made by Flexner at that meeting.

On April 1, 1908, Simon wrote to Holt saying that he would like to submit his application for a new grant before the next Board meeting. It was his intention to continue the work along the same lines with special reference to carcinoma and sarcoma and to study in greater detail the response of the carcinoma subject to inoculation and to vaccination with cancer material. Simon pointed out that with the complement fixation method, it was possible to demonstrate substances in the serum of cancer patients which in the presence of suitable cancer antigen were capable of fixing complement. He suggested that with this method, it might be possible in certain cases to make the diagnosis of malignant disease from the blood. Simon wanted to investigate the chemical mechanism involved in this question, to ascertain whether the method could be perfected so as to be of service in routine diagnosis, and to study the relation of such fixation to that which is observed in earlier cases. Simon had noted that cancer cells, when suspended in normal saline or Ringer's solution, rapidly underwent destruction at body temperature. Suspended in normal blood serum they could be kept at 37° for at least 72 hours without being destroyed. He said that while similar results were usually obtained in the case of serum from cancer cases, specimens may be encountered which exerted a most intense cytolytic effect upon homologous cells such that destruction was brought about within a few hours. The lytic effect, he thought, was best explained by the assumption that in certain cases of cancer, autocytolysins are formed in the body and that these cytolysins might be concerned in the complement fixation.

However, by January 1909, Simon wrote to Flexner that from his experience during the past months, nothing could be accomplished regarding complement fixation in the diagnosis of cancer. He obtained the reaction in about 60% of the cases under the most favorable conditions, but it was unreliable as a diagnostic test because syphilis interfered. Under the circumstances he felt that it would not be wise to follow up this line of work to any great extent. Thus, Simon, along with others who followed him, thought prematurely that

he had found a method for the diagnosis of cancer from the study of patients' blood serum.

Simon, however, was not discouraged by the failure of his test for the diagnosis of cancer. He immediately turned to the study of the defensive reaction of the body against its own cells and cell products, particularly in cancer. He accidently came across

a most remarkable behavior on the part of the blood serum which seems to be common to both syphilis and tuberculosis and which I have not met with under other pathological conditions although we have already studied over 150 cases. My point of departure was to ascertain the resistance offered by cancer cases to various hemolytic poisons. Starting with saponin, I found that the red cells apparently play a passive role but that the blood serum under normal conditions already possesses antihemolytic properties which are quite constant. In pathological conditions other than tuberculosis and syphilis, we find essentially the same conditions while in the two diseases mentioned the antihemolytic action of the blood serum so far as saponin is concerned is materially diminished.

Simon thought that this work lay outside the scope of his research grant and so queried Flexner as to whether or not he should proceed. He did not wish by any means to abandon his cancer work; on the contrary, he felt that with this new method of investigation, the cancer problem could be tackled from a new point of view. To this end, he was eager to study the relation of cancer serum to various types of hemolytic agents. Flexner, of course, replied that Simon was free to follow out the leads bearing on his work, even though they might not be precisely within the scope of the problem offered to the Board.

In a letter to Flexner on February 23, 1909, Simon once again repeated what he had done under the latest grant and asked whether in Flexner's opinion he might obtain a grant for a fifth year to pursue these areas and whether or not this grant might be of some higher figure. He had a new idea which was to ascertain whether any special group of aniline dyes could be shown to have a selective affinity for malignant cells in the living animal and, if so, whether it would be possible to influence these by substitution of toxic molecular complexes to the exclusion of the toxic effect upon normal tissue. What was needed from Flexner, in addition to a grant, was a supply of mice or rats with cancer.

Flexner's reply of February 24, 1909 read as follows:

I have looked over your program and am interested in the several things which you have stated in connection with cancerous conditions. Although your results may not be connective ones, I think that in the present state of our ignorance they will be valuable. I have also looked over your plan for the modification of aniline dyes in such a way as to endeavor to secure a selective affinity for cancer cells in the living animal, and I think that such studies would be interesting, although they may not lead to any positive results.

As regards the matter of continuance of your grant

by the Board of the Institute, on that point I can, I regret to say, help you not at all. The policy of the directors has been in the past not to continue a grant to one person indefinitely on the basis of changing subjects unless there have been very good reasons for doing so. In certain cases, where a large subject has been taken up and pursued during many years, with gradually accumulating results, there has been no difficulty whatever concerning the continuance of the grant. I might mention in that connection Dr. Novy's work on trypanosomes, etc., but in many other cases grants have not been continued beyond four or five years. Their withdrawal is not intended to signify that the work proposed is not promising work, but merely that in view of the fact that the sums at the disposal of the Directors, to be given out in the form of grants, are not large and that they are, therefore, changed about as circumstances indicate to be best. This does not mean that your own grant may not be continued, and I can see no reason why you should not apply for it, or even for an increase of it, if you think that wise. My own attitude toward your work has always been one of great interest and confidence.

Simon received a grant for the fifth year, after which his support from the Rockefeller ceased.

SUMMERS IN NOVA SCOTIA

After each winter's intensive work in his laboratory, Simon spent the summers in Nova Scotia in an effort to restore himself to normal health. He acquired a house in Chester and became much attached to this region, never tiring of singing its praises. It was to a large degree through his personal influence that a number of his patients and friends similarly migrated to this area for the summer. A large Baltimore colony which characterizes that locality must regard Simon as the pioneer who discovered and advertised its beauty. He and his wife enjoyed frequent cruises along the coast of Nova Scotia which served to familiarize them with the historical landmarks and the explorations of the early adventurers to this region. He apparently could discourse entertainingly of Champlain and de la Roche and the beauties and tragedies of the Acadian period.

Dr. George G. Finney, Sr., recalled his boyhood memories of Simon and the early migration of Baltimorians to Chester:

I was born in our house on the corner of Eutaw and Lanvale Streets in 1899. Dr. Simon lived and had his laboratory, as I remember, three doors from Lanvale Street on Madison Avenue (No. 1302) which was just a block from where I lived. This was an area that harbored quite a few doctors. Dr. H. M. Thomas, Dr. Halsted, Dr. W. W. Russell, Dr. W. S. Thayer, Dr. J. T. King, Dr. Howard Kelly and later Dr. Charles Austrian all lived in the area.

I got to know Dr. Simon because some sons of the above mentioned doctors used to play in that territory and we would often stop in at Dr. Simon's house. He was always very nice to us younger boys. He had a stern look in a way, but it never materialized as far as we were concerned. He had a peculiar mannerism that when he was talking he would make a noise as if he were clearing his throat but it obviously never cleared anything. Mrs. Simon was a very nice lady, born in Switzerland, who talked with a definite accent.

Dr. H. M. Thomas, Dr. Russell and my father, Dr. John M. T. Finney, Sr., were all good friends. I remember one day my father, Dr. Russell and Dr. Simon were talking together (or I think I remember because at this time I was only six years old) and my father said something about how he wished he could go to a nice place for summer vacation when he had the opportunity. Dr. Simon said that he knew the ideal place. It so happened that my father was invited to give a paper on pyloroplasty in St. John's, New Brunswick, the next July. Dr. Simon had purchased a place in Chester, Nova Scotia, in Mahone Bay and he said it was an ideal spot. He then asked my father to come across the Bay of Fundy and across Nova Scotia to visit him in Chester after my father delivered his paper. He also asked Dr. Russell to come along. My father, taking my older brother John, Jr., with him, went to Nova Scotia, gave his paper, and then went to Chester. Simon's house was on a point of land in what was called the Back Harbor of Chester. There was a little two-acre island in the middle of the bay there. There are other islands around in Mahone Bay which is roughly 5 by 10 miles in diameter. When my father saw that little island named Little Fish from Dr. Simon's vantage point, he said, "That is the kind of place that looks good to me." There was a house on the island and a wharf. Dr. Simon then told him what he had heard, namely, that a General Bingham who was then police commissioner of New York City owned the island, had peripheral vascular disease and had lost a leg and didn't know if he would be able to get in and out of boats anymore. The story finishes by my father renting the island for July and August 1907 without even consulting my mother—which might have been a mistake. He also rented with the option to buy. My mother and father with their four children spent those two months in Chester. All the family were delighted. The island was bought with the house and all the furnishings, lock, stock, and barrel, for $5,500. That island is still owned by the Finney family and my parents always felt that Dr. and Mrs. Simon had done them a wonderful favor in every way (Figs 2 and 3).

As I mentioned earlier, Mrs. Simon was born in Switzerland. When World War I came on, both Dr. and Mrs. Simon were definitely pro-German during the three years before the U.S. entered the war. There were all kinds of stories that circulated around Chester about seeing lights from Dr. Simon's house out into the ocean sending messages to German submarines and other wild tales. Dr. Simon one summer, I think 1915, was visited by a young Swiss student who was interested in flora and fauna. He was seen late one evening up in a tree not far from the village by a very suspicious native and since he had a flashlight with him that was thought to be further evidence that messages were being transmitted to the submarines.

As a result of these summer excursions to Nova Scotia, Simon's health continually improved and he was soon able to increase his scientific activity in the laboratory and to prepare new editions of his manual (Fig 4). He developed a national reputation as an authority on clinical diagnostic methods which led to his appoint-

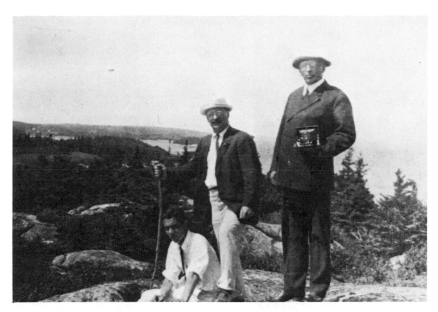

Fig 2.   Finney and Simon in Nova Scotia
Courtesy of Mrs. Stewart Lindsay

ment as the faculty member in charge of instruction in this subject at the College of Physicians and Surgeons of Baltimore. He was later made professor of clinical pathology and experimental medicine in this school (and later in the University of Maryland when the two schools merged); pathologist of the Union Protestant Infirmary and Hospital for the Women of Maryland; and clinical pathologist to the Mercy Hospital of Baltimore. Simon was a master of his subject and a devoted and enthusiastic teacher. His laboratory instruction was supplemented by bedside examinations in the hospital and one can imagine that his students went out into practice with a thoroughly sound knowledge of the methods of clinical diagnosis.

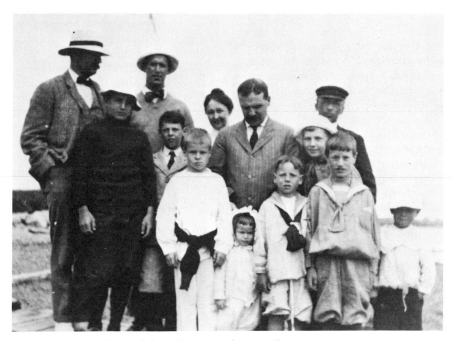

Fig 3.   Some members of the Baltimore colony in Chester.
Left to right: Dr. W. W. Russell, J.M.T. Finney, Jr., Dr. Henry N. Shaw, Charles R. Smith, George G. Finney, Sr., Helen Gross, J.M.T. Finney, Sr., Mary Finney, William G. Hoffman, Jr., Eben Finney, Charles Simon, Roswell Russell, unknown
Courtesy of Mrs. Stewart Lindsay

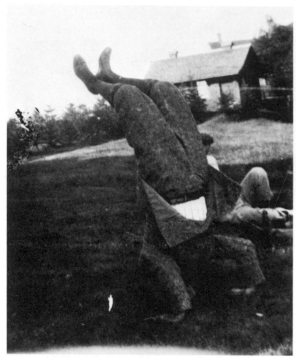

Fig 4.   Simon was well ahead of his time in the methods he used to provide mental relaxation.
Courtesy of Mrs. Stewart Lindsay

OTHER PUBLICATIONS

In 1912 Simon wrote a volume, which he dedicated to Paul Ehrlich, entitled *An Introduction to the Study of Infection and Immunity: Including Chapters on Serum Therapy, Vaccine Therapy, Chemotherapy and Serum Diagnosis for Students and Practitioners.* In this book, Simon pointed out that the enormous progress of medical science during the previous 25 years had been in great part the outcome of the experimental investigation of the interrelation between the macroorganisms and microorganisms during infection. He noted that immunology, while still in its infancy, had already yielded results of such great practical value and of such far-reaching biological significance that the time had come when the general practitioner, who would understandably follow that portion of the current medical literature which "may be said to represent the truly romantic side of modern medicine," should familiarize himself with the essential basis upon which the new science of immunology had been established. The first 11 chapters presented a picture of the conflict taking place when the opposing forces of the invading and the invaded organisms were brought together. The second part of the book, which dealt with the practical application of immunological studies to treatment and diagnosis, emphasized the principles involved and furnished an idea of the general character of immunological technique. No attempt was made to be exhaustive and only representative methods were considered.

In 1919 Simon published a small volume entitled *Human Infection Carriers: Their Significance, Recognition*

and Management. Interest in this subject was renewed with the outbreak of World War I, when attempts were made to guard troops against epidemics. Simon wrote that there had developed an ever-growing demand for men trained in the recognition of carriers by laboratory methods. A request from the Surgeon-General's Office that medical students be thoroughly drilled in the epidemiological aspects of the infectious diseases, including the laboratory side of the question, had created the problem as to what department should provide this training. At the University of Maryland School of Medicine and the College of Physicians and Surgeons of Baltimore, the carrier question was handled by the department of clinical pathology of which Simon was the director. Lack of communication between clinicians and laboratory workers had been a constant source of regret to Simon and he postulated that this was the reason that essentially no sanitary work was either demanded or conducted in the majority of the hospital laboratories. He noted that in institutions in which infectious diseases, which were apt to result in the development of the carrier state, were treated, no examination was made to determine this prior to the discharge of the patient. His book dealt with the problem only in connection with diseases of bacterial origin or those which were thought to be due to the activity of a filterable virus and in which healthy human carriers were known to play a role in their dissemination. The maladies discussed were cholera, diphtheria, typhoid and paratyphoid fever, dysentery, epidemic meningitis, poliomyelitis, *pneumococcus* pneumonia, certain streptococcal infections (such as camp septicemia, bronchopneumonia, septic sore throat, erysipelas and puerperal fever), influenza, and the pneumonic form of plague. Under these headings the various phases of the carrier problem were discussed, i.e., the occurrence of active and passive carriers, the duration of the carrier state, the numerical relation between patients and carriers, the habitat and the virulence of the organisms, the mode of infection, concrete examples illustrating the danger of the carrier to others, the recognition of the carrier with the description of the laboratory methods involved, and the management of the carrier from the standpoint of the public health officer. He also summarized the most important state laws, municipal ordinances and federal interstate regulations dealing with the carrier problem. It is of interest that, at the time, influenza was still thought to be due to the bacillus which had been described by Pfeiffer in 1892. As a result, it was believed that carriers could be identified by the detection of Pfeiffer's bacillus in the sputum or in throat cultures.

SIMON'S PERIOD AT THE SCHOOL OF HYGIENE AND PUBLIC HEALTH

Simon's life changed dramatically with the establishment of the School of Hygiene and Public Health of The Johns Hopkins University in 1918. Although he was not affiliated with the University at the time of the founding of this new school, he had been consulted as an adviser in connection with the medical phases of the work in parasitology. From that moment on, his interest in this new school and in its department of zoology became a consuming one.

Simon had had a fruitful association with the University of Maryland for a number of years, but in 1919 he found it necessary to leave this school because of his pro-German sympathies prior to the United States' entry into World War I. Outspoken about his convictions, he had provoked anger and antagonism among his colleagues which made it impossible to continue his work there. Simon had, of course, known Welch during his period on Osler's staff and had dealings with Welch when he received his research grants from the Rockefeller Institute. He had also known Howell, who was an associate professor of biology while Simon was enrolled in the Chemical-Biological course. Recognizing Simon's plight, they arranged for his first appointment as a voluntary assistant in The Johns Hopkins School of Hygiene and Public Health (1919–1920). The new environment in which research was a major activity was tailor made for Simon's scientific outlook. He gave to the department more and more of his time and participated as a teaching assistant in the courses of medical zoology during those early years. He was lecturer in medical zoology from 1920 to 1922 (Fig 5).

The development of Simon's interest in filterable viruses may have been stimulated by Welch who was well aware, as a result of his chairmanship of the Board of Scientific Advisors of the Rockefeller Institute, that this was a subject of growing importance. Other evidence of interest in virology at Johns Hopkins was seen in the plans for the new pathology building of the school of medicine which was constructed in 1922 after the original pathology building was destroyed by fire. In the new building, a special room with a skylight was designated for work with plant viruses. William G. MacCallum, professor of pathology, and his colleague Oppenheimer worked with vaccinia. Several observers had recognized minute granules in vaccinia and had observed the inclusions (guarnieri bodies) in the epithelial cells. MacCallum and Oppenheimer separated the granules from the rest of the vaccinia by differential centrifugalization. Oppenheimer washed these granules free of all adherent material and found them to be infective. Later Craciun and Oppenheimer were able to cultivate the washed granules in tissue cultures for many generations. MacCallum wrote an excellent review entitled "Present Knowledge of the Filterable Viruses," which was published in the journal *Medicine* in 1926.

However, Howell stated clearly in his memorial note on Simon that Simon's virus work at Johns Hopkins was entirely due to the latter's own initiative. Moreover, Thomas M. Rivers dedicated his classic monograph on

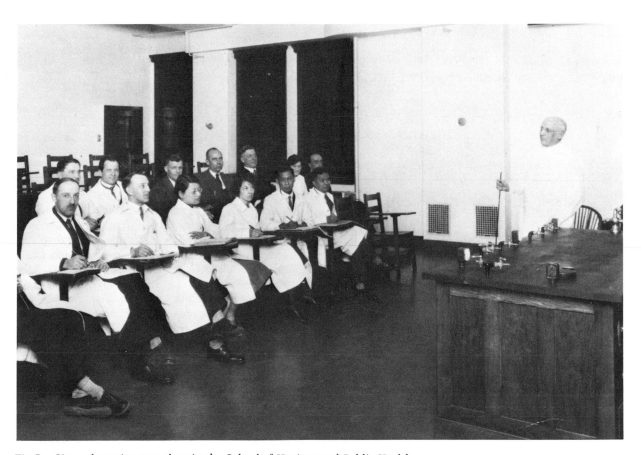

Fig 5.   Simon lecturing to a class in the School of Hygiene and Public Health.
From the Archives of the Johns Hopkins Medical Institutions

filterable viruses, which was published in 1928, as follows: "To the memory, Charles E. Simon, in evidence of appreciation of his leadership and foresight in the development in the United States of the first Department of Filterable Viruses." Rivers had known Simon in Baltimore before Rivers began his work in virology. He knew of Simon's interest and followed his activities closely. The two remained friends and kept in close contact after Rivers joined the staff of the Hospital of the Rockefeller Institute in 1923 and began his own career in virology. Rivers also said of Simon: "Although Simon was an elderly man he was one of those who in the United States very early appreciated the future of virus research."

That Simon was attuned to the importance of virology is evidenced by his review on "The Filterable Viruses" published in the *Physiological Reviews* in 1923. That he was chosen to write this also demonstrates that he had rapidly acquired a national reputation for his knowledge in this area. The nature of filterable viruses, of course, was not too clear at that particular juncture and consideration of various ramifications of this subject occupied a considerable portion of Simon's review. One aspect was the question of the corpuscular character and size of viruses. He stated that mere filterability could hardly be regarded as sufficient grounds for assuming that the viruses represented a homogeneous group and he pointed out the important observations of Beijerinck who had expressed the belief that the virus which caused the mosaic disease of tobacco was a "contagium vivum fluidum," and had come to the conclusion that the virus was not corpuscular, but present in solution. Later investigations made in connection with various other viruses had brought forth no evidence to suggest that any of them were not of a corpuscular nature. Another question was whether or not the filterable viruses were animate or inanimate. A third question was the taxonomic position of the animate filterable viruses. (For example, at that time it was not clear whether the rickettsial organisms should be classified with the filterable viruses.) Simon discussed the relation between filterable viruses and specific cell inclusions which by that time had been noted in several infectious diseases including mollucum contagiosum, epithelioma contagiosum and variola. He summarized the recent investigations on the role of filterable viruses as disease-producing agents, including (a) the supposed relationship of the herpetic virus as the causative agent of epidemic encephalitis; (b) *B. pneumosintes* (Olitsky, Gates) and its relation to epidemic influenza; (c) recent investigations into the etiology of measles; (d) trachoma and inclusion blenorrhea; and (e) filterable viruses in plant and insect diseases.

THE COURSE IN FILTERABLE VIRUSES

Simon organized the first course in filterable viruses in 1922. In the School of Hygiene and Public Health catalogue for 1922–1923, course 5 in the Department of Zoology is listed as follows:

Filterable viruses, Medical zoology 5, Credit 1/2 major, Dr. Simon. Three mornings per week during one-half of one trimester. The aims of this course are: (1) to acquaint the student with that important group of microorganisms which is collectively known by the name of the Filterable Viruses and with certain other pathogenic agents of indeterminate taxonomic position; (2) to familiarize the student with those methods which have been successfully employed in the search for and in the study of these minute forms of living matter; (3) to enable the student to recognize those pathological changes in the tissues of the host that are diagnostic of the corresponding diseases; and (4) to call attention to those methods of control which are based upon a knowledge of the biological properties of the organisms under consideration.

The course consisted of lectures, laboratory exercises, conferences and prescribed readings. The lectures dealt with the general techniques employed in the search for, and in the study of, filterable viruses, their biology, their mode of dissemination and infection and their tissue tropism. Among the diseases then known to be caused by filterable viruses which were discussed were rabies, poliomyelitis, variola, vaccinia, alastrim, trachoma, mumps, measles and dengue. The etiology of scarlatina was not yet clear, and the exact position of the agents causing Rocky Mountain spotted fever and typhus fever, although designated as rickettsia, had not received a final taxonomic classification. The laboratory exercises included experience with the various methods for determining the presence of filterable organisms, methods of concentrating them, methods of isolating the viruses of certain diseases by inoculating them into laboratory animals, the examination of macroscopic and microscopic preparations of pathological lesions, and the study of intermediate hosts.

Fortunately, one of the laboratory manuals for the course in filterable viruses for 1927 had been saved by Joseph Hobbs and was made available by his widow. It is a complete, approximately 60-page mimeographed set of laboratory exercises and special instructions. The course began on October 6, 1927 and the final examination was given on December 21, 1927. During that period, there was a three-hour laboratory session on three afternoons a week. Following each session, there was a lecture related to the day's subject matter. In order to demonstrate the intensity of the laboratory course, the detailed outlines for the sessions of October 24, 26, 28 and 31 are presented (See Appendix I). Simon's intense Germanic approach to this course is illustrated by the written quizzes given on February 11, 1924 (which Hobbs had inserted into the manual) and on March 11, 1927, and the final examination given on December 21, 1927 (See Appendix II).

Simon's course was a popular one with the students, and he and his assistants and special students published a number of papers on the diagnosis of smallpox, the experimental study of measles, the cell inclusions in varicella, the formation of the guarnieri bodies and the origin of malignant growth.

Simon not only organized what was perhaps the first formal course and laboratory in filterable viruses, but, through correspondence or personal visits, he came into contact with all the leading workers in the field in various parts of the world and obtained from them specimens of different kinds of viruses which were used in his classes and in his investigative work. He received materials from Theobald Smith, Peyton Rous, James B. Murphy, Simon Flexner, Alexis Carrel, Thomas Rivers, and others. How he obtained the help of these scientists is brought to light by his correspondence with Peter K. Olitsky and others (19).

In a letter written on November 29, 1922 to Peter Olitsky, Simon spoke of his plans for the first course that he gave:

Our course is to extend over six weeks, three mornings of four hours each. I am, of course, very anxious to bring in your influenza work and was wondering whether you would be so kind as to assist me with some necessary material. I thought the most practical demonstration would be to produce the disease in the rabbit by intra-tracheal insufflation of the culture and to show the organism in the smear. . .

Then comes the question of typhus. What would you recommend as a practical exercise or demonstration and could you help me with material in this connection also?

(Simon was always looking for material for the new *American Journal of Hygiene*, of which he was managing editor and to this letter a postscript is attached: "Incidentally, could you not let me have a paper sometime for our journal?")

Olitsky agreed to come to Baltimore to participate in the course and to bring with him as much material as he thought would be illustrative of the subject. Simon wrote to Olitsky again on December 23: "The class so far as we can now tell may be composed of 14 students who can all be classified as postgraduates. About half of them are medical graduates and the other half students in their last year's work for the doctor of science degree. They have all had courses in bacteriology. Will you perhaps let me have a little outline of what you plan to do on these two days. The hours which are available are from 9 to 1 and you can have as much of that time as you like. As to assistants, Mr. Scott and I could attend to that."

On December 14, 1922, Simon wrote to Simon Flexner giving the following information about the course:

I enclose for you a tentative outline which will give you an idea of what we will try to cover in the few weeks which this year are at my disposal. Any suggestions that may occur to you will, of course, be most welcome.

You will note that the course starts on February 6 and ends on March 13. . .

On the subject of poliomyelitis I was anxious to show the students your coccoid bodies in culture, and have them examine sections of both monkey and human cords. Could I get such material from you? The sections we can, of course, prepare ourselves.

When I left Basel, Dorr gave me some of his

supposed encephalitic virus. I saw this "in action" in his laboratory but unfortunately it had become inactive by the time it reached our laboratory.

On December 27, 1922 Olitsky wrote Simon further about his contemplated participation in the course:

My plan is as follows:

March 6. Influenza. Your program covers the subject completely; no changes in it are necessary. However, may I trouble you to provide a lantern for the numerous slides I will take with me. I will provide each student with a culture of *B. pneumosintes* and possibly of group organisms (See Addendum Paper No. IX in *Journal of Experimental Medicine* for November.) I should also like to have one or two full-grown rabbits to demonstrate intratracheal injection. In general, this is the procedure: a talk from 9 to 10, then laboratory work on the examining of cultures, etc., ending up with demonstrations and methods of cultivating and discussion.

March 8. Typhus Fever. I shall follow your program as closely as possible.

You are generous to allow me the free use of the time. I am not very strong and feel that the presentation of these two courses will require all my energy. May I request that no other plans, socially or professionally, be made?

I shall bring with me all the necessary materials so please do not trouble yourself with any preparation except to provide a rabbit and a lantern.

October 23, 1923 finds Simon writing to Olitsky again asking for his participation in the second course:

I am preparing for this winter's course in the filterable viruses, which has been enlarged to a full trimester starting January 2. The problem again comes up what to do with the class in connection with influenza. Could you supply me with material this year? I will gladly promise that none of it shall leave the laboratory and no investigations will be carried on with any of your material. . . .

I read your paper on the etiology of common colds with a great deal of interest, and I am very much indebted to you that you allowed this virus to remain a truly filterable one, and one that did not become a bacterium.

In Olitsky's reply of October 26, he indicated that he could not leave the Institute but would be glad to send material. He wrote: "Would you please send me a tentative curriculum and the number of your students, together with a list of what you would like to have. If you would do this well in advance of the date when the class begins, it would give both of us a chance to get materials in order."

In his reply of December 15 to Olitsky, Simon said:

. . . my plan for the influenza exercise is the following: the students are to syringe out each other's noses and filter the washings. They are then to make cultures from the filtrate and to inoculate some rabbits intratracheally. I thought it would be a good plan at that time to interpose some material containing *Bacterium pneumosintes*, to observe their rabbits for awhile and then to kill them and to examine the lungs.

In connection with typhus I thought it would be of

interest to show the students the wide distribution of the Rickettsias, as you did last spring. Dr. Nicholson wrote me at that time that he hoped to have an extra supply of sections later on, and that he would let me have some for my class.

Olitsky replied:

... I will send you influenza and typhus materials and will include some of Drs. Cowdry and Nicholson's slides.

I think that your plan is splendid. I would suggest using Ringer's solution for nasopharyngeal washings instead of saline solution, plating filtrate on rabbit blood agar plates and incubating for 7 days anaerobically. The students will then be interested in attempts to find some of the Group I to III of the filter passers. These occur in normal persons. They should be warned to make a distinction between contusion of the lung from inflammation when examining rabbits' lungs after intratracheal inoculation. Our cultures are now saprophytic so they would be of little use to you. I hope that we may obtain a virulent strain before February...

How tight a hand Flexner held on the affairs of the Rockefeller Institute is revealed in correspondence of April 27, 1923 when Simon wrote Olitsky requesting his photograph: "I do not wish to embarrass you at all with any request which may make a call on your pocket book, but do not forget to send me a copy whenever the opportunity should arise. Tell Dr. Flexner what we want. I really think the Institute should bear that expense." There is a pencil note in the margin of the letter saying: "I am willing to pay the expense if you approve sending Dr. Simon my photograph. PKO." Obviously, Olitsky showed the request to his chief, Simon Flexner.

As requested, Simon sent Olitsky a list of the lectures and reports for the course in 1923–1924 and also the laboratory outline (Tables I and II).

Another example of Simon's vigorous effort to obtain current and relevant material for his course is illustrated in the following correspondence between Thomas M. Rivers and one of Simon's postgraduate students, Joseph Hobbs, and between Hobbs and the H. K. Mulford Company:

9–24–27

Dear Hobbs:

Dr. Simon requested that I send him some Virus III for class work—If you will let me know just when you need it I'll send down two rabbits inoculated in the skin and testicles. That is about the only safe way to get it to you as it does not stay active for long at ordinary temperatures (20–37°C) outside the animal body.

Please let me know 10 days ahead of the time you need the virus and I shall be glad to see that you get it.

Sincerely yours,
T. M. Rivers

11–18–27

Dear Hobbs,

I sent two rabbits, 2148–2151, inoculated today in testicles and skin with Virus III. They will be ready for use on 21st or 22nd.

They were sent by express so be on the lookout for them.

Sincerely yours,
T. M. Rivers

11–19–27

Dear Hobbs,

I am afraid the rabbits I sent you are not good—I made transfers yesterday and sent you two of four rabbits inoculated. The material that was used for inoculation was cultured and this morning there is a heavy growth of bacteria in the tubes. Of course contaminating bacteria come in at times when serial passages are made and of course they had to come in just at this time—a time that I wanted everything to go right.

I'll get some new ones ready and send them to you but I'm afraid it will take at least two weeks to be sure all things are as they should be.

Sorry that this had to happen and hope it won't inconvenience you too much.

Sincerely yours,
T. M. Rivers

October 20, 1927

Mr. Joseph R. Hobbs
School of Hygiene and Public Health
615 N. Wolfe Street
Baltimore, Maryland

Dear Sir:

Replying to your favor of October 18th regarding the visit of Dr. Charles E. Simon to our laboratories at Glenolden on November 28, the date is perfectly satisfactory to us, but we have written to Dr. Simon stating that

TABLE I

Lectures and Reports in Course in Filterable Vira
School of Hygiene and Public Health
The Johns Hopkins University

February 6.	Historical Introduction. Dr. Simon
February 8.	Nature of the Vira. Dr. Simon
February 10.	The D'Herelle Phenomenon. Miss Langwill Mosaic Disease in Plants. Mr. Scott
February 13.	Relation of Vira to Specific Cell-Inclusions. Dr. Simon
February 15.	General Biological Characteristics of the Vira. Dr. Simon
February 17.	Foot and Mouth Disease. Mr. Rawson Insect borne Vira. Mr. Hoffman
February 20.	Rabies. Dr. Simon
February 24.	Rabies. Dr. Simon
February 27.	Poliomyelitis. Dr. Simon
March 1.	Encephalitis Lethargica and Herpes. Dr. Simon
March 3.	Influenza. Mr. Scott
March 6.	Small-pox. Dr. Simon
March 8.	Small-pox. Dr. Simon
March 10.	Trachoma. Dr. Simon and Miss Ben-Harel
March 13	Typhus Fever. Dr. Simon

Dr. Simon will also lecture on measles at some time during the course.

TABLE II

Laboratory Outline for the Course in the
Filterable Vira
School of Hygiene and Public Health
The Johns Hopkins University
February 6–March 13, 1922

Filters

Examination of various filters and ultra-filters.
Demonstration of bacteria-retaining ability of Berkefeld filters.
Demonstration of colloidal suspension-retaining ability of ultra-filters.

Hühnerpest

Inoculation of chickens with Hühnerpest virus.
Observation of course of the disease.
Demonstration of pathogenic agent in the blood with ability to pass a Berkefeld filter.
Inoculation of chickens with the filtrate.

Sheep-pox

Inoculation of sheep with sheep-pox virus.
Observation of course of the disease.
Autopsy.
Transfer of virus from nodules of sheep-pox to skin and cornea of rabbits with production of a lapine.
Transformation of the lapine to a vaccine.

Epithelioma contagiosum

Inoculation of chickens with the virus of epithelioma contagiosum.
Observation of course of the disease.
Examination of klatch preparations of contents of vesicles for free strongyloplasms.
Examination of diseased tissues for cell-inclusions.

*Examination of Tissues and Smears for Strongyloplasms,
Chlamydozoa and Cell-Inclusions*

Strongyloplasms and Cell-inclusions of molluscum contagiosum (human).
Strongyloplasms and Cell-inclusions of epithelioma contagiosum (chickens).
Negri bodies and Babes-Koch coccoid bodies (dogs).
Guarnieri bodies (human and rabbits).
Kleine-Schiffmann bodies (geese).
Herpes bodies (human and rabbits).
Borrel bodies (sheep).
Prowazek bodies (human).
Polyhedral bodies (caterpillars).
Da Rocha-Lima bodies (human).

Mosaic Disease

Inoculation of young tobacco plants with the virus of mosaic disease.
Observation of course of the disease.

Rabies

Topographical examination of normal brains.
Examination of smears of rabies material for Negri bodies according to Lentz.
Examinations of smears of rabies material for Babes-Koch coccoid bodies according to Giemsa.

there will be no calves producing Smallpox Vaccine at that time; and as we understand that he is particularly anxious to have this class view the vaccinated animals, we have written him, thinking that he will probably prefer to postpone the visitation until after the first of the year. However, if it is decided to adhere to your selection of November 28th, it will be satisfactory to us as there will be other activities that will be of interest.

After leaving the train at Chester, arriving at 9:56 A.M., the trolley can be used to Glenolden, leaving at frequent intervals. This would make you arrive at about 10:30, and there will be somebody to receive you when you get there and conduct the class through the buildings and grounds.

Very truly yours,
H. K. Mulford Company
Department of Visual Education

It is clear that as the interest in the field of virology extended, Simon's laboratory became a potential source of individuals trained in this area. Indeed, many of Simon's students went to other institutions where they established similar activities. On July 12, 1924 Simon wrote to Peter Olitsky: "Nay, unfortunately, I know no one at present whom I could send to you. Scott just finished his Research Council year with me, and has gone back to his old place after having turned down three attractive offers. The members of last winter's class have either left and gone to their respective homes and positions or they are still working at the school. I should be very glad indeed to keep in contact with you in reference to this matter. . . ."

THE DOCTOR OF SCIENCE DEGREE IN FILTERABLE VIRUSES

Simon had three students who received the degree of Doctor of Science in Filterable Viruses. These were the first such degrees granted in this country. These graduate students helped Simon in conducting the course for undergraduates and spent long hours preparing the material for the laboratory course.

The first of these students, Joseph Mehollin Scott (Fig 6), received his degree in 1923. After obtaining his B.S. from Mount Union College, Alliance, Ohio, in 1913, Scott went to Michigan where he earned his M.S. in 1918. He enrolled in the University of Michigan School of Medicine but after two years realized that, because of his severe asthma, he could not endure the rigors of medical practice. From 1916 to 1918 he was chairman of the biology department at Dakota Wesleyan University. He enlisted in the Sanitary Corps of the U.S. Army as a second lieutenant in April 1918. He was sent to the Rockefeller Institute for a six-week course and then to Camp Devens, Massachusetts, during the great influenza epidemic of September 1918. With Leslie H. Spooner and Elmer H. Heath, Jr., he wrote a report of the epidemic which was published in the *Journal of the American Medical Association* on January 19, 1919. He conducted extensive research on influenza at the Saint Nazaire Debarkation Center until August 1919 when he

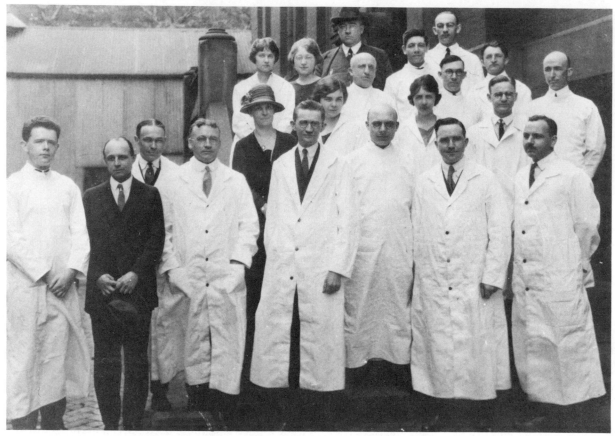

Fig 6.   Department of Medical Zoology, School of Hygiene and Public Health, Johns Hopkins University, May 9, 1924.
Left to right: Bottom row, Andrews, Duggar, R.M. Hegner, Cleveland, Taliaferro, Faust, Root; second row, Joseph M. Scott,
Mrs. Hegner, McNally, Lucy Taliaferro, Howard B. Andervont; third row, Coventry, Deems, Charles E. Simon, Herrick,
Bauer, Boyd; top row, Metcalf, Sandground, Hoffman

was discharged from the service. In 1918 he was elected
Milton Jay Lichty Professor of Biology at Mount Union
College; he held this post until his death in 1946.

Scott received his doctorate in filterable viruses
from Johns Hopkins while on a two-year leave of absence
from Mount Union. His dissertation was "A Critical
Study of the Reaction of the Rabbit Cornea to Inoculation with Variola and Varicella Material." (A varicella
epidemic was in progress in Baltimore and material for
smallpox was supplied by the Colorado State Board of
Health.) In 1924 Scott received a National Research
Council Fellowship in Medical Science to continue his
research under Simon.

After receiving his degree, Scott had several attractive job offers: as assistant professor of bacteriology
at Columbia; in zoology at the University of California at
Berkeley; and with Theobald Smith at the Rockefeller
Institute for Medical Research. He declined these offers
(The letter he received from Smith [Fig 7] provides some
insight into Smith's opinion of the field of filterable
viruses at that time) and decided to return to his old post
at Mount Union. Although he had received no support
from that college, he felt that he owed it a great deal and
realized that he preferred teaching and associating with
eager young people. Despite the fact that he had no time

for research, he kept abreast of new developments by
attendance at scientific meetings and was an active
member of the American Association for the Advancement of Science. He reorganized the laboratory of the
Alliance City Hospital, serving as director from 1924 to
1940. He trained young women college graduates as
medical technicians before such courses were offered in
teaching hospitals. Five of these women later graduated
from medical school. Under Scott's leadership, the biology department was noted for the number of its graduates who became physicians or research workers in
science.

One of Scott's students, Howard Bancroft Andervont, was Simon's second assistant in research and
teaching on filterable viruses (Fig 6). Andervont was
born in Canton, Ohio, on March 8, 1898. He attended
public schools there and then enrolled at Mount Union
College, where he helped to support himself by working
in steel mills. It was Scott who awakened his interest in
biological science and who recommended him to Simon
when he graduated with a degree of bachelor of science
in 1923. Andervont did three years of graduate work with
Simon, receiving his doctor of science degree in 1926.
His thesis was on the relationship between cowpox virus
and vaccinia virus.

May 13, 1924

Dr. Joseph M. Scott
School of Hygiene and Public Health
Baltimore, Maryland

Dear Doctor Scott:

I am sorry that you have made up your mind not to come to us next year. You will understand that our appointment for one year is a tentative appointment and is designed to determine whether the incoming staff member will fit himself to our conditions.

So far as the program of filterable viruses is concerned, I think that it would be unwise for anyone to spend all his time upon what are called filterable viruses inasmuch as they probably belong to a variety of types which are simply beneath our microscopic vision. A better program would be to study infectious diseases and select the one whose etiological factor has not yet been determined because of the probability of its being an ultra-microscopic organism. In order to determine causation it is necessary to study diseases not only in the laboratory but also under normal conditions in the field in the young as well as the old. In this way suggestions come for the laboratory problems. Keep me in touch with your plans and work, and we may perhaps take the matter up again another year.

Please remember me kindly to Doctor Simon and tell him that I have not forgotten that I promised to send him a slide of the rabbit parasite. Please also say to Doctor Lange that I have been inconvenienced in various ways since my return but that I shall try to find a section of bovine tuberculous tissue for her in the near future.

Sincerely yours,

Theobald Smith

Fig 7. Letter to Joseph M. Scott from Theobald Smith.
Courtesy of Mrs. Joseph M. Scott

Andervont recalled his time with Simon:

When I came to the School of Hygiene, the department was located in one of the old medical school buildings. (The Biology Building)[3] I think it was on the second or third floor. The bacteriology department was on the floor above or below it. There was one large room where we assistants worked. There were 4 or 5 of us. There was a series of small rooms which were used as student labora-

[3] In 1919 the Advisory Board of the School of Hygiene and Public Health took two significant actions. First, it agreed to support consolidation of the libraries of the School of Hygiene and Public Health with those of the School of Medicine and the Johns Hopkins Hospital if a suitable building could be obtained along with funds for its maintenance. Second, it strongly urged upon the Trustees "the importance of proceeding with the erection of a new building for the school as speedily as possible." A Committee appointed to explore ways of obtaining more space on a temporary basis recommended that the old biological laboratory at the southeast corner of N. Eutaw Street and Druid Hill Avenue be used for the departments of bacteriology, protozoology and medical zoology. The move to East Baltimore when the new building was completed was in the autumn of 1925. The activity in filterable viruses occupied two rooms on the 9th floor of the new building and some additional space on the 4th floor.

tories, research laboratories, and/or office space. It was obvious that the building was not constructed for the type of research that was done there. There was no satisfactory space for keeping animals, and to work with virus diseases one had to use experimental animals in those days. The animals were kept down in the basement. My predecessor, Dr. Scott, had done his research on measles in rabbits. My assignment was to work on fowl plague, better known as Hühner, which was a highly contagious and fatal infection for chickens. Unfortunately, this work had to be discontinued because it was discovered that Simon had imported the fowl plague virus illegally, to say the least, into this country, without the knowledge of the Department of Agriculture. It's a matter of record that the assistant (Andervont) to the head of the virus department at the School of Hygiene had taken this highly contagious and fatal virus out to his home in Ohio where he had transferred it at regular intervals (every 3 or 4 weeks) during the vacation period and had luckily buried the carcasses of the chickens. Upon Dr. Simon's suggestion, they were always buried at least 2 feet deep. When this venture was discovered by the Department of Agriculture, Ransom, the head of the department, interviewed myself and Dr. Simon. As I recall, we were interviewed separately. This is on the record in the J.A.M.A. of that period—about 1925—as a news item. The procedure for preserving virus-infected material in those days was to keep it in 50 percent glycerine and water. I don't think we even bothered to sterilize the mixture; we just dropped the brain in and we would transfer the virus at regular intervals, 3 or 4 weeks, and apparently there was no effort made to determine how long it would survive under these conditions. Chicken plague may have survived for years; we didn't know. But we had to keep it going because Dr. Simon wanted to use this virus in his course. Fortunately, there were no chickens in the neighborhood of our home so no damage was done. I have no idea how Dr. Simon procured this virus from abroad. My next assignment dealt with the virus of epithelioma contagiosum.

The chief responsibility of Simon's assistant was to help with the course and get all the materials ready. It took an awful lot of work, especially in virology where Dr. Simon would insist upon every student using a Berkefeld filter to show that the virus would come through and produce the disease when inoculated into another animal. The vaccinia virus was perfect for showing that this could be done. So when you had about 30 students and every student had to filter his own virus, you had a real job getting ready for that part of the course. Other than that, it was always a pleasure, really. I didn't work with any virus in the laboratory other than epithelioma contagiosum in chickens or the vaccinia virus. I was supposed to have worked, of course, with the myxoma virus (myxomatosis of rabbits) when we got it, but that was given up because it was too contagious and we couldn't keep animals separate. All this work was done in the old building. When we got to the new building, things were entirely different. The virus of rabbit myxomatosis was sent to Dr. Simon from abroad; it came via boat to New York; then from New York it was hand carried by the conductor on the train to Baltimore. Dr. Simon himself went down and got the virus at the station.

The first course in virology was given in the old laboratory. It would start out with a general description of viruses and then a series of lectures on the diseases known to be caused by viruses, their characteristics, and a review of the important investigations going on in that field. The whole time in the old building I can't remember a single student complaining about the inadequacy of the course. It was all brand new to at least 90 percent of us. Dr. Simon made no effort to conceal the fact that, in his opinion, within a matter of one decade or two at the most, every medical school in the country would have a department of filterable viruses. This, of course, didn't materialize because the virologists were soon absorbed by the bacteriologists. Simon would bring in outside lecturers at the slightest provocation. One lecturer was a young officer from the Public Health Service by the name of Roscoe R. Spencer. He had just completed his work on the development of a vaccine against Rocky Mountain spotted fever, which is, of course, a rickettsial disease. In the new building our location was jokingly referred to as "next to heaven" because we were in two small rooms presumably built as storage rooms on the roof of the present School of Hygiene. Between these two small rooms was all the elevator apparatus. The two rooms were probably twice as large as this room (20 × 18). That gave us a lot of space compared to what we had had. There was one small room in between the long corridor which was used as Dr. Simon's office. He had a separate office there but not one in the old building. The virus research work consisted of taking the material that presumably was carrying the virus, grinding it up with a mortar, diluting it adequately, and passing it through filters to prove it was filterable. The epithelioma contagiosum virus, or chickenpox, the one I worked with to get my degree, was kept in glycerine.

Dr. Simon was the editor of the *American Journal of Hygiene;* he did all the work himself with no assistance. He read all the papers and did all the correspondence. He just loved that kind of work. When we went over to the new School of Hygiene, he got his own secretary—Edna Kuehn.

The members of the Rockefeller Institute for Medical Research in New York all knew Simon and about the virus work going on at the School of Hygiene. During my tenure, practically every one of them came down on at least one or two occasions a year to stop in and talk to Dr. Simon and the rest of us about the work in virus diseases—Thomas Rivers, Peter Olitsky, James Murphy. I don't think Rous ever came down. There weren't many people in the country interested in viruses back in 1924 and 1925.

Simon was typical of the scientists of his generation. He wasn't only a medical man; he played the drums in the Baltimore Symphony Orchestra. Mrs. Simon would sit in the audience and worry about whether he was going to miss the cue. Every day was an interesting day around Dr. Simon. He was the medical officer of the School of Public Health, before we had gone over to the new School of Hygiene building. One of the usual events that would take place within a few weeks after the opening of school would be that a young lady or usually two of them together would come into the laboratory where Dr. Simon and I were working seeking medical advice from him. Simon would say: "What is it?" They would reply: "We've got whelps on our legs." Dr. Simon would say: "Let's see them." Dr. Simon would take one look and would say: "Oh, bedbugs. Just change the place where you're staying." Some of the people from the Middle West thought bedbugs were poison; they were just horrified.

One very unusual job I had concerned Mrs. Simon. I was to be careful to see to it that before Dr. Simon left the laboratory at night he took off the white gown he worked in. Otherwise, he would come home with the white gown sticking out about 6 to 8 inches beneath his overcoat. As far as Mrs. Simon was concerned, it was a major job. She was Swiss by birth. I remember Simon telling the story about Sir Arnold Theiler who was also Swiss by birth. Dr. Simon had the pleasure of taking Theiler to his home for dinner one night and introducing him to Mrs. Simon who greeted Sir Arnold in Swiss. He used to tell that story over and over and how Sir Arnold was so happy. Later, when I was at Harvard, I met Sir Arnold's sons, Hans and Max. Hans was in Tyzzer's department and Max was in Strong's department. I got to know them very well. It was there that Max got his yellow fever virus into the mouse by using the intracerebral route for inoculation. In his first paper, he kindly gave me credit for the idea, as I had gotten the herpes virus into the mouse by this technique.

(Andervont gives Simon the full credit for originally suggesting localized inoculation of viral material intracerebrally—a technique that had an important impact on virological work at that time.)

Simon, of course, went to Nova Scotia every summer; he just couldn't stand warm weather even though he was a native of Baltimore. No one could work on top of that hot building in the summer. We would move all our paraffin blocks out of there and down to other parts of the building with cooler rooms. In the new building I worked with mice, rabbits, and chickens. Most of my work was being done with skin inoculations. Intracerebral inoculations were done after I went to Harvard. The reason for the mice being used at Harvard was that Dr. Lloyd Felton was running titration experiments for his pneumococcal antibodies on mice. I used the control mice after he had finished with them for my work with herpes virus. I got the herpes virus from Dr. Flexner at the Rockefeller.

I remember one story involving myself and Hobbs, who succeeded me as the assistant to Simon. We were doing some work with the Rous sarcoma virus and we were on the roof of the new School of Hygiene building taking the feathers out of the chickens with no other purpose in mind but that we would put them in an autoclave and have some chicken for food. Who should come out suddenly but Dr. Welch and Dr. Goodnow (President of the Johns Hopkins University at that time). Dr. Welch showed him the view and on the way out asked us what we were doing. We said we were working on the Rous sarcoma virus and explained the purpose and the results we were getting. When they left to get the elevator, Dr. Welch let Dr. Goodnow go first, turned and said: "I hope it tastes good, boys."

Everytime I talked with Dr. Howell or saw him, I admired him. A man with a wonderful personality—he was just a pure gentleman. Hegner (Fig 6) and Cort were the "big shots" and were just as nice as could be.[4] Rivers

---

[4] In 1922 Robert W. Hegner was associate professor of protozoology and William W. Cort was associate professor of helminthology in the Department of Medical Zoology. Hegner was promoted to full professor the following year and Cort in 1926 when helminthology became a separate department as did filterable viruses.

was a delightful man. Hegner had a daily luncheon to which the assistants were invited. I think every well-known parasitologist in the world in the course of a year or two had lunch with us and got up and said a few words afterwards.

Dr. Simon foresaw the importance of tissue culture work in virology and wanted me to learn how to do tissue cultures from Warren Lewis and his wife. I worked with Mrs. Lewis almost exclusively, but when you worked with one Lewis you were really working with both of them because he would come in the laboratory and talk all the time. Mrs. Lewis became interested in the absorption of the Rous tumor virus by certain chemical compounds. Our laboratory at Hopkins was not suitable for tissue culture work; you had to stop it every summer because of the heat. I had the Rous virus; Mrs. Lewis got that going in tissue culture. That's where I learned about macrophages.

Simon always told me: "Andervont, if you want to make a success in science, don't get married." One day when he and I were working in the laboratory, Dr. Hegner came in. Simon turned to him and said: "I've just been telling my young friend Andervont never to get married if he wants to make a success." Hegner looked at him and said: "But you got married." Simon replied, "Well, that was different." Osler didn't marry until he was well in his forties—and Simon worshipped Osler.

My wife and I were guests for Thanksgiving dinner at the Simon home in 1926; it was our first social meeting with the Simon's. Mrs. Andervont was carefully quizzed as to her activities; as to whether she spent any money outside of the household. They were much relieved to find out that she was working and was not a drain on her husband financially. Simon was a master host; perfect, absolutely perfect. Hobbs was an inbred New Englander, and when Hobbs came to the house, Simon threw open the door and said: "Oh, Mr. Hobbs, come in." Hobbs came in looking dignified; Simon took his coat and said: "Well, Mr. Hobbs, is your belly empty?"

Simon had been exposed to x-rays while in practice which gave him a severe burn on his gluteal region. He carried a little rubber circle to sit on in hard chairs. After many years he found a remedy for the problem. He secretly entered one of the hospitals in the Baltimore area and after a few days called me. I went over and talked with him. After talking about the laboratory work, he said: "Now, Andervont, I want you to do something for me." He turned over on his stomach, pulled up his gown and showed me his rear end. "I want you to draw a picture of what you see there." This was after he had removal of the scar and skin grafts. After I showed him the sketch, he said: "Are you sure you saw all those things? What was this color? What was that color? My God," he said, "they're telling me the truth."[5]

After receiving his doctorate, Andervont remained at Johns Hopkins for a year on a Carnegie Foundation Fellowship. He then accepted an instructorship with Dr. Milton J. Rosenau, who was professor of preventive medicine at Harvard University. Dr. J. W. Schereschewsky, assigned from the U.S. Public Health Service, was a member of Rosenau's department. Schereschewsky was instrumental in persuading the Surgeon-General of the Public Health Service that cancer was a public health problem. Upon Rosenau's retirement in 1930, Andervont became the first professional staff member of Schereschewsky's Office of Cancer Investigations. Andervont remained with the Public Health Service for the rest of his professional career. The Office of Cancer Investigations at Harvard became part of the National Cancer Institute when it was established in 1937, and was moved from Boston to the National Institutes of Health in Bethesda in 1939. Andervont was in charge of biological research at the National Cancer Institute until 1961 when he relinquished his post as chief of the laboratory of biology and became editor of the *Journal of the National Cancer Institute*.

Virus research continued to be one of Andervont's major interests. He showed that herpes virus of man could be transmitted to mice by intracerebral inoculation and thereby provided the means of studying this human virus in an animal. Max Theiler used this method in his studies on the action of yellow fever virus in mice. The following is the introduction of Theiler's first publication in the *Annals of Tropical Medicine and Parasitology* in 1930:

> The study of the etiology of a disease is greatly facilitated by the discovery of an experimental animal susceptible to the virus of that disease. The finding by the West African Yellow Fever Commission of the Rockefeller Foundation (1928) that the Indian monkey Macacus Rhesus is susceptible to the virus of yellow fever has been productive of a great deal of research with fruitful results. Rhesus monkeys, however, are rather expensive and at times the supply is limited. The finding of a common laboratory animal susceptible to the virus of yellow fever would be a great advantage.
>
> It is generally conceded by all workers that the common laboratory animals—rabbits, guinea pigs, rats and mice—are not susceptible to the virus of yellow fever when injected by the usual routes.
>
> The French workers Lasnet (1929) and Laigret noted in yellow fever patients neurological symptoms. Laigret suggested that the central nervous system of yellow fever patients should be tested for the presence of virus.

---

[5] This problem with the x-ray burn had been on Simon's mind for some time. Evidently he could not get a definitive answer as to what should be done or else he was skeptical of his surgeon's recommendation, for the following query appeared on p. 306 of the JAMA for January 24, 1925:

ROENTGEN–RAY BURNS

To the Editor: I was so unfortunate as to receive a roentgen-ray burn some time ago for which I have been vainly seeking relief. There must be many physicians who have been similarly unfortunate. Possibly something of benefit to all might result from a collective study of the experience of many cases, and I should be very glad indeed if any who share my opinion will communicate with me. If a sufficient number will do so, I shall tabulate the results.

Some of the points that should be given especial consideration are (a) the size, location, type and duration of the wound, and (b) the result of treatment of whatever kind. From the available literature no information of special value can be gleaned, and I accordingly feel that a study as proposed might be worth while.

Charles E. Simon, M.D., Baltimore
Resident Lecturer in Medical Zoology,
  Johns Hopkins University School of
  Hygiene and Public Health

It was decided to test the common laboratory animals by intracerebral injection. Familiarity with the work of Andervont (1929) with herpes virus and mice, and the simplicity of his technique, suggested mice as the first choice.

Thus, Andervont provided an important link in the chain of events which led Theiler to receive a Nobel prize for his work in developing a yellow fever vaccine.

It was but a short step from an interest in viruses as related to cancer to the development of a method of concentrating by absorption on charcoal the Rous sarcoma virus that infects fowl. Andervont made it possible in this way to obtain consistent production of viral tumors in fowl when previously negative and poorly reproducible results were common. Thus, some 25 years before the present intense interest in viruses as a cause of human cancer, Andervont developed a sustained interest in the importance of studying the viral etiology of cancer. Also, in his early work on the immunology of transplanted cancers, he recognized the importance of genetic factors as well as the utility of genetically homozygous strains of mice in cancer research. He made significant contributions related to the milk-transmitted mammary tumor agent of Bittner in mice.

Another of Andervont's important lines of investigation came from the early studies by the Harvard group on the induction of cancer in animals by chemical agents, particularly polycyclic hydrocarbons. Andervont was a pioneer in the development of biological methods of studying the experimental induction of cancer with chemicals.

For 20 years Andervont was also administratively responsible for, and guided the research of, the largest group of investigators in the National Cancer Institute. The work of this group encompassed tissue culture, electron microscopy, genetics, radiation biology, cell physiology, cell biology, tumor virology, and the etiology of spontaneous leukemia. This group was responsible for many advances including (1) the discovery of the Stewart-Eddy polyoma virus which produces multiple tumors in a number of animal species; (2) the discovery of the Moloney mouse leukemia virus; (3) the development of quantitative techniques for the study of tumor viruses; (4) the role of hormones in the experimental induction of cancer; (5) the first cloning of a mammalian cell in tissue culture; and (6) the first conversion of normal to cancerous cells in the test tube.

Andervont served as president of the American Association of Cancer Research in 1955 and received the Distinguished Service Award of the Department of Health, Education and Welfare in 1961.

Simon's third and last postgraduate student was Joseph Raymond Hobbs (Fig 8). Hobbs was born in Belmont, Massachussetts, on February 16, 1904. He attended schools in Weston, and graduated from the Massachusetts Institute of Technology in 1925. He joined the Department of Filterable Viruses in 1926. His letter of appointment from Simon, written on May 19, 1925, read: "I have your letter of application and your credentials. In a few days I shall write you some details

regarding the work. I trust Filterable Viruses will become as dear to your heart as they are to mine." Hobbs worked primarily with the myxomatosis virus in rabbits and was shouldered with the conduct of the undergraduate course after Simon became ill in the latter part of 1926. He received his degree of doctor of science in filterable viruses in 1928, his thesis being "Studies on the Nature of the Infectious Myxoma Virus of Rabbits."

Hobbs then decided to study medicine and graduated from the Harvard Medical School in 1932. After serving an internship at the Newton-Wellesley Hospital, he started practice in Williamsburg, Massachusetts, in 1933. His practice was interrupted during World War II when he served in the Army from 1943 to 1946. He resumed his practice in Williamsburg and also practiced in Northampton for many years. Hobbs was active in public medical affairs and served as a member of the Hampshire County and the Massachusetts Medical Societies. He was a staff member of the Cooley Dickinson Hospital, the Holyoke Soldiers Home, and the Hampshire County Hospital. He also served on the Williamsburg Board of Health. In 1973, the town of Williamsburg dedicated the annual town report to him.

TEXTBOOK ON FILTERABLE VIRUSES

At the time of his death, Simon was engaged in writing a book on filterable viruses. Fortunately, Howard Andervont and Joseph Hobbs saved a number of the

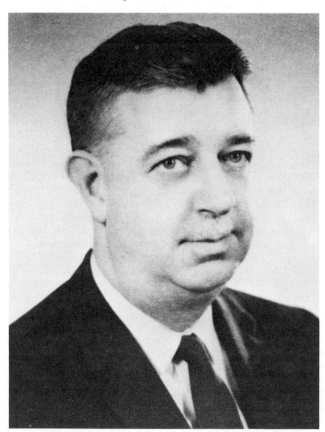

Fig 8. Joseph Raymond Hobbs
Courtesy of Mrs. Elizabeth Hobbs

chapters prepared for this textbook. They are in manuscript form and show many corrections and alterations in Simon's almost indecipherable handwriting.

In the first chapter, Simon defined filterable viruses and gave a historical summary of the work in the field. He stated:

> Viewed in retrospect the number of infectious diseases which have been traced to the activity of filterable viruses in the short time which has elapsed since their discovery, is truly astonishing. We are evidently dealing with a group of pathogenic agents which occur widely distributed in nature, and it does not seem unnatural to suppose that further investigations will lead to the discovery of still other representatives of the same type and of yet others that may be innocuous. Bearing in mind the great multitude of non-pathogenic bacteria and protozoa which occur in nature and the great disproportion which seems to exist between their number and that of disease producing forms, one naturally wonders whether similar conditions may not exist in this world of ultramicroscopic organisms also.

Table III presents the list of diseases caused by filterable viruses, with the names of the respective discoverers, chronologically arranged, which was to appear in the textbook.

In the next chapter Simon discussed the general characteristics of the filterable viruses including their development on artificial media. That he was well read on the subject is indicated by his reference to the work of Parker and Nye, who successfully cultured the vaccine virus in testicular cells in culture. Simon commented on the viability of viruses outside of the body, including the effect of drying, the effect of temperature, the behavior toward chemicals and chemical disinfectants, and behavior toward cytolytic agents and light, and he discussed the behavior of viruses toward adsorbants as well as the virulence of the viruses.

Simon was concerned with the nature of the filterable viruses in Chapter 3 and he presented a classification of filter passing agents which is shown in Table IV.

In the fourth chapter he dealt with the parasitism of the filterable viruses, discussing tissue tropism extensively and classifying the viruses on the basis of the presence or absence of tropism as shown in Table V. He defined the filterable viruses proper as corpuscular matter, not of ordinary bacterial or protozoal type, which is essentially characterized by its minute size—by virtue of which it can pass the ordinary anti-bacterial filters—and its apparent ability to reproduce itself either *ex ao ipso* or through the cooperation of its animate host. He discussed the endocellular existence of the tissue-tropic viruses, stating that while it was possible that some of the organotropic and tissue-tropic viruses may lead an extracellular existence, there was evidence to suggest that others were true endocellular parasites. He pointed out that Lipschütz had applied the term "strongyloplasms" to the visible intracellular forms. He stated that in this respect at least this particular group of viruses differed markedly from the pathogenic bacteria,

TABLE III

Diseases Caused by Filterable Viruses

A. *Diseases peculiar to man*

Molluscum contagiosum—Juliusberg, 1905
Dengue—Ashburn and Craig, 1906
Comon warts—Ciuffo, 1907
Pappataci fever—Doerr, 1908
Variola—Casagrandi, 1908
Trachoma—Bertarelli, 1908
Mumps—Granata, 1908
Poliomyelitis—Landsteiner and Levaditi, Flexner and Lewis, Leiner and Wiesner, 1909
Measles—Anderson and Goldberger, 1911
Alastrim—de Beaurepaire, Aragao, 1911
Inclusion blenorrhoea—Botteri, 1912
Herpes simplex—Grueter, 1913. Loewenthal, 1919
Common colds—Kraus, 1917. Gordon, 1919

Diseases affecting man which may be due to filterable viruses

Encephalitis epidemica
Varicella
Zona
Condyloma acuminatum
Psoriasis

B. *Diseases which may affect both man and animals*

Hoof and mouth disease—Loeffler and Frosch, 1896
Rabies—Remlinger and Riffat Bey, 1903
Vaccinia—Negri, 1905
Certain tumors of fowls—Carrel, 1925

C. *Diseases peculiar to vertebrate animals*

Pleuropneumonia of cattle—Nocard and Roux, 1898
South African horse sickness—McFadye, 1900
Chicken plague—Centanni and Savonunzi, 1902
Epithelioma contagiosum—Marx and Sticker, 1902
Sheep pox—Borrel, 1902
Rinderpest—M. Nicolle and Adil Bey, 1902
Virus septicemia of blackbirds—Centanni and Savonunzi, 1903
Hog cholera—De Schweinitz and Dorset, 1903
Infectious anemia of horses—Carré and Vallée, 1904
Distemper of dogs—Carré, 1905
Catarrhal fever of sheep—Spreull, 1905
Heartwater of sheep—Robertson and Theiler, 1905
Agalaktia contagiosa—Celli and Blasi, 1906
Stomatitis bovis papulosa specifica—Ostertag and Brugge, 1906
Chicken leukemia—Ellermann and Bang, 1908
Guinea pig plague—Petrie and O'Brien, 1910
Meningo-myelo-encephalitis—Roemer, 1911
Myxomatosis of rabbits—Sanarelli, 1911
Virus septicemia of rats—Novy, 1911
Nairobi disease of sheep—Montgomery, 1911
Infectious chicken sarcoma—Rous, 1912
Equine distemper—Bemelmann, 1913
Virus III disease of rabbits—Rivers and Tillett, 1923
Salivary virus of guinea pigs—Cole, 1926

some of which also may be found enclosed in cells, but evidently not as parasites. Simon also commented on mixed infections, noting the tendency of some viruses to become associated with secondary bacterial infections and citing the association of the virus of hog cholera and bacillus suipestifer.

TABLE IV

Classification of Filter Passing Agents

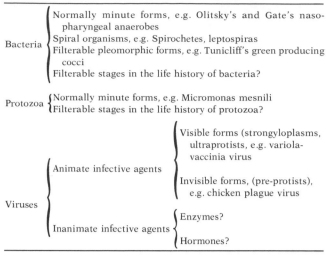

Bacteria	Normally minute forms, e.g. Olitsky's and Gate's naso-pharyngeal anaerobes Spiral organisms, e.g. Spirochetes, leptospiras Filterable pleomorphic forms, e.g. Tunicliff's green producing cocci Filterable stages in the life history of bacteria?
Protozoa	Normally minute forms, e.g. Micromonas mesnili Filterable stages in the life history of protozoa?
Viruses	Animate infective agents { Visible forms (strongyloplasms, ultraprotists, e.g. variola-vaccinia virus Invisible forms, (pre-protists), e.g. chicken plague virus Inanimate infective agents { Enzymes? Hormones?

In Chapter 5 Simon clearly and critically discussed the chlamydozoal cell inclusions. He provided a nomenclature for cell inclusions and presented a classification of the virus-inclusions as well as a detailed discussion of their general morphology and the techniques for their demonstration.

The last chapters dealt with various viral diseases as shown in Table VI.

SIMON AND THE AMERICAN JOURNAL OF HYGIENE

In 1921 The Johns Hopkins School of Hygiene and Public Health decided to establish the *American Journal of Hygiene* as an organ for the publication of technical research in public health and preventive medicine. The journal was under the editorship of William Henry Welch with a list of distinguished scientists as associates, and Simon was selected as managing editor. As one can imagine with Welch as editor, the actual labor of inaugurating and caring for every detail connected with the journal fell mainly upon Simon's shoulders. He took up this work with his usual enthusiasm and devotion and was obsessive in his attention to the selection and editing of the papers. Under his guidance, the journal became one of the leading outlets for the publication of scientific research in the field of hygiene. All of Simon's co-workers in this endeavor gave him the chief credit for its success.

SIMON—THE MAN

In the memorial for Simon, who died on November 8, 1927, written for the *American Journal of Hygiene*, William Howell had the following to say about this remarkable man:

Impulsive and emotional by nature, he entered into everything that interested him with great intensity. He

TABLE V

Classification of Viruses As to Tropism

I. *Viruses showing no evidence of any special tropism, or of tropism of limited extent only (Septicemic group). This group comprises the viruses of the following diseases:*

(a) *affecting man:*	(b) *affecting animals:*
Measles	Rinderpest
Pappataci fever	S.A. horse sickness
Dengue	H.W. dis. of sheep
	Catar. fever of sheep
	Chicken plague
	Septicemia of blackbirds
	Myxomatosis of rabbits
	Hog cholera
	Infectious sarcoma of fowls

II. *Viruses showing evidence of well defined tropism, with comparatively little or no tendency to a generalized distribution:*

1. *Epitheliotropic group:*
   Molluscum contagiosum
   Verruca vulgaris
   Condyloma acuminatum
   Trachoma
   Inclusion blenorrhoea
   Herpes simplex (in man)

2. *Dermotropic group:*
   Variola
   Alastrim
   Vaccinia
   Paravaccinia
   Sheep pox
   Horse pox
   Epithelioma contagiosum
   Hoof and mouth disease
   Stomatitis bovis papulosa specifica
   Myxomatosis of rabbits (in parte)
   Cole's guinea pig virus

3. *Neurotropic group:*
   Rabies
   Poliomyelitis
   Encephalitis epidemica?
   Chicken plague (in geese)
   Poliomyelitis of guinea pigs
   Herpes simplex (in guinea pigs and rabbits)

4. *Haemotropic group:*
   Leukemia of chickens
   Infectious anemia of horses
   Rabbit myxomatosis

5. *Organotropic group:*
   Pleuropneumonia
   Agalaktia contagiosa
   Parotitis

was no Laodicean. His convictions on all matters of importance were strong, and he held it to be the part of cowardice to conceal his opinions, religious, political or otherwise, if they happened to run counter to those of the majority. At the beginning of the war he suffered some harsh criticism on this score, since his early life in

TABLE VI

Chapter Headings for Simon's Textbook of
Filterable Viruses (1927)

I   *The filterable viruses*

Definition
Historical
List of diseases caused by filterable viruses with names
    of respective discoverers, chronologically arranged

II   *General characteristics of the filterable viruses*

Development on artificial media
Viability outside the body
    Effect of drying
    Influence of temperature
    Behavior towards chemicals (A)
    Behavior towards chemical disinfectants (B)
    Behavior towards cytolytic agents (C)
    Behavior towards light
    Behavior towards adsorbants
The virulence of filterable viruses

III   *The nature of filterable viruses*

Classification of filter passing agents

IV   *Parasitism of filterable viruses*

Tissue tropism
Classification
    I Viruses showing no evidence of any special tro-
       pism, or of tropism of limited extent only (sep-
       ticemic group)
    II Viruses showing evidence of well-defined tropism,
       with comparatively little or no tendency to a
       generalized distribution
Endocellular existence of tissue-tropic viruses
Mixed infections

V   *The chlamydozoal cell inclusions*

Nomenclature
    Occurrence
    Classification of the virus-inclusions
General morphology
General technique for the demonstration of the chlam-
    ydozoal cell inclusions

VI   *The d'Herelle phenomenon*

Views regarding the nature of the phage

VII   *The d'Herelle phenomenon (the phage in disease)*

The bacteriophage and immunity
    (a) d'Herelle experiments with the viewpoint of
        cure. . . .
    (b) attempts at active immunization

VIII   *The Twort phenomenon*

The d'Herelle phenomenon

IX   *Small pox*

X   *The diagnosis of small pox*

Paul's method
Paschen's method
Allergic skin reactions in the diagnosis of small pox
The prevention of small pox
Preparation of the small pox

XI   *Pappataci fever and dengue*

XII   *Rabies*

XIII   *Hog cholera*

XIV   *Herpes simplex*

XV   *Mosaic disease*

XVI   *Parotitis*

XVII   *Trachoma*

XVIII   *Poliomyelitis*

XIX   *Molluscum contagiosum and verrucae vulgaris*

XX   *Typhus fever*

XXI   *The infectious tumors of chickens I*

XXII   *The infectious tumors of chickens II*

XXIII   *Myxomatosis of rabbits*
Rabbit virus III of Rivers and Tillett

XXIV   *Heart water*

Germany had given him an affection for that nation which he was at no pains to disguise; in fact, he openly proclaimed his sympathies whenever and wherever the subject was discussed. But it should be added that when this country went into the war he stood with his own people, for he was first of all a loyal American. Generally speaking, political affairs made little appeal to him. His chief and absorbing interest was in science. The greatest achievement for him was to add something of importance to human knowledge. To work at some problem in his science and to keep in touch with the work of others gave him his greatest joy. . . He could rail in extravagant terms at the deceitfulness of man. . . But his heart was warm and gentle, his sentimental side was easily touched, and no one was more ready with help and sympathy for those in distress.

In his will Simon stated his wish for a memorial service at the School of Hygiene and Public Health. This was fitting. Simon was an agnostic and his devotion to the School of Hygiene at Johns Hopkins and to his research there made the building in which he had worked so energetically his temple. Howell's remarks on this occasion were informal and were not published.

THE FATE OF SIMON'S DEPARTMENT OF FILTERABLE VIRUSES

After Simon's death, the department of filterable viruses was placed under the charge of Roscoe R. Hyde, associate professor of immunology, with Joseph R. Hobbs and Raymond E. Gardner, a candidate for the doctor of science in filterable viruses, as his assistants. In 1928, as mentioned, Hobbs received his doctorate; in 1929, Hyde was appointed professor of filterable viruses; and in 1930, Gardner received his doctorate and became an instructor in the department.

The department of filterable viruses, as described in the 1930–1931 catalogue, consisted of Roscoe R. Hyde, associate professor; R. E. Gardner, instructor; and Herold R. Cox, student assistant. The basic course in filterable viruses continued to be offered and an advanced course was available for students to work on an assigned problem in cooperation with some member of the department, with written reports setting forth the progress of the work done at the close of the trimester. There was also an opportunity for research for students who had completed both of these courses and whose preliminary training qualified them for independent investigation. Hyde also conducted a Journal Club, which met weekly throughout the year, for the advanced students in the department. Here topics of current interest in the virus field were discussed.

The following subjects were under consideration for the 1930–1931 session: (1) living matter in the colloidal state; (2) normal and pathological studies of the living cell as revealed by genetic analysis; and (3) autocatalysis and the theory of enzymes. It was stated that "the problems that confront the student of the filterable viruses are the classic ones of the origin, the structure, the evolution and the nature of life. Students who offer filterable viruses as their major subject will familiarize themselves with the life and works of those who have made outstanding contributions to these problems."

In 1932 Roscoe Hyde was appointed professor of immunology. Under his leadership, the department of filterable viruses became part of the department of immunology. The course in filterable viruses and the opportunity for research continued. In 1939 Hyde, whose title at that time was professor of immunology and director of the laboratories of immunology and filterable viruses, with the assistance of Raymond E. Gardner, published a laboratory outline of the filterable viruses which was undoubtedly a bringing up to date of the laboratory course which had been started by Simon. In the introduction, Hyde made the following tribute: "We are greatly indebted to the late Charles E. Simon who opened the way for these studies by establishing in this university the first department of filterable viruses in the United States."

ROSCOE R. HYDE

Early in his career, Roscoe Hyde had taught in the department of zoology and physiology at the Indiana State Normal School. He had obtained his Ph.D. in genetics at Columbia University under the tutelage of Thomas Hunt Morgan. Hyde had two daughters, both of whom graduated from The Johns Hopkins School of Medicine: Dr. Martina Hyde (class of 1937) who died in 1969, and Dr. Margaret Hyde Moore (class of 1939) to whom I am indebted for the following comments:

My father was working with fruit flies, and kept jars of them all over the place when one day a mutant appeared in one of the bottles in the kitchen. It was duly described, named *drosophyla hydei*, and its genetic explanation carefully given. It has become a very famous fly. My father came to Johns Hopkins in 1917 in the department of immunology. At that time the School of Hygiene was located in downtown Baltimore near the office of the

Afro-American Newspaper. It was an old red brick building; the labs were a bit dark, the drawers of the desks were full of cockroaches, probably because the animals were kept handy. My father had bottles of his fruitfly strains in the laboratory feeding them dried bananas which we kids all had to taste each time we visited.

When my father (in 1927–28) took over the department of filterable viruses, it was located on the top floor of the new School of Hygiene building on Wolfe Street—sort of in the attic which was like an architectural afterthought. I remember well his eagerness to carry on the excellent work of the laboratory. Later the department merged with immunology and occupied the sixth floor, one half of which was devoted to virus teaching and research. The animals were kept in the back center separated area, with the animal caretaker Hans, a willing German-speaking worker devoted to their care and understanding practical matters related to the research work. My father was professor of immunology and filterable viruses from 1932 to 1943 when he died, probably from a pulmonary embolism, following an operation for a small carcinoma of the intestine. He was 59 and was in some of his best productive years.

Much of his earlier work was in the field of genetics which served to focus his interest in the interior of the cells and led to his passionate regard for searching out the reason for rapid cell growth in tumors; it also schooled him for dealing with a factor he could not see under the microscope. I always wanted to see viruses, but he said that while he would like to be able to show me one, it made little difference to him as you could know them even better by what they do. He did show us inclusion bodies, filters, animals and tissues. I thought it all very thrilling and in our West Arlington home he was considered by the neighborhood a hero who would one day discover a cure for cancer. Several friends near home—the pharmacist, the family doctor, and a chemist who worked for American Cyanamid—often talked over the back fence about cancer research, the discussion lasting as long as it took father to smoke one of his long cigars.

From 1914 through 1922 he published numerous papers in the field of genetics, counting flies by the hundred thousands; he introduced, for example, a paper on a multiple allelomorph system in 1916. After 1922 when he was in the department of immunology his papers reflect his changing orientation. He wrote then on the complement deficient guinea pig, on anaphylaxis as an immunological phenomenon, heparin and anaphylactic shock, heterophile antigen, experimental purpura, and with students and doctoral candidates, much work was done under his direction.

In 1929 his interest turned more directly to virus disease and he studied the myxoma virus, epithelioma contagiosum, bacteriophage, which had also had Dr. Simon's attention. He wrote his first paper on virus disease while in the department of filterable viruses in 1930. It was entitled "The Behavior of Certain Filterable Viruses when Subjected to Cataphoresis." Also in 1930 a student, Raymond E. Gardner, wrote a long study on "Immunity to Transplantable Rat Tumors," and for several years the papers were devoted to the study of immunity to virus diseases, particularly animal tumors. One student (Herold Cox) worked with Hyde to develop a new filter using collodion membranes and to clarify the methods of pore size calculation with a view to measuring virus particle size. Later studies were directed toward transmission of viral diseases, using the myoma virus in rabbits and the influenza and rabies viruses.

The last paper he wrote was with Gardner and, interestingly enough, it related all of the areas of his previous research interests. It suggested the possibility that the rabbit fibroma virus may be transformable into infectious myxomatosis.

Herold R. Cox held a Lilly Research Fellowship while he was a candidate for the doctor of science degree. Commenting on his period in the department of filterable viruses, Cox stated:

I came from Indiana in 1928 to work with Hyde. I must admit that during the time that I was at Johns Hopkins, none of us knew very much about the virus field. Dr. Hyde was an immunologist and geneticist by training and he and Gardner were much interested in working with transplantable tumors in rats, hoping to secure some worthwhile leads in the tumor field. I came to Hopkins from Indiana with no background whatsoever in the biological or medical sciences since I had had four years of training in chemistry, four years in physics, and five in math. To acquire some proficiency in the biological sciences, I was required to take the medical school courses in anatomy and physiology, biochemistry and pathology and to take courses in elementary bacteriology and protozoology in the school of hygiene. Actually, the work I did to secure the doctor of science degree at Hopkins was primarily in the field of physics and mathematics because I got interested in ultrafiltration and developed a mathematical formula that allowed me to determine the diameter of pores in collodion membranes which could be used to roughly determine the particle sizes of colloidal particles or viruses that passed through the ultrafilter membranes. Now, of course, all this type of work has been supplemented by electron microscopy. Tom Rivers' textbook on *The Filterable Viruses* was published while I was at Hopkins, and that, of course, stimulated a lot of interest in the field, but actually none of us in the department at that time (Hyde, Gardner, or myself) knew any more about the field besides what we read.

Actually, when I went up to New York in 1932 to work with Dr. Peter Olitsky, Dr. Olitsky called Dr. Jerome T. Syverton and myself into his office and told us that he had the viruses of Barna's disease, poliomyelitis, vesicular stomatitis and Herpes (simplex) as glycerinated specimens in the ice box, but he added that he didn't have any idea as to what we should do with them: that we were free to work with them until we got some ideas as to what we wished to do. So that is how I really got started in the virus field.

Thus, Charles Simon's influence on the development of virology in this country was widespread, extending far beyond the confines of the Department of Filterable Viruses which he had established at Johns Hopkins. The work that he accomplished in the laboratory, the learning he imparted to his students, and the inspiration which he gave to such persons as Thomas Rivers clearly mark him as a pioneer in American virology.

ACKNOWLEDGMENTS

I wish to thank Ms. Carol Bocchini for her assistance in the preparation of this essay; Mrs. Stewart Lindsay for allowing me to use some of her photographs; Dr. Frederik Bang and Dr. Ernest Stebbins for providing resource information; and the following for their generosity in sharing their experiences with me: Mrs. Ruth Scott, Mrs. Elizabeth Hobbs, Dr. Howard B. Andervont, Dr. George G. Finney, Sr., Dr. Margaret Hyde Moore, and Dr. Herold Cox. I am indebted to the American Philosophical Society and the Rockefeller Archive Center for access to their material concerning Charles E. Simon.

REFERENCES

1. Andervont HB: Is the formation of Guarnieri bodies an exclusively mammalian response to infection with the vaccine virus? Am J Hyg 6: 618, 1926
2. Andervont HB: The relationship of the epithelioma contagiosum virus of fowls to the vaccine virus. Am J Hyg 6: 719, 1926
3. Andervont HB: On immunity of fowls against the Carrel indol tumor. Am J Hyg 7: 786, 1927
4. Andervont HB and Friedenwald JS: A case of vacciniform blepharitis due to an atypical herpes virus. Bull Johns Hopkins Hosp 42: 1, 1928
5. Andervont HB and Simon CE: On the origin of the so-called pellucid areas which develop on agar cultures of certain spore-bearing bacteria. Am J Hyg 4: 386, 1924
6. Andervont HB: Personal communication
7. Craciun EC and Oppenheimer EH: Vaccinia virus in tissue cultures. Bull Johns Hopkins Hosp 37: 428, 1925
8. Finney GG Sr: Personal communication
9. Hobbs JR: Studies on the nature of the infectious myxoma virus of rabbits. Am J Hyg 8: 800, 1928
10. Hobbs JR: The occurrence of natural and acquired immunity to infectious myxomatosis of rabbits. Science 78: 94, 1931
11. Hobbs E: Personal communication
12. Howell WH: Dr. Charles E. Simon (1866–1927). Am J Hyg 8: 1, 1928
13. Hughes SS: The Virus: A History of the Concept. New York: Science History Publications, 1977
14. Lewis MR and Andervont HB: The serial transmission of chicken tumors by means of injection of the white blood cells and the plasma. Am J Hyg 6: 498, 1926
15. Lewis MR and Andervont HB: The inactivation of the chicken-tumor virus by means of carmine. Bull Johns Hopkins Hosp 40: 265, 1927
16. Lewis MR and Andervont HB: The inactivation of the chicken tumor virus by means of aluminium compounds. Bull Johns Hopkins Hosp 41: 185, 1927
17. Lewis MR and Andervont HB: The adsorption of certain viruses by means of particulate substances. Am J Hyg 7: 505, 1927
18. Lewis MR and Andervont HB: The inactivation of the chicken-tumor virus by means of calcium compounds. Bull Johns Hopkins Hosp 42: 191, 1928
19. Library of the American Philosophical Society: Correspondence between Peter Olitsky and Charles E. Simon and between Simon Flexner and Charles E. Simon
20. MacCallum WG and Oppenheimer EH: Differential centrifugation. A method for the study of filterable viruses as applied to vaccine. JAMA 78: 410, 1922
21. MacCallum WG: Present knowledge of the filterable viruses. Medicine 5: 59, 1926

22. MacCallum WG and Moody LM: Alastrim in Jamaica. Am J Hyg 1: 388, 1921

23. Rivers TM (Ed): Filterable Viruses. Baltimore: Williams and Wilkins, 1928

24. Rockefeller Archive Center. Correspondence between Charles E. Simon and members of the Board of Directors of the Rockefeller Institute.

25. Scott R: Personal communication

26. Scott JM and Simon CE: Experimental measles. I. The thermic and leucocyte response of the rabbit to inoculation with the virus of measles and their value as criteria of infection. Am J Hyg 4: 559, 1924

27. Scott JM and Simon CE: Experimental measles. II. On the occurrence of protective antibodies in the blood of rabbits, following inoculation with blood or nasopharyngeal secretion from cases of human measles. Am J Hyg 4: 725, 1924

28. Scott JM and Simon CE: The diagnosis of smallpox by the Paul method. Am J Hyg 3: 401, 1923

29. Scott JM and Simon CE: Experimental measles. III. On the fate of the measles virus in the inoculated rabbit and its viability outside the body. Am J Hyg 5: 109, 1925

30. Simon CE: A further contribution to the knowledge of the opsonins. J Exp Med 9: 487, 1907

31. Simon CE: Meningococcus septicemia. Demonstration of the meningococcus in the blood smear. JAMA 48: 1938, 1907

32. Simon CE: Recent research into the pathology of malignant disease. Int Clin II (18th series): 287, 1908

33. Simon CE (Assisted by Melvin E and Roche M): On auto-antibody formation and antihemolysis. J Exp Med 11: 695, 1909

34. Simon CE (Assisted by Wood MA): The inhibitory action of certain anilin dyes upon bacterial development. Am J Med Sci 147: 524, 1914

35. Simon CE: The Abderhalden-Fauser reaction in mental diseases; with special reference to dementia praecox. JAMA 52: 1701, 1914

36. Simon CE: A case of yeast (monilia) infection of the lung. Am J Med Sci 143: 231, 1917

37. Simon CE: Giardia enterica: A parasitic intestinal flagellate of man. Am J Hyg 1: 440, 1921

38. Simon CE: A critique of the supposed rodent origin of human giardiasis. Am J Hyg 2: 406, 1922

39. Simon CE: Further observations of lamblia intestinalis infestation and its treatment. South Med J 15: 458, 1922

40. Simon CE: The filterable viruses. Physiol Rev 3: 483, 1923

41. Simon CE: The filterable viruses and their nature. Sci Monthly 23: 407, 1926

42. Simon CE: The virus of herpes simplex. Int Clin III (37th series), 123, 1927

43. Simon CE and Beck MD: A study of the indol tumor of Carrel in reference to Gye's hypothesis regarding the origin of malignant growths. Am J Hyg 6: 659, 1926

44. Simon CE and Judd CCW: Acute lymphatic leukemia: On the occurrence of the corynebacterium lymphomatosis granulomatosae. JAMA 55: 1630, 1915

45. Simon CE and Lamar RV: A method of estimating the opsonic content of blood and other fluids. Johns Hopkins Hosp Bull 17: 27, 1906

46. Simon CE, Lamar RV and Bispham WN: A contribution to the study of the opsonins. J Exp Med 8: 651, 1906

47 Simon CE and Scott JM: On the occurrence of cell-inclusions in the rabbit cornea after inoculation with the vesicular contents and nasopharyngeal secretion of varicella cases. Am J Hyg 4: 675, 1924

48. Simon CE and Scott JM: The Paul test in the diagnosis of small pox. J Lab Clin Med 10: 562, 1925

49. Simon CE and Thomas WS: On complement-fixation in malignant disease. J Exp Med 10: 673, 1908

50. Weinstein L and Chang T: Viral infections: An overview. Am J Med Sci 272: 301, 1976

APPENDIX I

Filterable Viruses
October 24, 1927

I. Laboratory exercises: Dr. Simon and Mr. Hobbs

1. Filter a specimen of city sewage, after passage through the disposal plant, through a Berkefeld filter and examine the filtrate for the presence of the bacteriophage, using the intestinal bacteria, Str. erysipelatus and St. aureus.

2. Was a phage present in the feces, meconium and forest soil examined, and for which organism was it most active? Draw typical appearance. Construct a table showing the virulence of any phages which you have obtained, in reference to the various bacteria against which the material has been tested, using the notations given in your sheet of special instructions.

3. Examine the cultures of your vaccine specimens. If any glassy or eroded colonies are present, wash off the entire surface of the corresponding slant with 10 c.c. of bouillon; filter through a sterile Berkefeld candle and test the filtrate against St. albus (Twort).

4. Make transfers of all your bacterial cultures to new agar slants.

5. Heat any broth tubes that have cleared partially or entirely in connection with experiment 2 (supra), for 30 minutes at 56°C. (in a beaker of water) to destroy any remaining organisms, and add about 10–15 drops to the turbid control tube (c) of the same lot, after having transferred one half to a sterile (c¹) tube; reincubate.

6. Allow one of the B. coli X tubes which has cleared wholly or in part to remain in the incubator until the next meeting.

II. Lecture: Cell inclusions. Dr. Simon

Filterable Viruses
October 26, 1927

I. Laboratory exercises: Dr. Simon and Mr. Hobbs

1. To demonstrate the fact that the phage is reproduced gradually when in contact with susceptible bacilli, proceed as follows: Add to a tube of bouillon a sufficient quantity of an emulsion of colon bacillus X to render it definitely turbid. Inoculate this tube with 1 c.c. of a 10^7 dilution of a corresponding phage, mixing it well. Incubate at 37°C. Every hour transfer one drop to an agar slant and spread it. Number the tubes. Incubate for 24 hours. The first tube will probably show no plaques, the second may show a few, the third more and so on.

2. What has happened to your coli X tube, corresponding to exercise 6 of the last meeting? Make an agar slant culture and incubate for 24 hours.

3. What was the result of experiment 5 of the last meeting. What does this experiment teach?

4. Filter one of the coli X tubes in which lysis has occurred wholly or in part through a Berkefeld N filter and keep the filtrate sterile until the next meeting.

5. Transfer your coli X and all the other bacteria with which you are working to new agar slants.

6. *The structure of the phage is corpuscular (discontinuous)* Set up 10 test tubes, each containing 9 c.c. of saline. Number them from 1–10. To 1 add 1 c.c. of phage containing bacteriophage coli X d'Herelle and mix. Transfer 1 c.c. of this mixture to tube 2 and so on. Dilutions from 10^1 to 10^{10} are thus obtained. Set up another set of 10 tubes and add 9 c.c. of a definitely turbid emulsion of dysentery bacilli, freshly prepared in broth. To each of these tubes add 1 c.c. of the 10^5 dilution of the phage filtrate. Incubate at 37°C. After 48 hours examine the tubes. You will note that complete bacteriophagia has occurred in a few tubes and none in the rest.

Filterable Viruses
October 28, 1927

I. Laboratory exercises: Dr. Simon and Mr. Hobbs
1. Was there any phage in the city sewage? If so for what organisms had it any affinity? Construct table of virulence.
2. Was there a lytic principle in the vaccine washings?
3. Note the results obtained in experiment 6 of the last meeting. Was the phage non-corpuscular, bacteriophagia should have occurred in all tubes.
4. Prepare a suspension in bouillon for two agar slants (a and b) of a 24 hour growth of the Shiga bacillus (d'Herelle). Use 10 c.c. of bouillon per agar slant. Transfer the washed off and emulsified bacilli of one tube (a) to a sterile test tube. Add one drop of the corresponding phage (d'Herelle). Allow bacteriophagia to proceed at 32°C. until complete lysis has apparently taken place (5 hours approximately). Centrifugalize the contents of the other tube (b) at high speed for one hour; decant the supernatant fluid into a bichloride jar and examine smears from the last drop for bacteria. Stain with Loeffler's blue. What do you find? Make transfers from tube (a) to 3 broth tubes and to 3 agar slants (spread well) daily for 10 days using a drop for each tube. Incubate at 37°C. and note the findings from day to day.

II. Lecture: Illustrated—cell inclusions.

Filterable Viruses
October 31, 1927

I. Laboratory exercises: Dr. Simon and Mr. Hobbs
1. What was the outcome of number 4 of last time?
2. Determine the titre of your anti-dysentery (d'Herelle) phage, using dilutions of 1:1000 to 1:1,000,000. To this end set up five tubes, each containing 9 c.c. of broth. Inoculate each with 10 drops of B. dysentery (Shiga) emulsion. Number your tubes. Add 1 c.c. of phage to tube 1, mix well, transfer 1 c.c. of the mixture to tube 2, 1 c.c. from tube 2 to tube 3 and so on. The 1 c.c. removed from tube 4 is discarded. Tube 5 receives instead 1 c.c. of sterile broth (control). Incubate to the end of the morning. Then smear agar slants with a drop from each tube. Incubate until the next period. (Careful disinfection of used glassware.)
3. Continue with experiment 5 of last meeting. We expect that all of the inoculations corresponding to the first seven days will remain sterile; that on the eighth day the dissolved culture has become slightly turbid; that some of the cultures corresponding to the 9th day show a growth which appears agglutinated in the broth. Do not forget to make daily

transfers and examinations. How do you interpret the result?
4. Add 9 volumes of 96 per cent alcohol in a test tube to 1 volume of anticoli X filtrate and allow the mixture to stand until the next meeting.

II. Lecture: Chicken tumors I.

APPENDIX II

Filterable Viruses
February 11, 1924
Written Quiz

Please write on any five of the following topics.
1. The contributions of these investigators to the subject of filterable viruses. a. Iwanowski. b. De Schweinetz and Dorset. c. Ellermann. d. Lipschütz. e. Sir Arnold Theiler. f. MacCallum. g. Twort. h. von Prowazek. i. G.F. White. j. Doerr. k. Beach. l. Loeffler and Frosch. m. Peyton Rous. n. Baur. o. Bechhold.
2. The nature of the filterable viruses.
   a. Corpuscular character and size.
   b. Animate or inanimate nature.
   c. Taxonomic classification.
3. Cell inclusions.
   a. Significance of cell inclusions according to the chlamydozoon doctrine.
   b. Groups of cell inclusions. Examples of each.
4. The bacteriophage.
   a. Historical.
   b. Sources of the phage.
   c. Nature of the phage.
   d. Isolation of a phage.
5. The mosaic disease of tobacco.
   a. Nature of the disease. Other plants affected.
   b. Nature and properties of the virus.
   c. Transmission of the disease.
      Experimental transmission.
      Natural transmission.
6. Hühnerpest. (Chicken plague).
   a. Symptoms and course.
   b. Method of inoculation.
   c. The virus.
7. Lipschütz' classification of the filterable viruses on the basis of tissue tropism. Examples of each class.
8. a. Association of viruses with bacteria in disease. Examples.
   b. Relationship between traumatism and proliferation of viruses. Examples.
9. Filters.
   a. Types of filters.
   b. Relative porosity of the types of filters.
   c. Preparation of materials for filtration and necessary controls.
10. a. Viriferous insects. Examples.
    b. Tenacity of viruses in general.

Written examination in Filterable Viruses
March 11, 1927

Answer any five of the following questions:
1. What essential contributions to our knowledge of the filterable viruses do we owe to the following investigators: Iwanowski, Beijerinck, Frosch and Loeffler,

Borrel, Ellermann, Lipschütz, v. Prowazek, Rous, Negri, Guarnieri.

2. Discuss the significance of cell inclusions in respect to their specificity. Name the different groups (according to Lipschütz) and give examples of each.
3. Discuss the nature of the so-called infectious tumors of fowls.
4. Discuss the etiology of trachoma.
5. Discuss the Paul test in detail.
6. Discuss the herpes-encephalitis problem.

Department of Filterable Viruses
Final Examination
December 21, 1927

Answer first question and any other five questions.

1. Examine four sections, naming tissues, describe inclusions present, if any, and classify according to Lipschütz' scheme.

In the case of sections 3 and 4, discuss prophylaxis of disease represented.

2. What essential contributions to our knowledge of the filterable viruses do we owe to the following investigators: Iwanowski, de Schweinetz and Dorset, Ellermann, Lipschütz, Sir Arnold Theiler, v. Prowazek, Rous, Doerr and Bechhold.
3. Discuss the nature of the so-called infectious tumors of fowls.
4. Discuss the etiology of typhus fever.
5. Discuss the etiology of trachoma and the significance of the Prowazek-Halberstaedter bodies.
6. Describe the Paul test in detail.
7. Give a consideration of the herpes encephalitis problem as it stands today.
8. Discuss the association of viruses with bacteria in disease.
9. What is the significance of the cell inclusions?
10. Give a brief consideration of virus diseases conveyed by insect vectors.

12.

Lewis Hill Weed: Dean of the School of Medicine and the Second Professor of Anatomy

Nearly every scientist who finds success in research is sooner or later asked to assume a position of executive or administrative leadership. Lewis Hill Weed was no exception and during the latter part of his career he gave an outstanding performance as organizer and director of the Division of Medical Sciences of the National Research Council. He was so successful at this that many are not aware that this protégé of Harvey Cushing was, particularly in his younger years, a brilliant investigator and an effective leader of a research group.

Lewis Weed was born in Cleveland, Ohio on November 15, 1886, the son of a successful ironmaster and banker whose family descended from early Connecticut settlers in the Western Reserve. At Yale, Weed graduated near the top of his class, receiving an A.B. in 1908 and an M.A. in 1909. He was also an excellent student at the Johns Hopkins School of Medicine, receiving his M.D. in 1912. As a student at Hopkins, he attracted the attention of Harvey Cushing, who when he accepted the offer to become the Moseley Professor of Surgery at Harvard and Surgeon-in-Chief at the new Peter Bent Brigham Hospital, invited Weed to go with him. Weed accepted, and as Arthur Tracy Cabot fellow in surgery, he began his studies on the origin and circulation of the cerebrospinal fluid, studies which captivated Weed's research interest throughout his active career.

After two years in Boston, Weed accepted a faculty position in the Department of Anatomy at Johns Hopkins. During World War I he was commissioned in the Medical Corps of the Army and assigned to direct an army neurosurgical laboratory at Johns Hopkins. His success in this venture and his important research contributions made him the obvious choice for the professorship of anatomy at Hopkins when Franklin P. Mall died in 1917. With the help of Florence R. Sabin, who already held pro-

fessorial rank in the department, Weed organized an "enthusiastic, competent faculty—almost too successfully, indeed, for they were rapidly called away to head departments elsewhere." Weed continued the great Mall tradition of training teachers and investigators. Among his distinguished pupils and colleagues were George Wislocki, who became Professor of Anatomy at the Harvard Medical School; Louis Flexner, who became Professor of Anatomy at the University of Pennsylvania; Adolph Schultz, who held the chair of Physical Anthropology at Zurich; and Marion Hines, who became a professor in the Department of Anatomy at Emory University.

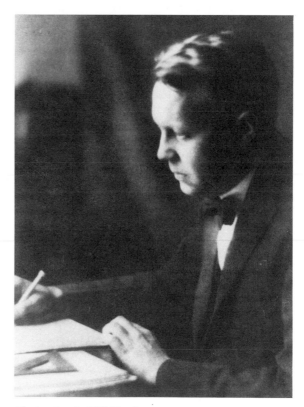

Fig 1. Lewis Hill Weed

Reprinted from the *Johns Hopkins Medical Journal* **139**: 77, 1976.

In 1923, at the age of 37, Weed was made Dean of the School of Medicine, and in 1929, its Director. During his administration, the school made many important advances. He was effective in stimulating research throughout the school not only by his skill at getting financial support but also by the personal stimulus which he supplied to the members of the faculty. His greatest contribution in terms of facilities was the building of the Welch Medical Library in which the libraries of the School of Medicine, the Hospital, and the School of Hygiene and Public Health were merged, and in which the newly created Institute of the History of Medicine was housed. Weed was an enthusiastic supporter of the Institute of the History of Medicine under the leadership of William Welch and Henry Sigerist, and was obsessed with the need for good libraries—a belief in which he was undoubtedly influenced by Welch, Osler, Kelly and Cushing.

Despite the great demands which his administrative duties at Hopkins placed on him, Weed still found the time to pursue in earnest the research which he had begun as a fellow at Harvard.

RESEARCH ON THE CEREBROSPINAL FLUID

The cerebrospinal fluid was first effectively described by Magendie in 1825. Since that time, many investigators have been intrigued with the study of its origin, distribution and reabsorption. It was an important area of study as knowledge of this physiological function was essential to progress in brain surgery and also provided an introduction to a very broad field of physiological anatomy, which encompassed the general character of the body fluids, the tissue spaces in which they reside, and the mechanisms by which they are produced and reabsorbed. Weed was fascinated by the subject and for two decades made important contributions to our knowledge of the cerebrospinal fluid.

SOURCE OF THE CEREBROSPINAL FLUID

In 1897, reports by Claisse and Levy of a case of internal hydrocephalus associated with hypertrophy of the choroid plexuses directed renewed attention to these intraventricular plexuses as the source of cerebrospinal fluid. Dandy and Blackfan gave additional support to this view when they experimentally produced an internal hydrocephalus by occlusion of the aqueduct of Sylvius. Harvey Cushing's observation of exudation of a clear fluid from a choroid plexus exposed on exploration of a porencephalic defect added further substantiation of the hypothesis.

Weed succeeded in providing more tangible proof of the intraventricular elaboration of the fluid when he demonstrated that a definite and sustained outflow of cerebrospinal fluid could be obtained by catheterization of the third ventricle through the aqueduct of Sylvius. The outflow from such a catheter was similar in amount to the fluid obtained from a cannula in the subarachnoid space, leading to the conclusion that the major portion of the fluid is produced within the cerebral ventricles. Later experiments by Dandy provided evidence not only that production of the fluid is intraventricular but also that the choroid plexuses are the responsible structures. He was able to produce a unilateral internal hydrocephalus by obstructing one foramen of Monro; extirpation of the choroid plexus in such an obstructed lateral ventricle prevented the development of an internal hydrocephalus.

From an entirely different approach, Weed provided corroborative evidence in favor of the choroidal origin of the fluid in his embryologic observations. In this study of the development of the cerebrospinal spaces he showed that the first extraventricular expulsion of the cerebrospinal fluid occurred simultaneously with the first tufting and histological differentiation of the ependymal cells to form the choroid plexuses.

His classic monograph on the embryonic development of the cerebrospinal spaces in pig and man was published in 1917. These investigations were primarily based on intensive microscopic study and the use of skillfully performed experimental injections. This work was beautifully illustrated by James Didusch, a pupil of Max Broedel's, and was published by the Carnegie Institution of Washington. In 1922 the Department of Embryology of the Carnegie Institution appointed Weed as one of its research associates and from then until 1935 supported his work by an annual grant.

Weed had pointed out in 1914 that the choroid plexuses must not be considered the sole elaborators of the cerebrospinal fluid. He presented anatomical evidence indicating that the perivascular spaces also pour a certain amount of fluid into the subarachnoid space, where this fluid mixes with the liquid produced in the cerebral ventricles.

Aside from their established function as efficient fluid-retainers, the cells lining the subarachnoid space are of interest because of their changing morphology under different physiological conditions. Weed was the first to note that these mesothelial cells phagocytized carbon granules introduced into the subarachnoid space and that when phagocytic, the cells increased in size.

A major problem in this area is the relationship of the dura mater to the process of cerebrospinal fluid circulation. The areas of penetration of the dense fibrous tissues of the dura by the arachnoid represent points of fusion between these two membranes. The most frequent of these areas of penetration are the arachnoid villi (prolongations of the arachnoid membrane) so that the arachnoid mesothelial cell comes to be directly beneath the vascular endothelium of the great dural venous sinuses. Weed identified these structures in adult man, in infants, and in the common laboratory animals. These villi are covered by typical arachnoid cells, usually of a single layer but often forming whorls. The arachnoid villi are normal structures, the great enlargement of which in adult life results in the formation of the well-known Pacchionian granulations. The cerebrospinal fluid circulates everywhere about the central nervous system. These channels are all closed with a specialized fluid-retaining cell, so that a true circulation of fluid may be maintained.

ABSORPTION OF THE CEREBROSPINAL FLUID

Of great experimental interest has been the study of the mechanisms of absorption of the cerebrospinal fluid. Harvey Cushing's observations on mercury and nonabsorbable gases led him to hypothesize a valve-like mechanism for drainage into the venous channel—an idea which was later disproved. Dandy and Blackfan in 1913 concluded that the absorption of cerebrospinal fluid was a "diffuse process from the entire subarachnoid space," for with the spinal subarachnoid space isolated from the cranial, they found a "quantitative absorption proportionately as great as from the entire subarachnoid space." The evidence for this statement was based largely on the excretion by the kidneys of phenolsulphonephthalein after its introduction into the subarachnoid space. A very rapid absorption into the blood stream occurred under such environmental conditions.

It was with these physiological contributions as a background that Lewis Weed began his anatomical studies of the absorption of the cerebrospinal fluid. He utilized an experimental approach in which a subarachnoid injection of a true isotonic solution of a nontoxic foreign salt, capable of subsequent precipitation in situ for histological examination and not diffusely staining cellular material, could be made in the living animal under pressures slightly above normal. His experiments were carried out over periods of several hours in living anesthetized animals, with introduction of the isotonic foreign solution—potassium ferrocyanide and iron ammonium citrate—into the lumbar subarachnoid

space; subsequently the central nervous system, still enclosed in the meninges, was fixed in an acid medium. Precipitation of the foreign salt as Prussian blue permitted adequate histological identification of the pathways taken. Histological examination demonstrated that the solution had not penetrated any of the cells lining the subarachnoid space; the precipitated granules adhered to the surfaces of the cell but were not within the cytoplasm. He found that the foreign solution had passed directly into the venous sinuses by way of the arachnoid villi into which the precipitated granules could be traced from the cerebral subarachnoid spaces. These granules of the foreign solution were found within the mesothelial cells covering the villi and the endothelial cells lining the venous sinuses, as well as within the lining of the venous sinuses, thus demonstrating, in his view, the essential pathway of absorption.

In addition to this major venous absorption through arachnoid villi directly into the great dural sinuses, an accessory drainage by way of the lymphatic system was demonstrated. Weed could find no valve-like structures such as those described by Cushing. He also believed Dandy and Blackfan's conception of a diffuse absorption by the vessels of the subarachnoid space untenable, for in no case were the mesothelial cells covering these vessels penetrated by the foreign solution. In reviewing the field in 1922, Weed believed the absorption of the cerebrospinal fluid to be a twofold process, chiefly a rapid drainage into the great dural sinuses, and in small part a slow indirect escape into the true lymphatic vessels.

CEREBROSPINAL FLUID PRESSURE

Weed, working with P. S. McKibben, also made important observations on the pressure of the cerebrospinal fluid. They reported an initial average of 119 mm of Ringer's solution in cats anesthetized by intratracheal ether and an extreme constancy of the cerebrospinal fluid pressure under experimental conditions. Later with Hughson, Weed reported an average pressure of 119 mm of Ringer's solution for 77 cats under ether. The fluctuations in the pressure under the experimental conditions were very slight.

All of the conceptions of the maintenance mechanism of cerebrospinal fluid pressure were based primarily upon the rigid character of the bony coverings of the nervous system. The idea that the cerebrospinal axis is situated within a "closed box" to which the physical laws of such a system apply was first advanced in 1783 by Alexander Monro. Monro believed that the substances of the brain, like that of other solids of the body, are nearly incompressible and are "enclosed in a case of bone" assuring the constancy of the intracranial blood content. The further development of this hypothesis by Kellie in 1824 led to wide acceptance, and the Monro—Kellie doctrine with but few alterations has served as the basis upon which the physiology of the intracranial contents has been interpreted. As further extended by Burrows, this hypothesis is stated as follows: "The whole contents of the cranium, the brain, the blood and this serum (cerebrospinal fluid) together, must be at all times nearly a constant quantity." Work done by Weed and Hughson demonstrated the essential truth of the doctrine that "the bony coverings of the central nervous system constitute within tested physiological limits inelastic and rigid containers; the ordinary physical laws of a 'closed box' may therefore be applied to the cranium." Appreciating the importance of variability in volume of the constituents, Weed and McKibben stated the hypothesis as follows: "The cranial cavity is relatively fixed in volume and is completely filled by brain, cerebrospinal fluid and blood; variations in any one of the three elements may occur, compensation being afforded by alteration in the volume of one or both of the remaining elements."

With the cranium and vertebral columns serving as rigid containers, the relation of the intracranial vascular pressures to the pressure of the cerebrospinal fluid was a matter of considerable importance. Weed and Hughson devised a simple method for recording intracranial venous pressure in the superior sagittal sinus as it emptied into the torcula. Their procedure possessed the distinct advantage of permitting direct observation of the effect of the manipulative procedure upon the pressure of the cerebrospinal fluid due to venous obstruction in the cranium. With such technical controls, Weed and Hughson were able to show that in essentially every case the pressure of the cerebrospinal fluid was considerably above that of the sagittal sinus. They also showed that alteration in intracranial venous pressure effected alterations in the pressure of the cerebrospinal fluid in the same direction but of lesser magnitude. Conversely, it was shown that within the physiological limits tested alteration in the pressure of the cerebrospinal fluid caused changes of lesser extent but in the same direction in the sagittal venous pressure. In view of his own and other experiments Weed felt that the normal pressure may be largely determined by the balance between the constant new production within the cerebral ventricles and the absorption into the dural sinuses; this pressure of the cerebrospinal fluid becomes dependent also upon intracranial arterial and venous pressures, not only because of the relation of these latter pressures to the production and absorption of the fluid, but because of the constancy of volume of the intracranial contents.

MODIFICATION OF CEREBROSPINAL FLUID PRESSURE

One of the most important areas of research engaged in by Weed was that of modification of the pressure of the cerebrospinal fluid. In 1919 he and McKibben reported that the pressure of the cerebrospinal fluid could be markedly altered by the intravenous injection of solutions of various concentrations. It was shown that such administration of a strongly hypertonic solution lowered the pressure of this liquid to an extreme degree, frequently producing negative values; with hypotonic solution (distilled water) a prolonged rise in the pressure of the fluid was obtained. Ringer's solution in large doses produced a temporary increase in the pressure of the cerebrospinal fluid, followed quickly by a return to the normal level. Accompanying these changes in fluid pressure were marked alterations in the volume of the brain, the hypertonic solution producing a small shrunken brain while the hypotonic solution caused an outspoken swelling of the brain-substance. The experimental changes in brain volume were particularly pronounced in animals in which the cranial cavity had been opened by trephining.

These findings were abundantly confirmed and soon were applied clinically. Cushing and Foley demonstrated that similar alterations in the pressure of the cerebrospinal fluid could be brought about by the ingestion of hypertonic and hypotonic solutions. Later experiments by Weed and Hughson confirmed the initial work in detail and presented data showing the general systemic and intracranial vascular alterations effected by such agents.

Pharmacological attempts were also made to modify the rate of outflow of cerebrospinal fluid. That certain substances may modify the rate of outflow of cerebrospinal fluid from a cannula introduced into the subarachnoid space was first demonstrated by Capeletti in 1900. Dandy and Blackfan obtained cerebrospinal fluid by introduction of a special cannula through the atlas and found marked accelerations in output of cerebrospinal fluid after ether. Seeing that there were limitations to this technique in that the normal channels of absorption were intact and the intracranial pressure was reduced to the resistance of the needle, Weed and Cushing catheterized the third ventricle and studied the outflow from the catheter whose resistance was established at approximately the normal pressure of the fluid. Under these circumstances they showed that posterior lobe extract from the hypophysis increased the outflow of cerebrospinal fluid in contrast to the findings of Dandy. However, Weed and Cushing saw that there were still limitations of this outflow method of study and that although their modifications had introduced a control for some of the sources of error, others were still present.

Lacking a true lymphatic system, the nervous tissue apparently makes use of its perivascular pathways for fluid elimination. The ultimate connection of these perivascular channels with potential spaces about each nerve cell indicates the close relationship between the cerebrospinal fluid and the nervous system. In addition to these rather obvious fluid spaces about the nerve cells, there is evidence that this fluid system is intimately connected with the general tissue channels through the ground-substance of the brain. The general direction of flow of this fluid under normal conditions is toward the subarachnoid space; under certain conditions this direction of flow may be reversed. The first of the conditions under which this flow is reversed is cerebral anemia. The second condition is brought about by the intravenous injection of strongly hypertonic solution. This phenomenon was first noted by Weed and McKibben who supplied a foreign solution of sodium ferrocyanide and iron–ammonium citrate to the subarachnoid space when the cerebrospinal fluid pressure was approaching zero. This foreign solution was subsequently found "to have passed from the subarachnoid space along the perivascular channels into the substance of the nervous system, reaching the interfibrous spaces in the white matter and the pericellular spaces in the gray." These observations indicated that under the influence of the intravenous injection of a strongly hypertonic solution, the dislocation of a considerable quantity of cerebrospinal fluid into the nervous system occurred. Further work by Weed showed that with the increase of osmotic pressure of the blood due to the intravenous injection of hypertonic solution, the cerebrospinal fluid was aspirated into the shrinking nervous system along the perivascular channels and also through the ependymal lining of the ventricle. Along these channels under this extraordinary osmotic pull, actual absorption of the fluid into the vessels of the nervous system took place. The findings suggested a reversal, following the injection of the hypertonic solution, of the normal processes; the osmotic pressure of the bloodstream under these conditions seemed to be a determining factor in the absorption of the cerebrospinal fluid. Weed concluded that diffusion also played a role in the process. Thus, Weed's work did

much to elucidate the "closed box" concept of Monro and Kellie.

ADMINISTRATIVE ROLE

In the later stages of his career, Weed was called upon more and more frequently to advise other schools and laboratories about appointments and educational ventures. After the death of Dr. Welch, Weed to a certain extent took his place, particularly within the Johns Hopkins sphere of influence outside Baltimore. He always followed with a keen interest the subsequent careers of men and the fate of the institutions to whom he had rendered advice.

In 1939 Weed became chairman of the Division of Medical Sciences of the National Research Council. Shortly after this, the probability of American entry into the war led to a great expansion in the work of this division and Weed had to shed most of his responsibilities at Hopkins. Weed's executive skill and his knowledge of the personalities of American scientific medicine were essential to the success of his work on a national as well as an international scale. As the scientific work related to the war expanded, the Division of Medical Sciences developed a relationship to the Office of Scientific Research and Development, and Weed became vice-chairman of the OSRD Committee on Medical Research. Thus he had a major role in planning the medical programs fostered by the OSRD and the NRC for wartime purposes. Among these were the search for improved drugs in the treatment of malaria, the production of the new antibiotics, improvements in blood transfusion and blood substitutes and studies in aviation medicine.

Weed's achievements before and during the war were recognized by the award of honorary degrees from 11 universities in the United States and England, the Presidential Medal of Merit and the Order of the British Empire, and by his election in 1942 to the American Philosophical Society. From his own viewpoint, the most meaningful tribute was the award of the LL.D. *honoris causa* from Johns Hopkins on February 22, 1951. On that occasion, his former colleague, George Corner, said of Weed: ". . . beginning his career in the dissecting room, a seeker of scientific knowledge in the dismembered human frame, this man has become a leader and counselor of those who heal the broken bodies of men, who guard our health in war and disaster and in time of peace unite themselves in constructive research for the welfare of our race."

Weed continued his important administrative responsibilities at the NRC after the end of World

War II. In 1949 he developed a chronic cough with hoarseness and loss of weight. Convinced that he had an incurable cancer of the larynx, he refused medical examination and continued to work until his progressive weakness forced him to enter the Johns Hopkins Hospital. There it was discovered that his symptoms were not due to a laryngeal carcinoma but were associated with tuberculosis of the lung and larynx. He went immediately to Saranac where with rest and antibiotic treatment his lesions were completely healed by the end of a year. At this point he retired from his official position and settled in Reading, Pennsylvania. He maintained his interest in scientific administration by participation in board meetings of the Carnegie Institution of Washington, the Institute for Advanced Studies at Princeton and the Yale Corporation. Toward the end of 1952 he developed symptoms of heart failure and died suddenly on December 21 of that year.

In a biographical memoir written for the American Philosophical Society, George Corner gave a penetrating summary of Weed's personal qualities: "Lewis Weed possessed strong powers of organization and command, tempered by a scientist's curiosity, by appreciation of cultural values, and respect for learning in every field. His offices and laboratories were smoothly managed. Teaching was well organized along broad modern lines. His lectures were forcible and clear; in the give and take of conversational teaching he was apt to be disconcertingly searching. To his staff and other collaborators in research he set an example of enthusiasm and persistence in the quest for new facts. Within any group which he himself organized to work with him there was always mutual loyalty and affection. Men who served with him competently were rewarded by lifelong friendship. At home in the spacious apartment presided over most hospitably for many years by his mother, Weed was the perfect host—a generous provider of good food and lively talk, and an expert judge of whiskey.

"On a larger stage, however, Weed's cooler side was more apparent, especially to those who did not know him well. Never shaken by outward circumstance, private uncertainties or domestic strains, he developed a genial air of confidence in his own wisdom which revealed itself in conversation and at the conference table more often than he knew. He did not easily put up with the timid counsels of less assured or more obsequious men. He was too honest to court favor or to modify his own judgments merely to gain support. Against shrewd and able opposition, which he enjoyed meeting, his principal weapon was the truth as he saw it, expressed with urbanity, and when he saw fit, with a dash of sarcasm; but an adverse majority decision was accepted without rancor . . . In the conduct of large affairs he took the lead, therefore, by mental strength and skill and organization rather than by the milder arts of inspiration and persuasion."

ACKNOWLEDGMENT

I wish to thank Ms. Carol Bocchini for her editorial assistance.

REFERENCES

1. Clark JH, Hooker DR, and Weed LH: The hydrostatic factor in venous pressure measurements. Amer J Physiol 109: 166, 1934

2. Corner GW: Lewis Hill Weed. American Philosophical Society Yearbook, 1952, p. 375

3. Cushing HW and Foley FEB: Alterations on intracranial tension by salt solutions in the alimentary canal. Proc Soc Exp Biol Med 17: 217, 1920

4. Flexner LB and Weed LH: Factors concerned in positional alterations of intracranial pressure. Amer J Physiol civ: 681, 1933

5. Fulton JF: Lewis Hill Weed. Yale J. Biol. Med. 25: 215, 1952

6. Kellie G: On death from cold and congestion of the brain. Edinburgh, 1824

7. Langworthy LH: Lewis Hill Weed. Trans Amer Neurol Assoc 78: 301, 1953

8. Magendie F: Recherches physiologiques et cliniques sur le liquide cephalorachidien. Paris, Mequignon-Marvis Fils, 1842

9. Monro A: Observations on the structure and functions of the nervous system. Edinburgh, W. Creech, 1783

10. Sachs E and Belcher GW: The use of saturated salt solution intravenously during intracranial operations. JAMA 75: 667, 1920

11. Weed LH: A reconstruction of the nuclear masses in the lower portion of the brain stem. Monograph, Carnegie Inst., Washington, 1914, Publ. No. 191

12. Weed LH: The development of the cerebrospinal spaces in pig and man. Monograph, Carnegie Inst., Washington, 1917, Publ. No. 225

13. Weed LH: The experimental production of an internal hydrocephalus. Carnegie Inst., Washington, 1919, Publ. No. 272, p. 427

14. Weed LH: The cerebrospinal fluid. Physiol Rev 2: 171, 1922

15. Weed LH: Experimental studies of intracranial pressure. Res Publ Assoc Res Nerv Ment Dis 8: 24, 1927

16. Weed LH: Positional adjustments of the pressure of the cerebrospinal fluid. Physiol Rev 13: 80, 1933

17. Weed LH: Certain anatomical and physiological aspects of the meninges and cerebrospinal fluid. Brain 58: 383, 1935

18. Weed LH: The National Research Council and medical preparedness. JAMA 117: 180, 1941

19. Weed LH and Flexner LB: Further observations upon the Monro-Kellie hypothesis. Bull Johns Hopkins Hosp 50: 196, 1932

20. Weed LH and Hughson W: Systemic effects of the intravenous injection of solutions of various concentrations with especial reference to the cerebrospinal fluid. Amer J Physiol 58: 101, 1921

21. Weed LH and McKibben PS: Pressure changes in the cerebrospinal fluid following intravenous injection of solutions and various concentrations. Amer J Physiol 48: 512, 1919

13.
Warfield Monroe Firor: A Surgeon for All Seasons

Warfield M. Firor was born in Baltimore, Maryland on November 7, 1896. From his first day as a student at The Johns Hopkins University in 1913 he has served his university well in many different capacities. An outstanding student, he received his A.B. in 1917 and his M.D. from The Johns Hopkins University School of Medicine in 1921. For over half a century, he has contributed not only as a superb surgeon, but as an outstanding teacher, an excellent administrator and an effective investigator. A deeply religious man, by his own example he has served as a stimulus and a career model for many young students of medicine and numerous surgical residents.

MEDICAL SCHOOL AND RESIDENCY TRAINING

His interest was directed at an early stage to surgery, since at that time it appeared to offer more opportunity for beneficial therapeutic intervention than did medicine. His attraction to surgery was no doubt, in significant measure, the result of his contacts during medical school and during his internship with William S. Halsted, professor of surgery. Firor has given a description of his student days and internship in an interview with Peter D. Olch of the History of Medicine Division of the National Library of Medicine (February 1967) and also in an unpublished essay entitled "Comments About the Surgical Chiefs at the Johns Hopkins Hospital Between 1918 and 1938." Firor's first contact with Halsted was in the Professors' Friday Clinics for the medical students, which were very formal. Halsted would come into the amphitheatre followed by the resident. The resident would call two students to the floor and introduce them to the professor. The patient was brought in; Halsted would question him about his illness and then do a brief physical examination. Firor was impressed by his gentleness, thoroughness and precision in the conduct of the examination. Halsted would then turn to the students and ask them to make their own examination. After the patient had been taken from the amphitheatre, Halsted would question the students about their examination; the entire clinic was conducted by the Socratic method. At no time did he lecture or address the entire student body. In fact, Firor commented, any student who did not

Reprinted from the *Johns Hopkins Medical Journal* **146:** 16, 1980.

happen to be in the first two or three rows would not hear what the professor said. This method of teaching reflected Halsted's belief that surgery could not be taught in a classroom; that surgeons were trained. His effort was directed toward setting an example and not imparting specific surgical information.

These clinics were quite thorough and were considered severe. The students were afraid to be called down as they were certain to be cross-examined by the professor. Always before the termination of the clinic, Halsted would call attention to the books which he had brought in before the clinic began, each book having a pertinent reference mark in it. Many of Halsted's clinics dealt with the fundamental aspects of physiology in relation to surgery. He frequently emphasized the historical development of the subject at hand, and the students were left with the impression that they had seen a great gentleman, a very erudite scholar and a meticulous surgeon in action.

Firor's next contact with Halsted was on the surgical wards where the professor made rounds on a weekly basis with the students. Halsted never appeared hurried and at times would discuss a single point for the entire hour in order to emphasize it. Firor was again impressed by Halsted's gentleness in dealing with patients. As a student, his last contact with Halsted occurred when he substituted for one of the surgical interns and had the opportunity to "scrub" on Halsted's team. Firor recalled an operation for bilateral herniorrhaphy which took three hours, during which time Halsted demonstrated those points in technique which contributed so much to his fame: meticulous handling of all tissues, accurate dissection, and complete hemostasis. Halsted did not leave the operating room when the major part of the surgery was finished and turn over the closure of the wound to the assistant. Halsted himself closed the wound with the same care and thoroughness with which he had performed the entire operation, even remaining to see that the dressings were applied precisely as he wished.

One of Firor's most vivid recollections was the amount of attention given to aseptic technique: "For instance when we scrubbed, we then soaked our forearms and hands in potassium permanganate and took that off with acetic acid. We then soaked again in a bichloride solution and put our gloves on in bichloride so that if an accident occurred and a needle punctured a glove there would be a layer of antiseptic material. That 'wet technique' as it was called, was not used anywhere else as far as I know but it exemplified Halsted's insistence on an approach to perfection in technique." This "wet technique" was used until Dean Lewis became professor of surgery. In fact, after Lewis arrived, Firor insisted on using it for about a year and finally was told by the operating room nurse that he was the only one in the hospital for whom they had to get out all of the necessary paraphernalia; he, too, switched over to the "dry technique."

The students who wished an internship in surgery applied in early December. The most desirable appointment in surgery was the one in the Hunterian Laboratory because the student who received this position was automatically kept on as an assistant resident.

Notice had been given that these appointments would be made along with the other internship appointments. However, before the remainder of the students had a chance to apply, one member of the class announced that he already had been given assurance of the position. Firor called Halsted at his home, not knowing that this was unheard of, and was disturbed to find out that Halsted had been told that there had been only one applicant. Firor was asked to come to Halsted's office the following day, at which time the secretary told him that the professor was not feeling well but wished him to come to his home. The butler ushered him into the library, and to Firor's amazement Halsted had looked up all the information about him in the dean's office. When he found out that Firor had been a patient at Saranac for treatment of tuberculosis he tried unsuccessfully to discourage him from applying for an internship. However, appointments were made strictly according to class standing and as Firor was entitled to an internship on that basis, he did not withdraw his application. The following year, the resident indicated to Firor that Halsted was reluctant to keep him on as an assistant resident because of Firor's history of tuberculosis. Halsted gave Firor the appointment when Firor pointed out that he was the only intern who had not missed any time from his duties and that for a period of three weeks had done all of another intern's work as well as his own.

DANDY'S SECOND NEUROSURGICAL RESIDENT

Firor was the second full-time resident on the neurosurgical service at Johns Hopkins (1923–1925), Frederick Reichert being the first. Prior to that time, Dandy had been assigned one of the assistant residents on the surgical service who worked part-time with him and part-time with other surgeons. Firor's period with Dandy began on July 5, 1923 and ended on January 29, 1925.

Shortly before this, Dandy had discovered ventriculography. Firor remembered the third patient in whom Dandy had injected air, a patient on whom Dr. Cushing had performed a subtemporal decompression but had been unable to locate the tumor. Dandy aspirated over 200 milliliters of cerebrospinal fluid from the lateral ventricle and replaced this with air. Following the

x-rays, he attempted to aspirate as much of the air as possible, but very little had passed beyond the third ventricle and through the aqueduct into the fourth ventricle. He told Firor to tap the lateral ventricle every two hours because he was afraid that the air would be irritating and that the patient would develop increased intracranial pressure, which she did. The ventricle was decompressed for almost four weeks before the professor was able to remove the tumor in the third ventricle, which had been beautifully visualized by the ventriculogram.

It was during Firor's period as neurosurgical resident that the first recovery room was organized. Three beds were set aside in one corner of the operating floor for this purpose. If the patient could afford private duty nurses, they attended the patients while in this recovery room. If not, one of the nurses from the operating room was called. It was a one-man show, manned in the beginning by Firor, who would frequently stay up all night with the critically ill patients operated on by Dr. Dandy during the day. After Firor finished his residency, Deryl Hart took over and continued the operation of this early recovery room. At times, general surgical patients were also admitted to this three-bed unit.

FIROR'S SERVICE UNDER DEAN LEWIS

Dean Lewis came to Baltimore as Halsted's successor in August 1925. In May 1926 Firor was appointed chief resident in surgery and served until September 1927. During the spring of his second year as resident, Lewis asked him to stay on for an additional year. When Firor told Deryl Hart that he had been invited to do this, Hart threatened to resign, pointing out that he had been waiting for six years for the residency. When this was reported to Lewis, the latter in his gruff way replied: "Tell him to leave. Nobody threatens me." Firor said, "Dr. Lewis, he is not threatening you. The facts are that he's three years older than I, we were classmates and he's trailed me all through this residency. I do not want it on my conscience that I did him out of the residency, so I will not accept the appointment next year." Lewis then added: "Will you stay on full-time?" Firor's reply was, "Yes." Lewis then said: "Good, I'll made you an associate professor." This was a little out of the ordinary but one month later Firor received his appointment as an associate, the former title for "associate professor." He went to Lewis and asked what he wanted him to do. Lewis replied: "I want you to write your own ticket. Put yourself down for whatever courses you want to give, be around to help me when I need it and do any investigative work you please." Fortunately, Firor's friends had given him $10,000 to use for investigative work the year he was resident. So in September 1927 when the residency had been completed, he began work in the Hunterian Laboratory (Fig. 1).

Firor decided to organize four elective courses. One of them was operative surgery and every Wednesday afternoon he would operate in the amphitheatre to instruct the students. While an assistant resident in charge of the accident room and admissions, Firor had to take care of all fractures because Halsted insisted that frac-

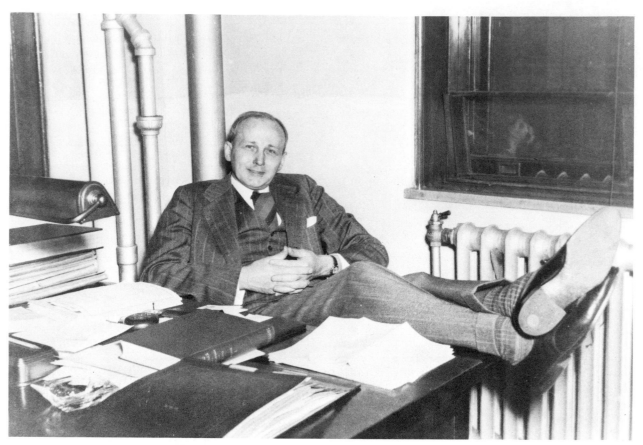

Fig 1.   Warfield M. Firor in the springtime of his career at Johns Hopkins.
From the Alan M. Chesney Medical Archives, The Johns Hopkins Medical Institutions.

tures belonged to the general surgeons and not to the orthopaedic surgeons. Knowing nothing about fractures, he persuaded George Bennett to give an elective course with him one afternoon a week on that subject. He did this primarily to learn something about fractures himself. Later on, when Firor was acting head of the department, he arranged with George Bennett to transfer all fractures to the orthopaedic service, provided that service would take one of the surgical assistant residents for six months and train him in this subject. The most important elective course that he set up came as a result of his experience with Dandy. During Firor's first year as neurosurgical resident, Dandy was not married. At that time, Dandy would invariably come back to the hospital after dinner to go over the x-ray films that had been taken that day. He would see things that no one else detected, making associations that nobody else thought of. Firor soon recognized that a major factor in Dandy's success was his incessant inquisitiveness. He was not asking other people questions; he was simply bombarding his own mind with questions. This so impressed Firor that when Lewis asked him to stay on full-time and teach, he put himself down for a simple elective entitled "Surgical-Pathological Conference," the objective of which was to teach students to ask themselves questions, not merely to make the correct diagnosis or learn surgical pathology. Firor gave this course for over 20 years.

The method was to provide the abstract of a case history without giving the students all the essentials that would make the diagnosis evident. Copies were distributed to the students before the session. In class Firor would go over the record, word by word, asking the significance of each symptom and its causes. By that method of continuous questioning the class would finally get to the end of the case and each student would commit himself to a single diagnosis, as would Firor. Then the correct diagnosis would be revealed. The course was very popular, and soon a similar one was organized in several other medical schools. Firor's fourth teaching assignment in this early period consisted of regular ward rounds one morning a week as well as substituting for Dr. Lewis on ward rounds during the professor's frequent absences.

INVESTIGATIVE WORK

In 1924 Harvey B. Stone and Firor published their study of absorption in intestinal obstruction. The stimulus for this work came from a patient who, after an appendectomy, developed paralytic ileus. For eight days there were no toxic symptoms, but on the ninth day the patient developed acute crampy abdominal pains, visible peristalsis, began to vomit material of a distinctly intestinal character, and for the first time developed fever and tachycardia. The appearance of these symptoms was thus synchronous with the increased intestinal activity and suggested that increased intra-intestinal pressure might have resulted in the absorption of toxic substances. The pressures of the contents of normal and obstructed bowels were found to be greatly different. Stone and Firor then studied pressure in isolated obstructed loops of small bowel. Using India ink they demonstrated increased absorption into the lymphatics when there was complete obstruction, as opposed to absorption in the normal state or in only partial obstruction. These findings also provided concrete evidence that toxin does not pass through a suspended living loop of bowel unless there is increased intra-intestinal pressure. From this well-designed series of experiments, they concluded that distention is an important element in the absorption of toxins not because it leads to vascular disturbances and subsequent necrosis, but because it results in increased intra-intestinal pressure. Great pressure may exist within obstructed loops even without gross distention. Recent studies of intestinal obstruction have tended to emphasize the loss of fluid and diminished circulating blood volume as responsible for the circulatory collapse of these patients, rather than the absorption of "toxins" from the obstructed bowel.

The period 1927–1938 was Firor's most active time in the laboratory. At the suggestion of Dean Lewis and also as a gesture of cooperation with the members of the Department of Pharmacology who were interested in liver function, Firor devised a method for removing the dog's liver in one stage. Up to that time, a three-stage operation had been described; this operation had not been satisfactory. After the operation the dogs were studied by G. S. Eadie of the Department of Pharmacology.

Following the epidemics of influenza, numerous cases of chronic empyema were encountered and the treatment was far from satisfactory. Firor felt that if one could produce this disease in dogs it would provide an experimental tool in which studies of the best therapeutic approach could be made. This he succeeded in doing, publishing his results in 1930.

EXPERIENCE IN INDIA

Firor's investigative work was interrupted in 1930, when he went to India for a year under the auspices of the Presbyterian Board of Foreign Missions. A friend, Steven Clark, had invited Firor to go to Cooperstown, New York as Director of Surgery at the Mary Imogene Bassett Hospital at a salary precisely ten times that which he was receiving at Johns Hopkins. In view of the fact that there would be little opportunity for investigative work and a rather small clinical load, he declined the post. When Cyrus McCormack, president of the International Harvester Company, heard that Firor had declined the Cooperstown offer he sent for him and offered to pay all of his expenses if he would go to India for a year. Although having initially refused to give Firor's wife health clearance, the Mission Board was willing to accept the arrangement on these terms. Firor was assigned to a

large hospital in Miraj, in western India. On arrival, it was suggested that he spend a year learning the language, but since he and his wife were to be there for only a year, this did not seem a reasonable course to pursue. As a result, cases were delegated to him which none of the surgeons there were able to handle, including all of the neurosurgery, spinal grafts for tuberculosis of the spine, carcinomas of the breast, and subtotal thyroidectomies. Firor was assigned an assistant resident, whom he trained and who later became the head surgeon at the hospital.

RESUMPTION OF RESEARCH

On his return from India, Firor met Arthur Grollman, who had just returned to Johns Hopkins after a fellowship year abroad. Exchanging pleasantries on the street corner, they soon decided to join forces in a study of the adrenal cortex from which Swingle and Pfiffner had just extracted a hormone which they considered vital for life. Grollman and Firor made arrangements to get adrenals from the slaughterhouse nearby and freeze them. Their first problem was to work out a mouse assay. Firor soon had his own animal quarters and his own diener so that it was quite easy for them to keep a colony of several hundred mice on which Firor would do bilateral adrenalectomies. Firor gives credit to Grollman for all of the important aspects of this work, which resulted in the publication of a series of some ten papers which are listed in the references.

Firor's modesty and generosity in acknowledging Grollman's contributions is typical. An anecdote further demonstrating these qualities in Firor stems from this period. Grollman and Firor were to present a paper at a meeting of the American Medical Association in June 1933. In typical fashion, Dean Lewis stuck his head in Firor's doorway every day for two weeks before that meeting, saying each time: "I want you to knock their eyes out." Firor did not have the faintest idea what he meant. It turned out that Lewis knew that there would be a committee from the University of Illinois at that meeting in search of a professor of surgery and that one of the possible candidates was Firor. What Lewis wanted was for Firor to read the paper, and to do it in such a way that the committee would be persuaded to offer Firor the professorship. Firor not having been told of this objective and the particular studies having represented Grollman's part of the work, Grollman was the one who delivered the paper in Atlantic City. Dr. Lewis was furious. Firor did not get the job, which went instead to Warren Cole.

It is unusual for a surgeon to become a member of the American Physiological Society before he becomes a member of the American Surgical Association, but this Firor did. He was frequently sought as a research collaborator by other groups in the medical school. In 1932 he became interested in the problem of hypophysectomy and at the request of Dr. Hartman of the Carnegie Institution, he devised a method for removing the pituitary gland from monkeys, an operation which had not previously been performed successfully. The method which he devised was a very simple one. He made a tiny opening in the dura mater at the point where the stalk of the pituitary descends. He next inserted a small cannula into this opening and connected it with a glass tube, at the other end of which was a suction pump. In this manner, suction could be applied, resulting in successful extraction of the pituitary, which when it hit a large glass bulb in the suction tube, remained intact so that it could be carefully examined histologically. Thus the glass bulb interposed between the aspirating tube and the water suction pump acted as a trap in which one could catch the specimen. It was possible to empty the sella thoroughly without producing the slightest bleeding. Dr. Ferdinand C. Lee examined all of the specimens showing the region of the sella turcica and overlying brain and from which serial sections had been prepared. He could find no remnants of the hypophysis, including the infundibulum.

In the same year Firor examined the relationship between the pituitary body and pregnancy by studying the effects of removing this gland at various periods of gestation. He demonstrated that the hypophysis is essential for ovulation and for the life of the corpus luteum in the rabbit. Without the hypophysis, implantation either does not occur or, if it occurs, does not persist. Thus in rabbits, the hypophysis is essential for the continuation of pregnancy.

In a subsequent study with S.R.M. Reynolds, Firor studied the uterine motility of hypophysectomized and pregnant rabbits. In the first group of experiments an effort was made to determine whether, following hypophysectomy, the corpora lutea of pregnancy lose their ability to counteract the effect of estrin on uterine motility following hypophysectomy and so in this respect cease to be functional. A second series of experiments was planned to determine the period of pregnancy at which the corpora lutea ceased to inhibit the response of estrin by obtaining motility records directly from gravid uteri in the unanesthetized rabbits. Thus, these experiments were performed under circumstances in which the hormonal and morphological conditions were essentially normal. They were able to demonstrate that in rabbits hypophysectomized on the fifth or sixth day of pregnancy or pseudopregnancy, the corpora lutea lose within 48 hours their power to inhibit typical uterine contractions induced by estrin; that in unanesthetized pregnant rabbits the uterus is refractory to the motility-inducing action of estrin until the 26th day of pregnancy, but on the 27th day the injection of estrin leads to abortion and death; that the corpus luteum functions at a high level as regards maintaining uterine quiescence, until about the middle of the fourth week of gestation, and is no longer functioning in this regard by the end of the fourth week.

No one had previously devised a technique for hypophysectomizing rabbits. It occurred to Firor that the approach should be through the orbit and he worked out a method of sucking out the hypophysis by puncturing the very thin wall in the posterior part of the rabbit's orbit.[1] Firor believes that his studies on the effect of

---

[1] This ingenious technique fascinated Max Brödel so much that he volunteered to illustrate it. His original drawings are now in the National Library of Medicine.

hypophysectomy on pregnancy represented the best of his investigative work. In the rabbit, ovulation occurs after copulation. If one hypophysectomizes a rabbit within three hours after coitus, ovulation does not occur. If one hypophysectomizes in the first week, implantation does not occur. If one performs the operation after the first week, development is stopped and the rabbit aborts. And if one waits until two days before delivery before doing the hypophysectomizing, the rabbit aborts. Thus every phase of pregnancy, from ovulation to delivery, is under the control of the hypophysis.

One of the most important research contributions made by Firor has never been properly recognized. Firor demonstrated that in a hypophysectomized dog, the adrenal does not hypertrophy. Firor's approach was simplicity: Firor would take out one adrenal, weigh it, hypophysectomize the animal, wait for three months and then weigh the remaining adrenal. His results showed that in a hypophysectomized animal, there was no increase in weight, whereas in the control animals that were not hypophysectomized the remaining adrenal would double in size. This might be considered as the earliest demonstration for the existence of an adrenocorticotropic hormone.

In the early 1930s Dr. John J. Abel redeveloped his interest in vividialysis and asked Firor if there was any technique by which he could circulate the blood through tubes without its clotting. Firor's answer was: Why not do it directly animal to animal? As a result, he developed a technique of end-to-end anastomosis between the carotid artery and the jugular veins of dogs so that there was cross-circulation. Then the kidneys were removed from one of the animals. When these experiments were reported, the Society for the Prevention of Cruelty to Animals rented a window on Charles Street in which they placed a huge sign which indicated that Firor was torturing dogs. They based their objection on the fact that one pair out of 40 developed hematuria, and after the word hematuria in their display, they wrote "Painful urination." For over a month this unsought publicity continued. It worried Dean Lewis far more than it worried Firor. In another effort, Pyrex tubes were used, but by that time Dr. Abel's interest had shifted to another problem. He had been elected president of the American Association for the Advancement of Science and took off an entire year to write his presidential address on bacterial toxins.

RESEARCH ON TETANUS

In the process of preparing this paper, Abel decided that the work of Meyer and Ransom was incorrect in concluding that tetanus toxin passes up the nerves from the periphery to the central nervous system. This theory had been accepted since 1904 and Abel reasoned that it was inconsistent in nature for a toxin to use such a neural route of transport. This started a series of experiments in which Firor cooperated. Firor devised a technique for the accurate injection of minute amounts of tetanus toxin into various parts of the dog's spinal cord. By this procedure, it was possible to produce pure reflex motor tetanus without the slightest evidence of muscular rigidity. As little as 1/2,000th of an intravenous lethal dose placed in the medulla sufficed to bring on reflex motor spasms of the pharyngeal muscles. The intraspinal injection of 1/400th or more of the usual intravenous lethal dose of tetanus toxin was always followed by the death of the animal, despite the fact that the toxin was placed in a nonvital center, such as the lumbar cord. The explanation that death resulted from an upward passage of the toxin was untenable because transection of the cord above the site of injection did not prevent death. Similarly, division of all sensory and motor pathways below the lesion was without effect. The death of the animal could not be caused by a multiplication of the tetanus molecule and subsequent reabsorption because the presence in the circulating blood of 100 neutralizing doses of antitoxin did not prevent a fatal outcome. One explanation for these results was that the tetanus toxin was altered in the spinal cord to form a secondary substance which in turn was responsible for the death of the dog. It was clear that a similar dose of toxin in other organs of the body did not cause death.

FURTHER WORK ON THE ADRENAL GLAND WITH GEORGE THORN

In 1938 Firor began a collaboration with George Thorn in his studies of desoxycorticosterone. They demonstrated that carefully prepared tablets of crystalline desoxycorticosterone acetate would maintain an adrenalectomized dog in excellent condition for periods of several months or more. (They had devised a method of implanting the tablets subcutaneously.) From time to time, they removed the pellets, weighed them and then reimplanted them, showing that over a prolonged period the hormone was absorbed at a fairly constant rate. Therefore, it was possible to establish the number of pellets which, when implanted, would correspond to a given dose of the hormone-in-oil injected subcutaneously once a day. The equivalence could be established by measurement of the electrolyte balance. If this could be maintained, then there was correspondence between dose and response. Firor and Thorn succeeded in applying this method to the treatment of patients with Addison's disease, for which they received a gold medal from the American Medical Association. The patient could, by this technique, be provided with a continuous and effective source of hormone for a period of 8 to 12 months. The small incision which was made at the time of implantation of the pellets served as a useful marker of any change in the patient's tendency toward hyperpigmentation. Later a technique of trochar insertion of the pellets eliminated the need for any operative procedure. They noted that the pellets, when removed for weighing, were always surrounded by a capsule and could be "shelled out" like peas. It was clearly this fibrotic capsule which resulted in the delayed absorption of the crystalline hormone.

BOWEL STERILIZATION WITH SULFONAMIDES

Firor initiated the introduction of sulfonamide derivatives for sterilization of the bowel in patients undergoing operation on the colon. In September 1940 Marshall and his co-workers published their studies with sulfanilylguanidine. Their paper described the method of preparation and the properties of this compound. Their experiments demonstrated that this new sulfonamide compound, when given orally, was less toxic than sulfapyridine or sulfathiazole. These studies established two facts of possible significance for surgeons. They showed that although sulfanilylguanidine is fairly soluble in water, it is poorly absorbed from the intestinal tract; and second, that the concentration of coliform bacteria in the feces of mice is greatly reduced after the oral administration of the drug. These observations led Firor and A. F. Jonas to use this drug in the preparation of patients who were to undergo operations upon the colon. In a paper entitled "The Use of Sulfanilylguanidine in Surgical Patients," they reported their experience with this drug in 12 such cases. Firor's interest in this subject was stimulated by a report of a surgeon in Toledo, Ohio, who immunized the peritoneal cavity against coliform organisms prior to operation. The idea occurred to Firor that use of one of the recently introduced sulfonamides might be simpler and just as effective as immunization. Firor went to E. K. Marshall, Jr. and asked if he could prepare a paste with sulfanilamide for application around the suture line in left colon resection to curtail the spread of coliform organisms. It so happened that when Firor entered his office Marshall was reading the page proofs of an article on sulfanilylguanidine. He lent the proofs to Firor, who returned the following day enthusiastic about making the trials with this new drug.

The 12 patients reported by Firor and Jonas, who had colon operations while receiving this sulfonamide derivative, were considered as only an initial step in a far-reaching clinical study. They felt, however, that they could contrast the postoperative progress of each patient receiving sulfanilylguanidine with the progress that might have been expected had the drug not been given. From this point of view, it was highly probable that at least two patients would have died if the concentration of coliform bacteria had not been reduced before operation. In addition, it was almost certain that without the use of the drug the intestinal wounds in three other patients would have failed to heal *per primam*. Of the remaining seven patients, the progress of only two could be regarded as significant in estimating the value of the drug in large-bowel surgery. These were two cases upon whom open anastomoses were successfully performed without the slightest evidence of subsequent infection. Judging from the convalescence of these patients, their impression was that the drug was a real adjuvant in colonic surgery.

Bacterial counts were performed each day on fresh stool specimens of a series of Firor's patients who had colostomies. All ten patients given sulfanilylguanidine developed sterile stools, subsequently enabling him to do a closed anastomosis without the slightest sign of infection. About this time, Edgar Poth came to work with Firor. In laboratory studies he found that Marshall's conclusion, that sulfanilylguanidine was poorly absorbed, was erroneous. The explanation for the fact that no significant blood levels could be demonstrated after administration of the drug was that it was absorbed and excreted within two hours. Soon they discovered that this drug caused a toxic reaction in many patients receiving it. They were able to obtain 20 different congeners from pharmaceutical firms for further trials. Poth found that sulfathalidine, which he synthesized, was best for patients who were constipated, while sulfasuxidine was best for those who had diarrhea.

Firor made isolated loops of bowel in dogs and reconstituted the continuity of the bowel. Ordinarily a closed loop obstruction causes death within two to four days. By the injection of sulfasuxidine into such a blind loop, the dog would live for weeks and months, secreting mucus into the loop until it became an enormous mass. Firor would then inject coliform organisms into the loop and within two or three days all of the toxic symptoms of intestinal obstruction would develop. This result seemed excellent evidence that the cause of death in intestinal obstruction was bacterial.

The successful completion of the studies on intestinal antisepsis with sulfonamides was due in large degree to the skill of Edgar J. Poth, who laid the foundation for the experimental work by constructing an apparatus for accurately feeding dogs a fixed amount of drug at regular intervals. Firor and Poth noted that when succinyl sulfathiazole was given by mouth in adequate amounts and at proper intervals, the contents of the gastrointestinal tract were profoundly altered. The stool became soft and odorless and the amount of flatus was diminished. These changes reflected the alterations that took place in the bacterial flora. They gave succinyl sulfathiazole to more than 120 patients. With quantitative studies of the number of coliform bacteria in the stool, they demonstrated that in almost every instance the ingestion of adequate amounts of this compound lowered the concentration of *E. coli* to less than 100 per gram of wet stool.

ACTING CHAIRMAN OF THE DEPARTMENT OF SURGERY

During the 1930s Firor began to operate on an increasing number of patients, at first, principally because all of the medical students and nurses sought his help when they needed surgical attention. In 1937 he decided to give up his full-time status and to share an office with Halsey Barker around the corner from 11 E. Chase Street. Just when arrangements had been almost completed, Dean Lewis became ill and Firor was asked to assume the role of acting department chairman. Because his practice grew so rapidly, he set up a small suite of examining rooms on Halsted 5. Soon others were permitted to use these facilities and it was there that James Bordley, III first established the Private Outpatient Clinic (POPS). Firor's heavy duties as acting chairman of surgery brought his investigative career to an end.

As acting chairman, Firor remembered the great benefit which he derived from the degree of responsibility given to him by Dean Lewis. In the summer of 1939,

Firor offered Edward S. Stafford, who was just beginning his period as resident in surgery, the same opportunity he had been offered by Lewis. Thus, when Ferdinand Lee left to become professor of surgery at the University of Georgia, Stafford suddenly found himself in charge of the Hunterian Laboratory and the Outpatient Clinic. He was responsible for Firor's teaching and patients when Firor was out of the city, with, as before, Harvey Stone to call on in case of need. Stafford recalls: "He was absolutely marvelous in his treatment of me as a resident; never failing to be helpful and always willing to back me up. He depended on me to request help when I needed it."

FIROR AND THE JEKYLL ISLAND CLUB

The Jekyll Island Club was formed in 1896 by a group of wealthy men who wanted a vacation place where they could be isolated. They built a clubhouse and an apartment house. They had a physician from the Roosevelt Hospital (in New York City) there during the season, which was usually two months, February and March. When Roy McClure, a Johns Hopkins graduate, was sent down from the Roosevelt Hospital while an assistant resident in surgery there, he was so popular that when he returned to Baltimore later to be the surgical resident (May 1914–March 1916), the Jekyll Island group wrote to Halsted requesting that Roy McClure be made available again as the doctor. Halsted knew many of the members of the Jekyll Island Club and his sister was a frequent visitor there, so he consented. When McClure went to the Henry Ford Hospital as surgeon-in-chief he turned the Jekyll Island assignment over to Walter Dandy, who went down for six successive years. Being on the part-time staff, he was able to charge fees for the work which he did there. In 1923 Dandy sent Firor down for six weeks. As the season was then three months, Frederick Reichert went for the last six weeks.

During that first visit in 1923 the manager of the Jekyll Island Club developed painless jaundice and Firor brought him to Baltimore. The surgeon who operated on him thought that he had a carcinoma of the pancreas but refused to tell the patient. At that time, Firor was the surgical assistant resident in charge of the Marburg service. Seeing that the man was unhappy over the evasive responses of his surgeon, Firor told the gentleman in a straightforward way that he had a mass in the head of the pancreas, that it was probably malignant, but that there was still a chance that it was benign. Firor explained that if the mass was malignant his life expectancy was only about 18 months. If benign, his life span was indefinite, as they had created a biliary shunt. Actually, the mass turned out to be benign and the patient lived for many years. Firor's candor impressed the man greatly so he insisted on Firor's coming back to Jekyll Island the following year. That second year that Firor was at Jekyll the president of the club, Walter B. James, a former professor of medicine at Columbia University's College of Physicians and Surgeons, had a coronary occlusion. Firor took care of him, largely at James's direction, and he recovered sufficiently to return to New York.

His excellent care of Dr. James endeared Firor to the Jekyll Island residents and they insisted that he return each year. Dean Lewis kindly requested the Trustees of the university to waive the rule that full-time faculty could not augment their salaries, thus permitting those who went to Jekyll Island to keep the money which they earned while there. This income was more than the yearly sum which Firor received as a full-time associate professor.

One of the members who no longer had a use for the house which he owned on Jekyll Island gave it to the club and Firor was asked to design it as an infirmary, thus filling a real need. The house was a substantial two-story structure and finally, in 1929, the second floor was remodeled to provide living quarters for club physicians. There were quarters for a full-time nurse and a pharmacy where drugs and other equipment could be stocked. Dean Lewis permitted Firor to go to Jekyll Island each winter for six weeks, since Lewis always went away in the summer for three months, during which time he left Firor in full charge of the department.

Firor had many interesting experiences at Jekyll Island with financiers of national prominence. The caddy master at Jekyll developed a severe myocardial insufficiency and the various women on the island provided nurses for him for several weeks. When the end of the season came, Pierpont Morgan asked Firor to breakfast one morning and said: "Firor, if you will give the time I will pay to have Ernest taken all the way to Ottawa in a private compartment." He gave Firor $3,000 to cover the expenses of the trip. Firor put the patient in a hospital in Ottawa and had $1,500 left over. He told the family that this would cover the hospital bills during the remainder of the illness. When Firor wrote to Morgan about the matter, he received a personal note in reply congratulating him on knowing how to dispense money.

Morgan, in Firor's experience, was a very warm person. One day while standing on the dock he said: "Firor, what are you going to make out of that boy of yours?" Firor replied: "I'm going to let him be whatever he wants to be." "That's right," Morgan said, "I had four children and I tried to teach them two things—self control and a sense of proportion." Firor then said: "Mr. Morgan, a sense of proportion depends on your standard of values." "You are right," replied Morgan, "and I put spiritual values ahead of everything else." Then Firor added: "By the way, do you know Francis Thompson's poem 'In No Strange Land'?" "No," Morgan replied and then said: "Come up to my apartment and tell me about it." So Firor introduced him to Francis Thompson's poem. The next year when he came to Jekyll Island, Morgan told Firor that he had obtained a first edition, then added: "They're wonderful but some of them I don't understand." This exchange between Morgan and Firor exemplifies the friendly atmosphere that existed at Jekyll Island. Everyone ate in the same dining room and each family had its own table. Members would give dinner parties by inviting other members to come over and sit at their tables. Firor developed many close friends there, and one year three different members came to him and

said: "I've just given $100,000 to that place of yours." Firor replied, "What for?" They said, "We all go to Dr. Wilmer and we adore him. When we heard that there's going to be an institute we each chucked in $100,000 toward the Wilmer Institute."

A frequent visitor to Jekyll Island was Lucy Warthin James. When Dr. Lewellys Barker became a member of the club she attended as his guest and Firor was asked to dinner. Lucy Warthin James had given The Johns Hopkins Hospital $600,000 for the building of the new Women's Clinic (a building which has recently been demolished). At that time Dr. Thomas S. Cullen was in charge of gynecology. The plans for the clinic were shown to him the night before the final contract with the builders was to be signed. Cullen went over the plans and sent them back with a note "Approved under duress." It turned out that the operating room suite for gynecology was smaller than the one in the building used for gynecology that had been provided by Howard Kelly (a building on the site of the present Wilmer Insitute). Cullen and the other members of the staff in gynecology continued to voice their dissatisfaction; they all closed ranks and refused to move into the new building when it was completed. Dr. Welch finally went to the Rockefeller Foundation and obtained $100,000 to add a new floor to the building so that the gynecologists would occupy it. As soon as Firor was introduced to Lucy Warthin James at dinner she said: "Oh, you're just the man I want to talk to. You can tell me all that happened about the new Women's Clinic which I endowed." Firor demurred, saying that he was just an assistant resident and that it did not seem proper for him to discuss the controversy that had taken place. She promptly told Firor the whole story and then added that if there had not been a quarrel about the matter, she would have given another $600,000.

FIROR AND RESIDENCY TRAINING IN SURGERY

Throughout his career, Firor maintained a continuing interest in residency training in surgery. In a paper published in 1965 in the *Review of Surgery*, entitled "Residency Training in Surgery—Birth, Decay and Recovery," he traced three distinct phases labeled as introduction, expansion with deterioration, and regulation. The concept of prolonged periods of training in specialty services in university-affiliated hospitals originated in Germany. It was introduced into this country when The Johns Hopkins Hospital opened in 1889. The Medical Board of the Hospital asked Drs. Osler, Halsted and Kelly to present their views on the best method of appointing interns. In response, Osler presented a report dealing with the larger question of appointment of resident physicians and interns. The first paragraph read as follows:

> The resident physician. It would be well to use for this officer the term first assistant at the medical, surgical and gynecological clinics respectively. Ultimately, we should look forward to having second assistants, as at the German clinics. These men should, as now, be salaried. They

should be selected with the greatest care by the staff, with the approval of the Medical Board and of the Trustees. They should be appointed annually, and it is expected that these men will remain for an indefinite period so long in fact as they do their work satisfactorily.

Perhaps the one special advantage which the large German hospitals have over corresponding American institutions is the presence of these highly trained men who remain in some cases 3, 5, or even 8 years and who, under the professor, have control of the clinical material.

Osler's recommendations were accepted, but this innovative method of training in surgery, medicine and gynecology attracted so little attention that 15 years later, Halsted thought it appropriate to state the following in an address at Yale University: "Although we now have in the United States five or six moderately well endowed medical schools with a university connection, the problem of the education of our surgeons is still unsolved. Here I may be permitted to instant conditions which evolved in a natural way at the Johns Hopkins Hospital, where the plan of organization of the staff differs from that which obtains elsewhere in the country. It was our intention originally to adopt as closely as feasible the German plan which in the main is the same for all the principal clinics of the German universities. A house surgeon or first assistant as he is called in Germany, is selected after several years of service from a number of well-tried assistants. There is no regular advancement from the bottom to the top of the staff." An important factor in the slow appreciation of the value of this method may be found in the status of surgery in the 1890s and early 1900s. Surgery at that time could be described as unscientific and purely empirical. Any licensed doctor was allowed to operate. A knowledge of anatomy was deemed far more important than knowledge of surgical technique. Dexterity and rapidity in operating were the hallmark of greatness. An additional factor was the retiring manner of Halsted, who made no effort to promote or to publicize his school of surgery, the cardinal features of which were: (1) close association of the resident with the professor; (2) harsh competition for the top position; (3) indefinite tenure; (4) responsibility for the total care of all charity patients; (5) teaching of the house staff; and (6) participation in research.

The great benefits accruing from such a long period of discipline with responsibility in an institution devoted to teaching and investigation had to be demonstrated before interest was aroused and imitation began. The system spread mainly through the men who had participated in the original program. The first surgical residency in a private hospital was initiated by Dr. J. M. T. Finney, Sr. at the Union Protestant Infirmary in Baltimore. In 1907 Stephen T. Watts left Baltimore to be professor at the University of Virginia and organized a three-year residency there. In 1912 Cushing went to the Peter Bent Brigham Hospital in Boston and introduced a duplicate of the Baltimore program in which he had been resident from 1900 to 1903. In the next decade Gatch did the same in Indianapolis; McClure in Detroit; Goetsch in Brooklyn; and Brooks in St. Louis. In 1922 Heuer and

Reid instituted a superb residency at the Cincinnati General Hospital.

It took over 30 years to develop approximately ten Halsted-type surgical residencies, but by 1939 the American Medical Association directory listed 203. Between 1889 and 1939 it had become popular to lengthen the period of hospital training, by one or at most two years; the term "residency" was used indiscriminately for any training after the internship year. One of the reasons for this explosive increase was the influence of the recently organized specialty boards and the special privileges accruing in military and civilian practice from board certification. Another was the steadily rising standard of medical education with the concomitant attraction to men anxious to secure the best possible preparation. During this interval, of course, the vast increase in medical knowledge and techniques challenged the young surgeon to learn more about his chosen specialty than was possible through the previously standard rotating internship. The popularity of this system of postgraduate training eventually led to deterioration in the concept of surgical residency until the term came to mean any period spent in a hospital after internship, regardless of whether the trainee had supervision, responsibility, or operating experience. Thus there were more than 500 so-called surgical residencies listed as approved by the A.M.A. by 1950. More than half of these had been approved without inspection.

Shortly after election to the American Board of Surgery, Firor urged the Board to define its own standards for an acceptable residency. This plan was agreed upon, and he was given the assignment. His description of a four-year graded residency was published in *Surgery, Gynecology and Obstetrics* in October 1951.

The first paragraph of this article reads as follows: "A four year graded residency in general surgery is not merely four years of training, nor does it denote a prescribed and rigid program of activity. It is regrettable that the only two components in a residency which can be measured are the number of operations performed and the duration of the training period. The intangible factors of a residency are more significant although harder to evaluate. These include: (1) the professional competence and the integrity of the senior staff and their ability and willingness to teach; (2) the responsibility given the resident; (3) the attitudes of enquiry pervading the service; (4) the opportunity afforded the resident for study, investigation and teaching." At that time Firor emphasized that the complexities of modern surgery made four years after internship the minimal period for adequate preparation for the practice of general surgery. This was evident when one thinks of the rapid expansion of knowledge in such subjects as anesthesia, bacteriology, physiology, chemotherapy and biophysics, all of which influence the care of the surgical patient.

The second requirement for improving surgical residencies was to get the cooperation of competent surgeons to check and verify compliance with the Board's standards. To do this, Firor sought the aid of members of the American Surgical Association; he also persuaded the

Board both to form its own Residency Review Committee, and not to accept the lists already published by the A.M.A. and the American College of Surgeons. To eliminate the confusion of all three organizations inspecting residencies (the Residency Review Committee; the A.M.A. and the College), Firor was able after months of struggle to get the Regents of the College to join the other two. Thus, the first Residency Review Committee in the country was formed; this group was known as the Conference Committee on Graduate Training in Surgery.

Despite the formation of this joint committee in 1947 and the active participation of the American College of Surgeons in all of its functions, the College continued to publish its list of "Approved Residency Programs" independently until the mid-1970s. This may give some indication of the difficulty Dr. Firor and his associates encountered in bringing the Joint Conference Committee on Graduate Training in Surgery into being and in making it the effective body it is today. Firor's formation of the Joint Conference Committee was an outstanding contribution and was an important factor in his election to the presidency of the American Surgical Association in 1963. Firor's efforts toward the upgrading of surgical training have left a durable imprint upon the surgical care of patients worldwide (Fig 2).

MONTE FIROR AS A HUMAN BEING

Dr. Firor is a very religious man. He served as an elder of the Franklin Street Presbyterian Church and taught religion at the Gilman School. His relationship with patients was always excellent and his gentleness and thoughtfulness endeared him to them. In 1961 he wrote an editorial in *Postgraduate Medicine* entitled "The Last Mile," in which he discussed the problem of the patient who is inflicted with an incurable disease or is nearing the end of life. Serious illness has many concomitants in human beings.

Their actualities in our daily practice, and the purpose of this editorial is to urge all who read it to give critical consideration to their own way of helping the patient and the relatives when specific therapy fails. When this occurs the physician can adopt one of three courses of action: (1) avoid the situation by referring the patient to the family doctor; (2) maintain an optimism that is full of cheerful, but false, prognostication; or (3) explain to the family the improbability of curing the patient and the necessity of directing all one's efforts toward the alleviation of physical and mental suffering. More precisely, this means that it's just as much a physician's duty to help the patient to die comfortably when death is inevitable as it is his duty to prolong life while there is hope of recovery. The alleviation of physical suffering is relatively easy if the physician is not a fool. Unfortunately, there are many physicians who refuse opiates to patients with incurable maladies because the patients might become addicted! What nonsense!

From experience, I am convinced that another very important aspect in the handling of terminal illness is to

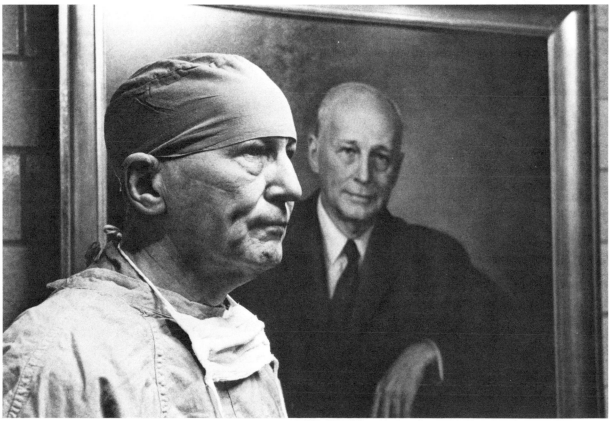

Fig 2.   Warfield M. Firor in the autumn of his career at Johns Hopkins.
From the Alan M. Chesney Medical Archives, The Johns Hopkins Medical Institutions

advise against the use of treatments designed solely to prolong existence. Useless transfusions and forced feedings are unjustifiable. Occasionally this may require a firm stand on the part of the physician, but more frequently the needless postponement of death is the result of the physician's fear of criticism.

The alleviation of mental suffering is an altogether different matter and often demands the utmost patience, perception and sacrifice on the part of the physician. Just to walk along with the patient and family day after day, so that they do not feel deserted, is one of the finest ways to help. Paradoxical as it may sound, it is in helping patients to die comfortably that the ministry of healing can sometimes achieve its greatest height.

Warfield M. Firor—surgeon, physiologist, creative scholar—exemplifies everything that the true physician should be in his relationship with patients and with the society in which he lives. His long career in the service of mankind in the fullest sense casts the image of excellence on the University and Hospital he has been affiliated with during his professional career. He is from every viewpoint—a surgeon for all seasons.

ACKNOWLEDGMENTS

I wish to thank Edward S. Stafford and William P. Longmire, Jr. for their help during the preparation of this essay.

REFERENCES

1. Abel JJ: On poisons and disease and some experiments with the toxin of *B. tetani*. Science 79: 121, 1934
2. Abel JJ., Firor WM and Chalian W: Researches on tetanus. IX. Further evidence to show that tetanus toxin is not carried to central neurons by way of the axis cylinders of motor nerves. Johns Hopkins Hosp Bull 63: 373, 1938
3. Approved residencies and fellowships in surgery. JAMA 113: 856, 1939
4. Chesney AM: The Johns Hopkins Hospital and Johns Hopkins University School of Medicine. Baltimore: The Johns Hopkins Press, Volume 1, p 161, 1943
5. Day HG, Kruse HD and Firor WM: Application of paired feeding method to studies of chemical changes in the blood of dogs following suprarenalectomy. Am J Hyg 25: 269, 1937
6. Firor WM: The use of plaster in the treatment of fractured femurs. Bull Johns Hopkins Hosp 35: 412, 1924
7. Firor WM: Torula infection of the central nervous system. Int Surg Dig 2: 3, 1926
8. Firor WM: Cervical adenitis due to Bacillus fusiformis. Johns Hopkins Hosp Bull 47: 378, 1930
9. Firor WM: The experimental production of chronic empyema in dogs. Proc Soc Exp Biol Med 28: 70, 1930
10. Firor WM: Experiments in cross circulation. Am J Physiol 96: 146, 1931
11. Firor WM: A review of crossed circulation experiments. N Engl J Med 204: 157, 1931
12. Firor WM: Hypophysectomy in the monkey (Macacus rhesus). Johns Hopkins Hosp Bull 50: 33, 1932
13. Firor WM: Hypophysectomy in pregnant rabbits. Am J Physiol 104: 204, 1933
14. Firor WM: The treatment of Addison's disease by the implantation of synthetic hormone. Ann Surg 111: 942, 1940
15. Firor WM: Intrathecal administration of tetanus antitoxin. Arch Surg 41: 299, 1940
16. Firor WM: Toxin-antitoxin reactions in experimental tetanus. Johns Hopkins Hosp Bull 67: 92, 1940
17. Firor WM: Intestinal antisepsis with sulfonamides. Ann Surg 115: 829, 1942
18. Firor WM: Observations on the conversion of normal into malignant cells. Ann Surg 121: 700, 1945
19. Firor WM: A four year graded residency. Surg Gynecol Obstet 93: 496, 1951
20. Firor WM: The story of the Hunterian Laboratory. Surgery 32: 485, 1952
21. Firor WM: A critical review of the treatment of mammary carcinoma. Surgery 46: 996, 1959
22. Firor WM: The last mile. Postgrad Med 29: 554, 1961
23. Firor WM: Residency training in surgery—Birth, decay and recovery. Rev Surg 22: 153, 1965
24. Firor WM and Eadie GS: The effect of epinephrin on muscle glycogen in the absence of the liver and a modification of the operation for liver removal. Am J Physiol 94: 615, 1930
25. Firor WM and Gey GO: The study of malignant cells with phase difference microscopy. Ann Surg 125: 604, 1947
26. Firor WM and Grollman A: Studies on the adrenal. I. Adrenalectomy in mammals with particular reference to the white rat (Mus norvegicus). Am J Physiol 103: 686, 1933
27. Firor WM and Jensen HJ: Toxins of high intestinal obstruction. Am J Surg 13: 281, 1931
28. Firor WM and Jonas AF Jr: Researches on tetanus. VI. The production of reflex motor tetanus by intraspinal injections of tetanus toxin. Johns Hopkins Hosp Bull 62: 91, 1938
29. Firor WM and Jonas AF: The use of sulfanilylguanidine in surgical patients. Ann Surg 114: 19, 1941
30. Firor WM and Lamont A: The apparent alteration of tetanus toxin within the spinal cord of dogs. Ann Surg 108: 941, 1938
31. Firor WM, Lamont A and Shumacker HB Jr: Studies on the cause of death in tetanus. Ann Surg 111: 246, 1940
32. Firor WM and Poth EJ: Intestinal antisepsis with special reference to sulfanilylguanidine. Ann Surg 114: 663, 1941
33. Firor WM and Stinson E Jr: Total extirpation of the dog's liver in one stage. Johns Hopkins Hosp Bull 44: 138, 1929
34. Firor WM and Woodhall B: Hemophilic pseudotumor: Diagnosis, pathology and surgical treatment of hemophilic lesions in the smaller bones and joints. Johns Hopkins Hosp Bull 59: 237, 1936
35. Ford FR and Firor WM: Primary "sarcomatosis" of the leptomeninges. Bull Johns Hopkins Hosp 35: 65, 1924
36. Ford FR and Firor WM: Gliomatosis of the leptomeninges. Bull Johns Hopkins Hosp 35: 108, 1924
37. Grollman A and Firor WM: Studies on the adrenal. II. Extraction of cortical hormone from urine. Proc Soc Exp Biol Med 30: 669, 1933
38. Grollman A and Firor WM: Studies on the adrenal. III. The preparation of an active extract of the hormone of the adrenal cortex. J Biol Chem 100: 429, 1933
39. Grollman A and Firor WM: Studies on the adrenal. IV. The oral administration of the adrenal cortical hormone and the use of fresh glands therapeutically. Johns Hopkins Hosp Bull 54: 216, 1934
40. Grollman A and Firor WM: Studies on the adrenal. VII. The relation of the adrenal cortical hormone to the vitamins. J Nutr 7: 569, 1934
41. Grollman A and Firor WM: Studies on the adrenal. X. Experimental studies on replacement therapy in adrenal insufficiency. Johns Hopkins Hosp Bull 57: 281, 1935
42. Grollman A, Firor WM and Grollman E: Studies on the adrenal. V. The extraction of the adrenal cortical hormone from the inter-renal body of fish. Am J Physiol 108: 237, 1934

43. Grollman A, Firor WM and Grollman E: Studies on the adrenal. VIII. A simple preparation of the adrenal cortical hormone suitable for oral administration. J Biol Chem 109: 189, 1935

44. Halsted WS: The training of the surgeon. Bull Johns Hopkins Hosp 15: 267, 1904

45. Hartman CG and Firor WM: Is there a "Hormone of menstruation?" Q Rev Biol 12: 85, 1937

46. Hartman CG, Geiling EMK and Firor WM: The anterior lobe and menstruation. Am J Physiol 95: 662, 1930

47. Hartman CG, Geiling EMK and Firor WM: Menstruation and the anterior pituitary. Proc Soc Exp Biol Med 28: 185, 1930

48. Lamont A, Firor WM and Shumacker HB Jr: The "lethal dose" of toxin in experimental tetanus. Johns Hopkins Hosp Bull 67: 25, 1940

49. Marshall EK, Jr et al.: Sulfanilylguanidine: A chemotherapeutic agent in intestinal infections. Johns Hopkins Hosp Bull 67: 163, 1940

50. McClure RD and Szilagyi DE: Halsted—Teacher of surgeons. Am J Surg 82: 122, 1951

51. Meyer H and Ransom F: Untersuchungen über das tetanus. Arch f Exper Path u Pharmakol 49: 369, 1903

52. Poth EJ et al.: Succinyl sulfathiazole: A new chemotherapeutic agent. Arch Surg 44: 187, 1942

53. Reynolds SRM and Firor WM: Uterine motility in hypophysectomized and in pregnant rabbits. Am J Physiol 104: 331, 1933

54. Reynolds SRM, Firor WM and Allen WM: Relative effectiveness of progestin in hypophysectomized and normal rabbits. Endocrinology 20: 681, 1936

55. Shumacker HB Jr and Firor WM: Studies on the adrenal. VI. The interrelationship of the adrenal cortex and the anterior lobe of the hypophysis. Endocrinology 18: 676, 1934

56. Shumacker HB Jr, Firor WM and Lamont A: The therapeutic use of antitoxin in experimental tetanus. Surgery 8: 1, 1940

57. Shumacker HB, Lamont A and Firor WM: The reaction of "tetanus-sensitive" and "tetanus-resistant" animals to the injection of tetanus toxin into the spinal cord. J Immunol 37: 425, 1939

58. Stone HB and Firor WM: Absorption in intestinal obstruction; Intra-abdominal pressure as a factor. Trans South Surg Assoc 37: 173, 1924

59. Thorn GW et al.: Treatment of Addison's disease with pellets of crystalline adrenal cortical hormone (synthetic desoxycorticosterone acetate) implanted subcutaneously. Johns Hopkins Hosp Bull 64: 339, 1939

14.

Tuberculosis: The Study of a Specific Disease at Johns Hopkins

OSLER'S EARLY INTEREST IN TUBERCULOSIS

Among the multitude of Osler's interests, tuberculosis held a high place. His first recognition of the disease as a scientific problem came during his transition from Toronto to Montreal. He received a letter in 1870 from his mentor Dr. James Bovell, who had gone to the West Indies in the summer of that year. This letter related Bovell's efforts to confirm some of Villemin's findings by the inoculation of guinea pigs with "tubercle." It is evident from the letter that this subject had been a matter of discussion between the two men.[1]

As a senior medical student, Osler spent the summer of 1871 in Montreal where he came into close contact with Professor Palmer Howard; a lasting, almost filial relationship developed. That summer the problem of tuberculosis was under discussion, stirred up not only by the epoch-making work of Villemin but also by the radical views of Niemeyer, an exponent of the dualistic theory of the origin of phthisis. Osler wrote many years later: "Every lung lesion at the Montreal General Hospital had to be shown to him (Howard), and I got my first-hand introduction to Laennec, to Graves and to Stokes, and became familiar with their works." Both Bovell and Howard had been students at Dublin when Graves and Stokes flourished there.

In the spring of 1875 Osler was appointed Professor of the Institutes of Medicine, and early in 1876 a new position, that of pathologist, was created for him at the Montreal General Hospital. It was in the autopsy room there that he developed an important part of the foundation for his future career. In the published report of the first 100 cases for the year ending May 1, 1877, 32 cases of tuberculosis were included. Osler published a second report in 1880 on a selection of 225 autopsies; of the 42 cases given detailed description, only six included tuberculosis in some form.

In April 1880, Mr. Duncan McEachran, principal of the Veterinary College, presented a paper entitled "The Transmissibility of Tuberculosis from Animals to Man" at the Montreal Medico-Chirurgical Society. This paper related particularly to infection through milk. In his discussion of this paper, Osler noted how many thoroughbred cattle had inflammation of the lungs, ending in caseation, which was regarded by all veterinary surgeons as phthisis: "The chief end of this discussion should be a proper milk inspection, not only of dairies but of milk brought into the city."

Koch's discovery of the tubercle bacillus was announced in the spring of 1882. Three months later the *Journal of the Montreal Medico-Chirurgical Society* had a note to the effect that Professor Osler had demonstrated before the students the presence of the organism in the lungs of a man who had died of rapidly advancing tuberculosis.

In 1885 Osler was appointed to the staff of the old "Blockley"—the Philadelphia General Hospital, originally a large almshouse. Here there was a wealth of untouched clinical and pathological material for teaching and investigation. Osler took on this assignment with enthusiasm and did 162 autopsies, of which 48 were on cases of tuberculosis. From his prolific pen came many editorials pertinent to the medical interest of that particular era. Sixteen articles in all related to tuberculosis; two were original papers.

---

[1] Jean Antoine Villemin (1827–1892) was a French military surgeon who became a professor at the Military Medical School, the Val-de-Grace. His consuming interest was tuberculosis. In 1865 Villemin inoculated tuberculous material, obtained from a lung cavity of a patient who had just died of pulmonary tuberculosis, into a healthy rabbit. Another rabbit from the same mother was used as a control, and both were kept in identical conditions and were killed after 3½ months. The uninoculated rabbit was free from tuberculosis, but in the inoculated rabbit, the lungs were full of tuberculous tissue. This material was used to inoculate another rabbit, with the same result, and so on in six series. Villemin's first statement of this and other important experiments along the same lines received a cool reception when presented at a meeting of the Académie de Médicine at Paris in 1867.

Reprinted from the *Johns Hopkins Medical Journal* 141: 198, 1977.

OSLER'S WORK ON TUBERCULOSIS IN BALTIMORE

When Osler arrived in Baltimore in the fall of 1888, his interest in tuberculosis was firmly established. His long experience with the disease made him familiar with all of its forms, and he knew that one-fourth of those infected recovered spontaneously and another one-fourth overcame the disease after showing signs of it. He was therefore able to give a paper in 1891 on "The Healing of Tuberculosis" with an optimistic note in contrast with the prevalent hopeless outlook of the profession. In this paper, he referred to Trudeau's successful experiments in curing infected rabbits by turning them loose, and to his practical application of the knowledge derived from this experiment to his patients by creating a sanatorium for them where they could live out-of-doors under favorable conditions. In Cushing's opinion, this paper signalled Osler's actual enlistment in the crusade against tuberculosis.

Welch attributed to Osler credit for being the first to work out the home treatment of the disease. Practical measures for home treatment, including rest out-of-doors, were outlined in the first edition of his textbook in 1892. His chapter on tuberculosis was considered by reviewers to be one of the best. A decade later, Osler modestly wrote to his friend John Musser, "Personally I think the only good thing I have done in connection with tuberculosis (though I have written a good many papers) is the article in my textbook, which Pepper always said was the best thing I'd ever written." In Baltimore, Osler's clinical studies on tuberculosis began to appear, before the publication of the textbook, in the Johns Hopkins Hospital periodicals—the *Bulletin* and the *Reports*. There were 19 papers in all, apart from six relating to public health.

THE HOSPITAL RECEIVES ITS FIRST GRANT FOR RESEARCH

The first donation ever made to The Johns Hopkins Hospital for research was a fund for the study of tuberculosis, which was received on February 9, 1898. The creation of this fund was announced in the Ninth Report of the Superintendent of The Johns Hopkins Hospital: "Through the liberality of benevolent individuals, who desire that their names not be mentioned, the hospital has been furnished with a fund of $750 per year for five years to promote the study of tuberculosis. It is the desire of the donors of this liberal gift that tuberculosis be studied in all its aspects, as to causes, means of communication, prophylaxis and treatment. The Trustees anticipate great benefit from this work conducted on a scientific basis."

It is no secret that the anonymous donors were William Osler himself and some of his friends whose interest and sympathy he had enlisted. Osler referred to the donation as having been given by "a couple of ladies—God bless them—" because just at that time the ill health of students made it clear that their living conditions, no less than those of the consumptives who came to the dispensary, needed to be looked into thoroughly. In the early years of the Johns Hopkins a number of staff members died from tuberculosis. Among them were Henry Newell Martin, who had been slated to be the first professor of physiology in the medical school; John B. MacCallum, the genius who made such important discoveries relating to the structure of heart muscle; and hardest of all for Osler, John Hewetson. In a memorial notice for Hewetson, who died in 1910, Osler wrote: "I just had the sad news of his death, and wish to pay a brief tribute to his memory. Long practice has given me a fair control of my vasomotors, but my grip has never been sure when a letter or some incident brought suddenly to my mind the tragedy of the life of Jack Hewetson. As I write there comes the far away vision of a young face, frank and open, with the gray-blue eyes that look so true and a voice to match with a merry laugh—no wonder that everyone loved him! Three happy years he lived with us, growing into a strong, earnest worker, and contributing with Dr. Thayer an important monograph on malaria, and many minor papers. . . . In 1894 Dr. Hewetson went to Germany, and in Leipzig appeared the signs of pulmonary tuberculosis. He had had a pleurisy in Montreal, and the disease made rapid progress. He returned to California where his father lived and began to fight the long and losing battle which has just ended."

Welch and Osler were appointed to supervise the tuberculosis studies, and Charles D. Parfitt, a Canadian, was appointed to take charge of the dispensary work. Parfitt, who himself shortly became victimized by the disease, recorded that Osler saw a great opportunity in a field in which in North America there were as yet few workers. Osler wished to bring about the segregation and more intensive study of dispensary cases of the disease and to develop a laboratory in which the special culture of the tubercle bacillus could be undertaken and animal inoculation carried out in order to verify the recent work of Le Damany on pleuritic effusion. Osler had long been interested in serous-membrane tuberculosis. A large group of histories relating to this subject were also to be analyzed and a special library collected.

During the year 1898–1899, Osler also inaugurated the visiting of dispensary cases of tuberculosis in their homes. He was eager to discover the conditions under which these patients lived and to bring competent advice to them. He wisely believed that improvement in home conditions was essential to any effective treatment of the tuberculosis problem in Baltimore. Two medical students, Miss Blanche Epler in 1899 and Miss Adelaide Dutcher in 1900, volunteered successively to do this work, for which the Fund for Tuberculosis Study was used. This house-to-house visitation by these medical students was really the pioneer effort in "hospital social service." Two other students, Miss Elizabeth H. Blauvelt and Miss Ester Rosencrantz, continued this service for two more years. It then became evident to Osler that more systemized visitation of the tuberculosis families, by a person who could devote full time to the work, was needed. In order to realize his wish, Grace Revere Osler raised a fund for this purpose in 1902, and the first special nurse, Miss Reba Thelin, a graduate of The Johns Hopkins Hospital Training School, was employed in 1903. The value of visiting nurses was clearly demonstrated and the number of such nurses was rapidly increased through other agencies.

In the Sixteenth Report of the Superintendent of The Johns Hopkins Hospital (January 31, 1905), there appeared a report on special nurses for the outpatient department. Reference was made to the work of Miss Thelin in visiting tubercular patients who had been in the habit of coming to the dispensary. It gives a rather dramatic picture of life in Baltimore at that time and the discouraging setting it provided for patients with tuberculosis:

"In Baltimore we do not have the tenement evil, but we have unsanitary rooms which have no opening to the outside air, lighted upstairs by a skylight, sometimes a shaft, and downstairs by a window into the kitchen. . . . we have the same overcrowding that exists in other cities where families of from five to nine people are living in two rooms or even one. Among other families who have a little four-roomed house the difficulty frequently is a lack of beds and bedding, and we find four or five people sleeping in the same bed. Of course, these are usually two adults and their young children, but in two instances a family of three—mother, son and daughter, all adults—were found occupying the same bed. The nurse's duty in such cases is obvious—to get the consumptive into another room, or failing that, into another bed, away from the rest of the family. . . . The daily bath is even more difficult of an accomplishment in cold houses, with the hydrant often out of doors and no means of heating water except on the kitchen stove. Many people do not bathe at all in cold weather. One woman, whose brother died of consumption, attributed it to the fact that 'he would change his flannels and take a bath once a week, no matter what the weather was.'

"In the matter of diet, material assistance was rendered by the federated charities, who supplied one quart of milk and two eggs daily, as long as they were needed, but to drink a stipulated amount of milk and eat two raw eggs every day soon pall upon anyone. . . . The average working man seems to live on the best of everything the market affords while he has the money. . . . However, when their money is wasted, they come down to bread and coffee, usually black coffee at that, for the rest of the week . . . The children, from three to four months up, eat just what their parents eat.

"We are told 'the treatment of the disease consists principally in fresh air, food, and rest.' Here we confront the most difficult proposition of all. How is a man to rest when his family are dependent upon him for support. How is a woman to rest, when there is no one to keep the house tidy and attend to the children.

"It is often difficult to make the consumptive himself believe that his sputum is dangerous, but the family is generally ready and anxious to observe precautions. The sputum cups with filter papers, furnished by the Johns Hopkins Hospital, were very faithfully used, and, in the majority of cases, as faithfully burned. Some patients, however, did throw the filters into the gutters and backyards, and one economical woman dried the filter in the sun and used it again. For the spittoons, which many persisted in using, a solution of carbolic acid, or a saturated solution of washing soda, was used and the spittoon was frequently emptied and scalded . . .

"One can scarcely credit the degree of superstition still prevalent among many of these people, did one not know that many more enlightened people still consult 'mediums and spiritualists.' Of course the patent medicine fiend rides rampant and many are the dollars wasted in 'Father John's medicine,' the 'Guardian Angel' remedies, and mysterious little bottles which hold about ten drops and cost several dollars. It will take time to teach this class that fresh air works the cure."

In the autumn of 1899 Osler read his first paper on the "Home Treatment of Consumption" before the Medical and Chirurgical Faculty of Maryland. The great practical problem was, he said, how best to treat the 95 percent of patients who could not leave their homes. Dr. Charles S. Millet, the first to recommend the use of unlimited night air for the treatment of consumption, was invited to speak at this meeting. His advice was soon widely accepted.

Through the initiative of Osler, the Laennec Society was formally organized on October 30, 1900 to stimulate the study of tuberculosis. This was the first society to be devoted to such a purpose. The members met monthly and provided an important stimulus for the developing antituberculous campaign. The reports of the meetings were published regularly in the *Johns Hopkins Hospital Bulletin*. At the first meeting Osler spoke "On the Study of Tuberculosis," and Miss Dutcher, in a paper entitled "Where the Danger Lies in Tuberculosis," reported her study of the social and domestic relations of 190 tuberculous outpatients whom she and two other medical students had visited.

Also at this meeting, mention was made for the first time, by Dr. Joseph E. Gichner, of the need and desirability of a state sanatorium in Maryland. Knowledge of Trudeau's successful work had, toward the end of the 19th Century, encouraged the building of sanatoria for treatment of patients near their homes. One of these was established at Gravenhurst, Ontario, by the National Sanatorium Association and opened in 1897. Dr. J. H. Elliott, the director, was a long-time worker in the field of tuberculosis in Canada. Osler corresponded with him about patients in whom he was interested and became a contributor to the work of the Association from 1898 on—another example of Osler's far-reaching support of useful enterprises.

Osler was chairman of the American Committee at the International Congress on Tuberculosis, which was held in London in the summer of 1901. In addressing the Congress, he referred to the wide efforts already being given to antituberculous work in the United States, and he discussed public health, pathology and diagnosis. The most important event of this meeting was Robert Koch's address on the difference in transmissibility of human and bovine bacilli to man and cattle, which later produced so much discussion and research.

On April 19, 1901, at the invitation of William Osler, Dr. Lawrence F. Flick of Philadelphia delivered an address in Baltimore on "Registration of Tuberculosis." Philadelphia and New York had already inaugurated the registration of cases of tuberculosis. Osler urged that Maryland do likewise since only in this way could the location of cases be known to the health authorities, allowing them to take advantageous steps for the patient and the community. By the end of that year great interest in the tuberculosis movement had developed, and it was proposed that the Maryland legislature of January 1902 pass new laws relating to this area of public health medicine. To this end, a meeting was held under the joint auspices of the Maryland Public Health Association, the Medical and Chirurgical Faculty of Maryland and the Laennec Society. Osler's vigorous speech on this occasion made a great impact on the audience: "Mr. Chairman and my long suffering, patient, inert fellow citizens: . . . Now what is our condition in this city, and what are we doing for the 10,000 consumptives who are living today in our midst? We are doing, Mr. Mayor and fellow citizens, not one solitary thing that a modern civilized community should do. Through the kindness of a couple of ladies—God bless them!—I have been enabled in the past 3 or 4 years to have two of the medical students of the Johns Hopkins University visit every case of pulmonary consumption that has applied for admission to the dispensary of the hospital and I tell you now that the story those students brought back is a disgrace to us as a city of 500,000 inhabitants. It is a story of desolation, want and helplessness, and of hopeless imbecility in everything that should be in our civic relation to the care of this disease." He went on to advance strong arguments for registration, disinfection after death or removal, a state sanatorium for curable cases and a hospital for advanced cases, a sewerage system, and a hospital for contagious diseases.

The addresses at that meeting influenced the Maryland Assembly of 1902 to create a Tuberculosis Commission, comprising John S. Fulton, Henry Barton Jacobs, and William S. Thayer as chairman. This Commission, which accomplished a great deal, was responsible for the organization of the Maryland Society for the Prevention of Tuberculosis (December 1904), of which Dr. Jacobs was for many years the president. Osler presided at the meeting of organization.

In December 1903 Osler gave a lecture at the Henry Phipps Institute of Philadelphia entitled "The Home and its Relation to the Tuberculosis Problem." This address was characterized as being so scientific, practical and inspiring that it should be read by every physician. It included a historical survey showing the evolution of knowledge about the disease and referred to three important contributions relating to the disease from this country: that of Trudeau on the importance of early sanatorium treatment, that of Biggs on city organization and that of Flick in the demonstration of the dangers of home infection. Since not more than two percent of patients could take advantage of sanatorium treatment or climatic change, a sound treatment of the patient at home was of immediate importance. In concluding, he quoted De Quincy, who had compared the many predestined to tuberculosis to the blazed trees marked by the forester as ripe for the axe.

At John S. Fulton's suggestion, the Tuberculosis Commission sponsored a tuberculosis exposition to be opened in January 1904, which would show graphically the general incidence of tuberculosis, its methods of prevention and cure, its etiology and pathology, its relations to social and economic problems and a history of its study from the time of Hippocrates. Such an exposition for any single disease had never been attempted previously. The attendance, not only from Baltimore but from the counties and from outside the state, was far greater than anticipated. The interest of the public demonstrated that it was both expedient and practicable to permit the general public to have free knowledge of the scientific work in tuberculosis. Osler was the moving spirit in this successful undertaking, and it was he who invited the distinguished speakers.

The exposition was well timed because two unrelated groups interested in tuberculosis had been planning international gatherings to be held in the United States. Dr. S. Adolphus Knopf took advantage of this meeting of leaders in the anti-tuberculosis campaign to interest them in creating a truly national organization. Its formation was completed the following June in New York City. The first annual meeting of the National Association for the Study and Prevention of Tuberculosis was held at Washington on May 18, 1905 under the presidency of Edward L. Trudeau. Osler, as vice president, spoke about the important problem of educating both the profession and the public. Three honorary vice presidents were elected at that meeting—Grover Cleveland, Theodore Roosevelt and William Osler.

Following the 1904 exposition, the Maryland Assembly of 1904 passed laws requiring registration of tuberculosis in Maryland, and providing means and measures to be administered by the State Board of Health for the domestic prophylaxis of consumptives.

THE DONATION BY HENRY PHIPPS FOR THE STUDY OF TUBERCULOSIS

Through the liberality of Mr. Henry Phipps (Fig. 1) of Pittsburgh, the sum of $20,000 was given to the trustees of The Hospital in 1903 to increase the facilities of the outpatient department for the study and treatment of tubercular patients. It was the wish of the donor that one half of this sum "should be used to construct a separate dispensary for tubercular patients so as to render it possible to segregate these from other patients." It was his further wish that "the remaining $10,000 should be so invested that the income may serve to promote special work and investigation."

Mr. Phipps was a partner of Andrew Carnegie and had made his fortune in the manufacture of iron and steel. He had become interested in doing something to combat the ravages of tuberculosis, and in February 1903 had established in Philadelphia the Henry Phipps Institute for the Study, Prevention and

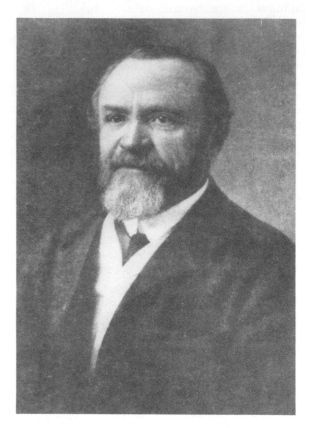

Fig 1.   Henry Phipps

Treatment of Tuberculosis under the direction of Dr. Lawrence F. Flick; a few months later he made his first donation to Johns Hopkins for the same purpose.

Harvey Cushing, in his biography of Osler, suggested that Osler, who had seen one of Mr. Phipps's children professionally, may have spoken to the father about the importance of the Philadelphia enterprise. But there is nothing in the records to show that he did, and there is certainly no evidence that Osler ever made any direct appeal to him for the support of work in tuberculosis in Baltimore. Indeed, the gift came as a great surprise to Osler, who was on his way to Europe when it arrived. Cushing related the informal way in which the donation was made: "In any event Mr. Phipps had come to feel that he would like to do something for Baltimore as well as Philadelphia. Having acquainted Dr. Flick of this intent, one evening early in June when at dinner in Philadelphia with the staff of the Institute, he excused himself, left the table for a moment, and returned with a small sheet of Club stationary partly torn in two on which he had scribbled, 'Pay $10,000 to Dr. Osler. (signed) Henry Phipps.' 'Would you mind taking this to Dr. Osler?' he said, 'and tell him that if he uses it well, I will send him more.' This slip, promptly taken to Baltimore by Dr. Flick, was forwarded to London by Dr. Welch where it was thought to be a hoax, and Brown, Shipley and Company forwarded it in turn to Paris, where its genuineness was recognized."

There was no doubt in Welch's mind about the genuineness of the offer, for he wrote the following letter of acknowledgment to Mr. Phipps on June 8, 1903:

Dear Sir,

Dr. Flick has been here today and has told me of your generous gift of $10,000 through Dr. Osler to aid our work in Baltimore in the investigation and prevention of tuberculosis. I wish to express to you his thanks and the thanks of Dr. Osler's colleagues for this important addition to our resources in promoting this line of research and work . . . The subject is one in which he and others among us are deeply interested. We have started in Baltimore a small hospital for consumptives and we hope to establish by public and private aid a sanitarium for early cases in the Blue Ridge Mountains in this state. A committee has been appointed by the Governor to investigate the local conditions in this state regarding tuberculosis . . . Your gift, therefore, is most timely and encouraging . . .

Very truly and respectfully yours,
William H. Welch

A second installment of $10,000 was sent by Mr. Phipps a few months later, thus making possible the continuation of the special study in tuberculosis which Osler had initiated several years previously.

The trustees of the hospital were greatly pleased and at their December 1903 meeting passed an appropriate resolution expressing their appreciation to Mr. Phipps. He replied as follows:

Dear Mr. Secretary:

The Johns Hopkins Hospital and University have taken so high a place by doing original and good work that they deserve all the gifts a liberal public can shower upon them, and I was only doing my little part when I sent my contributions . . .

Yours sincerely,
Henry Phipps

The new building for the study of patients with tuberculosis, the Phipps Tuberculosis Dispensary (Fig. 2), was completed in February 1905. As originally constructed, it was a two-story brick building, 40 by 36 feet, and was located on Monument Street, east of the original dispensary building with which it was connected by a one-story corridor. In order to provide space for it, the stable, one of the original hospital structures, was torn down. The first floor of the Dispensary had two waiting rooms, two history and examining rooms; the second floor had a large library and classroom, a nurses' room, a sputum room and two rooms for special research. At the opening of the Phipps Dispensary on February 21, brief addresses were given by Mr. Phipps, Dr. Osler, Herman M. Biggs of New York and Henry Barton Jacobs, president of the Laennec Society.

With the completion of this new building, it was possible for the first time to segregate the Dispensary patients found to be suffering from tuberculosis and to study them intensively in the clinic. Through the generosity of Mr. Victor G. Bloede, a well-known manufacturing chemist from Catonsville, Maryland, funds were provided that enabled the hospital to expand the program of home visiting of tuberculous patients by full-time nurses. Dr. Louis Hamman, who had assumed charge of the special work in tuberculosis in June 1904, was placed in charge of the Phipps Tuberculosis Dispensary when it was formally opened.

In 1907 Hamman reported on the first two year's work of the Dispensary. During the first year's operation, 639 patients were registered; during the second, 835. From two physicians and a nurse, the staff grew to ten physicians and three nurses. Of the three nurses, Miss Esther Spicer was supported through the funds supplied by Mr. Bloede; Miss LaMotte was supported by the private contributions secured by Mrs. Osler; and Miss Bond was supported by the Graduate Nurses' Fund. Their heavy task included a permanent visiting list of about 700 patients.

The main function of a tuberculosis dispensary, as Dr. Hamman viewed it, was the prevention of the spread of the disease, a campaign of prevention by education in the broadest sense. Hazen had accumulated figures that showed the importance of the home as a source of infection. It was impossible to follow Koch's suggestion to remove these cases to check the spread of the disease, but something at least could be accomplished by trying to render them relatively harmless. The second important aim of the dispensary was to help the individual patient. This required careful and efficient diagnosis so that the cases could be recognized in the earliest stages and placed at once under proper control. A return to the surroundings under which the disease was contracted inevitably meant relapse. A proper disposition of these early cases became possible during the second year of the clinic's operation through a close affiliation with the Eudowood Sanatorium. At the end of the second year much had been accomplished in terms of proficiency in diagnosis with the aid of the tuberculin test.

In December 1906 a small class of five or six patients was formed whose home conditions were to

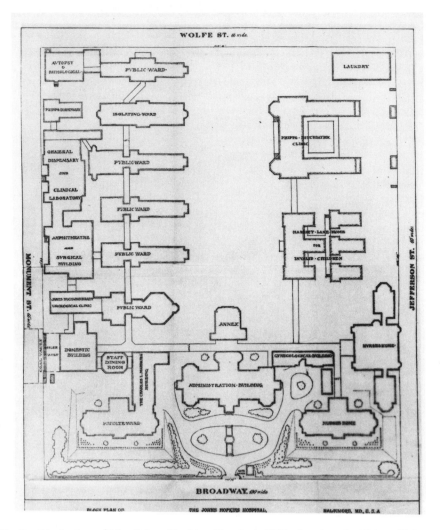

Fig 2. Block plan of The Johns Hopkins Hospital, 1921, showing the Phipps Tuberculosis Dispensary located on Monument Street between the Pathological Building on the corner and the General Dispensary.

be more vigorously controlled and their mode of life more carefully regulated. These patients were instructed in how to keep careful records of their temperature, pulse and symptoms preparatory to giving tuberculin injections. In January 1907 such injections were begun, only "old tuberculin" being used. This class of patients was gradually expanded to over 20 members. At the end of the report Hamman stated that Henry Phipps had "once more given proof of his broadminded generosity in a gift to us of $1250; $1000 to be used for laboratory work and $250 for the library in the purchase of books and journals on and relating to the subject of tuberculosis."

In a second report of the work of the Phipps Dispensary published in the *Johns Hopkins Hospital Bulletin* in 1909, Hamman noted that of the 2,512 patients registered during the first three years only 1,497 were cases of definite pulmonary tuberculosis, 480 were doubtful cases of pulmonary tuberculosis, and 325 were cases other than tuberculosis. He again emphasized the importance of careful and early diagnosis, and the invaluable aid of tuberculin.

In 1906 the Phipps Dispensary was formally selected as the examining station for Eudowood Sanatorium, and the resident physician, Dr. A. M. Forster, attended the dispensary three mornings a week to examine patients. At that time, only early cases were admitted to the Sanatorium; almost all of these cases were patients discovered and diagnosed in the Phipps Dispensary. A little later a similar agreement was entered into between the dispensary and the Jewish Sanatorium in Reisterstown. Dr. Smirnow, its resident physician, came to the Dispensary two days a week to select and examine cases for admission. These and other accommodations offered at the Municipal Hospital partly supplied the need for the case of ill patients but they were still inadequate to meet the demands; thus, the importance of devoting considerable time to the problem of the home treatment of patients unable to find accommodations in institutions.

The Phipps unit grew rapidly and soon was too large to function in its original quarters. How Mr. Phipps came to provide the funds needed to enlarge the clinic's quarters is best told in the following letter, which he wrote to Dr. Welch while en route to Europe in the summer of 1907.

Dear Dr. Welch:

I notice in the report of the Johns Hopkins Hospital, which you kindly sent to me, the following remarks in regard to the Phipps Dispensary: "The Phipps Dispensary is doing admirable work with its limited means, but unless it can secure more funds its work must remain limited, and it will be impossible to do as much as there is real need of." At your convenience please let one of your assistants write me how the fund has been expended and how much of this remains, and any details of the patients, etc. that you think might be interesting to me, with your views on the subject as to what you think should be done . . .

Yours sincerely,
Henry Phipps

P.S. In preparing the statement please have each month put separately, and where money has been paid to individuals for personal services, please tell the character of the service and the time devoted to the dispensary branch . . . It would also be interesting to know too [sic] the number of patients treated, and with what results, if this does not involve too much trouble.

Dr. Welch lost no time in taking action, and on July 5 wrote as follows to Dr. Hamman:

Dear Hamman:

I enclose a letter from Mr. Phipps which Dr. Norton may already have shown you.

I have no doubt that you and Dr. Norton will be glad to prepare such a statement as Mr. Phipps asks for . . .

Particularly important is Mr. Phipps invitation to submit to him a statement of the more urgent needs of the dispensary . . . I have written Mr. Phipps that I should be glad to do this after consultation with you

and others . . . Will you not make out as careful and detailed a statement of the directions in which improvements are especially urgent, with if possible at least approximate estimates of cost, and let me have it.

I must congratulate you upon the way in which you are developing the work of the dispensary . . .

Very sincerely yours,
William H. Welch

In October 1908 Mr. Phipps authorized an addition to the Tuberculosis Dispensary to be constructed at his expense. This addition took the form of a three-story building extending south from the existing two-story structure and cost $13,013 (Fig. 3). It more than doubled the size of the building and provided not only increased facilities for the examination of patients but also additional space for teaching and research. Construction began on November 14, 1908. Until its completion on May 1, 1909, the work of the Phipps Dispensary was carried on in temporary headquarters under Ward H.

Whether or not the fact that the Phipps Dispensary had sent an exhibit to the International Congress for Tuberculosis which was held in Washington, D.C. in September 1908, and had been awarded a prize of $1000 "for the best exhibit of a dispensary or kindred institution for the treatment of the tuberculous poor," had anything to do with influencing Mr. Phipps to make possible the enlargement of the Dispensary is not known.

Also in 1908, Mr. Phipps placed an additional sum of $6,250 at the disposal of the Dispensary. Five thousand dollars was to be used for general extension of the work of the Dispensary; $250 for books for the library; and $1000 to set up a laboratory for experimental research in tuberculosis. William Lorenzo Moss, a graduate of The Johns Hopkins School of Medicine and a former intern at The Hospital, was appointed director of the new laboratory on February 1, 1909. To assist Moss, an appropriation from the "Fund for the Study of Tuberculosis" was made to Dr. Walter W. Boardman of California, who took up his duties as a special research worker on January 17, 1910. Shortly thereafter Dr. George L. Brown was employed similarly. Table I lists the reports which appeared from the Phipps Dispensary between 1909 and 1912.

In the Report of the Superintendent for the year 1911, special reference was made to the work done by a voluntary assistant, Dr. H. Kennon Dunham of Cincinnati, in collaboration with Drs. Moss, Brown and Boardman, in the study of the early diagnosis of tuberculosis by means of x-rays. This work was painstaking in the extreme and continued for several months during the summer and autumn. Ar-

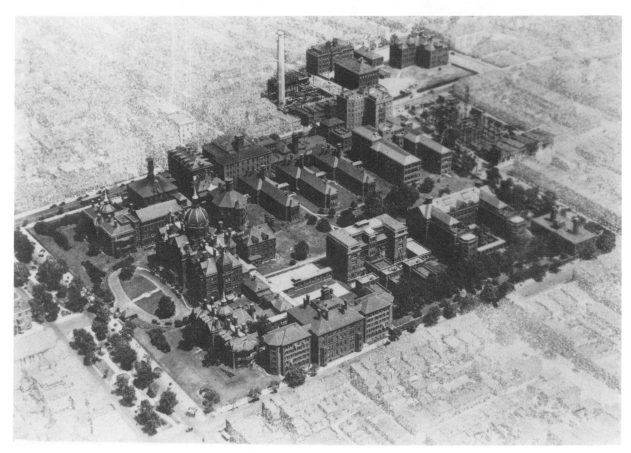

Fig 3. Aerial view of The Johns Hopkins Hospital, 1924, during the construction of the School of Hygiene and Public Health. The arrow indicates the Phipps Tuberculosis Dispensary located between the recently constructed Pathological Building (opened November 1923) on the corner of Monument and Wolfe Streets and the old General Dispensary which was not replaced until 1927.

TABLE I

PUBLICATIONS FROM THE PHIPPS DISPENSARY, 1909–1912

Author	Title	Journal, Date
Austrian, C.R.	The Ophthalmo-reaction in Typhoid Fever	Johns Hopkins Hospital Bulletin, January, 1912
Austrian, C.R.	The Production of Passive Hypersensitiveness to Tuberculin	Journal of Experimental Medicine, v. 15, 1912
Austrian, C.R.	The Effect of Hypersensitiveness to a Tuberculo-protein Upon Subsequent Infection with Bacillus Tuberculosis	Johns Hopkins Hospital Bulletin, v. 24, no. 263, January, 1913
Boardman, W.W.	The Use of Antiformin in the Examination of Sputum for the Tubercle Bacillus	Johns Hopkins Hospital Bulletin, July, 1911
Boardman, W.W. and Dunham, H.K.	The Calcification of the Costal Cartilages, the Cardio-thoracic Index and Other Signs of Pulmonary Tuberculosis	Johns Hopkins Hospital Bulletin, July, 1911
Dunham, H.K., Boardman, W.W. and Wolman, S.	The Stereoscopic X-ray Examination of the Chest with Especial Reference to the Diagnosis of Pulmonary Tuberculosis	Johns Hopkins Hospital Bulletin, July, 1911

TABLE I (*continued*)

PUBLICATIONS FROM THE PHIPPS DISPENSARY, 1909–1912

Author	Title	Journal, Date
Forster, A.M.	The Employment of Arrested Cases	Johns Hopkins Hospital Bulletin, August, 1909
Hamman, L.	The Use of Tuberculin in Treatment	International Clinics, v. 4, 1909
Hamman, L. and Wolman, S.	The Cutaneous and Conjunctival Tuberculin Tests in the Diagnosis of Pulmonary Tuberculosis	Archives of Internal Medicine, May, 1909
Hamman, L. and Wolman, S.	A Further Report of the Work of the Phipps Dispensary for Tuberculosis of the Johns Hopkins Hospital	Johns Hopkins Hospital Bulletin, August, 1909
Hamman, L. and Wolman, S.	Tuberculin Treatment Among Dispensary Patients	Johns Hopkins Hospital Bulletin, August, 1909
Hamman, L.	The Prevention of Tuberculosis	Journal of Outdoor Life, February, 1910
Hamman, L. and Wolman, S.	Cutaneous and Conjunctival Tuberculin Tests in the Diagnosis of Pulmonary Tuberculosis. Second Report	Archives of Internal Medicine, December, 1910
Hamman, L.	A Brief Account of the Development of the Specific Treatment of Tuberculosis	Journal of Outdoor Life, January, 1912
Hamman, L. and Wolman, S.	*Tuberculin in Diagnosis and Treatment*	D. Appleton and Company, New York and London, 1912
Hamman, L. and Sloan, M.F.	Induced Pneumothorax in the Treatment of Pulmonary Tuberculosis	Transactions of the National Association for the Study and Prevention of Tuberculosis, 1912
Knox, J.H.M., Jr., Moss, W.L. and Brown, G.L.	Subcutaneous Reaction of Rabbits to Horse Serum	Journal of Experimental Medicine, v. 12, no. 4, 1910
Moss, W.L.	Tuberculosis: A Plan of Study	Johns Hopkins Hospital Bulletin, March, 1909
Moss, W.L.	Studies on Isoagglutinins and Isohemolysins. Preliminary Report Preliminary Report	Ohio State Medical Journal, June, 1909 Transactions of the Association of American Physicians, 1909
Moss, W.L.	Studies in Isoagglutinins and Isohemolysins	Johns Hopkins Hospital Bulletin, March, 1910
Moss, W.L.	A Cutaneous Anaphylactic Reaction as a Contraindication to the Administration of Antitoxin	Journal of the American Medical Association, August 27, 1910
Moss, W.L.	Studien über Isoagglutinine und Isohamolysine	Sonderabdruck Internationales Zentralorgan für Blut und Serumforschung, Band V, 1910
Moss, W.L.	Paroxysmal Hemoglobinuria; Blood Studies in Three Cases	Johns Hopkins Hospital Bulletin, July, 1911
Moss, W.L. and Barnes, F.M.	Concerning the Much–Holzmann Reaction	Johns Hopkins Hospital Bulletin, July, 1911
Moss, W.L. and Gelien, J.	Serum Treatment of Hemorrhagic Diseases	Johns Hopkins Hospital Bulletin, July, 1911
Moss, W.L. and Brown, G.L.	Variations in the Leucocyte Count in Normal Rabbits, in Rabbits Following the Injection of Normal Horse Serum, and During a Cutaneous Anaphylactic Reaction	Johns Hopkins Hospital Bulletin, July, 1911
Wolman, S.	Marmorek's Serum in the Treatment of Pulmonary Tuberculosis	Johns Hopkins Hospital Bulletin, August, 1909

rangements were made for the continuation of similar studies by Dr. F. H. Baetjer, the associate in actinography in the Hospital, with Dr. Boardman as assistant.

Dunham, with the assistance of Dr. Boardman and Dr. Samuel Wolman, also made an investigation of the value of stereoscopic x-ray examinations in the diagnosis of tuberculosis.

HAMMAN'S INVESTIGATIONS IN THE PHIPPS CLINIC

When Hamman[2] was appointed director of the Phipps Dispensary Clinic, he began a series of investigations on the use of tuberculin in the diagnosis and treatment of tuberculosis. Beginning in 1908 he was aided in these studies by Dr. Samuel Wolman, assistant physician in charge of the clinical work of the dispensary. The work by Hamman and Wolman represents one of the pioneer investigations in the clinical use of tuberculin. Their conclusions are well expressed in the summary of their book: "(1) Tuberculin hypersensitiveness is a measure of resistance to tuberculous disease, (2) Nearly all adults have some tuberculin sensitiveness, (3) In a fresh invasion there is an increase in hypersensitiveness, (4) When an individual recovers and disease manifestations subside, hypersensitiveness subsides, (5) If the disease remains active the high level of hypersensitiveness persists and lasts until the body is overwhelmed and its resistance is broken down completely by the disease, then hypersensitiveness disappears, and (6) In rapidly advancing cases, absence of tuberculin sensitivity is an ominous sign!" These findings show how basic and pioneering their work was.

Samuel Wolman (Fig. 4) was born near Warsaw in Poland on June 17, 1880. He was brought to this country at the age of five. After attending the public schools in Baltimore he entered The Johns Hopkins University in 1899 and received his A.B. in 1902. Four years later he graduated from The Johns Hopkins School of Medicine. Although eligible for an intern appointment at The Johns Hopkins Hospital, he declined because of financial needs. Instead he accepted a part-time paid position in the Department of Medicine as an assistant to Thomas R. Boggs, who was in charge of the clinical laboratory of the hospital. After one year he joined Hamman in the Phipps Tuberculosis Clinic. For many years Wolman was a successful practitioner and teacher of medicine, continuing a fruitful association with the Johns Hopkins and the Sinai Hospital of Baltimore. He was president of the Maryland Tuberculosis Association from 1930 to 1945 and was an outspoken critic of health conditions in the city. He was a member of the Board of Directors of the National Tuberculosis Association from 1937 to 1942.

In addition to this work with Wolman, Hamman finished his report on serous membrane disease begun at Osler's instigation in 1903. This study was

[2] For a more complete discussion of Hamman's career, see Harvey A McG: Compleat Clinician and a Renaissance Pathologist: Louis Hamman and Arnold R. Rich. Johns Hopkins Med J 136: 212, 1975.

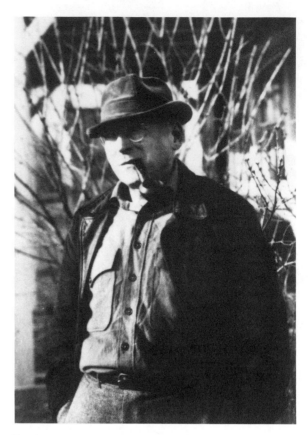

Fig 4.   Samuel Wolman
Courtesy of Dr. Abel Wolman

published in 1908 in the *Johns Hopkins Hospital Bulletin*. In 1909 Hamman and Wolman wrote "A Further Report on the Work in the Phipps Dispensary" which was also published in the *Bulletin*. Dr. Osler, then at Oxford, wrote of this report to Mr. Phipps as follows: "I suppose Dr. Hamman has sent you the number of the Bulletin with the last report ... Such good work." Certainly high praise from the Chief.

In 1913 Hamman and Martin F. Sloan reported their experience with induced pneumothorax in the treatment of pulmonary disease. They concluded that it was a harmless procedure when carefully performed. They found in three out of 20 cases that it was impossible to produce any pulmonary collapse owing to general pleural adhesions. Of 16 cases in which pneumothorax was successfully produced, in only seven was it complete. Of nine cases with induced pneumothorax existing for four months or longer, four developed pleurisy with effusion. They found that pneumothorax has, in most instances, an immediate and striking influence upon the cough and expectoration and that tubercle bacilli may disappear from the sputum. The constitutional symptoms abated more slowly. It was their opinion that induced pneumothorax would never become a routine method for the treatment of pulmonary tuberculosis; in selected cases, however, it offered a prospect of temporary and permanent relief when the usual methods of treatment had been unsuccessfully tried.

CHARLES R. AUSTRIAN AND THE PHIPPS DISPENSARY

In September 1911, William Moss resigned as director of the laboratory of the Phipps Dispensary to accept the position of assistant resident physician in The Johns Hopkins Hospital. He was succeeded on October 1, 1911 by Dr. Charles R. Austrian, who had recently been an assistant resident in the hospital. Dr. Hiram Fried was appointed assistant in the laboratory, and Dr. Edward V. Coolahan, in 1912, accepted a paid position to work in the Dispensary four mornings a week. Fried and Coolahan gave valuable aid in the clinical work, as well as in the laboratory investigations.

Austrian retained his position as chief of the laboratory for two years, after which the Dispensary re-engaged the services of William Moss. In 1914, owing to a rearrangement of the Dispensary budget, the laboratory was no longer a sub-department of the Phipps Dispensary, but became one of the laboratories of the biological division of the medical clinic. In that year, Moss resigned as chief of the laboratory.

During the two years in which Austrian headed the laboratory, he conducted a number of important investigations. He noted that the successful transference of hypersensitiveness to tuberculin from man to animals was the crucial evidence needed to substantiate the theory of von Pirquet, Richet, and others that the tuberculin reaction is a true anaphylactic phenomenon. A large amount of literature had already appeared on the subject, but the results of the experiments reported had been, for the most part, negative. In his studies, Austrian used the blood of a 44-year-old physician suffering from tuberculosis who had an extraordinarily severe reaction following the administration of old tuberculin by the cutaneous test of von Pirquet. He also had a very severe reaction to installation of old tuberculin into the left conjunctival sac. Austrian injected whole blood into a guinea pig in some experiments and varying amounts of serum from the same patient in other experiments. Two to four days later he injected an antigen composed of finely pulverized tubercle bacilli extracted for 70 hours with distilled water into the guinea pigs. The results of this series of experiments showed that guinea pigs could be passively sensitized to extracts of tubercle bacilli by the injection of the blood of a patient with a maximal grade of tuberculin hypersensitiveness. Austrian further demonstrated that whole blood was much more effect as a sensitizing agent than was serum. It seems likely that he was transferring sensitivity by transferring sensitized lymphocytes. Austrian concluded that tuberculin hypersensitiveness in man was a condition of true anaphylaxis and that in cases of tuberculin "idiosyncrasy," at least "sensibilisin" may be present in the circulating blood.

A second paper, "The Effect of Hypersensitiveness to a Tuberculo-protein upon Subsequent Infection with Bacillus Tuberculosis," appeared in the *Johns Hopkins Hospital Bulletin* in 1913. In these studies it was shown that in animals with pre-existing hypersensitiveness to the tuberculo-protein that was used, there was in the majority a diminished resistance to infection with tubercle bacilli of the human type; in a large number of cases no alteration of resistance was noted. From these facts it seemed clear to Austrian that hypersensitiveness to this protein was not protective against the small amounts of tubercle bacilli injected. He was cautious in drawing any far-reaching conclusions from his observations and summarized the results as follows: hypersensitiveness produced in guinea pigs and in rabbits by sensitization with a protein obtained from the bacillus tuberculosis, human type, by water extraction, exerted a baneful or a neutral influence on a subsequent tuberculous infection.

Another paper entitled "Hypersensitiveness to Tuberculo-protein and to Tuberculin" appeared in the *Johns Hopkins Hospital Bulletin* in 1913. Austrian noted that all the manifestations of typical hypersensitiveness to protein could be produced in guinea pigs by treatment with aqueous extracts of tubercle bacilli.

The passive transfer of hypersensitiveness from a tuberculous man to normal guinea pigs was successfully accomplished and positive results were likewise obtained when the serum of a sensitized animal was injected into an untreated one. The type of reaction in an infected host after the administration of minimum doses of tuberculin provided evidence justifying the interpretation of the tuberculin reaction as a manifestation of hypersensitiveness.

With Hiram Fried, Austrian published another paper in 1913 entitled "The Production of Passive Hypersensitiveness to Tuberculin." These experiments were made in order to determine if the blood or serum of tuberculous individuals with an average degree of hypersensitiveness to tuberculin would sensitize normal guinea pigs. Both the blood and serum of the patients were tested by this method and although many combinations of varying quantities of blood or serum with complement and antigen, and variations of the duration and the temperature of incubation were tried, no definite positive results were obtained.

Charles R. Austrian (Fig. 5) was born in Baltimore, Maryland, on May 28, 1885. He graduated from The Johns Hopkins University in 1904 with honors and then entered The Johns Hopkins School of Medicine. Almost immediately he came down with an attack of typhoid fever, which forced him to postpone the first year of work. He graduated first in his class in 1909. In September of that year he became a resident medical house officer in The Johns Hopkins Hospital. Following the completion of his internship, he was appointed assistant resident in the hospital. In 1914 he resigned as a member of the resident staff of the hospital and was appointed associate in medicine in the medical school. The records of the institution indicate that this was a full-time post and one of the first to be filled in a clinical department. The year 1914–15 was the first in which the full-time system in the clinical departments of the school was operative. In 1915 he resigned this post to enter the private practice of medicine.

Austrian retained his connection with the Phipps Tuberculosis Dispensary, however, and in 1915 was placed in charge of the Phipps Clinic, a position he held until 1917 when the Phipps was merged with the General Medical Clinic. He had progressive appointments on the medical faculty, achieving the rank of associate professor. He was also physician-in-chief of the Sinai Hospital in Baltimore from 1921 to 1944.

Austrian's greatness in medicine rested upon his superb skill as a clinician, but he always had an abiding interest in the development of medical knowledge and contributed to that development particularly in the early phase of his career. While still a student, he worked with Walter Jones in the field of nucleic acid chemistry, and formed an enduring friendship with that unique and engaging figure. However, Austrian's chief interest subsequently was in the field of infectious diseases, particularly in tuberculosis. He became an expert in the diagnosis of diseases of the chest due to his unusually acute sense of hearing, his talent in physical diagnosis, and his experience in the use of the x-ray. Much of this skill undoubtedly came from the many hours that he devoted to the examination of patients, first in the Phipps Dispensary and later in the chest clinic of the General Medical Dispensary. Austrian was in the direct line of the great clinicians who have graced The

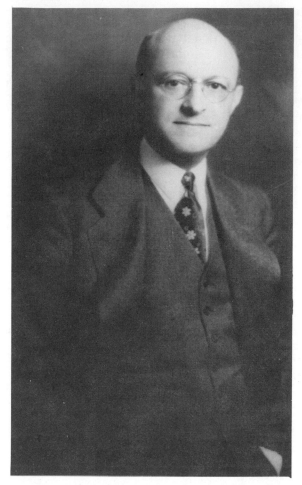

Fig 5.   Charles R. Austrian

Johns Hopkins Hospital's department of medicine, and his name deserves to be linked with the predecessors who set and maintained at the Johns Hopkins the tradition of careful clinical observation in the study and care of patients.

Austrian also took a great interest in the affairs of the local medical profession. He was president of the Baltimore City Medical Society in 1938 and president of the Medical and Chirurgical Faculty of Maryland five years later. He was a member of the Association of American Physicians, the American Clinical and Climatological Association, the Association of American Pathologists and Bacteriologists, and the Cosmopolitan Clinical Club. In World War I he served as a medical advisor to the state director of the Selective Service System and as a member of Medical Advisory Board #7 of the United States Army. He died on July 13, 1956.

ALLEN K. KRAUSE AND THE KENNETH DOWS TUBERCULOSIS RESEARCH LABORATORY

The Kenneth Dows Tuberculosis Research Fund was established at Johns Hopkins by a young man who himself was a victim of tuberculosis. Kenneth Dows (Fig 6) was born at Irvington-on-the-Hudson, on September 7, 1888. In his 18th year he developed symptoms of pulmonary tuberculosis; two years later, in 1909, he went to Arosa, Switzerland, and the next year to Davos. Although he improved and lived in reasonably good health until 1915, he was forced to pay close attention to his health for the rest of his life. In 1915, because of the conditions in Europe brought about by the war, he returned to the United States and settled in Denver, Colorado. He intended to return to Davos at the end of the war, but he developed malignant influenza in the first great wave of 1918–1919, and after less than a week's illness, he died in Denver on April 3, 1919.

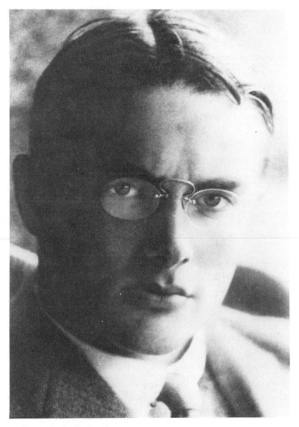

Fig 6. Kenneth Dows
From: Krause AK, Miller WS, and Willis HS: Studies on Tuberculous Infection, privately printed, Baltimore, 1928. Assembled from reprints of papers published in the *American Review of Tuberculosis*, 1919–1926

During his long struggle with tuberculosis, Dows became increasingly curious about the causes of the illness of which he was only one of countless victims. He studied the available literature on tuberculosis, visited most of the world's eminent physicians and found that knowledge concerning tuberculosis was heavy on opinion and weak on facts. Dows wanted to see this situation changed. He wanted to know how tuberculosis was acquired and how it acted within the body. Further, he wanted dissemination of accurate information on tuberculosis among physicians and the public. To these ends, the Kenneth Dows Tuberculosis Research Fund was established in 1916. A special research laboratory was organized with Dr. Allen K. Krause as director.

Allen Krause (Fig 7) was born in Lebanon, Pennsylvania, on February 13, 1881 into a Pennsylvania-German family whose forebears were invited by Willian Penn in 1681 to settle in that region. After graduation from high school at the age of 14, he studied for one year each with a lawyer, an engineer and a physician before entering Brown University in 1898. He graduated with an A.B. degree after three years and obtained his master's degree at age 22.

Krause then entered The Johns Hopkins School of Medicine, receiving his M.D. in 1907. His classmates regarded him as a non-conformist; a brilliant student of strong opinions. He spent a good deal of time with his thoughts and his books and was often absent from class. He could frequently be found at the corner emporium known as Louie's for shop talk over the beverage table. In spite of this, he graduated fifth in a class of 76 and was elected to Alpha Omega Alpha. Krause then joined Welch's department of pathology as an assistant. It was here that he showed the beginnings of his investigative interests.

About a year after his graduation from Johns Hopkins, Krause began to lose weight and strength and developed what he called "intercostal neuralgia." In December 1908, he became a patient in Trudeau Sanatorium, with bilateral tuberculosis. In this new environment, his symptoms vanished dramatically and he was soon up and about working with his books.

On March 30, 1909 he began a seven-year period of work at the Saranac Laboratory with Trudeau and E. R. Baldwin. Both men became his heroes, and he was soon engrossed in devising and executing experiments. It was through this work at Saranac that Krause gained his vast knowledge of tuberculosis and developed ideas and techniques that placed him in the top rank of research workers in this field.

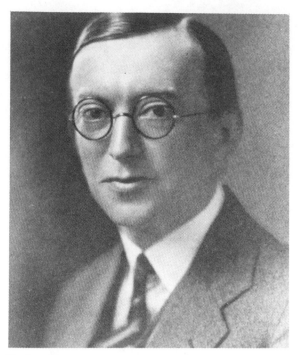

Fig 7.   Allen K. Krause

In 1910 E. R. Baldwin described in detail the manifestations produced in guinea pigs by treatment with aqueous extracts of tubercle bacilli. He demonstrated that a true sensitization could be produced with the watery extracts of this organism, the most striking being obtained when the preliminary injection was given into the peritoneum and when the intoxicating dose was injected by the post-orbital route. He stated that as little as 0.0008 grams of the dry protein was sufficient to sensitize a normal guinea pig; that probably even less was required, since 0.0004 grams sufficed to produce fatal sensitization in 22 days. Baldwin's paper contained valuable data and important new ideas about the nature of the tuberculous process.

Krause, in the following year, talked to the Laennec Society about his own work in this field. Among other things he discussed the routes best suited for sensitization and for intoxication, the optimal incubation period for the development of maximum hypersensitiveness, the preparations best adapted to the work and the quantitative interrelation of these factors. He found that sensitization could be obtained with 0.0005 grams of tuberculoprotein, that the shortest incubation period was six days and that the longest duration of the hypersensitized state was 286 days. He believed it probable, however, that sensitization lasts throughout the life of the organism. It was undoubtedly on the basis of

this visit to Baltimore that Krause was invited to be director of the Kenneth Dows Tuberculosis Research Laboratory in 1916 as well as physician-in-charge of the Phipps Dispensary.

When Krause arrived in Baltimore after seven years in Saranac Lake, he sought to fulfill a dream he had outlined in a letter to a friend:

"Once a man laid open his dream to his friend. As he did so, he engraved his medical credo and ambition in bold lines. His thought was threefold, namely: to push back the frontiers of our ignorance of tuberculosis; to arouse his fellow physicians to the importance of a fuller knowledge of tuberculosis; and to give his fellow lay citizens information of value about this disease.

"These were the points of the dream and plan: to study the why and how of the body's responses to the tubercle bacillus—why lazy first infection and rapid, abortive reinfection—why predominantly in lungs and why different in adults and children—why tubercle formation . . .

"To emphasize that other factors than the bacillus are important in the development of the disease tuberculosis.

"To inspire, guide and direct through students and through publications.

"To emphasize the value of the classics and, by critical translation and re-publication, to give them their proper place in the history and literature of tuberculosis.

"To point out medical achievements of our own countrymen.

"To encourage sanatorium men to keep abreast of medicine by spending time in general hospitals and to send general medical men to sanatoriums.

"To feed the public with the truth.

"To remember always that tuberculosis is only one of many diseases and to develop our interests accordingly."

In 1916, few medical schools in the United States had a tuberculosis service worthy of the name. With the exception of the Phipps Institute of the University of Pennsylvania, none had a well-equipped research laboratory for controlled experimental study correlated with a clinical service or a well-directed course of instruction encompassing the history of the disease, its diagnosis, its etiology and pathology, its behavior and treatment. The combination of the Phipps Dispensary and the Dows Laboratory became, technically at least, the tuberculosis service of the department of medicine with Allen Krause as director. In fact, the clinic was under the able direction of Charles R. Austrian, but the work of the clinic and laboratory was well coordinated and attracted many students. Through this coordinated effort, Krause availed himself of the opportunity to seek clinic manifestations bearing out the principles of his experimental work.

Unfortunately, the laboratory was opened only a short time before the United States entered World War I and did not get off to a good start. Three different physicians took a brief turn at "research." Most of the interested or capable men were either in the service or were swamped with routine work made doubly hard because so many were at war. The two dieners left on the same day for the army. One day while at Louie's, Krause learned of a young German tombstone maker in the neighborhood named Albert Lutz, who needed a new job because, as an alien, his activities and movements had been limited and he was unable to travel from his home to his place of work. Krause arranged an interview with him which ended by Lutz's joining the laboratory and becoming a perfect worker. Throughout much of the war the laboratory had no physician on its staff except Krause, but he performed enough work to justify continuation of the laboratory's support. At that time he had in preparation papers on "What is Tuberculosis?", "America's Work in Tuberculosis," "Studies on Lymphatic Transmission of Tuberculosis," "Chronic Protein Intoxication and Tuberculosis," "The Nature of Resistance to Tuberculosis," and others on the pathology of the disease. For one portion of the school year, Krause had three clinics, one lecture and one conference a week, and managed in addition to write 10,000 to 12,000 words monthly for a series of articles for the *Journal of the Outdoor Life.* He was secretary of the Laennec Society and of the Historical Club and managing editor of the *American Review of Tuberculosis.* Displaying to the full his limitless energy, he accepted in addition several invitations a year to speak at meetings.

Krause was an outstanding teacher. His complete knowledge of the history of tuberculosis added a fascinating aspect to his lectures, which he always delivered without notes. His first lecture was usually attended by the students in the course; his later ones were given to a capacity house. His lectures and writings led to many invitations to address societies and he became a headline attraction at many meetings.

In his laboratory teaching Krause always emphasized two important things: safety to the operator who must often handle living tubercle bacilli; and meticulous technique in the execution of procedures. He would put on his protecting gown and demonstrate step by step the proper maneuvers for the procedure on the day's agenda. This would be followed by a very informal quiz and then he would watch the student and help him until he proved his understanding of the process. An occasional student,

showing that he could perform the work safely and well, was taken in the laboratory family for more intensive study and research. Krause's rare gift in the laboratory was his capacity to formulate experiments, single and in series, to test a certain point, and then to execute them in complete detail. His reports were a tribute to good medical writing and he was also particular about the quality of his accompanying illustrations. Throughout the life of the Dows Laboratory there was always an able artist on the staff. The first of these was Dorothy Peters; the second, Hermann Becker, who had been brought to Baltimore by Max Broedel. The color drawings of these two artists added much value to the papers originating from the laboratory.

In the field of medical writing, Krause was a genius. His magnum opus, "The Anatomical Structure of Tubercle from Histogenesis to Cavity," which was delivered at the Fifth Conference of the International Union Against Tuberculosis, contained more than 15,000 words, but the total time required for writing it was only four and a half days. His bibliography consisted of 187 items. One hundred and sixty-two of these came from his pen during the period between 1909 when he was at his peak at Saranac Lake to 1929 when he left his active laboratory work in Baltimore—an average of eight papers a year, all of very high quality.

Almost simultaneously with the establishment of the Dows Fund and Krause's arrival in Baltimore, the National Tuberculosis Association created an official journal—the *American Review of Tuberculosis.* E. R. Baldwin, Krause's old colleague at Saranac, was the editor-in-chief and Krause accepted the position as managing editor. As such, he was responsible for the content, make-up and editorial policy. He began work at once and the first volume appeared in March 1917. Krause had great talent, of course, as an editor; he was so concerned to have the *Review* free from mistakes that he even verified the references in all the articles published in the first several volumes. At one point, he developed a fluctuating refractive error and photophobia that made it necessary for him to remain in comparative darkness for several weeks. During this period his secretary would sit for hours on end in a room lighted only by a small sub-stage lamp, reading page after page of manuscript and taking notes of the changes Krause wished to make. Throughout the 23 years of Krause's editorship, the quality of the journal remained high.

The Dows Fund was a five-year grant, which was renewed for two successive five-year periods. The last renewal in 1926 made no provision for further extension. When Krause received an offer in 1929 to become president and director of the Desert

Sanatorium and Institute of Research at Tucson, Arizona, he accepted, it being clear that although he could continue as associate professor in Baltimore, there would be curtailment of his laboratory program.

Krause's new position was essentially an executive one, but he continued to edit the *American Review of Tuberculosis* and spent a good deal of time lecturing. All of this occupied him well until his own health began to deteriorate and the inroads of the depression upon the Sanatorium became evident. Eventually he resigned and returned to Baltimore in 1936. He was given space in The Johns Hopkins School of Hygiene and Public Health to continue his editorial work, but within a few months, failing health confined him to bed. He died on May 12, 1941.

In 1931 the National Tuberculosis Association awarded him the Trudeau Medal. The citation clearly sets forth the esteem in which he was held by his colleagues: "As a pathologist of unsurpassed reputation, he has studied tuberculosis in all its forms and relations. As an author and editor of scientific articles and journals and as a lecturer to the laity, he has disseminated knowledge concerning the causes, treatment and prevention of tuberculosis, and in this connection has developed tuberculosis thought as much as any man in the country today. As a physician, he has stimulated the work of various antituberculosis agencies throughout the country, cooperated with other health organizations and promoted international relations in connection with health activities in the study and control of tuberculosis."

When the Carnegie building was erected in 1927, the Phipps Tuberculosis Clinic and the tuberculosis research laboratories were moved into that building, the clinic being designated as Medicine 3. The clinic had already begun to accept patients with all types of respiratory ailments and after a few years also accepted general medical patients. It was the forerunner of the present day chest clinic.

STUDIES FROM THE KENNETH DOWS TUBERCULOSIS LABORATORY

Allen Krause had the idea that the well-planned studies from the Kenneth Dows Tuberculosis Research Fund might be published in serial fashion in the *American Review of Tuberculosis* and then bound separately as a volume of research contributions from the Dows Laboratory. Krause discussed this plan with Mr. Dows. As mentioned, Dows was deeply interested in the etiology of tuberculosis and regarded researches in this direction and the widest possible dissemination of modern knowledge of tuberculosis as the two most important uses for his fund. He eagerly embraced the idea of issuing the

studies in the manner proposed by Krause, provided the studies proved to be productive and conditions seemed to warrant it. This method of publication involved a certain repetition and restatement of essentials that a complete revision and rewriting with all the material in hand would have avoided. However, the continued request for reprints as the articles appeared justified the appropriateness of the project. Only 250 of these handsomely bound volumes of the collected studies were put together.

The first article in this series of studies from the Dows Laboratory was "A Note on Experimental Tracheo-bronchial Node Tuberculosis Together with a Brief Consideration of Several Phases of Tuberculous Infection Suggested Thereby," by Allen Krause. In 1891 Trudeau had isolated a culture of human tubercle bacilli by passing through a rabbit material that had been obtained from the cadaver of a man who had died of miliary tuberculosis. At the time of isolation and for a short period thereafter there was exhibited what might be called standard virulence for guinea pigs; after two or three years of incubator existence, it underwent a very noticeable diminution in its capacity to infect these animals. Virulence did not diminish completely, however. From time to time attempts were made to enhance its virulence by means of successive animal passage, but these efforts were always unsuccessful. Krause worked with this bacillus for many years and never noticed any variation in its virulence. When bacilli were injected into an animal the changes which took place included a more or less general involvement of the lymphatic apparatus, advanced disease in the spleen and usually also in the liver, with surprisingly little tubercle in the lungs. Considering the slight amount of tubercle that was usually found in the lungs, the tracheo-bronchial lymph nodes as a rule showed relatively great changes.

The bacillus that Trudeau isolated, after it subsided in virulence, produced effects that differed in several ways from those caused by ordinary human bacilli. If inoculated only once even in relatively large doses, it never brought about the death of the animal. It never set up gross tubercle in the viscera such as the lungs, liver and spleen except in the few rare instances when pregnancy occurred before or after artificial infection. For the first several weeks all that would appear was enlargement of the lymph nodes draining the area in which the injection had been made. They would then gradually subside with a tendency for the nodes to return to their original size and consistency. Although the visibly infected structures seemed normal with the lapse of time, tubercle was never eradicated from the body during the normal life time of a guinea pig. Whenever the nodes were sectioned, they always revealed classical tubercle. Thus Krause produced in what is generally considered a highly susceptible animal a set of conditions that in many respects was comparable to that obtained in most human beings with tuberculous infection. He could now employ new approaches which would have been impossible in the more common experiments where the infection progressed and rapidly overwhelmed the animal.

Trudeau had already shown that such a self-limited infection did confer a high degree of resistance to artifical reinfection with more virulent microorganisms. Krause also found that in animals that had been infected with this culture, hypersensitiveness ran parallel and fluctuated with the course of visible infection; that as infection established itself and developed, hypersensitiveness increased; that the latter attained a maximum with the most advanced production of lesion and that it diminished with the retrogression of the pathological process.

In further studies Krause was impressed by the fact that nearly all of his animals showed involvement of the tracheo-bronchial nodes. In some instances the process had gone on to caseation with disintegration of tissue in the center of the tuberculous area. Thus he demonstrated that visible tuberculous changes in the tracheo-bronchial nodes can precede those in the lungs and can even exist without the latter. He believed that the same event occurred in human beings. This was in contrast to Ghon's views, expressed in his well-known monograph, that a tracheo-bronchial node lesion in human beings always arose from a pulmonary lesion. Ghon would have been treading on more solid ground had he advanced the thesis that infection, instead of lesion, of the lung preceded that of the tracheo-bronchial nodes. There is a difference between infection and lesion, if by lesion one means gross tubercle or its visible remains. Krause's general results showed a condition in which the visible tuberculosis was confined to the lymphatic system, while the more important viscera, through which the tubercle bacilli must have gone and in which some undoubtedly lodged, were spared.

He then posed the question of what this circumstance meant. He believed that students of the interaction between invading microorganisms and infected hosts had been slow to appreciate that perhaps the anatomical relations in the host determine the issue of infection and its subsequent development. Thus one can see that this laboratory was engaged in a new approach and was contributing greatly to the then meager knowledge of the pathogenesis of tuberculosis.

The next series of papers, by William Snow Miller, fit in well with the earlier studies. In "A Description of Plastic Models (Reconstruction) of a Conglomerate Tubercle and the Surrounding Structures in a Human Lung," Miller presented a clear picture of the normal structure of the lung, which he felt was essential before a study of any pathological process could be undertaken. It was a purely anatomical study and his descriptions and illustrations are classical. The tubercle from the human lung was situated just beneath the pleura but did not extend to that structure. The tubercle did not belong to any single system of air spaces. The deformity of the air spaces was in large measure due to the mechanical pressure exerted by the tubercle, or to the closure, in varying degrees, of the opening by which they communicated with the bronchial tree.

Another paper by Miller gave a vivid description of the lymphatics and the lymph flow in the human lung, showing that in both pleura and lung the flow is toward the hilum. He found that the lymphatics formed a rich plexus in the walls of the bronchial tree and that no lymphatics were seen in the walls of the air spaces beyond the ductuli alveolares. He showed that the deep lymphatics and the superficial (pleural) lymphatics were connected by a short vessel which followed that branch of the pulmonary vein which took origin from the pleura and passed along the interlobular septum. No lymphatics unconnected with lymph nodes were seen leaving the lungs.

In paper number 4, Miller presented his studies on "The Vascular Supply of the Lymphoid Tissue in the Rabbit's Lungs." This study was mounted because in the course of the overall studies of tuberculosis in the experimental animal it became desirable to obtain more exact information of the finer structure of the lungs of several experimental animals. Paper number 5, along the same lines, discussed "The Origin and Relationships of the Bronchial Artery in the Guinea Pig."

Paper number 6, by Krause, was a detailed study of "Tuberculosis in the Guinea Pig after Subcutaneous Infection, with Particular Reference to the Tracheo-bronchial Lymph Nodes." He found that in the tuberculous guinea pig gross lesion of the lung was not indispensable to the appearance of gross lesion in the tracheo-bronchial nodes. It was shown that the amount of involvement of the tracheo-bronchial nodes was directly related to the amount of tubercle that was present anywhere in the body. It was also shown that since under ordinary conditions the spleen is the most extensive depot of tubercle in the guinea pig, the condition of the tracheo-bronchial nodes usually reflected that of the spleen.

In the next paper Krause directed his attention to "Some Factors that Influence the Development of Tubercle in the Lymph Node of the Guinea

Pig." He found that in the guinea pig the existence of tubercle in a lymph node is contingent on the occurrence of lesion at a point peripheral to the node. The progression or retrogression of tubercle in this animal's lymph nodes was largely dependent on the progression or retrogression of the peripheral foci.

At the time the eighth paper appeared, on "Spontaneous Pneumokoniosis in the Guinea Pig" by Henry Stuart Willis, this whole series of studies on tuberculous infection had been in progress almost five years. Willis was a recent graduate of The Johns Hopkins School of Medicine who joined Krause in 1919 on a full-time basis. Together they formed the research team of the Phipps Tuberculosis Clinic. Thus far in the studies, in comparing the lung of the guinea pig to that of the rabbit, it had been found that the normal structure varied in so fundamental a way as to be decisive in determining differences of hematogeneous distribution to this organ in the two species. The data suggested the generalization that the origin and development of tuberculous infection in the guinea pig were particularly influenced by the lymphatic anatomy of several body organs. Krause believed it was important to try to influence and change what might be called the normal or natural localization of infection by altering the lymphatic system of animals by experiment. Willis undertook this investigation using various inorganic dusts as his experimental media. However, before presenting the results of his work, and by way of laying the foundation for it, he exhaustively investigated the pulmonary localization of inert foreign particles in guinea pigs that had naturally and without experimental interference acquired spontaneous anthracosis by reason of long confinement indoors. It was thought that such a study might throw light on some features of experimental anthracosis that had remained obscure because of technical obstacles.

Willis found that spontaneous pneumonoconiosis occurred in guinea pigs that had lived in a cage for a year or longer. The pigment was laid down under the pleura in spots and lines that marked off the secondary lobules. It was also found in the walls of bronchi and blood vessels, in lymph nodes and lymph masses throughout the lung. In the tracheo-bronchial nodes it was present in considerable quantity. Practically all of the dust was intracellular. Lymphatics transported the dust cells, but on section these vessels usually appeared empty.

Willis reported his observations on the influence of the inhalation of coal dust on tuberculous infection in guinea pigs in paper number 9. He found that coal dust accumulated slowly in the lungs of guinea pigs exposed repeatedly to its inhalation. It tended to become localized in the alveoli and alveolar walls, under the pleura at intervals, in the lym-

phoid tissue situated along the air and blood passages and at the hilum, and along the lymphatics in the adventitia of these tubes and vessels. Practically all of the dust became intracellular soon after inhalation. After infection, tubercle developed more abundantly in lungs of animals exposed to dust than in those of normal animals, the ratio being about 3 to 2.

"Early Dissemination of Tubercle Bacilli after Intracutaneous Inoculation of Guinea Pigs of First Infection" was the subject of the tenth paper. Willis showed that tubercle bacilli were disseminated rapidly from a point of inoculation in the skin of normal guinea pigs. Migration of bacilli from the site of inoculation was often accomplished within the first hour after their introduction, and some bacilli had always migrated from the area by three hours after inoculation. Bacilli always spread from a point in the skin of the side to the axillary and inguinal lymph nodes within 24 hours of their inoculation.

In the next study Willis described the "Early Dissemination of Tubercle Bacilli after Intracutaneous Inoculation of Immune Guinea Pigs." In marked contrast to the rapid dissemination of tubercle bacilli from a point of inoculation in the skin of normal guinea pigs, dissemination of bacilli was materially retarded in the skin of guinea pigs made allergic or immune by a previous infection. This finding was further confirmation of the hypothesis that specific immunity of tuberculosis is accomplished in part through a fixation of bacilli of reinfection by the rapid inflammatory response of the allergic reaction.

In the twelfth paper Krause addressed himself to the problem of "The Dissemination of Tubercle Bacilli in the Immune Guinea Pig, with a Discussion of Probable Factors Involved in Tuberculo-immunity." He believed that there were two possible explanations for the retardation and diminution of bacilli in immune animals: (1) they are brought about by specific immuno-lysins that destroy the bacilli, or (2) they result from the prompt interposition of a barrier, which checks, at least temporarily, the further spread of bacilli. He thought the evidence weighed against the mechanism of immuno-lysis of bacilli. It was more probable that upon being reinfected, the tissues of the immune guinea pig reacted promptly with some process that served to impede further passage of bacilli and that this process was the allergic exudative or inflammatory reaction which invariably set in upon reinfection of the tuberculous immune guinea pig that is otherwise normal.

In paper number 13 of the series, Willis described the tracheo-bronchial lymph nodes of the rabbit and their blood supply. He found that these lymph nodes were very small and relatively insignificant in view of the size of the rabbit's lungs. Their blood supply was derived from branches coming from a trunk originating from the subclavian artery on either side.

Krause, in the fourteenth paper, discussed "The Localization of Tuberculous Infection in the Rabbit, with Particular Reference to that in the Lung." After experimental inoculation of every kind, he found that in the rabbit the lungs are normally the organs most affected with tuberculosis. In this respect, the rabbit differs from the guinea pig. Within one hour after intravenous infection, tubercle bacilli were found in intrapulmonary lymphoid tissue. During the first four weeks after intravenous infection, tubercle was most prominent in the intrapulmonary lymphoid tissue, particularly that associated with bronchi. The most important determinant of this peculiarity of localization in the rabbit was the quantity of intrapulmonary lymphoid tissue and its blood supply. The contribution of these two factors insured direct infection of the lymphoid tissue by blood-borne bacilli, and the intrapulmonary fixation of bacilli that are being moved lymphatically through the lung.

In the final paper, Krause gave a detailed summary, analysis and application of the studies of tuberculous infection reported from the laboratory. The two major problems they addressed were: (1) Does the lymphatic system play a decisive part in the focalization of tuberculous infection, especially pulmonary infection. If so, what are its significant elements; and (2) How does tuberculo-immunity arrive at its effects, that is, less and more chronic disease; and through what agencies does it work. After a well-structured critical discussion of the results, Krause points out their possible relationship to the understanding of the pathogenesis of tuberculosis in human beings.

As a supplement to these papers, Krause published two of his studies on immunity to tuberculosis. The first study, with Dorothy Peters, was "A Description of Graphic Records of the Local Allergic and Immune Reactions to Tuberculous Reinfection in Guinea Pigs." The second, with Henry Stuart Willis, described "The Results of Virulent Reinfections in Tuberculin-reacting Areas (Skin) of Tuberculous Guinea Pigs." Krause concluded that if, because of an existing tuberculous infection, an animal (guinea pig) has acquired a given degree of allergy and immunity, both of these are reduced under the following conditions: (1) They are reduced at the site of an inflammatory tuberculin reaction for at least four days after the application of the tuberculin; (2) They are more reduced by inflammatory tuberculin reactions at places that are within the lymphatic drainage area of tuberculous foci than at places that are not so situated; (3) They are reduced to a greater

extent shortly (one to two days) after the application of tuberculin than later (four days after tuberculin). The part played by the inflammation of the allergic reaction, considered purely by itself, remained undisclosed.

Thus the studies that were carried out by Krause, Willis, Miller and their group under the Kenneth Dows Research Fund added greatly to the basic knowledge of how tuberculous infection behaves in the experimental animal.

During the 1920s another talented Johns Hopkins investigator was interested in the study of tuberculosis—Arnold Rice Rich.[3] Rich was interested in bacterial allergy and immunity and the relation between them. The concept of the day regarded the hypersensitive response as a protective one though it might result in tissue necrosis, the exaggerated inflammation being thought necessary to wall off the noxious agent. In tuberculosis the dictum was "the individual is as resistant as the shell of his tubercule." Rich and his co-workers were able to show, however, first in tuberculosis, then in syphilis and in other infections, that though hypersensitivity and immunity might develop simultaneously they were quite independent phenomena. The two could be dissociated in a variety of ways. Hypersensitivity might wane while resistance remained, and cellular barriers were easily penetrated when resistance was low. It was antibodies rather than cell walls that checked the spread of bacteria. It was therefore not necessary to pay the price of tissue necrosis to get resistance, and today much of our therapeutic effort is directed to eliminating the necrotizing effects of bacterial allergy.

These studies on tuberculosis led Rich to a series of studies on the nature of resistance to tuberculosis in general, and, later, to write a monograph and an outstanding textbook on this subject. One of his most significant contributions was the observation that bacterial allergy is a cellular phenomenon. The cells themselves are sensitized and retain this property when grown in tissue culture. This is in sharp contrast to anaphylactic hypersensitivity in which the ability to respond, as is well known, can be transferred with the serum. Rich subsequently went on to study the role of anaphylactic hypersensitivity in disease, particularly in reference to the so-called collagen diseases.

Krause and his associates developed the thesis that the large destructive pulmonary lesions of late tuberculous infection represented an immune re-

[3] For a more complete discussion of Rich's career, see Harvey A McG: Compleat Clinician and a Renaissance Pathologist: Louis Hamman and Arnold R. Rich. Johns Hopkins Med J 136: 212, 1975.

sponse of an allergic nature and that such a response tended to be protective and, in that sense, beneficial to the host. Rich interpreted his own experiments as indicating that, although the late destructive lesions of pulmonary tuberculosis were allergic in character, they did not play a significant role in protection and were detrimental rather than beneficial to the patient. Johns Hopkins was enlivened over these years by the informal debates of these two protagonists.

ACKNOWLEDGMENTS

I am grateful to Dr. Abel Wolman for providing information about his brother, Samuel Wolman. My thanks go to Carol Bocchini for her editorial assistance and to Patricia King for typing the manuscript.

REFERENCES

1. Adamson JD: Osler and tuberculosis. Univ Manitoba Med J 20: 119, 1949

2. Austrian CR: The production of passive hypersensitiveness to tuberculin: A preliminary report. J Exp Med 15: 149, 1912

3. Austrian CR: Hypersensitiveness to tuberculo-protein and to tuberculin. Johns Hopkins Hosp Bull 24: 141, 1913

4. Austrian CR: The effect of hypersensitiveness to a tuberculo-protein upon subsequent infection with bacillus tuberculosis. Johns Hopkins Hosp Bull 24: 11, 1913

5. Austrian CR and Fried H: The production of passive hypersensitiveness to tuberculin. Johns Hopkins Hosp Bull 24: 280, 1913

6. Cushing H: The Life of Sir William Osler. New York: Oxford University Press, 1940

7. Dutcher A: Where the danger lies in tuberculosis. Phila Med J 6: 1030, 1900

8. Hamman L: Notes from a brief report of the first two years work in the Phipps Dispensary for Tuberculosis of the Johns Hopkins Hospital. Johns Hopkins Hosp Bull 18: 293, 1907

9. Hamman L: A further report of the work on the Phipps Dispensary for Tuberculosis of the Johns Hopkins Hospital. Johns Hopkins Hosp Bull 20: 248, 1909

10. Hamman L: Osler and the tuberculosis work of the hospital. Johns Hopkins Hosp Bull 30: 202, 1919

11. Harvey JC: The writings of Louis Hamman. Bull Johns Hopkins Hosp 95: 178, 1954. (Contains the complete bibliography of Louis Hamman.)

12. Holt LE Jr: Presentation of the Kober Medal to Arnold Rice Rich. Trans Assoc Am Physicians 71: 40, 1958

13. Hurd H: Twentieth Report of the Superintendent of the Johns Hopkins Hospital for the year ending January 31, 1909. Baltimore: The Johns Hopkins Press, p. 14, 1909.

14. Hurd H: Twenty-first Report of the Superintendent of the Johns Hopkins Hospital for the year ending January 31, 1910. Baltimore: The Johns Hopkins Press, p. 36, 1910

15. Hurd H: Twenty-second Report of the Superintendent of the Johns Hopkins Hospital for the year ending January 31, 1911. Baltimore: The Johns Hopkins Press, p. 42, 1911

16. Krause AK: The anatomical structure of tubercle from histogenesis to cavity. Am Rev Tuberc 15: 137, 1927

17. Krause AK et al.: Studies on Tuberculous Infection. Baltimore: privately printed, 1928 (Reprinted from the American Review of Tuberculosis, 1919–1926)

18. Landis HRM: The pathological records of the Blockley Hospital. Int Assoc Med Mus Bull 9: 232, 1926

19. Long ER: Allen Kramer Krause, 1881–1941. Trans Assoc Am Physicians 57: 22, 1942

20. McEachran D: The transmissability of tuberculosis from animals to man. Can Med Assoc J 8: 453, 1880

21. Millet CS: The night air of New England and the treatment of consumption. Md Med J 43: 12, 1900

22. Parfitt CD: Osler's influence in the war against tuberculosis. Can Med Assoc J 47: 293, 1942

23. Pratt JH: Osler and tuberculosis. Int Assoc Med Mus Bull 9: 59, 1926

24. Report of the Maryland Association for the Prevention and Relief of Tuberculosis for 1907–8, p. 22

25. Turner TB: Heritage of Excellence. The Johns Hopkins Medical Institutions, 1914–1947. Baltimore: The Johns Hopkins Press, 1974

26. Willis HS: Allen Kramer Krause: A brief biographical story. Am Rev Tuberc 45: 595, 1942

15.

Snake Venom and Medical Research—Some Contributions Related to The Johns Hopkins University School of Medicine

The serpent beguiled me. . .
Genesis

Snake bites must have been among the first illnesses of man, leading to the fear of and veneration for serpents. Serpents and medicine have been symbolically associated since earliest recorded history. The coiled serpent around the headdress of the snake goddess of Crete, of some 4,000 years ago, was derived from the Egyptian Nekhebet, or birth-goddess. The Greek god of medicine, Aesculapius, whom the Greeks identified with the Egyptian Imhotep, was usually depicted with the sacred snake entwined around a rod. In the temples of Aesculapius, sacred serpents would creep over the sleeping patients; they were supposed to whisper the remedy into the patient's ear. The cult of Aesculapius was transplanted to Rome in the shape of a huge serpent. The snake still symbolizes medicine: the emblem of the profession is the staff of Aesculapius.

Watchers of religious snake dances in the American Southwest, and of snake charmers in the Egyptian temples, were filled with wonder at the natives' ability to handle venomous reptiles. Often, the snakes had been defanged or their lips sewn together. In general, however, the Indians and Egyptians immunized themselves by allowing young snakes with a small supply of venom to bite them. Older snakes were used later until full immunity was achieved.

Snake venom has been a tool in medical research since the middle of the 19th century and a number of important discoveries have resulted from these studies. Among the investigators involved, several have had a close relationship with Johns Hopkins.

Reprinted from the *Johns Hopkins Medical Journal* **142**: 47, 1978.

HENRY SEWALL AND THE DISCOVERY OF ANTITOXIN

Nothing was added to our knowledge of immunization between Mithradates, who was said to have become impervious to poisons by drinking the blood of ducks kept on a poison ration, and Jenner, who in 1796 first vaccinated for smallpox.

Between Jenner and Henry Sewall, there were a series of discoveries in microbiology which led to the experimental and comparative study of infection, and the cure and prevention of disease. Koch tracked down the anthrax bacillus, and he and Pasteur independently devised methods of inoculating animals against the disease; Pasteur went on to inoculate human beings against rabies with equal success. It was in 1887 that Henry Sewall performed his pioneer work which demonstrated the principle of antitoxin production by the injection of snake venom into pigeons.

After graduating with honors from Wesleyan College, Henry Sewall joined the staff of the new Johns Hopkins University in 1876. He worked as an assistant to H. Newell Martin, the first professor of biology at the University, who had trained primarily as a physiologist under Michael Foster and Thomas Huxley. In describing his first meeting with Martin, Sewall wrote:

Through the kindly offices of that sweet and gentle character, Dr. James Carey Thomas, a member of the original Board of Trustees of the University, an introduction was secured to Professor Martin, whose sufficient distinction it was to have been an associate of Huxley, that grand Napoleon of biologic science, who had already enthralled the youth of two continents. I called on Professor Martin at his rooms and my spirits were lightened when I saw a very young man—he was then twenty-eight and looked younger—who treated me at once something like a companion. He was scarcely of medium height, of slight but well developed frame. His head was rather small, the eyes blue and wide open, nose thin and fine, complexion fair and mustache blond. His dress was strikingly neat without being foppish. I cannot but fancy that Martin then was homesick and keen to relish the devotion of one not far from his own age. Martin accepted me as his assistant in the biological laboratory at a stipend of $250 for the first six months.

Sewall was to discover months later that there was no university appropriation for an assistant in the biology laboratory. Martin paid the salary out of his own pocket. The two young men developed a strong friendship which lasted until Martin's death in 1896.

If Sewall had gone to a regular medical school at that time, he would have wasted years studying systems and techniques that were on the point of being outdated. By going to Johns Hopkins, he received a basic training in the sciences of physiology and biology, upon which the new medicine would be based. He received that training from one of America's great physiologists who has been labelled by some as the "fountainhead" of physiology in America.

Sewall took his Ph.D. in 1879, but he spent a fourth year under Martin after a period of study abroad in Carl Ludwig's laboratory (Fig 1). Thus, he had ample opportunity to observe Martin at his scientific work, which included a two-year study of the action of the gastric juices. He saw Martin devise a unique technique for studying the isolated dog's heart by perfusing the coronary vessels. He watched him use this discovery to conduct investigations on the effects of various substances and conditions upon this vital organ, thus becoming one of the early experimental pharmacologists. By the time Sewall had left Johns Hopkins, he was fully capable of conducting experiments of his own design and had reported new discoveries which influenced later research. He demonstrated that a stimulus too mild to cause a reaction could nevertheless modify succeeding reactions. He established the source of the pepsin in gastric juice to be the chief or central cells. This investigation was particularly important because it combined histologic and chemical methods in an original way.

In 1881 Sewall was appointed to the professorship of physiology at Michigan, winning out over Charles Minot, another pupil of Ludwig's. During the spring of 1882 Sewall lectured three times a week on his subject without being able to give any laboratory instruction. At the end of the semester he consulted with the dean, Victor Vaughan, regarding a final examination of the students in his course. Vaughan

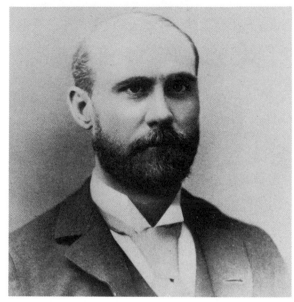

Fig 1. Henry Sewall
Reprinted, with permission, from: Webb GB and Powell D: Henry Sewall: Physiologist and Physician. Baltimore: The Johns Hopkins University Press, 1946

suggested that he make a trial run with three of the best students so that he might judge from their performance what the expectations should be for the rest of the class. After examining these three students, Sewall told them in no uncertain terms that they knew nothing about physiology and he predicted that none of them would ever make a success in medicine or in science. The three students whom he examined were Franklin Paine Mall, who later became professor of anatomy at Johns Hopkins; William J. Mayo, who developed into an internationally known surgeon; and Walter Courtney, later chief surgeon for the Northern Pacific Railroad.

Work on rattlesnake venom in America had begun as early as 1860, when S. Weir Mitchell of Philadelphia published a paper on the subject in the *Smithsonian Contributions to Knowledge*. This work was followed at intervals by other experiments which culminated in the well-known article by Mitchell and Reichert in 1886 on "Researches Upon the Venom of Poisonous Serpents." This paper, which was the starting point for numerous investigations in toxicology and in immunology, directed attention to the presence of so-called toxic albumins. Mitchell's description of his work presents a fascinating glimpse of how research ideas are generated and pursued.[1]

[1] After finishing his medical course in 1850 with a thesis "On the Intestinal Gases," Mitchell took a year of medical study in Europe. In Paris he liked the "lessons of Bernard in physiology" and recalled one remark of the great physiologist. "I said, 'I think so and so must be the case.' 'Why

In 1933 Sewall recalled how he became interested in this line of investigation:

My early training with Martin, a pupil and colleague of Huxley's and Foster's, found its lure in the mechanism of life in general, unhampered by shibboleths.

About 1880 Louis Pasteur was at his peak. I was fascinated with his feats of vaccinating animals by the inoculation of attenuated pathogens. But obviously that procedure had inherent dangers. It seemed to me that if one could get the metabolized excreta of germs, which could not reproduce, an animal inoculated with such products might be protected from the living deadly organism. But there was no bacteriology for me, though I had been closely associated with G. M. Sternberg who worked as a guest in Martin's laboratory.

About that time I read the classic essay of Weir Mitchell and Reichert on Snake Venoms and later found their technique most valuable. Then, as now, fancy found its stimulus in the field of analogy. I thought: Why should not one assume that the malignant microbe found its animal counterpart in the salivary cell of the snake's poison gland? Why should not the snake's poison, properly diluted, be inoculated into an animal in increasing doses with the prospect of protecting it against an otherwise deadly dose?

Well, the idea lay dormant for a long time. Meanwhile the tubercle bacillus had picked me for his game and I felt unequal to the strain of ordinary physiological research—but research there must be!

It was in the fall of 1887; I was going to Asheville for mid-winter to escape the northern blasts. Then it seemed I might start something in the line of the snake idea, which might work itself out while I was away! But where was I to get a live rattlesnake? By good fortune there was a blessed man in charge of zoology on the campus, Professor J. B. Steere, who had had broad field experience in South America, I believe. He promised to catch me rattlesnakes in Tamarack Swamp.

One day he came to my laboratory-shack under part of the seats of the upper lecture room in the Old Medical Building (at the University of Michigan). Steere brought a gunny-sack from which he emptied on the floor a half dozen massasaugas—little rattlesnakes a couple of feet long.

I won't bore you with the course of "nerve" culture I then entered before I could comfortably handle the creatures, but I succeeded by Weir Mitchell's technique in getting the snakes to spit into a capsule where I mixed the poison with glycerine. It was easy to find the lethal dose for pigeons and then to vaccinate. . . .

It is interesting to note that my close friend, V. C. Vaughan, in Ann Arbor and W. H. Welch in Baltimore, alone saw anything in the paper.

Frederick Novy has given a vivid picture of Sewall at work on the snake venom experiments. At

---

think,' he replied, 'when you can experiment? Exhaust experiment and then think.'" Young Mitchell carried home with him from France the idea of experiment. Of this method, he says: "It was my habit to get through work at three or four o'clock; to leave my servant at home with orders to come for me if I was wanted, and then to remain in the laboratory all the evening, sometimes up to one in the morning, a slight meal being brought me from a neighboring inn."

For four years of such leisure as he could snatch from building up a practice, he worked on his "Researches upon the Venom of the Rattlesnake." The "story of the perils and anxieties of this research embarrassed by want of help and by its great cost" is told in a short section of Mitchell's *Autobiography*:

At one time my scientific work was in the direction of comparative physiology among reptilians, and later, again and again, of researches on the poison of serpents; these were the foundation for more modern study of toxic albumins. My interest in these investigations began with the aid of Edward T. Reichert, Professor of Physiology in the University of Pennsylvania when my conception of the duality of venoms tempted me; and to this day I find it hard to keep out of it. . . .

I was lecturing on physiology in the Summer School when the late Dr. William A. Hammond, afterwards Surgeon General, mentioned to me that when in Texas he had used with success an antidote for snake poison known as Bibron's, a famous herpetologist in Paris. It turned out later that Bibron had never heard of the antidote. Just at this time a man offered to sell me a half dozen rattlesnakes. Instantly I became curious as to the truth of Hammond's statement and bought the reptiles. Several experiments convinced me that the antidote was valueless, and, my curiosity broadening in scope, I found that no one knew anything about the poison of serpents since Spallanzani, who had written nearly a hundred years before. Here was an opportunity, energized by the unfailing curiosity with which I have always regarded any problem in any of my lines of interest.

I set about examining the poison, physically and chemically, and for several years I gave up all my leisure to this work. That leisure was small or was won when other men were idling or had left town for their summer holidays. In fact, most of my work was done in summer and with great difficulty, on account of lack of money and time. Now here comes one of the peculiarities which I noted. Ideas about snake poison, how to do this or that, the phenomena it causes in animals, occupied my mind incessantly. I took it to sleep with me and woke to think about it, and found it hard to escape when in church or conversing with people. It is something like being haunted, this grip a fruitful research gets upon you. You come upon a difficulty, try to think a way out of it. This happens continually. You are like a cat at a mouse hole watching for the mouse. All sorts of things present themselves, are tested, accepted, rejected, or set aside, and at last experiments are made following some apparently fruitful idea.

The process is not very unlike that which is present when in fiction or verse you wait, watching the succession of ideas that come when you keep an open mind. And acquiring the habit of the open mind is not always an easy matter, especially if you have occupations outside of your work. In fiction and poetry, the form of expressing a thing has to be considered. In science, this is primarily of little moment, but always I find that I think best when, having come to a a meeting of the American Association for the Advancement of Science held in Denver, on June 25, 1937, he delivered a eulogy on Sewall, saying in part: "I had the real pleasure and satisfaction of assisting Dr. Sewall in connection with his work on venom immunity. It was only a little part of a play, as it were. It was in the spring of '87. One day several rattlesnakes were brought into the laboratory and the trick was to collect the venom to be used for inoculation. I might say that the laboratory of Dr. Sewall's was of the kind that you wouldn't use even for a dog house. The rooms were barely ten feet wide, and the slope of an amphitheatre above them left a six-footer walking space of only seven feet. We had never collected venom from a serpent, but we knew that the method was to take a porcelain crucible, cover, and a pair of forceps, and while one would hold the head of the snake, another would pry a capsule into his mouth, and as the fangs came down there would be deposited a couple of drops of venom. We tried it. I do not remember who had the end of the stick, but I do remember that the snake got loose. I think we broke all records in reflex action. Then, from our perches, we deliberated how to recapture the snake."

Sewall's paper was published in the *Journal of Physiology* in 1887 under the title "Experiments on the Preventive Inoculation of Snake Venom." Mitchell and others had found that pigeons were particularly sensitive to the influence of rattlesnake poison,

and these birds were therefore uniformly used in Sewall's experiments. The first symptom of action of the poison was a weakness in the legs, inducing the pigeon to sit down or to move with a tottering gait when forced to rise. A number of inoculations were made upon various pigeons to determine the minimal fatal dose of the venom, and then Sewall set out to determine whether repeated inoculations with subminimal but continually increasing doses of the venom would produce immunity against the fatal effects of unlimited amounts of the material and whether such immunity might be merely transient or persistent in character. He showed clearly that repeated inoculation of pigeons with sublethal doses of rattlesnake venom produced a continually increasing resistance to the injurious effects of the poison without apparent influence on the general health of the animals.

Sewall, in his production of antitoxin to snake venom in the pigeon, not only established a new fact, but also recognized its implications. In the preface to his paper, he wrote:

The following work was undertaken with the hope that it might form a worthy contribution to the theory of Prophylaxis, and the results obtained during the first stage of its progress are put forward at this time because of the impression that, perhaps, at least their practical significance may induce investigators more fortunately situated for the performance of such experiments to take up the same line

---

critical point, I state a theory which I am going to accept or reject as experiment decides. I must always write it out, sometimes again and again. This is a favorite method with me for fruitful thought. Above all, when engaged in any form of production, my mind is turned on to it as one winds a piece of machinery and waits to see it grind out results. I seem to be dealing with ideas which come from what I call my mind, but as to the mechanism of this process, beyond a certain point it is absolutely mystery. I say, "I will think this over. How does it look? To what does it lead?" Then there comes to me from somewhere criticisms, suggestions, in a word, ideas, about the ultimate origin of which I know nothing.

I may as well say a few words as to the later history of snake poisons. My early work carried me into the war and ceased when I became acting surgeon. I had completed a large quarto, which was published by the Smithsonian Institution in 1860. This enormously advanced the subject of snake venoms. . . .

In 1881 or 1882 my attention was again called to the subject by an extraordinary incident. At the time of which I speak, no one had imagined that the poison of serpents was other than a single poison, varied in different serpents. At dusk one day I was going up the steps of a house where I had once lived, and, being absorbed in thought, I took out my pass-key. Then remembering, I rang the bell. Happening to look down, I noticed the rug on which I stood, which was made of rope, one corner partly raveled and slightly resembling a serpent. Suddenly, there came the idea that the

poison of serpents must be a double and not a single poison. Whether this was the result of some past thoughts that had never risen into the region of consciousness, or was one of those swift decisions brought up by incident, I cannot say. It impressed me greatly. I went to my house, asked to have dinner put off, and for ten or fifteen minutes wrote my reasons why snake poison must be double.

The next day I asked the aid of Professor Reichert. We set about finding serpents, but it was five months before we succeeded in splitting the poison into two or more. This is now ancient history; it was, however, the foundation of all the work since then. With the exception of a brief but very elaborate paper on the effect of venoms on the blood, by Dr. Alonzo B. Stewart and myself, I have done nothing further, except that I wrote out a series of hints for researches which, greatly modified and pecuniarily and otherwise assisted by me, were worked out by Professor Simon Flexner and Dr. Hideyo Noguchi, with the highly satisfactory result now well known to the world of science.

One effect of the rattlesnake investigation was to bring its author a number of letters from men of science. Fayrer, in London, wrote him about them; while in Paris Dumeril expressed interest in "vos longues, savantes et instructives recherches." And there was always the gay, little Autocrat in Boston (Oliver Wendell Holmes), whose wit, during many years of interchange, played happily over the subject. A copy of *Elsie Venner* was sent to Dr. Mitchell with the message: "It's a little bit rattlesnaky as you will find out!"

of observation. I have assumed an analogy between the venom of the poisonous serpent and the ptomaines produced under the influence of bacterial organisms. Both are the outcome of the activity of living protoplasm although chemically widely distinct, the ptomaines belonging to the group of alkaloids, while the active principles of the venom, according to Mitchell and Reichert and to Wolfenden, are of proteid nature.

If immunity from the fatal effects of snake-bite can be secured in an animal by means of repeated inoculation with doses of the poison too small to produce ill effects, we may suspect that the same sort of resistance against germ disease might follow the inoculation of the appropriate ptomaine. . .

Thus, in anti-toxic, as distinguished from anti-microbic, immunity Sewall was the pioneer.

After publishing these results, Sewall was prevented by ill health from doing much further work on immunization. In the twenty years following his snake venom experiments, the scientific journals took but slight notice of them. T. Lauder Brunton seems to have been the only man in the 1890's who publicly recognized the significance of Sewall's work. It was not until 1905 that Sewall had any direct indication that his experiments were considered important by fellow scientists beyond the confines of the Michigan campus. In that year Roger Morris wrote to Sewall from abroad describing a visit to the medical clinic of Ludolf Krehl in Strasbourg: "After chatting for some few moments, he (Krehl) referred to some proof which lay before him on the table. It seems that a series of monographs is being published—by whom I cannot remember, I'm sorry to say—and he is writing the one on animal poisons. Having told him that I was from Ann Arbor, he immediately spoke of your work of which he could not say enough. He said the Germans had a tendency to pay too little attention to the work of foreigners, which everyone realizes, and then said to me, 'How does this sound?' reading from his proof substantially as follows: 'The foundation for all the work which has been done on animal poisons is to be found in the Arbeit of Sewall, done at Ann Arbor, Michigan, in 1887, the great significance of which was not fully realized until some years afterwards.' "

Three years later Sewall was to find in print evidence that his work was finally recognized. In 1908 Albert Calmette wrote in his authoritative volume on venoms: "So long ago as the year 1887 it was shown by Sewall, in an important paper on 'Rattlesnake-Venom' that it is possible to render pigeons gradually more resistant to the action of this venom by injecting them with doses at first very small, and certainly incapable of producing serious effects, and then with stronger and stronger doses. In this way, although these little animals are very sen-

sitive, he succeeded in making them withstand doses ten times greater than the minimal lethal dose." In the same year Calmette made a visit to the University of Michigan which was described by Victor Vaughan as follows: "Twenty or more years after Sewall had been compelled by ill health to give up his work with us, I received a call from a delegation of learned Frenchmen who introduced themselves by saying that *they had journeyed to Ann Arbor to see the place* where Henry Sewall had demonstrated that pigeons could be immunized to the venom of the rattlesnake, because they said that work had pointed out the way to the discovery of diphtheria anti-toxin."

Thus, in Henry Sewall, Johns Hopkins in no small measure repaid at least part of its debt to Michigan for such giants as Abel, Howell, Mall, and Hurd.

CHARLES B. EWING AND COMPLEMENT FIXATION

Interest in the anticomplementary activity of snake venom spans virtually the entire history of the study of complement. Only recently, however, has a reasonable explanation been produced for the otherwise enigmatic, highly specific interaction of a snake venom protein with mammalian serum, an enigma that had been puzzling scientists for some eighty years. The first chapter in this story takes us back to the work of Charles Beverly Ewing, a voluntary assistant in the laboratory of William H. Welch in Baltimore.

Charles Ewing was born in Jefferson City, Missouri, on July 11, 1858. In 1889, he became a major and surgeon in the United States Volunteers. He served in the Philippines, where he was chairman of the Board of Study for Tropical Diseases, and was later head of the Army Pathological Laboratory in Manila. At first his chief interests were in anatomy and surgery, but he later turned his attention to pathology, bacteriology, and microscopy. It was while he was stationed at Fort McHenry in 1893 that he worked as a volunteer in the pathology laboratory of William H. Welch and also took postgraduate courses at Johns Hopkins.

As a result of his experiences in the Philippines and in the Western United States, Ewing was impressed with the great loss of life from poisonous reptiles. Apparently at Professor Welch's suggestion, a series of experiments were conducted in the spring of 1893 to determine the action of rattlesnake venom upon the bactericidal power of the blood. Welch's attention had been directed to this subject by the work of Mitchell and Reichert, which had demonstrated that the poisonous properties of rattlesnake venom depended upon the presence of "proteid substances." From their monograph, as well as from previous observations, it was known that animals killed by rattlesnake venom decomposed with great rapidity, indeed, with such rapidity, that Formad, who had contributed to their monograph an appendix upon the pathological anatomy of animals dead of rattlesnake venom, believed this was evidence of the spontaneous generation of bacteria. Formad thought it impossible for the bacteria to make their way into the circulation and multiply so quickly. Formad's interpretation seemed improbable to Welch and he suggested to Weir Mitchell the importance of having this point investigated. Mitchell kindly gave Welch and Ewing some dried snake venom. However, they were fortunate enough to obtain a live rattlesnake of the diamond species, known as the *Crotalus adamanteus*, from which fresh venom was extracted and used in preference to the dried poison.

Welch and Ewing first addressed themselves to the question of whether the blood of animals killed by rattlesnake poison had lost any of its germicidal power. Injections of venom were given subcutaneously in all cases. A result which served their purpose admirably was that the blood either did not coagulate after death or coagulated only feebly and after a long interval. After death, the heart was exposed, and with sterilized instruments, 7 or 8 cc of blood was collected in a sterilized test tube and refrigerated. After 24 hours, the red blood corpuscles had settled; sometimes a small, soft, dark coagulant had formed and there was a layer of clear serum which was then pipetted off. The organisms used to test the germicidal powers of the serum were the bacillus coli communis and the bacillus anthracis. Using the bacillus coli, they inoculated 250,000 bacteria into normal serum. Immediately afterwards, there were 256 colonies; after 24 hours, only 157 colonies. In other words, there was not only no increase, but an actual diminution in the number of bacteria. After inoculating the serum from the animals who had received the venom, they found countless organisms after 24 hours, demonstrating that the blood of rabbits killed in one-half to three hours after subcutaneous inoculation of rattlesnake venom had lost its germicidal power. In the normal animal it was shown that temperature materially affected the bactericidal power of the blood, which increased with the rise of temperature from 38° to 40°C and then gradually diminished. The loss of the normal germicidal power after venom injection explained the varying rapidity with which postmortem decomposition developed. The blood at the time of death and even before death had lost all or nearly all power of resisting the invasion and multiplication of certain bacteria. The bacterial putrefaction normally present in the intestine developed with astonishing rapidity and, even before the animal was cold, produced this very rapid decomposition.

The results of these studies, which demonstrated that venom from some poisonous snakes destroyed the bactericidal activity of serum (the substance with which venom combined in the serum was complement), were published by Captain Ewing in the *Medical Record* in 1894. Bordet's work on complement for which he received the Nobel Prize (1919) was begun in 1898.

SIMON FLEXNER'S STUDIES WITH VENOM

The next contribution was made by Simon Flexner, another investigator trained in Welch's department of pathology, who, with Hideyo Noguchi, demonstrated in 1902 that snake venoms acted by destroying complement activity *in vitro*. In the introduction to their paper entitled "Snake Venom in relation to Haemolysis, Bacteriolysis and Toxicity," the following statement by S. Weir Mitchell appeared: "I have long desired that the action of venoms upon blood should be further examined. I finally indicated in a series of propositions the direction I wished the inquiry to take. Starting from these, the following very satisfactory study has been made by Professor Flexner and Dr. Noguchi. My own share in it, although so limited, I mention with satisfaction." Flexner and Noguchi wrote that the time seemed ripe for a further study of the physiological effect of venom upon the blood, upon bacterial life, and upon tissues, in the light of recent studies upon various kinds of immunity. They pointed out that convincing experiments by Ehrlich and Morgenroth indicated that (1) a special principle was concerned in agglutination—the so-called agglutinin; and (2) two principles, different in origin, were concerned in lysis. The first of these, which was stable, was the product of immunization. Because of certain combining properties possessed by it, Ehrlich and Morgenroth called it "intermediary body." The other principle, which they proposed to call "complement," was normally present in the body juices but easily destroyed by heat, and tended to disappear spontaneously when the fluids were removed from the body. This latter material had been labelled "alexin" by Bordet.

Flexner and Noguchi concluded from their studies that snake venom contained several intermediary bodies that showed specific affinities for certain complements. They also found that there was a "dissolving principle" for leukocytes which was distinct from that for red blood cells and that dissolution of venomized leukocytes required a complement-containing fluid as did red cells. In a final summary they stated: (1) all venoms when used in suitable quantities destroy the bactericidal properties of many normal blood sera; (2) the manner of this destruction consists in the fixation of the serum-complements by the venoms; (3) venoms have no action upon the intermediary bodies of serum; and (4) if the venom is incapable of uniting with the serum complement, as in *Necturus*, then the original bactericidal properties remain unaffected by the presence of venom.

The career of Simon Flexner, of course, was most important for the development of scientific medicine in America. However, never did a career in science begin more inauspiciously. When he arrived at Johns Hopkins in Baltimore in 1890 for postgraduate work in pathology, he had only a minimal knowledge of physiology and pathology, and his acquaintance with bacteriology was limited to a reading of Tyndall's *Floating-Matter of the Air.* William T. Councilman, who was Welch's principal assistant and who later became the first professor at Harvard Medical School to be appointed from another city, took Flexner under his wing and helped him to obtain necessary fundamental knowledge. Learning by the "apprenticeship method," Flexner soon acquired competence in gross anatomy and in the laboratory techniques of preparing slides and specimens. With this experience, he was able to undertake his first investigation, which was related to the diphtheria bacillus, in 1892.

After Loeffler's discovery of the diphtheria bacillus in 1884, there was considerable reluctance on the part of many to accept this organism as the sole cause of diphtheria in human beings. In some laboratories there was difficulty in cultivating the bacillus, and Loeffler had failed to demonstrate in guinea pigs the characteristic lesions found in human beings. Welch had had a difference of opinion over this matter with T. Mitchell Prudden, the professor of pathology at Columbia, and was eager to demonstrate in his own laboratory the nature of the histological changes produced in animals inoculated with living diphtheria bacilli and diphtheria toxin. Welch assigned the problem to Flexner, who quickly demonstrated in rabbits injected with diphtheria bacilli the characteristic lesions found in man and showed that such lesions could be produced equally well with a soluble toxin. His findings confirmed the etiological relationship of the diphtheria bacillus in the human disease and added much strength to the concept that the essential effects were produced by a soluble toxic agent.

This work is also of interest from another viewpoint. It led Flexner to an examination of the problem of "toxalbumin intoxication," in which he studied the effects of toxic products of various bacteria, as well as the corresponding toxins of castor and paternoster beans—ricin and abrin—in rabbits. Although the results of these investigations were substantive and led to his study with Noguchi on the effects of snake venom, it is noteworthy that during the course of this research, Flexner observed, but overlooked the importance of, the biological phenomenon of anaphylaxis. In 1909, Charles Richet of France recognized the significance of the anaphylactic reaction, an observation for which he received a Nobel Prize.

Flexner's development as a pathologist and bacteriologist proceeded so rapidly that when Councilman was called to Harvard in 1892, Welch appointed Flexner as associate professor of pathology in his place. In 1893 Welch received a request from the Governor of Maryland for help in relation to an epidemic of cerebrospinal meningitis which had developed in the Lonacoming Valley. Welch immediately sent Flexner and Lewellys Barker to investigate (Fig 2). Barker was responsible for the study of the clinical features of the epidemic and Flexner for the pathological aspects. In the course of these studies, Flexner isolated a meningococcus. He knew that Weichselbaum in Germany had isolated a similar organism in such an epidemic several years previously; nevertheless, he mistakenly assigned the diplococcus that he isolated to the class of pneumococci. The error probably came about because Flexner could get no laboratory proof by an *in vitro* cultivation. His laboratory was set up under poor sanitary conditions in a stable and his Petri dishes became so contaminated with hay bacilli that it was almost impossible to accomplish an *in vitro* cultivation of the fastidious meningococcus. However, in discussing this incident, Benison presents the interesting theory that one of the likely reasons for the error was Flexner's deference at the time to authority—the authority of position and the authority that scientific activity itself sometimes inadvertently creates. Benison notes that although Flexner knew of Weichselbaum's isolation of the meningococcus, he was also aware that Baumgarten, one of the leaders of German pathology, had been particularly critical of Weichselbaum's findings. Baumgarten, then in the midst of a debate in German medical journals with Elie Metchnikoff over the role of phagocytes in immunity, enjoyed an excellent public reputation. In the face of his essentially negative laboratory findings, Flexner found it easier to side with the older authority than to try to confirm the work of the younger Weichselbaum. Furthermore, in

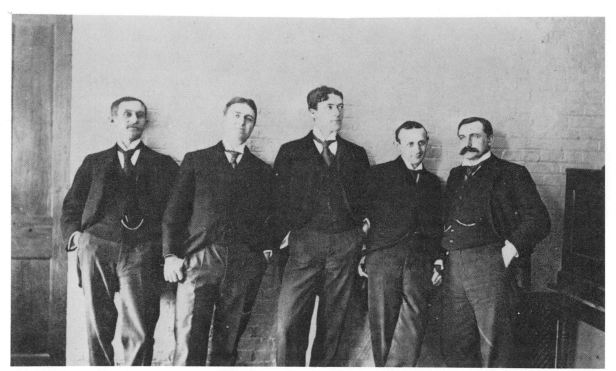

Fig 2.   Some younger members of the staff of The Johns Hopkins Hospital (about 1891–92). Left to right, F.P. Mall, W.S. Thayer, L.F. Barker, Simon Flexner, F.R. Smith.
From the Archives of the Johns Hopkins Medical Institutions.

Benison's view, the balance may have been tipped by work then being done in the department of pathology at Johns Hopkins. During the weeks prior to the epidemic, Welch had lectured extensively on pneumonia. Flexner, as Welch's chief assistant, had been absorbed in preparing slides of pathological specimens for these lectures. Under such circumstances it would be understandable that in an uncritical moment, he might classify the diplococcus he had isolated as belonging to the pneumococci.

In spite of this error, which might happen to any young worker, Flexner's experience in Maryland added to his developing skill as a pathologist. In order to enhance this skill, Welch arranged for Flexner to have a sojourn in Europe with periods of residence with such outstanding pathologists and bacteriologists as Friedrich von Recklinghausen and Karl Weigert.

Later during his Baltimore period, Flexner became less involved in the study of the pathological changes occurring in organs as a result of disease and shifted his interest to the more experimental aspects of pathology, i.e., determining the nature and causes of disease. While performing an autopsy on a case of acute pancreatitis in 1897, Flexner observed the extensive areas of fat necrosis in the abdomen. Suspecting that the lesions might be associated with a fat-splitting ferment secreted by the pancreas, but lacking the chemical know-how to study this, he sought help from John J. Abel, the professor of pharmacology who was a superb chemist. Utilizing the techniques provided by Abel, Flexner succeeded in demonstrating the presence of such a ferment. He later confirmed his observations by producing fat necrosis experimentally in laboratory animals.

In 1898, just eight years after his first arrival in Baltimore, Flexner was appointed professor of pathological anatomy. However, knowing that he had little hope of succeeding Welch, who was then only 50 years of age, Flexner recognized that the time had come for him to move. In 1899, as offers of professorships from the University of Buffalo Medical School, Jefferson Medical College and Cornell Medical School were received, Flexner began to consider the problem of a move seriously. At first he was inclined to accept the offer from Cornell, but when the chair of pathology at the University of Pennsylvania School of Medicine became available, he accepted this position in the belief that it offered him greater opportunity for development. At that time, unlike Cornell, the medical school of Pennsylvania was an integral part of the university and possessed a full preclinical faculty. In spite of early difficulties, Flexner successfully developed the Ayer Laboratories and trained a number of young investigators who came to work with him. Among these were Richard Pearce, Frederick Gay, Henry Bunting, Warfield Longcope, and Hideyo Noguchi. Throughout his period at Pennsylvania, Flexner was engrossed in problems relating to immunology, and experimental work in this area became one of the hallmarks of his department.

An important turning point in Flexner's career came in 1902 when he was invited to join William H. Welch, Theobald Smith, Christian A. Herter, L. Emmett Holt, T. Mitchell Prudden, and Herman M. Biggs in planning the organization of the Rockefeller Institute for Medical Research, of which he later became the first director. It is quite clear that this invitation to Flexner was made on the strong recommendation of William Henry Welch, who had, of course, developed a high regard for the outstanding abilities of his pupil.

Flexner maintained a lifelong friendship with Lewellys Barker with whom he was associated in the investigation of the epidemic of meningitis and who succeeded Osler as Professor of Medicine at Johns Hopkins in 1905. It was to Barker that Flexner turned for advice when the offer to head the Institute came. On February 29, 1902, he wrote to Barker as follows:

> This note comes to you in confidence; the matter being one about which I am greatly undecided and of which I am not speaking outside. But I wish you to know of it and if you have any word of advice or caution to give I shall be only too happy to know it.
>
> It seems that Mr. Rockefeller is now about ready to go forward with the foundation of the Institute in New York that bears his name...
>
> The proposition has been made to me tentatively to assume charge of the first department and become the central head, for a central or nominal head is deemed desirable. This would give me more or less dictation of the first organization of the Institute and of its policies although all will be done under the direction of the Board of Directors.
>
> Of course I am greatly attracted and flattered by the offer. I am, however, beset by many doubts. Am I the man for the place? Have I the originality to keep it going and the physical strength and temperamental qualities to carry it to a successful issue?
>
> The undertaking is so important for the future medical progress of this country and so vast in itself that I cannot but view it with some misgiving. I am thinking about it much and if I should follow my inclinations there is no doubt of my accepting. But is it best that I rather than another make this important start? You know me better than any other person, even perhaps, better than I do myself. You have seen me in many moods and as "naked" as at birth. Tell

me what your advice is—freely and without reserve and "from the heart." Anything you say I will understand.

> Let me hear from you as soon as you can conveniently.

Barker's reply was written on March 5, 1902.

Dear Flexner:

> The only three men who could be considered for the position are Theobald Smith, Herter and yourself and in my opinion you have more of the desirable qualities than either of the other two. You know enough to get the strongest men available around you and to give them a free hand and all the credit. Your love for scientific work is so great that there will be no danger of the prostitution of the fund and the opportunities to unworthy objects; your position in science is such that young and clever minds will be attracted to you, will have confidence in you and will work enthusiastically under you.
>
> My own opinion is that such a research institution ought to be in the medical faculty of a university. It is the fault of university presidents and Boards of Trustees that we are having research institutions endowed independently. It is because university authorities, though they talk of research and ask in a way for money for research, are not really convinced of its paramount necessity; they overestimate the importance of college work and a large number of students and in their hearts are not enough impressed with the value of expensive research institutions to think that wealthy men would give the money they require. The rapid springing up of endowed research institutions should teach a salutory lesson; if it does not the universities will become colleges and the research institutes will become the universities.... In the meantime as a real university position has been offered to you, the finest medical position in America, I should take it and I shall hope to see you develop in New York not only a Pasteur Institute or an Ehrlich Institute for the Study of General Problems but also a research hospital for medicine...

Flexner accepted the position in 1903 and the success of the venture under his leadership is one of the milestones in the evolution of medical science in the United States.

Since the paper by Flexner and Noguchi in 1902, the action of venoms on complement has been clarified. In 1912 Ritz showed that snake venom did not destroy either the first or second components of complement, the only components known at that time, and he, therefore, defined a third component. Some 50 years later, when it had become evident that this "third component" was complex and, in fact, consisted of several different proteins, Klein and Wellensieck demonstrated that venom attacked what is now known as C3. Nelson and Müeller-Eberhard and his colleagues characterized and isolated from snake venom the protein (cobra venom factor or CoF) which induced C3 cleavage and showed that this attack on C3 was not direct but required at least one normal human serum protein. Factor B of the properdin system was shown to be required for the CoF-mediated attack on C3. Initially there was controversy about whether a complex was formed between factor B and CoF. Götze and Müeller-Eberhard obtained evidence that the purified proteins formed an equimolar complex, but neither Alper and Balavitch nor Hunsicker, Ruddy and Austen could demonstrate such a complex. Evidence was later found that a complex of CoF and factor B does form in the presence of factor D. In whole serum only a small fraction of the factor B is involved. There is, thus, no CoF-binding protein distinct from factor B as was previously thought. The identification of a positive feedback loop within the properdin or alternative pathway of complement activation triggered by C3b, led Lachmann and Nicol to draw an analogy between the action of purified CoF and human C3b. Later, Alper and Balavitch presented evidence that cobra venom factor, the anti-complementary protein in *Naja naja* venom, is modified cobra C3 (the third component of complement). Antiserum to the cobra venom factor cross reacts with human C3. A protein in cobra serum reacts strongly with antiserum to the venom factor and the former protein, like human C3, is converted by incubation of cobra serum with endotoxin, hydrazine, or simple storage at 37°C. Incubation of cobra venom factor with cobra serum destroys the C3 cleaving activity of the venom factor in human serum, whereas human C3b inactivator is ineffective. Thus, the cobra venom factor appears to be a form of C3 (perhaps C3b); its potent action in human serum probably derives from its lack of sensitivity to human C3b inactivator. These observations supply what appears to be a reasonable explanation for the enigmatic, highly specific interaction of a snake venom protein with mammalian serum.

KELLY'S FAMOUS STUDENT DEMONSTRATION ON SNAKES

Members of the Johns Hopkins faculty have had an interest in snakes from other points of view. Perhaps one of the most exciting student demonstrations ever given in The Johns Hopkins University School of Medicine was that presented by Howard A. Kelly at a meeting of The Johns Hopkins Hospital Medical Society on November 6, 1889. The objective of the lecture entitled "The Recognition of the Poisonous Serpents of North America" was to impress upon the students the anatomical structure of snakes by which one could decide with certainty whether a given species under examination was or was not poisonous.

Kelly's interest in snakes went back to his boyhood, but his career as a gynecological surgeon had prevented his following this interest for more than 20 years. He stated that it was his pleasure to brush up the forgotten lore in order to put before the students certain facts that he thought all should master before graduation. He presented the students with a complete list of reference works regarding reptiles and then proceeded to describe in detail how snakes are distinguished from other species, including the frog family, lizards, and others. These descriptions were accompanied by live demonstrations, including one of gila monsters.

The demonstrations were unquestionably dramatic, as illustrated by the following quote from Kelly's lecture:

If the snake is living, as in the case of the copperhead which I now show you, he is apt upon touching the fang to throw one or both forward, projecting and erecting them as in striking; further if the edge of a saucer or a watch-glass such as I hold here is placed under the fang, a convulsive movement may be started by which the animal endeavors to thrust his fangs into the object and then rotates the maxillary bone inwards so as to bring them violently toward the gullet with the ejection of a few drops of the clear yellow poison. . . The poison fangs are shed from time to time; I show you one dropped a few days ago in my library by this large banded rattlesnake, which is also just about to shed the opposite fang, which I now remove. . . .

I have here three living rattlesnakes representing two species: the first two are specimens of *Crotalus horridus*, the banded rattlesnake; one of these, so black as to scarcely show any markings, comes from Central Pennsylvania, while the larger snake, 50 inches in length and 7¼ in circumference, is a beautiful specimen from Dr. Goss, in Georgia. . . . In order to emphasize the remarkable contrast between these poisonous vipers and some of the harmless snakes, which I shall produce presently, note that of the entire 50 inches but 4 inches is tail. All the rattles of this larger snake have been lost, so that when he vibrates his tail as now there is no sound whatever unless the end of the tail strikes a hard or dry surface; this disposes of the common notion that the number of rattles is any indication of the age of the animal; note also, as I open the mouth, that the fang of one side has been shed, and the other is just ready to drop into the watch-glass which I hold under it. . . .

I also show you here another beautiful *Crotalus*, received from Oklahoma, 43½ inches long, powerfully built in proportion to his length with six rattles which are vigorously agitated at the slightest provocation.

Kelly then went on to describe and demonstrate a number of harmless snakes which "through ignorance have acquired a bad reputation": "Here, for example, is a full-grown hognosed viper, or spreading, puffing or blowing adder (*Heterodon*) as it is often called, one of our most valuable serpents in the destruction of field-vermin, found over a wide geographical range, and everywhere in ill-repute as deadly poisonous, and yet perfectly harmless and most gentle and easily tamed. When first alarmed this snake flattens himself out until the upper part of his body and head are spread out like a thin skin and bearing a remarkable resemblance to the hood of a cobra. He then draws in wind and forces it out with a loud hissing noise presenting on the whole a most threatening and forbidding aspect. Even if you were to pick him up and he bit you, the bite would not amount literally to more than the pricking of a 'row of pins.' "

In closing the lecture Kelly stated: "I trust that this demonstration with the living forms before you will impress upon you the easily recognized differences between poisonous and non-poisonous forms so that you will feel yourselves not only equipped to decide in case of accident whether the bite of a particular snake is liable to be followed by dangerous symptoms, but that you will constitute yourselves as . . . defenders of the harmless snakes, which are not only of great economical value but aid as well in the destruction of the poisonous forms."

Not many professors today are capable of presenting such an exciting demonstration for the benefit of the medical students.

SNAKE VENOM AND NEUROMUSCULAR FUNCTION

Kelly's demonstration was followed by a talk entitled "On the Chemistry, Toxicology and Therapy of Snake Poisoning" by Thomas R. Brown. As fine a talk as it was, it must have been quite an anticlimax to Kelly's presentation.

Brown pointed out that in India in 1898, 21,901 human beings died from the effect of snake bite. In this enormous mortality, the most destructive snakes were, in the following order, cobra, krait, *Echis*, and daboia. The toxicity of the venom, he said, besides varying according to the species, varied markedly in the same species and variety. Some of the snakes from the Far East mentioned by Brown have since become important in medical research. Their poison, notably from the cobra and the krait, is the source of alpha-bungarotoxin. This material has a specific affinity for the motor end plate in skeletal muscle and has been an invaluable tool in studying the complexities of neuromuscular trans-

mission and in understanding the pathogenesis of myasthenia gravis.

Brown noted in his lecture that in cobra poisoning, there is an especially rapid destruction of the respiratory functions but the pupil of the eye is not affected; in the daboia poisoning, there is wide pupillary dilatation. There is also a greater tendency to convulsions in cobra poisoning. He suggested that the cause of death may be (1) general paralysis, especially paralysis of respiration; (2) tetanic arrest of the cardiac action, probably due to the action of the venom upon the cardiac ganglia; (3) a combination of these causes; or (4) secondary infections of various character, due to the destruction by the venom of the bactericidal power of the serum. He referred to Ewing's studies, which had shown that the normal germicidal power of the serum is entirely lost after poisoning with rattlesnake venom.

He also summarized the studies of Brunton and Fayrer, which revealed that cobra poison, besides paralyzing the reflex action of the cord, acts upon the nerve endings in the muscle as curare does. In their paper of January 22, 1874 presented to the Royal Society of London, Brunton and Fayrer stated:

> But if we find instances in which the muscles still retain their irritability almost unaltered, and respond readily to direct stimulation after they have ceased to contract on irritation of the motor nerve, we are justified in saying that the nerve is paralyzed; and such is the case in Experiment XLI.
>
> In Experiment XXV this action on the ends of motor nerves is all the more evident from the paralysis being most complete in the part where the poison was introduced.
>
> The action of the poison on motor nerves is illustrated by the following experiments performed by Bernard's method of ligaturing one leg of a dog before poisoning it. The poison is thus carried to every part of the body except the ligatured limb . . . the continuance of movement in the ligatured leg, after it had ceased in other parts of the body, indicates that the ends of the motor nerves have been paralyzed; and this is confirmed by the production of tetanus in the ligatured leg and absence of movement in the poisoned leg when the motor nerves are stimulated.

In addition, Brown cited the work of Ragotzi, who confirmed Brunton and Fayrer's findings and concluded that "failure of respiration is mainly brought about by this paralysis of the nerve-endings in muscle, and that the direct action of cobra-poison on the central nervous system is altogether subsidiary."

These important observations lay fallow in the literature for many years before their significance for medical research on neuromuscular diseases was fully appreciated.

THE PATHOGENESIS OF MYASTHENIA GRAVIS

Since the muscles of myasthenia gravis patients are easily fatigable (particularly in the head and neck) but recover strength with rest, work on this disease over many years has focused on the transmission of the nerve impulse at the neuromuscular junction. The work of Harvey, Masland, Lilienthal, Grob, and Johns provided convincing evidence that the abnormality in neuromuscular function was an inadequate response of the motor end plates (now referred to as the acetylcholine receptors) to the transmitter substance acetylcholine, which is released from the nerve endings with each nerve impulse. The presence of thymic hyperplasia and the demonstration of autoantibodies to muscle tissue by Strauss led to speculation that myasthenia gravis is an autoimmune disease in which antibodies result in this motor end plate dysfunction. This theory appeared to offer an explanation for both the muscle weakness and its alleviation by the administration of adrenal steroids and thymectomy as well as by anticholinesterases like neostigmine. It was postulated that the transient myasthenia seen in some infants of mothers with myasthenia gravis was caused by the crossing of the placenta by this antibody. Such an antibody would gradually be degraded in the infant with disappearance of the myasthenia gravis, which does take place within a few weeks.

Over the past few years this theory has been substantiated by the results of experiments that stemmed from two discoveries by scientists working on basic properties of membrane receptors. The first of these discoveries was reported from the National Taiwan University by Chang and Lee, who found that alpha-bungarotoxin was bound specifically by the acetylcholine receptor molecule. This toxin, which is structurally unrelated to acetylcholine and is found in the venom of a Taiwanese snake, has been used in the purification of acetylcholine receptors. Chang and Lee's work clearly recalls that of Brunton and Fayrer, who found in their experiments that in certain mammals cobra poison acts upon the nerve ending in the muscle just as curare does.

The second important discovery was made in 1973 when Lindstrom and Patrick of the Salk Institute found that when pure acetylcholine receptor was injected into rabbits, not only was antibody to acetylcholine receptor formed, but the animals became ill with symptoms much like those of myasthenia gravis. Attempts were then made to find a deficiency of acetylcholine receptor in patients with myasthenia gravis. At Johns Hopkins, Daniel Drachman and his colleagues, working with Fambrough of

the Carnegie Institute, showed that muscle biopsy specimens from four myasthenic patients had less than one-third as many alpha-bungarotoxin binding sites as normal muscle. Their data suggested blockade or loss of acetylcholine receptor but did not tell anything specific about the mechanism.

During 1974 and 1975 several groups demonstrated an antiacetylcholine-receptor antibody in the serum of myasthenic patients. Appel and his co-workers at Duke demonstrated that the globulin fraction from myasthenic sera inhibits binding of alpha-bungarotoxin to purified rat muscle acetylcholine-receptor substance. Engel and his group at the National Institute of Neurological and Communicative Disorders and Stroke used histochemical methods to show that myasthenic sera blocked the binding of alpha-bungarotoxin to the neuromuscular junction of human muscle biopsy tissue. In addition, Aharonov and his colleagues at the Weizmann Institute in Israel described complement fixation during incubation of myasthenic sera with purified human acetylcholine receptor. In 1975 Drachman and his colleagues demonstrated a connection between the defects of the neuromuscular junction and the antibody in myasthenic serum. They treated 15 mice with immunoglobulin from pooled human myasthenic sera. Although only one of the animals had clinical weakness, muscles from all of the treated animals had reduced alpha-bungarotoxin binding and reduced electrical activity, consistent with antibody blockade of acetylcholine receptor activity.

In 1976 work carried out in the laboratory of Albuquerque of the University of Maryland School of Medicine defined the electrophysiological and ultrastructural defects of human myasthenic muscle and the nature of the interaction of myasthenic sera with muscle. They provided the first direct evidence for the postsynaptic hypothesis of myasthenia gravis; namely, that human myasthenic muscles have greatly reduced sensitivity to acetylcholine and to electrical stimulation. In five patients with myasthenia, response of the intercostal muscles to acetylcholine was reduced by 30 to 80 percent relative to controls, and 50 percent of the muscle fibers were unable to generate an action potential when electrically stimulated. Heinemann and his co-workers incubated normal human fetal muscle *in vitro* with the immunoglobulin fraction from human myasthenic sera and found a 50 to 90 percent reduction in the response of the muscle to acetylcholine. Albuquerque and his co-workers, as well as Engel and his colleagues at the Mayo Clinic, have shown that the junctional folds and acetylcholine receptor sites of postsynaptic membranes are reduced in human myasthenic muscle and that the degree of reduction is correlated to a significant degree with the severity of the disease. Engel, working with Lambert at the Mayo Clinic, and Lindstrom and Lennon of the Salk Institute, have demonstrated further that the degree of synaptic membrane destruction correlates quantitatively with the reduction in electrical activity of the muscle, which would be expected if loss of acetylcholine receptor and destruction of membrane occur concomitantly by the same mechanism.

More recently, Drachman and his group, as well as others, have shown that human myasthenic sera increase the rate of degradation of acetylcholine receptor of cultured rat or mouse muscle cells by two- to three-fold. By analogy to other systems, these investigators conclude that binding of antibody to acetylcholine receptor causes internalization and proteolysis of the receptors.

The Mayo Clinic group has published evidence that another destructive mechanism may be involved as well. They prepared specific reagents to visualize immunoglobulin and one complement component, C3, with the electron microscope and reacted these reagents with muscle biopsy tissue from 12 patients with myasthenia. This was the first direct visualization of antibody and C3 attached to the motor end plates. They also found vesicles within the junctional space bearing antibody and C3 on their surfaces. Their conclusion was that antibody and complement damaged the postsynaptic membrane, following which there was release of fragments into the intercellular space.

ACKNOWLEDGMENT

I wish to thank Ms. Carol Bocchini for her editorial assistance.

REFERENCES

1. Abramsky O, Aharonov A, Teitelbaum D and Fuchs S: Myasthenia gravis and acetylcholine receptor. Arch Neurol 32: 684, 1975

2. Albuquerque EX, Rash JE, Mayer RF and Satterfield JR: An electrophysiological and morphological study of the neuromuscular junction in patients with myasthenia gravis. Exp Neurol 51: 536, 1976

3. Alper CA and Balavitch D: Cobra venom factor: Evidence for its being altered cobra C3 (the third component of complement). Science 191: 1275, 1976

4. Appel SH, Almon RR and Levy N: Acetylcholine receptor antibodies in myasthenia gravis. N Engl J Med 293: 760, 1975

5. Bender AN, Ringel SP, Engel WK, Vogel Z and Daniels MP: Immuno-peroxidase localization of alpha-bungarotoxin: A new approach to myasthenia gravis. Ann NY Acad Sci 274: 20, 1976

6. Benison S: Simon Flexner: The evolution of a career in science. In Institute to University. A Seventy-fifth Anniversary Colloquium—June 8, 1976. New York: Rockefeller University Press, 1977, p. 13

7. Brown TR: On the chemistry, toxicology and therapy of snake-poisoning. Bull Johns Hopkins Hosp 105: 221, 1899

8. Brunton TL and Fayrer J: On the nature and physiological action of the poison of Naja tripudians and other Indian venomous snakes. Part I. Proc R Soc (Lond) 21: 358, 1873

9. Brunton TL and Fayrer J: On the nature and physiological action of the poison of Naja tripudians and other Indian venomous snakes. Part II. Proc R Soc (Lond) 22: 68, 1874

10. Burr AR: Weir Mitchell: His Life and Letters. New York: Duffield and Company, 1930, pp. 73–77

11. Chang CC and Lee CY: Electrophysiological study of neuromuscular blocking action of cobra neurotoxin. Br J Pharmacol Chemother 28: 172, 1966

12. Drachman DB, Kao I, Angus CW and Murphy A: Effect of myasthenic immunoglobulin on acetylcholine receptors of cultured muscle. Ann Neurol 1: 504, 1977

13. Engel AG, Lambert EH and Howard FM: Immune complexes (IgG and C3) at the motor end-plate in myasthenia gravis. Mayo Clin Proc 52: 267, 1977

14. Engel AG and Santa T: Histometric analysis of the ultrastructure of the neuromuscular junction in myasthenia gravis and in the myasthenic syndrome. Ann NY Acad Sci 183: 46, 1971

15. Engel AG, Sujihata MT, Lambert EH, et al.: Experimental autoimmune myasthenia gravis. A sequential and quantitative study of the neuromuscular junction ultrastructure and electrophysiologic correlation. J Neuropathol Exp Neurol 35: 563, 1976

16. Ewing CB: The action of rattlesnake venom upon the bactericidal power of the blood serum. Med Record 45: 663, 1894

17. Fambrough DM, Drachman DB and Satyamurti S: Neuromuscular junction in myasthenia gravis: Decreased acetylcholine receptors. Science 182: 293, 1973

18. Flexner S and Noguchi H: Snake venom in relation to haemolysis, bacteriolysis and toxicity. J Exp Med 6: 277, 1902

19. Harvey A McG: Adventures in Medical Research: A Century of Discovery at Johns Hopkins. Baltimore: The Johns Hopkins University Press, 1976, p. 419

20. Kelly HA: The recognition of the poisonous serpents of North America. Bull Johns Hopkins Hosp 105: 221, 1899

21. Library of the American Philosophical Society. Selected letters from the Barker-Flexner and the Cole-Flexner correspondence.

22. Mitchell SW: Researches upon the venom of the rattlesnake, with an investigation of the anatomy and physiology of the organs concerned. In Smithsonian Contributions to Knowledge, Vol. 12. Washington, D.C.: The Smithsonian Institution, 1860

23. Mitchell SW: Experimental contributions to the toxicology of rattlesnake venom. New York Med J 6: 289, 1868

24. Mitchell SW: Observations on poisoning with rattlesnake venom. Am J Med Sci 59: 317, 1870

25. Mitchell SW and Reichert ET: Researches upon the venom of poisonous serpents. In Smithsonian Contributions to Knowledge, Vol. 26. Washington, D.C.: The Smithsonian Institution, 1886

26. Patrick J and Lindstrom J: Autoimmune response to acetylcholine receptor. Science 180: 871, 1973

27. Ragotzi V: Ueber die Wirking des Giftes der Naja tripudians. Arch f path Anat 122: 201, 1890

28. Rash JE, Albuquerque EX, Hudson CS, et al.: Studies on human myasthenia gravis. Electrophysiological and ultrastructural evidence compatible with antibody labeling of the acetylcholine receptor complex. Proc Natl Acad Sci 73: 4584, 1976

29. Sewall H: On the effect of two succeeding stimuli upon muscular contraction. J Physiol 2: 164, 1879–80

30. Sewall H: A note on the processes concerned in the secretion of pepsin-forming glands of the frog. Johns Hopkins University, Studies Biol Lab 2: 131, 1881–82

31. Sewall H: Experiments on the preventive inoculation of snake venom. J Physiol 8: 203, 1887

32. Toyka KV, Drachman DB, Griffith DE, et al.: Myasthenia gravis: Study of humoral immune mechanisms by passive transfer to mice. N Engl J Med 296: 125, 1977

33. Webb GB and Powell D: Henry Sewall, Physiologist and Physician. Baltimore: The Johns Hopkins Press, 1946

16.

The Conquest of Scarlet Fever: Some Johns Hopkins Contributions

So fatal have been the results, so fearful the ravages, so widespread the devastation of the disease, so interesting the period of life at which it commonly occurs, just as parental hopes are budding with promise, and the tendrils of affection entwining themselves most closely round the heart, that the very name is a signal of distress, and its introduction into the family circle is looked upon as the angel of death with an irreprievable warrant to destroy.

Caspar Morris (1851)

INTRODUCTION

A half century has passed since the problems which caused so much confusion in earlier times concerning the nature of scarlet fever were solved. If the earlier students of the disease had been able to solidify two important observations: first, that the rash of scarlet fever is due to a soluble toxin produced in the throat by the causal organisms; and second, that a permanent immunity to the rash is usually conferred by an attack without lessening susceptibility to subsequent infection with other types of the same group of hemolytic streptococci, many of the puzzles which later perplexed a number of competent observers would have been resolved even earlier. Major contributors to the resolution of these problems were graduates of the Johns Hopkins University School of Medicine and members of its faculty: Alphonse R. Dochez, Gladys Henry Dick, Walter P. Bliss and Konrad Birkhaug.

The descriptive terms "scarlet fever" and "scarlatina" were already in common use in the seventeenth and eighteenth centuries. "My little girl, Susan, is fallen sick of the meazles, we fear, or at least, of a scarlett feavour," said Samuel Pepys in his diary under the entry for November 10, 1664. For many years the disease was confused with measles, erysipelas, diphtheria and certain septic processes. Thomas Sydenham, who was among the first to employ the name "scarlet fever," clearly differentiated it from measles by his careful description of the disease as it appeared in London from 1661 to 1675, and thus laid the foundation of an accurate knowledge of its special characteristics. However, in spite of the advance made by the accounts of the disease given by Sydenham, Fothergill and Huxham, confusion still reigned in differentiating scarlet fever from other throat infections, such as diphtheria.

It was Armand Trousseau, the master French clinician, who gave the first account of scarlet fever in the modern sense. He pointed out the great differences in severity of various outbreaks: "Scarlet fever may not appear on the skin; it is not less serious on this account." He gave minutely accurate descriptions of the character and course of the rash and of the sore throat: "From the first day of the disease, the palate is red like the skin, and the tonsils are swollen and violaceous. There appear on the tonsils little white spots. They are different from the false membrane of diphtheria. They are pultaceous and appear to be secretions from the surface of the tonsillar ulcers. As the rash fades, the tonsils get rid of these patches, although they remain reddened and sometimes ulcerated: the disease is cured." Trousseau clearly distinguished the peeling of scarlet fever from the branlike desquamation of measles. In contrast to diphtheria, "scarlatina does not like the larynx." Trousseau also gave an accurate description of the postscarlatinal disorders: "I cannot repeat too emphatically that in scarlet fever one cannot consider the patients cured until a long time after the cessation of all morbid phenomena." He emphasized anasarca: "This accident occurs in convalescents not only if they have been exposed to cold or have committed some imprudence but even when they have remained quiet with the best of care and the most constant solicitude." The associated hematuria and albuminuria were discussed. Trousseau also differentiated the postscarlatinal "rheumatism," pleurisy, pericarditis, and endocarditis from the occasional suppurative lesions. He also came very close to understanding the implications of scarlatina without rash: "I have seen members of the same family who, having had the sore throat without eruption, were then immune to scarlet fever even though the others around them were more or less violently attacked (with scarlet fever)."

As the years passed, there were many excellent clinical and epidemiological studies which ensured the easy recognition of typical attacks of the disease and which furnished the essential data for useful quarantine regulations, but the causative organism of scarlet fever remained unknown. Experimental studies were pub-

Reprinted from the *Johns Hopkins Medical Journal* **147**: 53, 1980.

lished from time to time suggesting that the infective agent belonged to one or another of the principal groups of micro-organisms. Certain observers discovered inclusion bodies in leukocytes and in epidermal cells which they thought indicative of a protozoan cause for the disease. Finally, scientific opinion seized upon those mysterious living bodies commonly designated as filterable viruses as the most probable cause of the disease. This last view became widely accepted and was the usual etiology assigned in textbooks for many years, despite the fact that no real evidence was ever produced to show that such micro-organisms existed either in the pharyngeal secretions, tissues, or blood of an individual suffering from scarlatina.

During the years in which these various etiologies were proposed, with varying emphasis attached to one or another species of parasites from time to time, the constant relationship to this disease of one organism, the *Streptococcus hemolyticus* (present terminology, *S. pyogenes*), became more and more significant. As early as 1885 Crook reported the presence of streptococci in the blood and organs of individuals dying of scarlet fever. Friedrich Loeffler in 1884 found this organism to be present in certain types of "necrotic angina" associated with scarlet fever and was successful in isolating the germ in pure culture. By that time streptococci had also been isolated from patients with erysipelas and puerperal fever. From this time on no competent observer doubted the frequent or constant occurrence of streptococci in scarlet fever. The questions debated were whether these organisms were the primary cause of the disease, secondary invaders or incidental findings of no consequence at all. Obviously, these questions could not be answered convincingly until better methods of isolating and classifying streptococci were developed.

Hallier has been credited with being the first to isolate streptococci from the blood of scarlet fever patients. Examination of his paper, however, reveals that he was dealing with a mold; his drawings are quite conclusive, in that they show hyphae and conidia.

In trying to establish priority, it is always important to examine original reports. Pohl-Pincus has been spoken of in the literature as the first to describe streptococci in scarlet fever. What he did was to examine desquamated skin by direct smears and described cocci which were, in all probability, staphylococci. He produced no evidence identifying them as streptococci.

Bloomfield points out that when Dochez and George and Gladys Dick, some 30 years later, described the local growth of streptococci in the throat with production of a soluble toxin, not enough credit was given to the precise observations of Bergé (1893), whose conclusions were as follows: "1) Scarlet fever is a local infection. 2) The infectious agent which causes it is a streptococcus; in ordinary scarlatina the streptococcus grows in the crypts of the tonsils where it secretes an 'erythemogenic' toxin, the diffusion of which into the organism produces the exanthem and enanthem after the manner of certain known toxins. 3) In puerperal or in wound scarlatina the streptococci grow in the uterus or

in the wound." Bergé gave reasons for supporting these statements and the identity of acute streptococcal tonsillitis and scarlet fever, except for the rash, was pointed out. Bergé's final sentence shows him to have been many years ahead of his time: "As to the immunity conferred by scarlatina, it exists only against the rash because the tonsillitis, on the contrary, recurs frequently after scarlet fever." Had later workers fully appreciated these findings, much unnecessary effort would have been avoided.

Later writers also stated their unequivocal belief that streptococci were the cause of scarlet fever because in the disease these bacteria were constantly present in the throat, patients responded to specific serum therapy, and the rash was reduced by scarlatinal streptococcal vaccine. However, there were a number of authorities, including Jochmann, who disagreed with this view and therefore the subject remained unresolved.

Since serum therapy has played a major role in clarifying the problems of scarlet fever, it is important to mention the studies of Alexandre Marmorek. Marmorek concluded that strains of streptococci from human disease were all of a single type and that the streptococci of erysipelas, for example, were not the specific cause of the disease and could not be sharply differentiated from pyogenic streptococci obtained from an abscess. He thought that the type of disease produced depended on the portal of entry and virulence. All of this is of interest in view of the claims made years later that the streptococci of scarlet fever and of erysipelas were immunologically distinct, which in the end turned out to be incorrect. Marmorek immunized large animals, including horses, with increasing amounts of living virulent streptococci. The serum was used therapeutically in all sorts of streptococcal infections, including scarlatina, with encouraging but not conclusive results. However, the results were in fact much like those described by Blake with Dochez's serum some thirty years later, as we shall see.

Moser, in 1902, found that if the serum was given early in the disease, there was, especially in severe cases, remarkable improvement in well-being, suppression or rapid fading of rash, fall of temperature and pulse rate, and clearing of toxic symptoms. On the basis of his results, he raised the question of whether streptococci were not the real cause of scarlet fever and not just a combination with an unknown agent. In retrospect, Moser's work is essentially as impressive as that of Blake, using Dochez's serum, many years later.

The start of a useful subdivision of streptococci was made by Schottmüller in 1903. Schottmüller had introduced the technique of blood culture in 1897 and soon found that the appearance of colonies on blood-agar plates might be of diagnostic value. He observed that colonies of pathogenic streptococci showed a "characteristic circular light area around them. This light area, which results from the complete absorption of the hemoglobin, has an area of 2–3 mm." He clearly distinguished the green-producing non-hemolytic streptococci which he never found in scarlet fever or in pyogenic processes. This fundamental work on the subdivision of streptococci was elaborated later by J. Howard Brown of the Rockefeller Institute in his monograph on the *Use of Blood Agar for Study of Streptococci*. Brown later came to Baltimore to head the division of bacteriology (at that time, part of the department of pathology and not a separate department).

Further classification was attempted by numerous investigators, using as a basis of differentiation certain biochemical reactions. Holman, in 1916, using carbohydrate fermentation as a test, was able to demonstrate the existence of a number of separate fermentation types. Many efforts were also made to establish biological differences, especially among hemolytic streptococci, by means of serological methods which had proven successful in the study of the various types of pneumococcus and meningococcus. However, conflicting beliefs continued, and a definite opinion was not at hand as to whether or not separate biological types of *S. hemolyticus* existed. As late as 1918, Swift and Kinsella, using the complement fixation reaction as a test, made a series of observations on 28 strains of hemolytic streptococci from varying sources. They were unable to determine significant serological differences among these strains.

THE WORK OF ALPHONSE RAYMOND DOCHEZ AND WALTER P. BLISS

In 1918 Dochez, Avery and Lancefield undertook the biological study of a number of strains of *S. hemolyticus* obtained from a variety of pathologic conditions among the changing population of a large military establishment. The purpose of their investigation was to determine if there existed among the hemolytic streptococci diverse biological types, as is the case with pneumococcus and meningococcus. The specific test reactions which they used were those of agglutination and protection. These studies proved that there are separate biological types among hemolytic streptococci, just as there are among other apparently closely related groups of microorganisms. More than 68% of the strains investigated comprised six easily distinguishable serologic types.

In 1920 Walter Parks Bliss, an instructor in medicine at Johns Hopkins associated with the biological division of the department from 1919 to 1921, published the results of his study of the agglutination reactions of 25 strains of *S. hemolyticus* isolated from the throats of patients suffering from scarlet fever. Of these strains, 20 were agglutinated at equal titers by four separate immune sera prepared by the immunization of rabbits to individual strains of scarlatinal streptococci. With the exception of four strains, none was agglutinated by any of four antistreptococcal sera obtained by immunization of animals to strains of *S. hemolyticus* isolated from diseases other than scarlet fever. These facts suggested that certain hemolytic streptococci found in the throats of scarlet fever patients constituted a single biological group. In a second paper, Bliss found hemolytic streptococci in 100% of the throats of patients with scarlet fever during the first week of the disease. The average

length of time that these organisms were present in the throat varied from 10 to 20 days. Ten immune sera were prepared with different strains of scarlet fever streptococci and each of the sera agglutinated more than 80% of the strains isolated from scarlatinal throats. On the other hand, scarlatinal streptococci were not agglutinated by immune sera prepared from hemolytic streptococci isolated from other pathological sources. Serum from patients convalescent from scarlet fever agglutinated weakly, or not at all, the homologous strains of hemolytic streptococcus. The specificity of the agglutination reaction of scarlatinal streptococci was confirmed by absorption experiments. Scarlatinal antistreptococcic serum afforded some degree of protection against virulent scarlet fever streptococci but had no protective power against hemolytic streptococci from other diseases. In a study of a number of contacts with a case of scarlet fever, in only one instance was a scarlatinal type of hemolytic streptococcus recovered from the throat. It was his conclusion that the streptococci from scarlet fever comprised a specific type. Later work was to show that Bliss's view was incorrect, but it furnished a great stimulus to studies of the etiology of scarlet fever, including the definitive human inoculation experiments of the Dicks, which will be described later. Bliss's observations confirmed the earlier studies of Moser and von Pirquet. Later, Stevens and Dochez emphasized the rapidity with which specific agglutinating qualities were lost upon continued growth of these streptococci in artificial medium, and Eagles suggested that the same change may take place under the influence of the immune bodies formed by the scarlatinal subject during convalescence.

TRANSMISSION OF THE DISEASE TO ANIMALS AND MAN

Krumwiede, Nicoll and Pratt, in 1914, observed an accidental infection of a laboratory worker who sucked into her mouth a mixture of living streptococci containing *S. scarlatinae*. Three days later she developed a sore throat and subsequently experienced a typical attack of scarlet fever. Efforts to infect monkeys with the same streptococcus failed. In 1920, Dochez and Bliss, while studying the biological reactions of *S. scarlatinae*, observed in a dog infected subcutaneously with living organisms, the development of an intense general erythema followed later by desquamation. Attempts to reproduce this phenomenon in dogs resulted in failure. These failures seemed to be due to their inability to induce a local infection because of the low virulence of the organisms for the animals employed. Finally, Dochez and Sherman were successful in producing in guinea pigs and in young swine a series of manifestations comprising some of the principal phenomena of scarlet fever. Successful local infection was achieved by injecting melted agar subcutaneously and infiltrating the mass with a living culture of *S. scarlatinae*. Since by that time it was becoming evident that scarlatina had a certain resemblance to diphtheria, in that there is a local infection in the throat from which the specific toxic substance is distributed, they hoped that a similar absorption of toxic material would take place from the local area of infected agar. This proved to be the case, and guinea pigs and swine treated in this manner developed an erythematous rash, fever, leukocytosis and progressive loss of weight. From 8 to 12 days following infection, the swine had generalized scaly desquamation and the guinea pigs slight general desquamation and complete separation of the skin over the pads of the feet. This phenomenon could not be induced when hemolytic streptococci from sources other than scarlet fever were utilized.

THE CLASSIC STUDIES OF GEORGE AND GLADYS DICK

In 1921 George and Gladys Dick made a series of pharyngeal inoculations in man with certain organisms obtained from the throats of individuals suffering from scarlet fever. Among the organisms utilized for this purpose was *S. scarlatinae*. Though some of the volunteers experienced sore throats as a result of the treatment, no true instances of experimental scarlet fever resulted. In 1923 the Dicks repeated their efforts to produce scarlet fever in human volunteers with a hemolytic streptococcus obtained from the infected finger of a nurse suffering from wound scarlet fever. Five volunteers were inoculated by swabbing the tonsils and pharynx with 4-day-old cultures of the streptococcus in question. Three of these individuals remained without evidence of infection and one suffered from sore throat and fever without a rash. The fifth volunteer, however, who had been inoculated with the streptococcus grown for 3 weeks in artificial medium, experienced a typical but mild attack of scarlet fever beginning 44 hours after inoculation and characterized by sore throat, general malaise, nausea, fever, leukocytosis, a typical rash and albuminuria. Desquamation began on the hands and feet on the tenth day and was complete by the end of the fourth week. Subsequent inoculation of four of these volunteers with living unfiltered cultures of the original streptococcus resulted in the experimental production of another instance of scarlet fever. These observations were confirmed later by the Dicks with the experimental production of another instance of scarlet fever in an individual proven susceptible by the use of their skin test.

The production of experimental scarlet fever in human beings and in animals by inoculation with *S. scarlatinae* made it increasingly likely that this organism was the causative agent of the disease. The evidence in favor of the absorption from the area of local infection of a toxic substance which might be responsible for the clinical picture had again brought into the foreground the analogy with diphtheria.

THE ERYTHEMOGENIC TOXIN

Much evidence in favor of the existence of a soluble circulating poison in scarlet fever had come from the study of the so-called Schultz–Charlton extinction phenomenon. In 1918 these two observers discovered that if one injects into the skin of a scarlet fever patient with a bright red rash 1 ml of serum from a normal person, or from a patient convalescent from scarlet fever, after about 6 hours there is complete blanching of the rash over an area of from one-half inch to a few inches in diameter. On the other hand, serum taken from scarlet fever patients during the acute stage of the illness invariably gave negative results. These and later studies established that the serum of about 60% of normal adults possesses the capacity to blanch the rash in an active case of scarlet fever, that convalescent scarlatinal serum gives a positive rash extinction test in from 80 to 100% of instances, and that the serum during the active stages of scarlet fever never manifests blanching power. This reaction was first used as a diagnostic test of scarlet fever, and this phenomenon was later shown to result from neutralization of erythemogenic toxin by specific antitoxin.

Konrad E. Birkhaug performed a series of studies on scarlet fever and erysipelas while associated with the biological division of the department of medicine and the Sydenham Hospital in Baltimore.[1] He worked under the direction of Dr. Harold L. Amoss, who was at that time head of the biological division. In his first paper, Birkhaug found that serum from normal persons without a history of scarlet fever or general septic infection produced the Schultz–Charlton rash extinction phenomenon in four of six cases tested on the second day of the rash and in one of seven cases tested on the third day. Serum from convalescent scarlet fever patients produced the Schultz–Charlton rash extinction phenomenon in 24 of 27 cases tested during the first 60 hours of the rash, but did not cause blanching 70 hours after appearance of the rash. Dochez's serum produced the Schultz–Charlton rash extinction phenomenon in 40 cases (100%) during the first 60 hours of the rash. It continued to produce blanching 70 hours after the appearance of the rash, but did not blanch 80 hours later. This latter finding indicates that Dochez's serum possessed the same specific property found in normal and in convalescent serum but in considerably greater concentration.

ISOLATION OF THE TOXIN—THE DICK TEST

The observations of the Dicks on soluble toxins in scarlet fever were of fundamental importance in leading to the final understanding of the disease. Simultaneously with their work, Dochez expressed the view that the

[1] Birkhaug attended the Geofysic Institute in Bergen, Norway where he was born on October 12, 1892. He received his A.B. from Jamestown College in 1917 and his M.D. from Johns Hopkins in 1927. He was a Charlton Fellow in 1924–25 and was awarded the M.S. by the University of Rochester in 1927. In 1923–24 he worked at the Sydenham Hospital and was an assistant in medicine at Johns Hopkins in 1924–25. He then went to Rochester, N.Y. when the medical school was organized there, holding the rank of assistant professor (1926–1928) and of associate (1928–1932). He was a member of the Pasteur Institute of Paris (1932–1935) and received the Civic Award from the City of Rochester, N.Y. for his work on erysipelas.

"principal localization of the infection is in the throat in most instances and that there the streptococcus in question elaborates a toxin which is absorbed and produces the rash and general symptoms." Dochez's paper appeared three weeks after that of the Dicks and he deserves equal credit for establishing the streptococcus as the cause of scarlet fever. It was the Dicks, however, who first prepared a usable toxin from filtrates of cultures of streptococci obtained from scarlet fever patients. They showed that an intracutaneous injection of this filtrate practically never produced a skin reaction in people convalescent from scarlet fever or who had a history of a previous attack, whereas 41.6% of persons who had no history of scarlet fever showed a red area up to 5 cm in diameter in 24 to 36 hours. These positive tests could be inhibited by convalescent scarlet fever serum and positive skin tests were reversed after an attack of scarlet fever—the basis of the Dick test. They then raised the question of whether all the symptoms of scarlet fever could be due to this toxin. They injected toxin into healthy people who had never had scarlet fever and produced severe local reactions, fever, nausea, and in some cases, a rash, and found that the previously positive skin test had been reversed. They thought they had produced an active immunization but did not realize at the time that the immunity was primarily to the skin toxin and did not prevent scarlet fever without rash, i.e., streptococcal pharyngitis.

PREPARATION OF AN ANTITOXIN AND ITS CLINICAL USE

The next paper of the Dicks dealt with the production of an antitoxic serum by immunizing a horse, not with streptococci, but with the toxic filtrate of streptococcal cultures. More detailed reports on preventive immunization by injections of toxin were reported in a further paper, and soon a study from their laboratory appeared describing the use of their horse serum in clinical cases. They concluded that the antitoxin blanches the rash, lowers temperature and improves the general condition of many scarlet fever patients. If given early, the course of the disease was shortened and the incidence of complications and sequelae was greatly reduced. It was ultimately shown that the antitoxin acted on the rash and perhaps certain toxic symptoms, but did not have the antibacterial action necessary to eliminate the streptococcal infection and therefore did not furnish a complete cure of the disease. All of the work described above was amplified in two further papers by the Dicks. The important point in these papers was that not all strains of scarlet fever streptococci were equally good toxin producers. The Dicks also failed to substantiate the immunological identity of scarlet fever streptococci as observed by Dochez and his associates. Sheep immunized with two strains of streptococci which had produced experimental scarlet fever yielded sera which agglutinated the homologous organism in high concentration but gave no cross-agglutination reaction. This position was later confirmed.

The fundamental importance of all this work is not to be underestimated. It clearly brought into focus the question of what part of the disease was due to the soluble toxin and what part was the result of the local streptococcal infection in the throat.

The antiserum which Dochez produced by instilling scarlatinal streptococci into a mass of agar previously injected subcutaneously into a horse possessed the capacity to blanch the rash locally in scarlet fever, and when used therapeutically, caused a marked abatement of all the symptoms. Blake and his associates reported good clinical results with Dochez's antiscarlatinal horse serum. They laid stress on its value in diagnosis and described its capacity locally to blanch the rash in scarlet fever patients. Also, "the serum would appear to possess very marked curative properties." In some toxemic cases there was complete recovery within 24 to 36 hours.

Konrad Birkhaug also reported favorable results with Dochez's serum. In 37 cases of scarlet fever treated by intramuscular injections of serum from convalescent cases, it was demonstrated that a rapid improvement in the general symptoms and a slight fall in temperature and pulse rate occurred, but there was no effect upon the general rash and no shortening of convalescence or reduction in the incidence of septic complications during convalescence. A comparative study of 31 cases of scarlet fever showed that the intramuscular injection of Dochez's scarlatinal antistreptococcic serum in amounts of 40 cc administered during the first three days of the disease caused a prompt disappearance of the toxemia, a critical fall in temperature and pulse rate, prompt fading of the general exanthem, rapid reduction in leukocytosis, and rapid disappearance of the glandular enlargement. The Schultz–Charlton rash extinction phenomenon could be obtained with samples of serum withdrawn from patients treated with Dochez's serum shortly after its injection. A therapeutic dose of 40 cc of Dochez's serum brought about a clinical cure in moderately severe cases of scarlet fever, and the incidence of septic complications was low in the cases treated prior to the fourth day of the disease.

SCARLET FEVER SINE EXANTHEMATE

There were already many clinical observations of contacts with scarlet fever patients who developed sore throat without rash. It remained for Stevens and Dochez to isolate strains of streptococci from the throats of such patients and to prove by agglutination and absorption tests that they were identical in subjects with and without rash. They also showed that in the type of infection without rash the Dick test was negative, although the strain could be demonstrated to produce toxin, which, in turn, was neutralized by antitoxin. Throat infections without rash were found to occur in people who had previously had scarlet fever, although the organism was a S. scarlatinae and produced toxin. Stevens and Dochez concluded that scarlatinal antitoxin was an efficient therapeutic agent in scarlatinal throat infections without rash, a position which was not borne out by later observations.

The important question as to whether the soluble toxin of scarlatinal streptococci produced any clinical effects besides the rash was answered by Arthur L. Bloomfield and Lowell A. Rantz. They studied an outbreak of infection in young men in an army camp, presumably resulting from contaminated milk or food. Several hundred men were taken sick almost simultaneously with an acute streptococcic sore throat. It was shown that one strain—Type 15—was responsible. Approximately 25% of the patients had a typical scarlatinal rash; in most cases, no rash was seen. As far as they could tell, by clinical observation, there was no overall difference in the severity, course or complications in the two groups. It was their conclusion, in this outbreak at least, that the effect of the toxin was confined to production of the rash. It was hard to escape the conviction, however, that the hyperacute variety of scarlet fever with death from "toxemia" in the first few days must be due to other or more potent soluble toxins. This view was supported by the undoubted beneficial effects of antitoxic sera observed in such cases in the past. Arthur Bloomfield, a Johns Hopkins graduate, had his residency training in medicine in Baltimore and until 1926 was on the faculty, achieving the rank of associate professor. In 1926 he became chairman of the department of medicine at the Leland Stanford School of Medicine.

Thus, while the Dicks deserve credit for the final proof that the streptococcus is the cause of scarlet fever, it is generally accepted that the logical, progressive and systematic approach to the problem by Dochez and his associates was equally important.

Dochez, in closing his Harvey Lecture of 1925 on the etiology of scarlet fever, said:

> Have we now reached the end of man's long struggle to find the cause of this interesting, and at times, formidable and dangerous disease? Personally, I think we have. Belief that scarlet fever may be caused by a protozoan parasite, or by one of the mysterious ultramicroscopic viruses, must, I think, be discarded in view of the fact that the evidence brought forward in support of the causative relationship of such types of microorganisms to the disease is entirely unconvincing. On the other hand, can we say with certainty that scarlet fever is caused by a type of *Streptococcus hemolyticus*? Certainly a chain of evidence in favor of this organism has been patiently and progressively forged which is as strong as that in many diseases whose etiology is now accepted without discussion. The constant association of this organism with the primary and secondary manifestations of the disease, its specific character, its capacity to produce the experimental disease in man and in animals, the ability of human convalescent scarlet fever serum to neutralize the toxic effects of this streptococcus, the capacity of an antistreptococcus horse serum antitoxic in nature to counteract the specific toxic manifestations of the disease in man, and finally the isolation from Berkefeld filtrates of this streptococcus of a toxic substance which bears a specific relationship to immunity in scarlet fever, leaves little room to doubt that *Streptococcus scarlatinae* is the principal and probably only etiological agent of scarlet fever.
>
>   Let us therefore be optimistic and assume that a just reward has come to those many soldiers in the army

of science, too numerous to be mentioned in so short an exposition, and that another disease has been added to those about which the essential specific facts are known.

GLADYS HENRY DICK

Gladys Henry was born in Pawnee City, Nebraska in December 1881. She graduated from the University of Nebraska at the age of 18 and after an interval of graduate work, followed by teaching in high school, she entered the Johns Hopkins University School of Medicine, receiving her M.D. in 1907 (Fig 1). From September 1907 to September 1908 she was a medical house officer and the following year an assistant resident in medicine at Johns Hopkins. After a period of time in Europe, she went to the University of Chicago in 1911 and joined the staff of the McCormick Institute for Infectious Diseases. It was at the McCormick Institute in 1914 that she met and married George Frederick Dick. They began their collaborative research on the cause and treatment of scarlet fever, which culminated in the series of studies which have been described and which led to their receiving the Cameron Prize from the University of Edinburgh and the Mickel Prize from the University of Toronto.

George Frederick Dick was born at Fort Wayne, Indiana on July 21, 1881. He received his medical training at Rush Medical College, interned at Cook County Hospital and then did postgraduate work in Vienna and Munich before joining the staff of the McCormick Institute.

He served as a Major in France during World War I and later was head of the department of medicine at Rush. In 1933 he accepted the same post at the University of Chicago, serving until 1946.

STREPTOCOCCI IN ERYSIPELAS VERSUS SCARLET FEVER

In further studies on the biology of the *S. erysipelatis*,[2] Birkhaug showed that intracutaneous injection of agar inoculated with live *S. hemolyticus* for the production of immune bodies was found to produce an immune serum of a higher agglutination titer than that obtained by the intravenous or subcutaneous inoculation of dead or live hemolytic streptococci. Of 34 strains of erysipelatous hemolytic streptococci, 7 were employed for the production of 7 immune erysipelatous sera.

---

[2] Suitable techniques for the classification of beta hemolytic streptococci were not available prior to the use of extracts of these organisms in precipitin tests, a method introduced by Lancefield (J Exp Med 57: 571, 1933). Most bacteria isolated from humans with infections such as pharyngitis, scarlet fever and erysipelas and classified formerly as "*Streptococcus hemolyticus*," "*Streptococcus scarlatinae*" or "*Streptococcus erysipelatis*" would now be designated *Streptococcus pyogenes*, Lancefield's group A beta hemolytic streptococcus. The significance of studies, such as those of Birkhaug, seeking to distinguish streptococci causing different clinical syndromes by agglutination is doubtful in the light of more modern bacteriologic investigations.

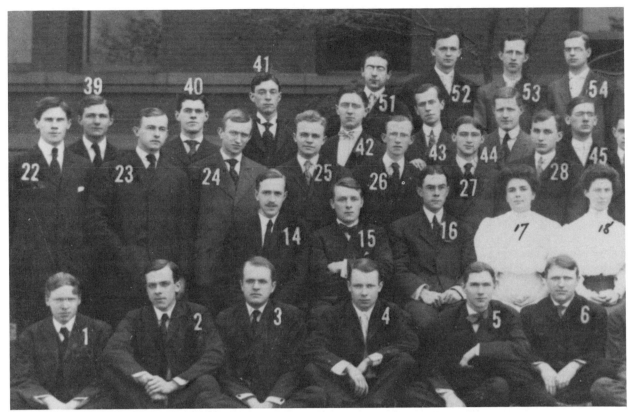

Fig 1.   Enlargement of a portion of the picture of the Class of 1907, The Johns Hopkins University School of Medicine. 17: G. R. Henry (Mrs. Gladys H. Dick), 39: A. R. Dochez.

From the Alan M. Chesney Archives, The Johns Hopkins University School of Medicine

Thirty-one strains of the 34 erysipelatous strains agglutinated with each of 7 immune erysipelatous sera. Of 45 strains of hemolytic streptococci isolated from sources other than erysipelas, 9, or 20%, were agglutinated by several immune erysipelatous sera. Eight of the 9 strains of *S. hemolyticus* agglutinated by the serum from rabbits immunized against erysipelatous strains were obtained from cases of nasal sinusitis. Agglutinin absorption was accomplished under the conditions of the experiments, with all the combinations of immune erysipelatous sera and strains of hemolytic streptococci of erysipelatous origin. These experiments indicated that it was possible to differentiate by immunological methods a group of hemolytic streptococci causing erysipelas from the group of hemolytic streptococci responsible for scarlet fever, on the one hand, and on the other, from the large series of miscellaneous hemolytic streptococci producing a variety of pyogenic infections.

In a study of the biology of the *S. erysipelatis*, Birkhaug demonstrated that at least 90% of the strains of *S. hemolyticus* isolated from erysipelatous lesions fall immunologically, as determined by the agglutination and absorption reactions, into one group. This group of hemolytic streptococci could be differentiated by the same methods from the type of hemolytic streptococci isolated from patients with scarlet fever.

ALPHONSE RAYMOND DOCHEZ AND HIS STUDIES ON RESPIRATORY DISEASE

A. R. Dochez was born in 1882 in San Francisco, California. His family migrated eastward and settled in Baltimore. Dochez received his A.B. from Johns Hopkins in 1903 and his M.D. in 1907 (Fig 2). Immediately after graduation, he entered the pathology laboratory at Johns Hopkins, where he spent a year studying the effects of feeding animals upon an iodine-free diet. He next became a fellow in pathology at the Rockefeller Institute in New York, working under Dr. Eugene Opie who was a member of the first graduating class of the Johns Hopkins University School of Medicine. Dochez's studies on proteolytic enzymes in the liver were published in a series of four papers. When the Hospital of the Rockefeller Institute was opened in 1910, Dochez was offered an assistant residency and also the position of bacteriologist to the hospital. Dochez remembered years later, with some amusement, having asked Noguchi if one could possibly become a bacteriologist in three weeks. There is no record of Noguchi's reply, but in any event Dochez did become a bacteriologist and during his active career contributed many important additions to the science of microbiology.

Dochez remained as an assistant resident and then

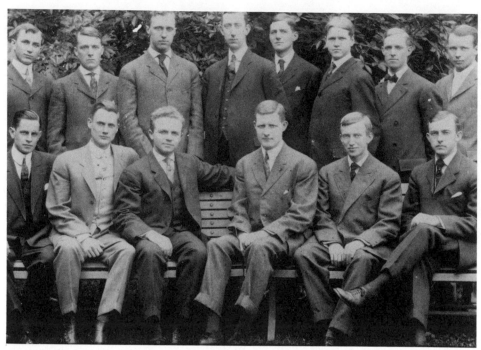

Fig 2. Members of the Pithotomy Club, Class of 1907, Johns Hopkins University School of Medicine. Top row, left to right: Shallenberger, Randall, Hopkins, Smith, Dochez, Clark, Boyd, Dernehl. Bottom row, left to right: Lyon, Bristol, Heuer, Guthrie, Krause, Hellenbrand.
Courtesy of the Pithotomy Club: From the Alan M. Chesney Archives, The Johns Hopkins University School of Medicine

as resident at the Rockefeller Hospital for a period of five years, during which time he collaborated in the famous studies instituted there on the subject of pneumonia by Rufus Cole, the director.

DOCHEZ'S STUDIES ON PNEUMOCOCCAL PNEUMONIA

Dochez's first important contribution was made in 1913, when he classified pneumococci by means of immunity reactions. In 1902 Neufeld described the phenomenon of capsular swelling (quellung) when pneumococci are mixed with antiserum. This phenomenon later turned out to be type-specific and was adopted as a quick method of identifying pneumococci in sputum. While this paper remains the classic study, Dochez and Gillespie clearly established by mouse-protection and agglutination tests that as many as 65% of pneumococci from patients with pneumonia fell into two distinct immunological types; that 14% more could be identified by cultural qualities as Type 3; and that only 22% fell into a miscellaneous group. The differentiation of these types served for years as the basis for developing specific therapeutic sera.

In 1915 Dochez and Avery extended these studies of Dochez and Gillespie and again found that about 75% of the pneumococci from cases of pneumonia fell into three groups. They reasoned that if these highly pathogenic strains were the same as the pneumococci so constantly present in the mouths of healthy people, infection should be essentially universal. They made a study

of the types of pneumococci in the salivas of healthy people, and almost without exception members of the three virulent groups which usually cause pneumonia were absent, while the pneumococci present were of the relatively avirulent heterologous types. In addition, they discovered that following acute lobar pneumonia the types causing the disease almost always disappeared from the saliva within a short time and were replaced by the usual mouth varieties. This very important study disposed of the idea which had been held for some time that pneumonia was always an autogenous infection with strains of essentially harmless pneumococci carried in the mouth and that some "resistance-lowering" factor permitted invasion to occur. They clearly established that infection usually resulted from a virulent strain which was not indigenous to the patients' upper air passages. In a later paper, they determined that healthy persons closely associated with individuals with lobar pneumonia harbor the disease-producing types of pneumococcus and that in every such instance the pneumococcus isolated corresponded in type with that of the infected individual. These observations of the existence of the carrier state of virulent pneumococci established a basis for understanding the mechanism by which lobar pneumonia spreads and maintains its high incidence from year to year. In addition, two workers at Johns Hopkins, Virgil P. W. Sydenstricker (M.D., Johns Hopkins, 1915) and Allen C. Sutton (M.D., Johns Hopkins, 1916), found, in a group of workmen living in very close contact among whom there was a high incidence of fixed-type pneumonia, that the presence of Type I and II pneumococci in the salivas of healthy men showed the remarkably high figure of 22%. Sutton, in collaboration with Charles E. Sevier (M.D., Johns Hopkins, 1916), made daily quantitative blood cultures on a consecutive series of patients with the disease. Ninety-three percent of the patients with persistently negative blood cultures recovered without complications. Of the patients with positive blood cultures, all with over 5 colonies/ml at any period of the disease died, except one with 20 colonies on admission who received serum therapy. This work showed clearly that bacteremia was not the cause of death, but that bacteremia was an indication that the powers of resistance of the patient against infection were breaking down; his immunological status, in other words, came to resemble that of the mouse, which notably has little resistance against pneumococcal infections. From these observations, Bloomfield drew conclusions as to the practical efficacy of serum therapy, "demonstrating that blood stream infection was the critical point and that as long as the blood culture was negative, the effects of serum were good; whereas if the blood cultures were positive, the results were poor regardless of the day of the disease." In other words, serum seemed to aid, up to a certain point, in preventing overwhelming infection, but beyond this, as in the mouse, it was impotent.[3]

Dochez's contribution to the field of pneumococcal pneumonia may be summarized as follows: 1) he established a biological classification of pneumococci into specific types; 2) he discovered (with Avery) the specific soluble substance which confers specificity, showing that it is of capsular origin and demonstrated its presence in blood and urine of patients during the acute stage of pneumonia; 3) he pointed to the importance of type-specific antibodies in the mechanism of recovery from lobar pneumonia which led directly to the production of antipneumococcal type specific horse serum (under the direction of Rufus Cole); and he demonstrated the efficacy of this serum in treatment. Antiserum remained the only effective therapy of pneumococcus pneumonia until the introduction of sulfapyridine.

DOCHEZ'S RESEARCH ON THE COMMON COLD

Dochez continued his clinical studies of respiratory disease while he was a Major in the Medical Corps in World War I. In 1919 he returned to the Johns Hopkins

[3] There was a tradition in the Osler Clinic at Johns Hopkins of describing disease on the basis of careful first-hand observation. Studies of malaria and of typhoid fever had already been made. In 1910, a valuable clinical study of pneumonia was reported based on the analysis of case records. (Chatard JA: An analytical study of acute lobar pneumonia in the Johns Hopkins Hospital from May 15, 1889 to May 15, 1905. Johns Hopkins Hosp Rep 15: 55, 1910) Other papers by various authors in the same volume deal with the pathological anatomy of pneumonia, the leukocytes in lobar pneumonia, terminal pneumonia, termination in recovery, pneumococcic endocarditis, pericarditis, empyema, thrombosis, arthritis, meningitis, and delayed resolution. Joseph Albert Chatard received his M.D. from Johns Hopkins in 1903.

School of Medicine as associate professor of medicine, and it was at this time that he began his studies of the streptococcus and its relation to scarlet fever; he continued these studies after he joined the staff of Columbia University in 1921 as professor of medicine.

After his studies of scarlet fever were completed, Dochez directed his interest to the common cold, which he pursued in his usual systematic fashion. He and his collaborators first studied the bacterial flora of the upper respiratory tract and clearly demonstrated that these bacteria were not of primary etiological significance. Other studies failed to incriminate the Gram-negative filter-passing anaerobes. He then turned his attention to the experimental transmission of the common cold to experimental animals and then to man. Dochez and his associates thus deserve full credit for reawakening interest in the search for a virus in the common cold. They worked first with monkeys in which they thought they had reproduced colds by installation into the nasal passages of filtered nasal washings from people with fresh colds. By a similar procedure, colds were produced in human volunteers in four of nine cases. They noted an abundance of pneumococci in the noses and throats of monkeys in the course of colds and thought that perhaps these grew on a "substrate of primary injury due to the filterable agent." In a later study, Dochez, Mills and Kneeland found that the virus survived for 13 days in the icebox. They then attempted to cultivate it in a medium which contained a chick embryo hash. After 12 to 15 subcultures, at intervals of 3 to 9 days, the material still produced colds in volunteers. They concluded that they had successfully grown an invisible agent. These studies were reported later in greater detail by Dochez, Mills and Kneeland. Still later, they described implantation of virus-containing material from a human cold on the chorio-allantoic membrane of the chick embryo and passage through a series of three eggs. Material from the third series produced a typical cold when tested on volunteers.

In a summary paper, Dochez, Mills and Kneeland reviewed the whole subject of "cold virus." They pointed out that unlike influenza virus it could not be established in ferrets but could in mice, and that it was generally inactivated at 56°F but well preserved in the icebox anaerobically. Thus they made initial inroads into an area of research in the pathogenesis of upper respiratory disease which has still not been completely solved. Attempts at cultivation of filterable agents at that time was difficult because the techniques were not adequate to propagate infectious agents indefinitely.

At the end of the 1930s Dochez found himself more and more involved in administrative work (Fig 3). In 1940 he was appointed chairman of the department of bacteriology at the College of Physicians and Surgeons, a post that he held for 9 years. Thus Dochez's studies resulted in major contributions in three separate areas and as O. T. Avery remarked when presenting to him the Kober Medal of the Association of American Physicians: "Throughout his studies there is unique continuity of thought centering in the dominant problem of acute re-

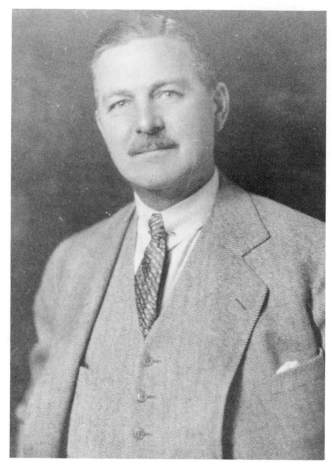

Fig 3.   Alphonse Raymond Dochez while a member of the faculty at the College of Physicians and Surgeons, New York City.
From the Alan M. Chesney Archives, The Johns Hopkins University School of Medicine

spiratory diseases. The results of his work are not random products of chance observation. They are the fruits of wise reflection, objective thinking and thoughtful experiments.''

During World War II, and for some time thereafter, Dochez served on a number of governmental boards and commissions including membership in the Office of Scientific Research and Development, the Board for Coordination of Malarial Studies, the Board for Control of Influenza and Other Epidemic Diseases, and the Hoover Commission on the Reorganization of the Executive Branch of the Government. He was the recipient of the Presidential Medal of Merit.

ACKNOWLEDGMENTS

I am indebted to Robert Austrian and Thomas B. Turner for their helpful review of the manuscript and to Patricia King for her secretarial assistance.

REFERENCES

1. Avery OT et al.: Acute lobar pneumonia; Prevention and serum treatment. Monograph Number 7, New York, Rockefeller Institute for Medical Research, 1917

2. Bergé A: Sur la pathogénie de la scarlatine. Compt rend Soc de biol 5: 1012, 1893

3. Birkhaug K: Studies in scarlet fever. Johns Hopkins Hosp Bull 36: 134, 1925

4. Birkhaug K: Studies in scarlet fever. I. Studies concerning the blanching phenomenon in scarlet fever. J Clin Invest 1: 273, 1925

5. Birkhaug K: A study of the biology of Streptococcus erysipelatis. Proc Soc Exp Biol Med 22: 292, 1925

6. Birkhaug K: Studies on the biology of the Streptococcus erysipelatis. I. Agglutination and agglutinin absorption with the Streptococcus erysipelatis. Johns Hopkins Hosp Bull 36: 248, 1925

7. Blake FG, Trask JD Jr and Lynch JF: Observations on the treatment of scarlet fever with scarlatinal antistreptococcic serum. JAMA 82: 712, 1924

8. Bliss WP: Hemolytic streptococci from throats of scarlet fever patients. Bull Johns Hopkins Hosp 31: 173, 1920

9. Bliss WP: Studies on the biology of streptococcus. II. Antigenic relationships between strains of Streptococcus hemolyticus isolated from scarlet fever. J Exp Med 36: 575, 1922

10. Bloomfield AL: The therapeutic value of Type I antipneumococcus serum. JAMA 81: 1437, 1923

11. Bloomfield AL: A Bibliography of Internal Medicine: Communicable Diseases. Chicago: University of Chicago Press, p 112, 1958

12. Bloomfield AL and Rantz LA: An outbreak of streptococcic septic sore throat in an army camp. JAMA 121: 315, 1943

13. Brown H: Use of Blood Agar for Study of Streptococci. Monograph Number 9, New York, Rockefeller Institute for Medical Research, 1919

14. Dick GF and Dick GH: Experimental inoculations in scarlet fever. JAMA 77: 782, 1921

15. Dick GF and Dick GH: Experimental scarlet fever. JAMA 81: 1166, 1923

16. Dick GF and Dick GH: The etiology of scarlet fever. JAMA 82: 301, 1924

17. Dick GF and Dick GH: Scarlet fever toxin in preventive immunization. JAMA 82: 544, 1924

18. Dick GF and Dick GH: A scarlet fever antitoxin. JAMA 82: 1246, 1924

19. Dick GF and Dick GH: The prevention of scarlet fever. JAMA 83: 84, 1924

20. Dick GF and Dick GH: Therapeutic results with concentrated scarlet fever antitoxin. JAMA 84: 803, 1925

21. Dick GF and Dick GH: Results with the skin test for susceptibility to scarlet fever. JAMA 84: 1477, 1925

22. Dick GF and Dick GH: Therapeutic results with concentrated scarlet fever antitoxin. JAMA 85: 1693, 1925

23. Dochez AR: A preliminary report upon the effects of feeding animals upon an iodine-free diet. Bull Johns Hopkins Hosp 19: 1, 1908

24. Dochez AR: The etiology of scarlet fever. The Harvey Lectures 20: 131, 1925

25. Dochez AR and Avery OT: Varieties of pneumococcus and their relation to lobar pneumonia. J Exp Med 21: 114, 1915

26. Dochez AR and Avery OT: The occurrence of carriers of disease-producing types of pneumococcus. J Exp Med 22: 105, 1915

27. Dochez AR and Avery OT: The elaboration of specific soluble substance by pneumococcus during growth. J Exp Med 26: 477, 1917

28. Dochez AR, Avery OT and Lancefield RC: Studies on the biology of streptococcus. I. Antigenic relationships between strains of Streptococcus hemolyticus. J Exp Med 30: 179, 1919

29. Dochez AR and Bliss WP: Biologic study of hemolytic

streptococci from throats of patients suffering from scarlet fever. JAMA 74: 1600, 1920

30. Dochez AR and Gillespie LJ: A biological classification of pneumococci by means of immunity reactions. JAMA 61: 727, 1913

31. Dochez AR, Mills KC and Kneeland Y Jr: Study of the virus of the common cold and its cultivation in tissue medium. Proc Soc Exp Biol Med 28: 513, 1931

32. Dochez AR, Mills KC and Kneeland Y Jr: Studies of the common cold. VI. Cultivation of the virus in tissue medium. J Exp Med 63: 559, 1936

33. Dochez AR, Mills KC and Kneeland Y Jr: Cultivation of the virus of the common cold in the chorio-allantoic membrane of the chick embryo. Proc Soc Exp Biol Med 35: 213, 1936

34. Dochez AR, Mills KC and Kneeland Y Jr: Filterable viruses in infection of the upper respiratory tract. JAMA 110: 177, 1938

35. Dochez AR and Sherman L: The significance of *Streptococcus hemolyticus* in scarlet fever. JAMA 82: 542, 1924

36. Dochez AR, Shibley GS and Mills, KC: Studies in the common cold. IV. Experimental transmission of the common cold to anthropoid apes and human beings by means of a filterable agent. J Exp Med 52: 701, 1930

37. Eagles GH: Significance of serologic grouping of hemolytic streptococci. Br J Exp Pathol 5: 199, 1924

38. Hallier E: Der pflanzliche Organismus im Blute der Scharlachkranken. Jahrb f Kinderh 2: 169, 1869

39. Holman WL: Classification of streptococci. J Med Res 34: 377, 1916

40. Jacobson LO: George F. Dick, 1880–1967. Trans Assoc Am Physicians 82: 32, 1969

41. Jochmann G: Die Bacterienbefunde bei Scharlach und ihre Bedeutung für den Krankheitsprocess. Ztschr f klin Med 56: 316, 1905

42. Kneeland Y Jr: Alphonse Raymond Dochez, 1882–1964. Trans Assoc Am Physicians 78: 21, 1965

43. Krumwiede C, Nicoll M and Pratt J: Attempts to produce scarlatina in monkeys. Arch Intern Med 13: 909, 1914

44. Loeffler F: Untersuchungen über die Bedeutung der Mikro-Organismen für die Entstehung der Diphtherie beim Menschen, bei der Taube und beim Kalbe. Mitt a d k Gsndhtsamte 2: 421, 1884

45. Marmorek A: Le Streptocoque et le sérum antistreptococcique. Ann Inst Pasteur 9: 593, 1895

46. Morris C: Lectures on Scarlet Fever. Philadelphia: Lindsay and Blakiston, p 1, 1851

47. Moser P: Ueber die Behandlung des Scharlachs mit einem Scharlach Streptococcenserum. Wien klin Wchnschr 15: 1053, 1902

48. Moser P and von Pirquet C: Agglutination von Streptococcendurch Pferdserum. Wien klin Wchnschr 15: 1086, 1902

49. Neufeld F: Ueber die Agglutination der Pneumococcen und über die Theorien der Agglutination. Ztschr f Hyg u Infektionskr 40: 54, 1902

50. Pohl-Pincus K: Mikrokokken an den Epidermisschuppen von Scharlachkranken. Centralbl f d med Wissensch 21: 640, 1883

51. Schottmüller H: Die Artunterscheidung der für den Menschen pathogenen Streptococcen durch Blutagar. München med Wchnschr 50: 849, 1903

52. Schultz W and Charlton W: Serologische Beobachtungen am Scharlachexanthem. Ztschr f Kinderh 17: 328, 1918

53. Stevens FA and Dochez AR: Biology of streptococcus. J Exp Med 40: 253, 1924

54. Stevens FA and Dochez AR: The occurrence of throat infection with Streptococcus scarlatinae without a rash. JAMA 86: 1110, 1926

55. Stevens FA and Dochez AR: The epidemiology of scarlatinal throat infections sine exanthemate. JAMA 87: 2137, 1926

56. Sutton AC and Sevier CE: A study of the bacteremia of lobar pneumonia. Bull Johns Hopkins Hosp 23: 315, 1917

57. Swift HF and Kinsella R: Classification of hemolytic streptococci. J Exp Med 28: 169, 1918

58. Sydenstricker VPW and Sutton AC: An epidemiological study of lobar pneumonia. Bull Johns Hopkins Hosp 28: 312, 1917

59. Trousseau A: Lectures on Clinical Medicine. Philadelphia: Lindsay and Blakiston, p 183, 1869

17.
G. Canby Robinson: Peripatetic Medical Educator

The career of G. Canby Robinson (Fig 1) coincided with a period which has been called "the golden age of American medicine." Robinson was not only influenced by the principal developments of this period, but was himself an innovator in the four major areas of academic medicine—patient care, scientific research, education, and administration. Since he played a key role in the organization of three important medical centers—Vanderbilt, Cornell, and Washington University—his influence on American medicine was widespread.

MEDICAL SCHOOL AT JOHNS HOPKINS

Canby Robinson's training and early experience fitted him well for the important positions he was to occupy. In his autobiographical sketch entitled *Adventures in Medical Education*, he gave an enlightening appraisal of his education at The Johns Hopkins School of Medicine from 1899 to 1903. He considered his experience during this time to be the most influential on his career.

When he entered Johns Hopkins, the school was beginning its seventh year. The heads of the departments were all relatively young and the spirit of youthful enthusiasm was in the air. There were 50 students in his class who came from all parts of the United States.

Their first experience was a course in anatomy, in which they devoted the first several months to the study of the names and shapes of bones, carefully dissecting and studying the human body and making drawings of sections of its various parts. Franklin Paine Mall, the professor of anatomy, gave independence and responsibility to the students, treating them as mature and well-trained college graduates. His remarks as he walked around the dissecting room casually looking over the shoulders of the students were frequently more philosophical than anatomical. In those days Mall had a splendid group of young associates who spent more time in small group teaching than did the professor. The senior of Mall's assistants was Ross G. Harrison who, a short time later, introduced the important technique of tissue culture. Harrison had charge of the course in microscopic anatomy. Another in the group was Charles R. Bardeen, a member of the first class at The Johns Hopkins University School of Medicine, who later became professor of anatomy and dean at the University of Wisconsin. He organized one of the first university medical schools in

Reprinted from the *Johns Hopkins Medical Journal* **143**: 84, 1978.

the Midwest and was a leader in medical education throughout his career. Others of Mall's assistants were Henry Knower who became professor of anatomy at the University of Cincinnati and Mervin T. Sudler who became professor of surgery and dean of the medical school at the University of Kansas. Also working with the students was Abram T. Kerr, who was doing research on the distribution of the nerves of the skin. He sought the help of the students in making special dissections and charts of the nerves of the bodies they were studying. Robinson's role in this research opened up the opportunity for him to work for a short period after his graduation in Kerr's laboratory when Kerr was professor of anatomy in the medical department of Cornell at Ithaca.

The students in anatomy worked in well-lighted rooms, each housing 8 to 12 students, which were clean and well ordered in contrast to the usual dissecting halls of that time. Robinson recalled that only once during the course was the serious tone of the dissecting room disturbed:

It was on a spring day when an Italian organ grinder took his stand beneath the open windows of our room. An unmusical classmate, either annoyed by the organ music or just looking for some fun, came to our table and took the spleen from our "body" and threw it down at the organ grinder. Unfortunately, an unnoticed policeman was standing nearby and picked up the spleen that had missed its mark. He brought it in to Professor Mall with the complaint that someone had thrown a "kidney" out of the window. After being assured by the professor that no "kidney" had been thrown out, he left, but Mall came immediately to the dissecting room with more than usual to say, and ordered those involved in the episode, from which the policeman's lack of anatomical knowledge had given a way out, to report immediately to his office. The thrower and his partner, my partner, and I, who had abetted the act, went together to his office to diffuse the blame and receive a scholarly discourse on proper behavior in a dissecting room, on public decency, and on the responsibility of scientists. And that was all. However, the student who threw the spleen was one of two students dropped from the class at the end of the year, not because of this episode but because it was a symptom of a crude personality which marked him off from the rest of his classmates.

The course in physiology consisted of well-organized lectures and demonstrations by Professor William H. Howell, supplemented by work in the laboratory in which the students performed experiments demonstrating important functions of the different organs.

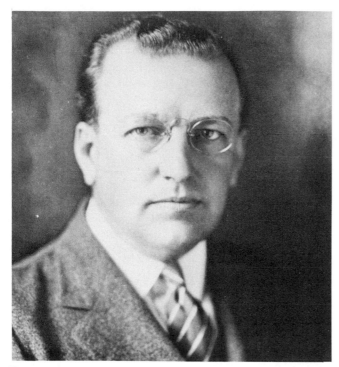

Fig 1.   George Canby Robinson
From the Alan M. Chesney Medical Archives, The Johns Hopkins Medical Institutions.

Robinson described Howell as a quiet, sympathetic man with an orderly mind who was a fine teacher. His textbook of physiology was widely used for many years in this country, going through 14 editions. The senior instructor was George P. Dryer, who soon became professor of physiology at the University of Illinois. Other young assistants, all recent graduates of the medical school, were Percy M. Dawson, later professor at the University of Wisconsin, Alfred B. Herrick, Percy G. Stiles and Joseph Erlanger. Erlanger, of course, had a distinguished career as a professor of physiology at Washington University in St. Louis and won the Nobel Prize with Herbert Gasser, another Johns Hopkins graduate, for work on single nerve fibers.

Physiological chemistry began in March and continued to June. It was taught by Walter Jones, who was then a young associate professor of chemistry under John Jacob Abel; he later became head of the newly organized department of physiological chemistry. Robinson depicted Jones as a spirited, and on occasion, a dramatic, talker. He demonstrated the vehemence that a scientific controversy could arouse, as he was at that time in the midst of a polemic with a professor in a German university and his arguments in support of his view bubbled over into his lectures, which gave them real life and interest for the students. One of Robinson's classmates, Arthur Loevenhart, was an advanced student of biochemistry who later became professor of pharmacology in the medical school at Wisconsin. When the subject of his previous research fitted into the course, Jones asked him to lecture to the class which shows the intimacy that existed among students and teachers in the medical school at that time.

The second year began with further studies in anatomy and physiology and with a course in bacteriology, taught by Norman MacL. Harris in the department of pathology, which occupied each afternoon until January. For the first two weeks the laboratory was in essence a kitchen, as the first part of the course consisted of the preparation of the various culture media which were to be used.

In January the course in pathology began under William H. Welch. This course was undoubtedly the best in the country at that time. Welch, who was in his early 50s, was fully interested in his teaching; he gave superb lectures and spent a great deal of time in the laboratory sessions discussing specimens being studied by the individual students. At the end of the course Welch called each student into his office and went over with him the microscopic sections that the student had to study as part of his final examination. Robinson clearly recalled this experience: Welch singled out one of his specimens and expressed enthusiasm about Robinson's description of it. This, of course, gave Robinson a tremendous stimulus and he left the room with the determination to do his best in medicine, if only to show Dr. Welch that he was worthy of this praise. What a fine example of the best approach to teaching and the value of encouragement properly transmitted to inspire students to do their best. Welch attracted many young men into the field of pathology. During Robinson's year in the department William G. MacCallum, Eugene L. Opie and Harry P. Marshall, all graduates of The Johns Hopkins Medical School, were the young instructors. MacCallum, who became professor of physiological pathology at Johns Hopkins, was called to Columbia University in 1909 as professor of pathology and returned to Johns Hopkins in 1917 as Welch's successor. Opie joined the staff of the newly organized Rockefeller Institute in 1904. In 1910 he became professor of pathology at the newly reorganized Washington University Medical School in St. Louis and later, as dean, he took a leading part in that University's outstanding development in medical education. In 1923 he became professor of experimental pathology at the University of Pennsylvania as well as director of the laboratory of the Henry Phipps Institute for the Study of Tuberculosis. In 1932, with the reorganization of the Cornell University Medical College, he was appointed professor of pathology and pathologist at the New York Hospital. Marshall became professor of pathology at the University of Virginia.

Robinson was assigned his first special project by MacCallum, who gave him a specimen of an unusual tumor removed from the neck of a recently autopsied subject suggesting that Robinson describe it, study it microscopically, and make drawings. After Robinson had done his best with the drawing he took it to Max Brödel who viewed it from various angles, upside down and sideways, and then said: "What is this, a hunting scene?" In spite of this initial setback, with Brödel's assistance the project reached its culmination. The tumor was recognized as a cyst originating from the thyroglossal duct of which only one case had been fully described previously. Thus, Robinson's first publication appeared in the *Bulletin of the Johns Hopkins Hospital* in 1902. It was clearly in pathology that Robinson's great stimulus occurred as a result of his close association with William Henry Welch and his brilliant group of young instructors.

The last of the laboratory courses in the second year was in pharmacology and toxicology under John J. Abel. Abel was primarily trained in chemistry and in contrast to Howell lectured in a reminiscent style, often referring to his unique seven years of peripatetic study with the leading medical scientists in various German universities. His talks as well as the laboratory course were not conducted very systematically, but his personality, his enthusiasm and his interest in his field of research made a strong impression on the students. Abel was the first professor of pharmacology in America, this subject having been newly imported from the German universities, and he was one of the most respected American medical scientists of his time.

Also in the second year the students began their clinical work with a course in physical diagnosis under William S. Thayer. The students, as in more recent times, first practiced the various examination techniques on each other, learning how to observe and how to employ palpation, percussion and auscultation before attempting these approaches on patients. When this time came, the class was divided into groups of 6 or 8 students, each with its own instructor. Robinson's group was directed by Henry Barton Jacobs. Jacobs was especially interested in tuberculosis and served as the first secretary to the National Tuberculosis Association when it was organized in 1904. The introductory course in surgery was given by John M. T. Finney who became one of the most prominent and beloved doctors in Baltimore, not only as a skillful surgeon, but also as an effective contributor to the community.

He and Thayer, in Robinson's opinion, were an outstanding duo "to guide the emotions and shape the attitude toward patients of impressionable students at the threshold of their clinical training."

All of the third year work was done in the Johns Hopkins Hospital under Osler, Halsted, Kelly, and J. Whitridge Williams (the latter had recently been appointed professor of obstetrics). This was a remarkable group of clinical teachers. During the mornings of that year groups of students worked in the various clinics of the outpatient department and attended the general clinics given in medicine and surgery by Osler and Halsted for third and fourth year students. Only in obstetrics were there systematic lectures. As depicted by so many of his students, the most memorable experience of the third year was, to Robinson, Osler's teaching in the dispensary. Three times a week he met the class at 12 o'clock for an informal discussion of patients which he called the "observation clinic." The students sat in two rows of chairs, a couch for the patient between them. Osler would come into the room with his buoyant enthusiasm and sit at the head of the couch, and a student would present the history of the case he had studied during the morning

under the guidance of an instructor. The patient would then be examined by Osler and the student. Although the primary objective was to teach the beginners how to look at, feel, and listen to a patient and how to observe the manifestations of disease, the students unconsciously learned much from watching the great physician—how he put the patient at ease with kindly words and jests, his delightful sense of humor, his keen analysis, and his literary and historical allusions. It was an extraordinarily effective way of teaching the doctor-patient relationship, an important lesson which Robinson said he and his classmates carried with them throughout their medical careers.

Osler, too, had an outstanding staff, all of whom later had distinguished careers in medicine. Among them were William S. Thayer, Henry M. Thomas, Thomas B. Futcher, Thomas R. Brown, and Louis P. Hamburger. Serving at that time on the resident staff were Thomas MacCrae, who became professor of medicine at the Jefferson Medical College; Rufus Cole, who organized and directed the Hospital of the Rockefeller Institute; Charles P. Emerson, subsequently professor of medicine and dean of the University of Indiana Medical School; and Campbell P. Howard, who filled the professorship of medicine first at Iowa and later at McGill where his father had been one of Osler's teachers.

In contrast to medicine, the weekly nonoperative clinics by Halsted tended to be over the heads of the students and Halsted was in their view a somewhat indistinct figure. Halsted's greatest contribution was his teaching of advanced students, especially those he selected for his resident staff.

The afternoons in the third year were largely taken up by two laboratory courses: clinical microscopy (Fig 2), conducted by Charles P. Emerson, who later wrote the first comprehensive textbook on this subject, and surgical pathology, taught by Joseph C. Bloodgood. Blood-

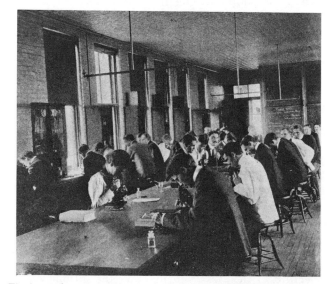

Fig 2. Laboratory class in clinical microscopy (1902), a course pioneered by William Osler.

good had pioneered the development of this field under Halsted's direction. The students also attended a few clinics and lectures on the surgical specialties including orthopedic surgery and ophthalmology. At the end of the afternoon they had special lectures by distinguished scientists from other cities, including Alexander C. Abbott of the University of Pennsylvania on hygiene (Abbott had formerly been in Welch's department); Robert Fletcher of the Surgeon-General's Library on medical jurisprudence, and Charles W. Stiles, the discoverer of the hookworm, on medical zoology. Lectures on the history of medicine were given at that time by John Shaw Billings, who played such an important role in the development of the medical school and hospital.

The work in the fourth year was devoted to the hospital wards where the students served as clinical clerks. The class was divided into three groups that rotated through medicine, surgery, and obstetrics and gynecology. This arrangement was one of Osler's great contributions which was followed by all of the other department heads. In medicine the students were an integral part of the hospital organization and had specific duties including taking the history, doing the physical examination, performing the simpler laboratory tests, and helping with surgical dressings. This brought a new spirit into clinical teaching and revived the best features of the old preceptor system. The students attended the ward rounds usually made each morning at 9 o'clock by the chief. At that time the students would present new cases assigned to them and participate in discussions of diagnosis and treatment. They spent the entire day on the wards either with patients or in the laboratories, having been prepared for the laboratory work by the course in clinical microscopy. One of Robinson's vivid memories was the lesson he learned in persistent diligence in the examination of patients. He searched for 20 days for tubercle bacilli in the sputum of a young girl before the organisms were demonstrated.

What a thrill for the students Saturday evenings at Osler's home must have been. At 8 o'clock seventeen members of the class taking medicine would gather around his dining room table and listen to an unsurpassed talk on medical history. After an hour or so light refreshments would be served and then the conversation would be directed toward the patients and the hospital wards, each student being asked to describe how his work was going. On several evenings there was a description of the 18th century and early 19th century physicians depicted in the famous Gold-headed Cane and on one evening Osler would also talk about his favorite book, Sir Thomas Browne's *Religio Medici* and show the students the more than 60 editions he had in his library. The fact that this great man would give up every Saturday evening from his busy life to this type of gathering with the students shows what a tremendous interest he had in medical education and is ample documentation of his greatness as a teacher.

On the surgical service Halsted rarely made morning rounds himself; they were frequently conducted by Harvey Cushing, who had just returned from a year of study in Europe. Cushing also conducted the afternoon sessions in surgical anatomy and in operative surgery on dogs. Hugh H. Young, who was just beginning his career in genito-urinary surgery, gave the instruction in that subject and there were a few lectures and demonstrations in otolaryngology, ophthalmology and dermatology. In obstetrics and gynecology the delivery of babies in the homes of poor patients was a valuable experience for the students and their initiation into practical medicine outside of the hospital. In gynecology Howard Kelly conducted operative clinics and gave a running commentary which was received enthusiastically by the students. Lectures in gynecology were given by William W. Russell, one of the early residents, and a course in gynecological pathology was conducted by Thomas S. Cullen who later succeeded Kelly as professor of gynecology. The only instruction in pediatrics consisted of a few lectures by William D. Booker who demonstrated cases of the contagious diseases of childhood. A course of lectures on psychiatry was given by Henry M. Hurd and at the end of the fourth year a few clinics were conducted by Henry J. Berkley at the Baltimore City Bay View Asylum.

In general, Robinson described the curriculum as being characterized by quality rather than by quantity and emphasized that there was a remarkable lack of external pressure on the staff and students. However, he indicated that everyone felt considerable internal pressure; that is, a drive toward high achievement and hard work which was natural in view of the general spirit of excitement that dominated Johns Hopkins in those early days (Fig 3).

Robinson contributed a number of stories about the character of the early professors, but most entertaining is the following about Howard A. Kelly: "He was a remarkable linguist; speaking, reading, and writing German, French and Spanish; speaking modern Greek; and reading the scriptures in Greek and Hebrew. He was a man of great energy and vigor as illustrated by a story that went around among the students. It was said that he rode a motorcycle to the hospital and, to save time, had arranged with the proprietor of a grocery store on his route that when he rode by with a shout, the grocer would telephone to instruct the hospital to start giving ether to the first patient he operated upon, for Dr. Kelly was on his way.... Once he was a watcher at the polls during a Baltimore election that promised to be unusually rough and corrupt. The occasion lived up to expectation. The brave Kelly's watchfulness was ended by the severe beating he received at the hands of thugs representing the ward heelers."

INTERNSHIP

Then as now, internship was a problem facing the senior medical students. Robinson described the tension in March of the senior year waiting for the announcement of the academic standing of students in the graduating class. The four students with the highest standing had first choice of internships in The Johns

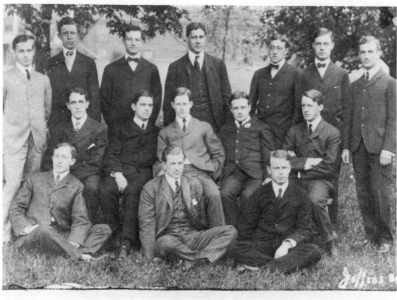

1903

Beadle Smith Gaenslin Goldsborough Brush Miller Hutchins
Chatard Bixler Watson Moulton Beidel
Marshall Robinson Haskell

Fig 3. Members of the Pithotomy Club, Class of 1903, Johns Hopkins University School of Medicine.
Kindly made available by the members of the Pithotomy Club.

Hopkins Hospital and usually chose the medical service under Osler. The next four were likely to choose the surgical service under Halsted. There were four internships in obstetrics and gynecology and several appointments in pathology or in special services, so that about 16 students at the top of the class of 50 had the opportunity of serving an internship in The Johns Hopkins Hospital.

Robinson found himself in the middle of the class, just one place below the last man on the list who wanted an internship at Johns Hopkins. He had equally poor success at other hospitals which offered good quality training. In the depths of his disappointment he consulted Warfield T. Longcope, a friend who had graduated from Hopkins two years previously, who was then resident pathologist at the Pennsylvania Hospital in Philadelphia. It was the custom at that hospital to appoint one resident every three months for a two-year service. Robinson was accepted as a qualified candidate for this position. However, having the summer to wait before he could receive an appointment at Pennsylvania, he went to Clifton Springs Sanitorium in the Finger Lakes district of New York to work with Dr. Martin B. Tinker who had just left the surgical staff at Johns Hopkins to open a surgical service there. (A few years later the medical service at Clifton Springs was modernized by Charles P. Emerson, who had been one of Osler's residents.) At Clifton Springs Robinson assisted Tinker with his operations and acted as his anesthetist, worked in the clinical laboratory and had charge of a few medical patients. At the end of the summer Robinson accepted an appointment to teach anatomy in the Ithaca Division of the Cornell University Medical College under his former instructor in anatomy at Hopkins, Abram T. Kerr. About two

months after Robinson arrived at Cornell, Longcope offered him a position as assistant in pathology. Longcope had just been made director of the Ayer Clinical Laboratory at Pennsylvania, replacing Simon Flexner who had been called to New York to organize the Rockefeller Institute for Medical Research.

THE AYER LABORATORY

At the Ayer laboratory, Robinson became interested in the museum which contained many rare specimens. He spent his evenings reviewing and arranging the specimens in an effort to revive the museum's catalogue. This work resulted in the finding of a fascinating case in which there was a tumor in the region of the bundle of His. His interest in this area of the heart had been aroused at Johns Hopkins by Erlanger's demonstration with his special clamp of the production of varying grades of heart block in the dog[1]. Records showed that

[1] Osler transferred his clinical interest in heart block to Joseph Erlanger in the hope that a trained physiologist could elucidate the problem further. Osler gave Erlanger a chance to study a clinical case and Part I of Erlanger's famous paper on this subject ("On the Physiology of Heart Block in Mammals; with a Special Reference to the Causation of Stokes–Adams Disease") deals with the tracings obtained from this patient (see references 8–10). Marey's cardiograph was used for the tracings of the heart's impulse, and the pulsations in the brachial artery were recorded with Erlanger's sphygmomanometer. The tracings on the patient showed at various times complete heart block and partial heart block. The syncopal attacks, he concluded, "are, in all probability, directly dependent upon a marked reduction of the ventricular rate." Erlanger then took

the patient he found in the museum who died in 1879 had had typical Adams–Stokes attacks marked by periods of unconsciousness and excessively slow heart beat, the cause of which was unknown at that time. The clinical record, written over 25 years previously, provided an excellent description of the patient's illness. Robinson reported the case in the *Bulletin of the Ayer Laboratory* and the paper attracted the attention of Professor Friedrich von Müller of Munich so that when he visited the Pennsylvania Hospital he asked Robinson to come to Germany and work in his clinic. This Robinson did after finishing his residency training.

After two and a half years in the laboratory, Robinson was appointed a resident physician beginning on July 1, 1906. The service started with three months in the clinical laboratory, followed by nine months on the three medical wards, three months principally on the ambulance, six months on the two surgical wards and the final three months in charge of the receiving ward.

During his period as resident pathologist and as resident physician to the Pennsylvania Hospital Robinson took full advantage of the pathological and clinical material which he had at his disposal for study. In 1904 he published a paper entitled "The Presence of Tubercle Bacilli in the Spinal Fluid in Tuberculous Meningitis with a Series of Cases from the Ayer Clinical Laboratory of the Pennsylvania Hospital." In those days it was somewhat of a new venture to study in the laboratory the spinal fluid from such cases. Robinson analyzed in detail fluids from 19 patients. Most remarkable was that in 19 spinal fluids tubercle bacilli were found 17 times, or in 89.5%. He defined clearly the fine cobweb-like coagulant which formed as a veil-like mass hanging down from the surface and spreading out towards the bottom of the tube. He compared the spinal fluid findings in tuberculosis with those in cases of epidemic cerebrospinal meningitis which he had previously reported. In 1905 he published a paper in the *Journal of Infectious Diseases* entitled "The Role of the Typhoid Bacillus in the Pulmonary Complications of Typhoid Fever," in which he pointed out that although the organism had been recovered repeatedly

from the lung there were in the literature but few cases in which the typhoid bacillus was demonstrated to have produced definite pulmonary lesions. From the study of three cases, he felt justified in concluding that the bacillus typhosus was capable of causing pulmonary abscess and gangrene in lung tissues already the seat of hemorrhagic infarction. That the organism may invade an infarcted area of the lung without causing abscess formation was shown by another case where the pulmonary artery was occluded by a thrombus, typhoid bacilli alone being isolated from the infarcted area. Also reported was a case of lobar pneumonia in which a pure culture of the B type of the paratyphoid bacillus was isolated.

Another subject which attracted his interest was the occurrence of acute endocarditis in patients with congenital malformations of the heart. He published an article entitled "The Relation Between Congenital Malformations of the Heart and Acute Endocarditis, with Report of Two Cases" in which he drew the following conclusions: (1) congenital malformations of the heart are generally considered to predispose to acute endocarditis; (2) the combination of acute endocarditis and congenital cardiac malformations is rare because comparatively few cases of congenital cardiac malformations reach the age at which acute endocarditis is most common. Most cases, showing both pathological lesions, die in young adult life; (3) the form of extensive congenital cardiac malformation which is most frequently attacked by acute endocarditis is that in which life is most prolonged; namely, obstruction to the pulmonary outflow with openings between the auricles or ventricles; and (4) the acute endocarditis most frequently attacks the right side of the heart in cases of congenital cardiac malformation.

A paper published in 1908 in the *American Journal of Medical Sciences* entitled "Gallop Rhythm of the Heart" reflects Robinson's interest in the use of physiological methods for studying the functional abnormalities of the heart. In the study, he made tracings using an apparatus similar to the polygraph described by Mackenzie. Simultaneous tracings were made from the apex beat, the jugular vein, and the carotid artery. He divided the gallop rhythms that he studied into presystolic and protodiastolic. Each form, he found, was associated with a characteristic cardiogram. He carefully recorded the time relationships in the cardiograms between the points where the two normal heart sounds and the extra sound of the gallop rhythm occurred.

---

the problem to the laboratory and in Part II ("On the Physiology of Heart Block in the Dog") he described the clamp which he devised whereby he could compress the A-V bundle; on the basis of his experiments he concluded that "in the dog the impulse which normally causes the ventricles to contract is conducted through the auriculoventricular bundle of His. By compression of this bundle all stages of heart block may be obtained." In Part III ("The Relation of Heart Block to Stokes–Adams Disease") Erlanger concluded: "All of the cardinal symptoms of Stokes–Adams disease may be duplicated by heart block resulting from a lesion in or near the auriculoventricular bundle of His and by this alone. No typical case of Stokes–Adams disease has been described in which heart block might not have been the cause of the trouble. It can be shown that all cases of Stokes–Adams disease which have been studied by sufficient accurate methods were cases of heart block."
The introduction of electrocardiography made it clear that certain cases of Stokes–Adams attacks are due to other disturbances of mechanism than classical heart block as illustrated by the case of Robinson and Bredeck (see reference 53).

SOJOURN IN EUROPE

Unexpected opportunities often appeared in those days. While Robinson was working on the surgical service, one of his patients with exophthalmic goiter was advised to go to Switzerland to have his thyroid removed by Theodor Kocher, the world's leading thyroid surgeon. Robinson was asked by the attending surgeon to accompany the patient and in the summer of 1907 spent five weeks in Switzerland, where he had interesting contacts with Kocher and met other members of the distinguished faculty at Bern, including Sahli in medicine, Kronecker in physiology and Langerhans in pathology.

In October 1908 Robinson went to Munich to work in the clinic of Friedrich von Müller. Since Müller set an example of how to organize a medical clinic which was followed later in the United States, it is worthwhile to record Robinson's description of how it functioned:

I was much impressed by his clinical lectures which he gave every morning at 9 o'clock before about 200 students who crowded his auditorium. Each lecture began with the presentation of a patient who served as the focal point of the discussion to follow. After the medical history had been read, the diagnosis was often announced, and an examination of the patient, including the demonstration of physical signs, the simpler laboratory tests, and instrumental examinations, was made by the professor or an assistant before the class. A projection lantern, charts, drawings, and diagrams were freely used and the students were given as complete and clear a description of the case as possible. Treatment was always discussed, and recent contributions of pharmacology were sometimes explained. The best feature of Müller's teaching was the prominent place he gave to pathology ... Many of the specimens shown to illustrate bodily changes caused by the disease under discussion were from cases he himself had studied both clinically and anatomically ... Bacteriology was also brought into close relation to the study of patients ... He always had a thorough understanding and detailed knowledge of the disease illustrated by the case presented. He seemed to know just what points he wished to emphasize and did it in a masterly way, at times approaching the dramatic. The sincerity and directness of his teaching were very stimulating. Müller's lectures made one feel that he was a great teacher because they were based on his incessant, broad, and intense study of internal medicine and its allied sciences. His teaching went far beyond his lectures to undergraduate medical students for it included the direction of advanced students in various fields of study and research. This necessitated not only a thorough knowledge of present day medicine but an ability to see future possibilities so that promising problems for investigation could be suggested and the most likely method of solution advised. His knowledge of the various branches of the medical sciences was such that he knew when one branch might borrow from another and he was able to coordinate many fields successfully.

Müller's clinic represented an outstanding example of the true university spirit which bases teaching primarily on research. The clinical lecture was the core of medical instruction and the opportunity to learn by hearing and seeing was developed to its highest degree. However, this method had one fault: the chance to learn from doing—so well practiced in British medical schools, and, more recently, so extensively developed in America—but seldom available to Müller's students.

While in Germany, Robinson met George Draper (with whom he was to be associated later at the Rockefeller Hospital) and they studied the presphygmic period of the heart. With the help of Ernst Edens, Müller's assistant who studied the heart and circulation, they worked out a method of measuring the time between the beginning of the contraction of the heart and the first evidence of the pulse in the arteries.

RETURN TO PHILADELPHIA

Robinson then returned to Philadelphia where in June 1909 he began the practice of medicine, establishing his office in a small house on 15th Street between Spruce and Pine where Warfield Longcope and Charles Mitchell of the Pennsylvania Hospital staff took him into their bachelor quarters. He was appointed clinical pathologist at the Presbyterian Hospital of Philadelphia and his first assignment there was to construct and equip a clinical laboratory in an abandoned ward and to provide the facilities required to carry out the clinical tests and examinations that the staff of the hospital needed. He also taught at the University of Pennsylvania Medical School.

During this period he published a paper in the *Archives of Internal Medicine* in May 1910 entitled "Blood Pressure in Epidemic Cerebrospinal Meningitis." Because of the intimate relation that had been shown by Cushing and others to exist between intracranial pressure and blood pressure, it was thought that a series of observations on the blood pressure in cases of epidemic cerebrospinal meningitis would prove interesting, especially when the effect of withdrawal of the cerebrospinal fluid was considered. Robinson concluded that his observations afforded no definite evidence that increased intracranial tension caused an increased blood pressure in meningitis unless it was late in the disease when internal hydrocephalus may have developed as a result of blocking of the foramina of the fourth ventricle.

Although he expected to remain in Philadelphia permanently, his plans were abruptly changed when in the spring of 1910 he was offered the opportunity to be the first resident physician in the new Hospital of the Rockefeller Institute for Medical Research. This appointment opened the way for an academic career in medicine and he quickly accepted.

COLE'S FIRST RESIDENT AT THE ROCKEFELLER HOSPITAL

Robinson reported to the Hospital of the Rockefeller Institute on September 1, 1910. George Draper, the first assistant resident appointed to the staff, arrived on the same day. Miss Nancy P. Ellicott[2] was to be superintendent of the hospital and her assistant, Miss Mary B. Thompson,[3] was to be in charge of the nursing service. Both had been recruited from The Johns Hopkins Hospi-

[2] Miss Nancy P. Ellicott was a graduate of the Johns Hopkins Hospital Nursing School in 1903. After graduation she assumed charge of Ward H in the Johns Hopkins Hospital and then of Ward B. In 1905 she became superintendent of nurses at the Church Home and Infirmary and in 1907 was appointed superintendent of that hospital where she remained until April 17, 1909. Then she accepted the superintendency of the Rockefeller Hospital in New York City; she held this position until her retirement on May 1, 1938.

[3] Mary B. Thompson was a graduate of the Johns Hopkins Hospital School of Nursing in 1904. She became superintendent of the training school for nurses at the Church Home and Infirmary from which position she resigned in 1908. In the following

tal. Within a few weeks Homer F. Swift and Henry Marks arrived from Europe and Alphonse Raymond Dochez moved over to the hospital from the Institute laboratories to complete the initial resident staff. Francis H. McCrudden assumed direction of the chemical laboratory and a short time later Arthur W. M. Ellis and Francis W. Peabody joined the resident staff (Fig 4).

At the time of Robinson's arrival, the Hospital was nearly completed and equipped, but the organization of the medical service was an enormous task which faced him and his colleagues. This included designing clinical record forms, temperature charts and admission forms as well as all the other details needed to put the hospital in readiness for its opening on October 17, 1910.

The next endeavor was to get access to the patients required for the clinical studies to be carried out. In order to facilitate the referral of the desired patients an effort was made to provide for the public, and in particular the medical profession, an understanding of the objectives and the plan of operation of the hospital. A statement was published by the Rockefeller Institute explaining that the hospital planned to study

> disease as it actually appears in human beings, under conditions equally favorable to treatment and to scientific observation. A common motive actuates the Institute as a whole, namely, that of advancing knowledge and of securing more perfect means of preventing and healing disease. Thus the work of the laboratories and hospital is unified. Their common aim and the physical connection of the different buildings with each other, often admits of the same problems being studied both in their biological or pathological and in their clinical aspects. In the organization of the scientific staff of the Institute, the principle has been recognized that the ultimate purposes of medical research and discovery may be greatly served by the study of biological and chemical problems that, as such, may appear remote from medical application. It has not thus far been the purpose of the Institute to choose rare and strange diseases in preference to those more prevalent or familiar, on which to spend its resources. On the contrary, the diseases now under investigation . . . include many of those which are regarded as the chief scourges of mankind . . . The director issues bulletins from time to time informing physicians of the diseases chosen for investigation. While making the fullest use of its opportunities for observation and study, the Institute recognizes at all times the paramount right of the patient to receive the most effective treatment within the power of the attending physicians.

George Draper and Robinson began research on the heart and circulation, continuing the same approach they had used while in Munich. Their major thrust was on methods by which the functional capacity of the heart might be measured. At that time the type and extent of the disease present in the heart could be reasonably well determined but it was little more than guesswork to conclude how much the efficiency of the diseased heart was

impaired in maintaining the circulation, and to what extent the work of the heart should be limited by reducing physical activity in order to prevent symptoms of heart failure. They had made some progress when their attention was diverted by the arrival from Germany of the electrocardiograph. They found that putting this complex instrument for recording the action of the heart into operation was a formidable problem. Fortunately they were able to enlist the help of Dr. Horatio B. Williams, a physicist in the department of physiology at Columbia who had already set up an electrocardiograph at that institution. With his help the instrument became functional on March 5, 1911. Robinson and Draper's work over the next two years with the electrocardiograph contributed significantly to the development of knowledge concerning irregularities in the heart beat.[4]

In 1912 Francis R. Fraser and Frederic M. Hanes joined Robinson's resident staff, and Florentine Medigreceanu came to work in the chemical laboratory. After two years Fraser accepted an appointment at Columbia under Warfield Longcope, then professor of medicine in the College of Physicians and Surgeons. Later he returned to London to become the first full-time professor of medicine in the medical school of St. Bartholomew's Hospital. Hanes, a Johns Hopkins graduate with excellent training in pathology at Columbia, had a relatively short period at the Rockefeller, and later became professor of medicine at Duke.

On July 1, 1912 Robinson's service as senior resident physician ended but he continued on the staff as an associate. During that period he did experimental studies, principally with John Auer who also was a graduate of Johns Hopkins, in the physiological division of the Institute.

WASHINGTON UNIVERSITY SCHOOL OF MEDICINE

In the spring of 1913 Robinson accepted a position as associate professor of medicine at Washington University in St. Louis. He succeeded Roger Sylvester Morris, who had been recruited to St. Louis from Baltimore, where he had been a pupil of Osler and Thayer, by

---

year she was appointed assistant superintendent of nurses at the new Hospital of the Rockefeller Institute in New York. She still occupied that position as late as May 1924. She was decorated by the French Government for her war work during World War I. She died in July 1936.

[4] Among Robinson's published papers while in New York were the following: With George Draper: "Studies With the Electrocardiograph on the Action of the Vagus Nerve on the Human Heart: I. The Effect of Mechanical Stimulation of the Vagus Nerve; and "Studies With the Electrocardiograph on the Action of the Vagus Nerve on the Human Heart: II. The Effects of Vagus Stimulation on the Hearts of Children With Chronic Valvular Disease."

There were four papers which Robinson published alone: (1) "A Study With the Electrocardiograph of the Mode of Death of the Human Heart" in which he recorded ventricular fibrillation; (2) "The Influence of the Vagus Nerves on the Faradized Auricles in the Dog's Heart;" (3) "The Relation of the Auricular Activity Following Faradization of the Dog's Auricle to Abnormal Auricular Activity in Man;" and (4) "The Influence of the Vagus Nerves Upon Conduction Between Auricles and Ventricles in the Dog During Auricular Fibrillation."

With John Auer: "Disturbances of the Heart Beat in the Dog Caused by Serum Anaphylaxis" (1913).

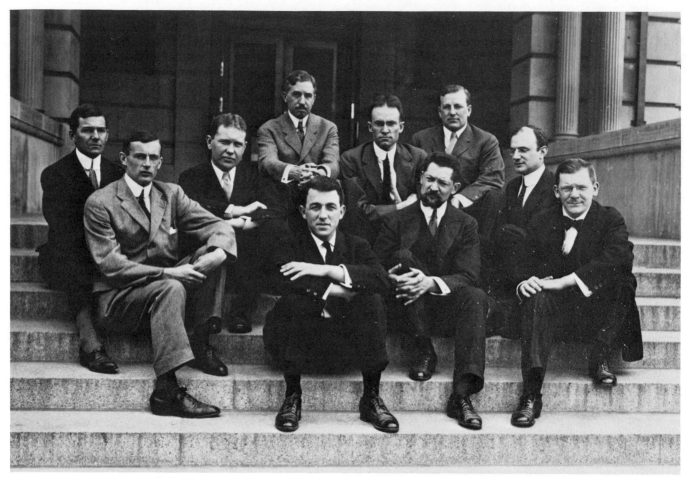

Fig 4.   The first resident staff of the Hospital of the Rockefeller Institute for Medical Research (1912). (Left to right, A. R. Dochez, A. Ellis, F. W. Peabody, Rufus Cole, H. Marks, G. Draper, F. Medigreceanu, G. Canby Robinson, H. F. Swift, F. McCrudden).
Reproduced with permission of the Rockefeller University Archives.

George Dock. Morris arrived at Washington University in 1911, after spending two summers in the clinic of Friedrich von Müller in Munich and serving for a short time as associate in medicine at Johns Hopkins. He left St. Louis in 1912 to become director of medicine at the Clifton Springs Sanatorium in New York.

Robinson had had essentially no teaching experience so that he learned, so to speak, by being thrown into water and told to swim. He had prepared himself during the previous summer to teach the course in clinical chemistry and microscopy, a subject in which his predecessor had become particularly proficient during his stay in the clinical laboratory in Baltimore under Thomas Boggs. This was an important course for the third year students since it was aimed at giving them the practical knowledge for making the laboratory examinations of blood, excreta, and other specimens of value in clinical diagnosis. Robinson also had responsibility for the diagnostic laboratory of the hospital medical service and instructed students in the laboratory work connected with their ward patients. As associate physician to the hospital, he took a small part in the care of ward patients and in the teaching of the fourth year students who served as clinical clerks. He was also in charge of the

medical outpatient clinic and of the teaching of clinical medicine to third year students during their assignments there.

During the spring trimester, after the laboratory course was completed, Robinson conducted the course in physical diagnosis for second year students, introducing them to the methods of examining patients. He had been strongly impressed by his experience under Osler of the importance of teaching students at the beginning of their contact with patients to develop their senses of seeing, feeling and hearing as carefully and methodically as possible.

Besides this extensive teaching responsibility, Robinson was to give an elective course in electrocardiography for undergraduates and graduate students. The medical department had purchased an Edelmann string galvanometer two years previously. It had been set up by J. S. Brotherhood, resident physician during 1910–11, but had been stored after Brotherhood's departure. After many hours of work Robinson was able to restore it to an operational state and to organize an electrocardiographic service.

Robinson took a special interest in organizing the laboratories of the medical department which were on the second floor of the building housing the dispensaries and the department of pathology and bacteriology. Here were laboratories for chemical, bacteriological and physiological research, closely related both to the patients and to the teaching laboratory of clinical chemistry and microscopy. Robinson was particularly concerned with the physiological division, where he continued his studies of the heart. The electrocardiograph was reassembled and various members of the resident staff worked with him on special cardiac problems: Hugh McCullough, who later had an outstanding career in pediatrics in St. Louis and Chicago; Drew Luten, who continued for many years as one of the leading teachers of the school; Joseph E. Bredeck, who later served as the Commissioner of Health in St. Louis; Fred J. Hodges, who became professor of radiology at the University of Michigan and then at Chicago; and George R. Herrmann, who became professor of medicine at the University of Texas after a period with Frank Wilson at Michigan. Robinson's outstanding associate was Frank N. Wilson who was appointed an instructor in medicine in 1916. Later, as a professor at the University of Michigan, Wilson became a national leader in electrocardiography, being the first to develop the precordial lead.

In 1914 the General Education Board made a grant to Washington University to establish medicine, surgery and pediatrics on a full-time basis. The plan was put into effect on July 1, 1916 with George Dock as full-time professor of medicine, Fred T. Murphy, professor of surgery, and William McKim Marriott, who had been recruited from Johns Hopkins, professor of pediatrics. Robinson became part of this full-time plan.

Robinson conducted a good deal of research while he was at Washington University. During 1915–16 he published six papers, three of which were clinical papers dealing with auricular fibrillation. One study concerned the action of the vagi on the heart in paroxysmal tachycardia. Another, published in the *Journal of Experimental Medicine*, was entitled "The Influence of the Vagus Nerves Upon Conduction Between Auricles and Ventricles in the Dog During Auricular Fibrillation." In 1916 he reported on "The Relation of Changes in the Form of the Ventricular Complex of the Electrocardiogram to Functional Changes in the Heart" and with S. Simon in 1917 published a paper on "Recurrent Transient Complete Heart Block" in the *Journal of the Missouri Medical Association*. Also in 1917 Robinson and J. F. Bredeck wrote two papers on ventricular fibrillation in man with cardiac recovery in which they were the first to report syncopal attacks in connection with bouts of ventricular fibrillation (see footnote 1). The following year he discussed the heart in diphtheria, and, with Frank N. Wilson, described two cases of heart block showing unusual features and reported a quantitative study on the effects of digitalis on the heart of the cat. Robinson published several other papers concerned with cardiac arrhythmias.

During World War I, Robinson was active in efforts to provide for rehabilitation of physically handicapped soldiers. He became interested in this area as a result of his deep concern with medical social service and he served on the first area committee of the Federal Board for Vocational Education, the initial governmental effort to rehabilitate disabled veterans. He also joined a group to organize and operate the St. Louis Placement Bureau for Handicapped Men headed by Mrs. Sydney I. Schwab, whose husband, the professor of neurology in the medical school, had developed a successful service for psychoneurotic soldiers overseas. In an effort to make this problem more generally known to and appreciated by the medical profession Robinson presented a paper at the annual meeting of the Missouri Medical Association in May 1918.[5] The development of occupational therapy as a phase of the rehabilitation program was one of Robinson's primary interests during the war years. Under the guidance of a committee made up of the medical faculty, the social service department at Washington University, and the St. Louis Junior League which financed the project, a security workshop was established at the Barnes Hospital. As a result of this the Missouri Occupational Therapy Association was formed to develop a school where occupational therapists could be trained for work in a number of St. Louis hospitals. In May 1919 Robinson attended the International Conference for the Disabled in New York where he presented a paper on occupational therapy in civilian hospitals, giving an account of the various rehabilitation projects in the St. Louis area.

Robinson served temporarily as dean of the Washington University School of Medicine while Philip A. Shaffer, who had succeeded Eugene L. Opie as dean in 1915, was serving in the Army during World War I. After Shaffer's return from his tour of duty, however, he asked to be relieved of the deanship and Robinson was appointed to the position. During his tenure, pharmacology, which had not been an independent department, was left without a head when Dennis Jackson was called to the University of Cincinnati in 1919 as professor of pharmacology. An appeal to the General Education Board resulted in a grant of $150,000 to establish an independent department and Mr. Edward Mallinckrodt generously contributed $150,000 in matching funds. The department was designated as the Edward Mallinckrodt Department of Pharmacology and E. Kennerly Marshall, Jr. was appointed professor in 1919. Marshall had a thorough training in chemistry, and held both the Ph.D. and M.D. degrees from Johns Hopkins where he was associate professor of pharmacology under John J. Abel. Also during this time, Evarts A. Graham was appointed a full-time professor of surgery.

By the fall of 1919 the University was back on its normal operating level after the hectic days of World War I. Robinson was able to concentrate more fully on his administrative duties as well as to participate in the care of patients. He found time to study the effects of

[5] Robinson, G. C.: The responsibility of the medical profession to the crippled soldier. J. Missouri Med. Assoc., 15: 250, 1918. Robinson, G. C.: The responsibility of the profession toward the disabled soldier. J. Kansas Med. Soc., 18: 185, 1918.

digitalis in patients as well as in the laboratory. However, he was soon faced with another major decision when he received an offer from the Vanderbilt University to direct the reorganization of its medical school. He resigned from Washington University to accept this challenge on July 1, 1920.

After Robinson's acceptance of the position at Vanderbilt Medical School, it was evident that several years would be required to design and build a new plant and that the reorganization of the faculty should wait until progress had been made in planning the facility.[6] The nearly four years that this process took, Robinson spent working at Johns Hopkins. However, he made frequent trips to Nashville to discuss plans with the architects and with Chancellor Kirkland of Vanderbilt University.

PROFESSOR, PRO TEMPORE, AT JOHNS HOPKINS

When he returned to Baltimore in the fall of 1920, Robinson began some studies on the blood gases in the full-time chemical research division in the department of medicine, which was at that time directed by Walter W. Palmer. Robinson also took part in establishing the *Journal of Clinical Investigation*, serving as editor-in-chief for the first few years after its inception.

After the death of Theodore C. Janeway in 1917, William S. Thayer, who had been Osler's right-hand man since the opening of the medical school, accepted the professorship. However, Thayer did not assume his active duties until 1919; in the interim he served on a Red Cross mission to investigate typhus fever in Poland and also served as chief medical consultant of the American Expeditionary Forces in France with the rank of Brigadier General. During the war, the full-time system was held in abeyance and the medical department was ably directed by Louis Hamman. On his return, Thayer gathered a promising group of younger men active in medical research, including Walter W. Palmer and Alphonse R. Dochez, who directed the chemical and biological laboratories, respectively. Edward F. Carter was in charge of the physiological laboratory and Allen K. Krause, who was an associate professor, was a leader in research in tuberculosis.

The younger men in the department of medicine under Thayer included Arthur L. Bloomfield, who had been resident in medicine and was later to become professor at Stanford; Dana W. Atchley, a Johns Hopkins graduate who became a professor at Columbia; Robert F. Loeb who was to become famous for his studies on the adrenal glands; William S. Ladd; Francis R. Dieuaide;

[6] Only one new appointment had been made, that of John P. Peters as associate professor of medicine. Peters accepted the appointment with the understanding that he would be given leave of absence from Vanderbilt, on salary, to spend a year in the Rockefeller Institute Hospital where he worked during 1920–21 with Donald D. Van Slyke. During that period he met Francis Blake, who was soon to become head of medicine at Yale. Peters was offered a position at New Haven which he accepted before the facilities at Vanderbilt were finished.

and Hugh J. Morgan who later became professor of medicine at Vanderbilt. There was also a distinguished group of part-time physicians in the department who participated actively in the teaching and patient care responsibilities, including Lewellys F. Barker, Thomas B. Futcher, Thomas R. Brown, Louis P. Hamburger, Thomas R. Boggs, Louis Hamman and Charles R. Austrian. However, there was deep antagonism which divided the younger men into the so-called research and clinical groups. It was a situation that disturbed Thayer greatly and one which he had great difficulty in coping with. The department was deeply shaken in the spring of 1921 when Thayer resigned saying that he did not enjoy his administrative duties and wished to make way for the appointment of Walter W. Palmer to whom the professorship was then offered. Palmer was at that time receiving offers from all over the country and he finally accepted the professorship at the College of Physicians and Surgeons at Columbia. When he left for New York, he took with him Dochez, Atchley, Loeb and Ladd. At the same time, Verne R. Mason and Henry M. Thomas, Jr. retired from the house staff to enter practice and Hugh J. Morgan accepted an appointment on the staff of the Rockefeller Institute Hospital. Thus, the department lost its major core.

A search committee for a new professor was organized. In the minutes of the Advisory Board of the Medical Faculty of the Johns Hopkins University School of Medicine for June 17, 1921, the following note appeared:

> Professorship of Medicine.
> On behalf of the committee appointed to consider the professorship of medicine Dr. Welch reported that it seemed inadvisable to appoint a professor at this time as the chances of obtaining a desirable man would be much greater next year. He then recommended that Dr. G. Canby Robinson, professor of medicine at Vanderbilt University, be borrowed from that institution and asked to serve as acting head of the department for the coming year, with the understanding that the regular incumbent would be appointed before the expiration of that period. After some discussion, the report was accepted.
> On motion, Dr. Welch, the superintendent of the hospital and the dean of the medical school were empowered to appoint an advisory committee for the department of medicine after consultation with the acting head of that department.

When Robinson assumed his duties as acting head on July 1, 1921, only Carter and Krause were left of the associate professors and in addition Henry S. Willis who worked with Krause in the tuberculosis section and Clyde G. Guthrie who was in charge of clinical pathology. Clearly, Robinson's first task was to replenish the ranks in his department. He recruited Alan M. Chesney from Washington University to be head of the biological division. Chesney, a Johns Hopkins graduate and former member of the resident staff of The Johns Hopkins Hospital, had had an excellent training in bacteriology at the Hospital of the Rockefeller Institute; he later became dean at Johns Hopkins. Robinson appointed William S. McCann to head the chemical division. McCann had been

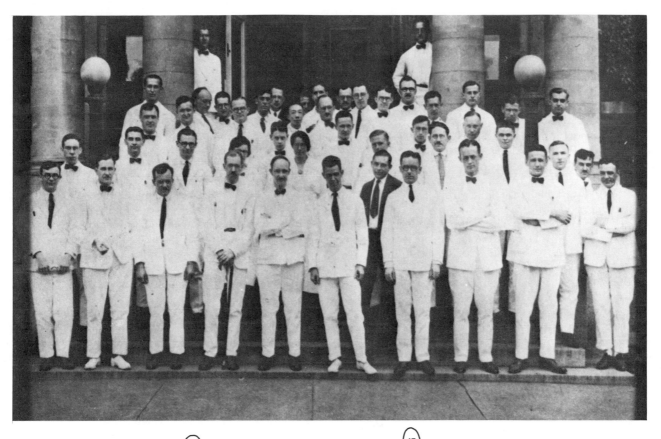

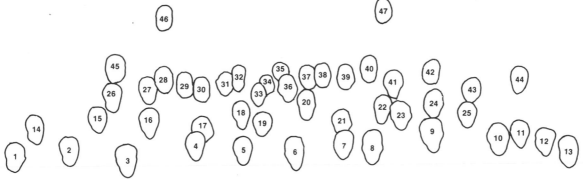

1. B. D. Lewin	17. Helen Vincent	33. Ko-chi Sun
2. Jay McLean	18. H. L. Higgins	34. W. P. Sadler
3. Horace Stewart	19. K. Dodd	35. Larry Kubie
4. C. S. Burwell	20. Tom Gay	36. Isaac Y. Olch
5. Emile Holman	21. A. R. Felty	37. Grant Ward
6. F. H. Cathrall	22. E. N. Van Dyke	38. H. M. Tiebout
7. Nathan Herman	23. H. Casparis	39. Deryl Hart
8. Leo Brady	24. J. H. Kite	40. Dan Eagle
9. R. K. Ghormley	25. David Smith	41. Bill Sisson
10. Frank Boone	26. Dorsey Brannon	42. Monty Firor
11. W. W. Gray	27. Fred Allen	43. Wm. Rienhoff
12. Karl Schlaepfer	28. Cleon Mason	44. Fritz Reichert
13. R. Roger Hannon	29. M. M. Zinninger	45. Geo. Gardner
14. A. S. Warinner	30. J. P. Molloy, Jr.	46. P. B. MacCready
15. A. A. Weech	31. Trevor Owen	47. E. C. Andrus
16. Harry Haggart	32. R. G. Craig	

Fig 5.   The resident staff of The Johns Hopkins Hospital, 1921–22. Sidney Burwell was the medical resident during Robinson's year as professor. This was the first year that the hospital furnished white uniforms to the residents.
From the Alan M. Chesney Medical Archives, The Johns Hopkins Medical Institutions.

working at Cornell Medical College in the Russell Sage Institute (in New York) where he had obtained excellent training under Graham Lusk and Eugene DuBois. An important problem was the appointment of the resident physician. There was no one in Baltimore at the time who had had sufficient experience to fill this position, but no one had ever been brought in from the outside. On the recommendation of Roger Lee and Paul D. White of Harvard, the position was offered to C. Sidney Burwell, a Harvard graduate who had trained at the Massachusetts General Hospital and who had just returned from a Red Cross mission to Latvia. This proved to be an outstanding choice as Burwell had excellent clinical training, fine clinical judgment, and an appealing sense of humor. Burwell later joined the faculty of Vanderbilt when Robinson returned there to take up his position as professor of medicine. The house staff under Burwell was organized with five assistant residents and four interns from the class of 1921. The assistant resident physicians were Robert R. Hannon, Francis R. Dieuaide, Nathan B. Herman and A. B. Hodges. The house medical officers included E. C. Andrus, Trevor Owen, William H. Resnick and Richard W. TeLinde (Fig 5). Krause, Carter, Guthrie and Chesney formed the group of full-time associate professors and Guthrie was made the director of the outpatient department in charge of teaching third year students. McCann became a full-time assistant professor. In addition there were three instructors: Henry S. Willis, C. Sidney Burwell and John G. Huck; and four fellows: Harold J. Stewart, who later became professor of medicine at Cornell and an outstanding cardiologist, was Bingham Fellow in Medicine; Edward A. Greenspon was a May Fellow in Medical Research; Alfred C. Kolls was also a fellow in research; and David M. Schulman was Charlton Fellow in Medical Research. Other members of the staff of medicine during Robinson's tenure in 1921 who later became outstanding in the annals of The Johns Hopkins School of Medicine were: Frank R. Smith, Paul W. Clough, and Walter A. Baetjer, associates in clinical medicine; and Arthur L. Bloomfield, Albert Keidel, Sidney R. Miller, Eveleth W. Bridgman and Thomas P. Sprunt, associates in medicine. Among the part-time instructors were J. Hall Pleasants, J. Albert Chatard, Harry Lee Smith, Samuel Wolman, John T. King, Jr., John H. King, Mary A. Hodge, Edward V. Coolahan, Martin F. Sloan, Ernest L. Zimmerman, Harry M. Robinson, Eugene J. Leopold, Ernest H. Gaither, J. Earle Moore, Henry M. Thomas, Jr., Jacob Cohen and Leslie N. Gay.

During that year Robinson succeeded in enlisting the cooperation of the departmental staff composed of some of his own teachers, a number of his contemporaries and classmates, as well as a significant group of younger men. Their desire to strengthen the medical department and their affection and sentiment for the medical school and hospital worked together as cohesive forces. This resulted in a strengthening of the department which had been brought close to chaos and probably salvaged the full-time plan. It was certainly excellent on-the-job training for Robinson as he had in Baltimore the opportunity to teach and conduct clinics, to administer a

department, to gain experience in choosing men and in coordinating their work, and to serve on the Advisory Board of the medical school and of the hospital, learning from the inside just how the Johns Hopkins University School of Medicine was operated.[7]

In addition to his formidable administrative tasks at Hopkins, Robinson also produced worthwhile research. As professor pro tem, he continued his work on the gaseous content of the blood which he had begun the previous year under Walter Palmer. He was assisted by his resident physician, C. Sidney Burwell, with whom he worked later after Burwell joined the staff in Nashville. They published several papers together, the first being on a method for the determination of the amount of oxygen and carbon dioxide in the mixed venous blood of man. The second paper was entitled "The Gaseous Content of the Blood and the Output of the Heart in Normal Resting Adults." In 1923 Burwell and Robinson presented a paper before the American Society for Clinical Investigation entitled "The Gases of the Mixed Venous Blood." There were other papers published by Robinson during his Baltimore period including one which appeared in the *Social Service Quarterly* in January 1922 entitled "The Influence of Social Service in the Hospital." He wrote a

---

[7] John B. Youmans,† who served as a fellow in medicine (neurology), has recalled the atmosphere in the Department of Medicine during Robinson's tenure: "My opinion of Dr. Robinson's performance during the time I was there was and remains highly favorable. When I arrived I found a feeling of refreshing change in the department, the school and the hospital. A new interest, a new anticipation of important and helpful changes, a sense of new direction and leadership and an eagerness to get on with new programs. Instead of a 'holding operation,' there was an advance to a new ground.

"Dr. Robinson showed a continual interest in the work of the individual members of the staff, at least the younger ones, and I suppose of the more senior ones as well. He kept informed of their research and other interests. He introduced weekly meetings of the staff of the department at which records of patients discharged (or who died) during the week were reviewed. The attendance included the house officers, some more senior faculty, and, of note, the social worker assigned to the department. The assignment of the social worker impressed me after my experience at the Massachusetts General Hospital.

"I do not remember any contact with social service when I was a student at Hopkins. Dr. Robinson was interested in enlarging and improving the neurological division. He proposed a position involving neurology, psychiatry and pathology and asked me to consider the position. For various reasons I declined. It was later filled by Dr. Frank Ford.

"As regards my research, I remember no specific grant for material, supplies or equipment. I worked with Dr. Kolls in pharmacology and we used the equipment and supplies of that department." (Youmans, J. B. and Kolls, A. C.: Quantitative studies with arsphenamine: I. Colorometric method for the estimation of arsphenamine in blood and tissues. Johns Hopkins Hosp. Bull., 34: 149, 1923; II. Distribution and excretion after intravenous injection. Ibid, p. 181.)

† John B. Youmans, personal communication, May 3, 1978.

At the end of his year in neurology, Youmans joined the faculty at the University of Michigan School of Medicine and later served again under Robinson at Vanderbilt.

monograph on "The Therapeutic Use of Digitalis" which was published as the first article in the new journal *Medicine*, just established under the editorship of David L. Edsall and John Howland. In addition he took part in a symposium at a meeting of the Southern Medical Association and his talk there entitled "The Use of Full-time Teachers in Clinical Medicine" was later published in the *Southern Medical Journal*.

VANDERBILT MEDICAL SCHOOL AND HOSPITAL

By June 1922 the basic work in designing the new Vanderbilt Medical School and Hospital had been completed. Since it would take three years to construct the plant, Robinson went abroad to study hospitals and medical schools and to gather ideas about medical education in other countries. In Denmark he was especially attracted by the arrangements in the university hospitals. Here he saw beds for ward patients divided into groups of four while still retaining a large number in one administrative unit. This plan he felt had clear advantages over the long open wards which were then in general use in the United States. This type of arrangement was incorporated in the new Vanderbilt facilities and eventually became a new feature of far-reaching influence on hospital design in this country.

During the first half of 1923 the building plans were completed and groundbreaking ceremonies were held on October 22, 1923. No complete description can be given of the complex structure that for the first time in this country assembled under one roof the departmental laboratories and a teaching hospital of a medical school. However, it would be worthwhile to discuss some of the features of the plant that made possible the implementation of certain principles of medical education. The medical school was located on the main campus of the university so that it could benefit from the general cultural atmosphere of the university and the members of the faculty would be able to cooperate with the basic departments of chemistry, biology, physics and so forth in education and research. A new educational feature was the provision of space and facilities for research in the clinical departments, so that investigations related to the study of patients could be closely correlated with the preclinical departments. In order to foster research that would not be confined to a single department, thought was given to correlating the teaching and research of the laboratory and the clinical departments. In the department of medicine, for example, the laboratory of clinical bacteriology adjoined the department of bacteriology; the laboratories of medical chemistry and physiology led into the departments of biochemistry, pharmacology and physiology; and the laboratory of surgery was next to the departments of anatomy and pathology. These special arrangements were designed to break down barriers between departments so that the influence of the medical sciences might be felt constantly by the clinical staff and students throughout their course and the knowledge and training gained in the laboratories would be carried into medical practice. It was hoped that this arrangement would serve also to keep laboratory teachers aware that the ultimate aim of medical education is the application of their sciences to the practice of medicine.

The architectural design and the engineering details were carried out with understanding by the architect, Henry R. Shepley. His work at Vanderbilt was the beginning of other important contributions to medical school and hospital design which culminated some eight years later in the outstanding buildings for that era of the New York Hospital and Cornell Medical College.

The full-time faculty members in the clinical departments were not formally restricted as to remuneration from private practice, the available funds being insufficient to allow higher salaries for the professors of medicine and surgery than for the professors in the laboratory departments. There was an understanding, however, that those receiving full university salaries would confine their practice to Vanderbilt University Hospital. The members of the faculty continuing in private practice were designated by the term *clinical* in the titles of their appointment. The arrangement for the full-time staff operated successfully, as those so appointed were taken up so fully with their teaching, research and administrative functions that none of them, at least in the early years, had any interest in outside medical practice, and no rivalry ever existed between those in practice and those giving their full time to the university.

Robinson was particularly fortunate in having Sidney Burwell and Hugh Morgan as the two associate professors of medicine; both were well trained not only in the art and science of medicine and teaching, but also in research. No better person could have been picked to head the initial house staff than Tinsley Harrison, a virtual dynamo both in teaching and in research. Two years later John B. Youmans, an unusually able administrator and physician, was added to the staff, and became director of the outpatient service in charge of the teaching there. The research laboratories of the medical department consisted of the physiological division under Burwell, the infectious disease division under Morgan and the chemical division under Harrison (thus showing the influence of Barker's arrangement which he initiated at Johns Hopkins in 1905). Each hospital assistant resident devoted half of his time to one of the laboratories, a pattern which Cole had established at the Hospital of the Rockefeller Institute. This plan of organization attracted excellent young men to the hospital staff, as it afforded opportunities for training in clinical medicine and in research which were at that time rarely available in the South or, for that matter, in any other part of the country. Studies were conducted on the mechanism of heart failure and on the action of drugs on the output of the heart, observations being made on patients, and, with the cooperation of the surgical department, on experimental animals. Problems of the physiology of the blood were studied in cooperation with the department of anatomy; long-term studies on latent syphilis were ini-

tiated; and arthritis, thyroid disease and other metabolic disorders were also investigated.

Robinson published very little while in Nashville, undoubtedly owing to the pressures of his administrative duties. In 1926 there were two papers; one on "The Community Organization for Social Welfare" and another on "The Measurement of the Cardiac Output in Man and Its Variations." Two publications followed the next year: "The Disturbances of Cardiac Function Leading to Heart Failure" and the Jerome Cochran Lecture before the Alabama Medical Association which was entitled "Mechanism and Treatment of Heart Failure."

In 1928 Burwell and Robinson published a note on "The Cardiac Output of a Single Individual Observed over a Period of Five Years." In the following year there were three publications, the first entitled "A Case of Coronary Occlusion, Association with Ventricular Paroxysmal Tachycardia." The other two papers, which described the new developments at Vanderbilt, appeared in the Rockefeller Foundation publication, "Methods and Problems of Medical Education."

SOJOURN IN NEW YORK

An invitation to leave Vanderbilt was first presented to Robinson at the October 1925 meeting of the Association of American Medical Colleges when Walter Niles and John Hartwell of Cornell University Medical College outlined to him the plan for bringing the Cornell Medical College and the New York Hospital together. Robinson indicated that he did not want to leave Vanderbilt, but one year later he received a letter asking him to come to New York for a conference about the matter. He was again asked to undertake the direction of this new project and was informed that land had already been purchased adjacent to the Rockefeller Institute. After much soul searching, Robinson decided that he was being offered a great opportunity for which much of his previous experience had provided an unusual preparation. A great point in favor of his going was that the plans for the new plant were already being drawn by the architectural firm in Boston with which Henry R. Shepley, who had cooperated so effectively with Robinson in the design of the plant at Vanderbilt, was associated. In March 1927 Robinson accepted the directorship of the New York Hospital–Cornell Medical College Association with the understanding that he would remain at Vanderbilt for another year, cooperating in the architectural and other planning in New York as was needed.

The Cornell University Medical College was founded in 1898, its inception being the result of a disagreement which led part of the faculty of the New York University and Bellevue Hospital Medical College to resign and organize a new school. This group retained the interest and backing of Colonel Oliver Hazard Payne who had been a generous benefactor of the Bellevue School previously. Colonel Payne, an associate of John D. Rockefeller in the early days of the oil industry, was a wealthy bachelor who became interested in supporting medical education through his friends Louis A. Stimson and H. P. Loomis, who were part of the dissenting Bellevue group. In April 1898 the trustees of Cornell University accepted the offer of this group to form a medical college of the university which opened in the fall of 1898 with 245 students, most of whom had transferred from the New York University and Bellevue Hospital Medical College. It occupied a rented building on the Bellevue Hospital grounds and used the Loomis laboratory which had been given by Colonel Payne to the Bellevue School, and had been assigned by legal action to the dissenting group of the faculty, ultimately to become the property of Cornell University. Payne provided funds for the erection of a medical school building and in the fall of 1900 the college occupied its new quarters on First Avenue, between 27th and 28th Streets, opposite Bellevue Hospital.

During the first ten years of its existence only graduation from high school was required for admission to the medical college. But in 1908 admission was restricted to graduates of approved colleges and to college seniors who would receive a bachelor's degree after completion of the first year in the medical school. This change caused an immediate drop in enrollment, only 11 students being admitted. At about this time the faculty was strengthened and the laboratory teaching modernized by the appointment of a number of distinguished scholars as professors, including Robert A. Hatcher in pharmacology, Graham Lusk in physiology, Charles R. Stockard in anatomy, Stanley R. Benedict in biochemistry and William J. Elser in bacteriology and immunology. By 1918 most of the original faculty had retired. Walter L. Niles became dean and a number of new appointments were made that put the clinical departments under the control of younger men such as Lewis A. Conner as professor of medicine and Oscar M. Schloss as professor of pediatrics. By 1928 the college had become organically associated with the New York Hospital. The formal agreement signed by the officers of the hospital and the university in June 1927 was the culmination of negotiations carried on for several years. The agreement stipulated that the hospital would erect a new general hospital "with all the usual equipment and accessories including a suitable out-patient department, ample pathological and research laboratories, and other facilities as needed, and, on plans approved by representatives of the university, accommodations for the instruction of medical students." The university would be granted every facility for teaching and research within the hospital consistent with the welfare of patients. The university agreed to build, maintain, and conduct new medical college buildings as part of the combined program and to confer the degree of doctor of medicine only on students educated in accordance with the requirements of the Association. The agreement defined the joint undertakings by the hospital and the university which would continue their independent corporate existence and control. The work of the institutions was to be conducted under the New York Hospital–Cornell Medical College Association, directed by the joint administrative board composed of three governors of the hospital, three trustees or other representatives of the university, and a seventh member elected by the six appointed members.

The agreement specified that the functions of the board were to supervise the Association and to appoint a director. The director was to serve as the executive officer of the board and of the medical faculty, to act as dean of the medical college, and to represent the educational and research interests in the hospital. He was responsible for coordinating the work of the school with the activities of the hospital in such a way as to promote harmonious and effective cooperation in teaching, research and the care of patients.

The plans were developed without definite limitations being placed on the cost of construction and equipment. It was estimated that the contemplated plant, including land, buildings, and equipment, would cost $30 million. These estimates were made in the halcyon days of finance during the boom that preceded the stock market crash of October 1929.

Early in the planning process three principles were agreed upon. The first was that each department of the medical college and of the hospital should be as far as possible a self-contained institute or clinic incorporating all the facilities needed for its own use, and that these units should be correlated with one another so as to encourage natural cooperation and intellectual intercourse. The second principle was that facilities should be provided for a relatively small body of medical students and that extensive opportunities should be offered for research by the staff and by graduate students in order to cultivate the university spirit in all departments of the hospital and medical school. The third principle was that each clinical unit should provide space for the number of patients that teaching experience had shown to be the optimum for a well-conducted university clinic. The central hospital building was planned to contain wards that had 167 beds for medicine, 292 for surgery and the surgical specialties, 100 rooms for private medical and surgical patients as well as accommodations for 114 members of the resident staff.

It was decided that each division of the hospital would be headed by a chief of service who would also be the professor and head of the department in the medical school. Appointments were made with the understanding that the heads of all major departments would give their full time to the hospital and medical college without financial dependence on private practice. Eugene F. DuBois was appointed professor of medicine and physician-in-chief of the hospital and Oscar M. Schloss was appointed professor of pediatrics and pediatrician-in-chief. DuBois, a well-trained and scholarly physician entirely devoted to the academic aspects of medicine, was the director of the large medical service in the Cornell division of Bellevue Hospital. He had been an associate professor at Cornell since 1919 and had served since 1913 as medical director of the Russell Sage Institute of Pathology which had sponsored medical research in the field of metabolism. With DuBois's appointment to the New York Hospital, the Russell Sage Institute was transferred to a specially designed laboratory in the new hospital's medical clinic.

George J. Heuer, who had graduated from Johns

Hopkins in 1907 and had had extensive training under William S. Halsted, was called from the University of Cincinnati, where he had developed a splendid surgical department during his ten years as professor of surgery, to head the new department of surgery. The professorship of obstetrics and gynecology was filled by Henricus J. Stander who was associate professor in J. Whitridge Williams's department at Johns Hopkins. Stander had studied at Harvard where he conducted research in the chemistry of substances derived from tar and invented a process which led to a well-paying position in a subsidiary firm of the DuPont Company located in the Southwest. He obtained an M.S. degree in 1916 at the University of Arizona and accumulated enough money to enable him to enter Yale to study medicine. He received his medical degree in 1921, interned at the New Haven Hospital, and in 1922 went to Johns Hopkins to join the staff of the department of obstetrics. In 1931 William S. Ladd was appointed associate dean of the medical college. He was a Columbia graduate and was in its department of medicine when appointed to Cornell. He had served on the Johns Hopkins medical staff with Walter W. Palmer and had gone to New York when Palmer left Baltimore to become head of medicine at the College of Physicians and Surgeons.

By June 1931 the 13 professors had been appointed as heads of departments of the medical college to take up their full duties in the fall of 1932. During that year consideration was given to the organization of the hospital staff around this core of full-time teachers, assisted by a large group of physicians and surgeons in private practice who would devote part of their time to the hospital and medical school. The organization of the large resident staff posed a problem for the chiefs of the services as the graded residency system (interns, assistant residents, and resident physicians and surgeons) was to be introduced. This system, originated by Osler at Johns Hopkins, was then generally recognized as the best method of training leaders in medicine.

Miss Anna D. Wolf was appointed director of nursing effective October 1, 1931, allowing her nearly a year to organize the nursing school and nursing service of the hospital. Miss Wolf had an exceptional educational record, having graduated from The Johns Hopkins School of Nursing and holding a master's degree from Columbia University. After serving on the Johns Hopkins staff, she was appointed superintendent of nursing in 1919 at the Peking Union Medical College in China where she organized a nursing service and a school of nursing. In 1926 she was appointed as associate professor and director of nursing at the University of Chicago Clinic; here she developed courses in teaching and administration for nurses. In December 1932 the entrance requirements of the School of Nursing at Cornell was increased to two years of college work and the quality of the curriculum was elevated in order to make a graduate eligible for a bachelor's degree from the college in which she had completed two years of study. However, as a result of the financial depression, these advanced requirements proved impractical and in 1934 it was necessary to re-

duce the admission requirements to high school graduation. It was not until 1942, two years after Miss Wolf had
resigned to become the director of nursing at Johns Hopkins, that the original plan of the university school was
put into effect.

One can see in all of these steps that were taken in
putting together this great medical center in New York
that the experience which Canby Robinson had obtained
in his peripatetic career as a medical educator was bearing fruit. Unfortunately, some of his plans were curtailed
when the unprecedented financial collapse ensued. As a
means of cutting the cost of operating the hospital, the
number of beds to be put into use was reduced by about
300 and the equipment for a number of floors was omitted. Restrictions had to be placed on departmental programs and a general feeling of insecurity pervaded the
hospital as it did elsewhere during the early days of the
depression. It was an unfortunate event to occur during
the launching of this great medical project for which
many people had such high hopes and expectations. In
this setting in which more and more decisions had to be
made to impose financial restrictions, Robinson's position as director became untenable. Arrangements were
made for his retirement on October 1, 1934.

In assessing the deterioration which occurred at
the medical center during the depression, Robinson believed that one of the most important factors was the
weakness in the original plan of administration of the
New York Hospital–Cornell Medical College Association. The top of the organization failed to hold together
under the strain of a serious financial crisis because authority and responsibility for the Association as a whole
were not centralized. The director of the Association was
responsible for the educational activities and the administration of the medical college, but had no authority
or responsibility for the administration of the hospital
and took no part in its financial operations. The two corporate bodies, the hospital and the university, delegated
authority to the joint administrative board, of which the
director was not a member.

Within a short time after his "retirement," Robinson was invited to serve for five months as visiting professor of medicine at the Peking Union Medical College
during the leave of absence of Francis R. Dieuaide, who
was professor of medicine there. The opportunity came
at a most appropriate time for him, for it gave him the
chance to return to the teaching of bedside medicine and
to participate in the administrative and intellectual activities in a department of medicine.

THE SOCIAL ASPECTS OF MEDICINE

After Robinson's return from China in 1935, he decided to devote himself to the study of the social aspects
of medicine, a subject which had interested him for many
years as a result of his experience in a number of medical
centers. In all of these centers, he noted that the personal
and social problems of patients constituted an important
factor of illness which was being neglected to a large
degree, both in the care of hospital patients and in the

teaching of medical students. He was one of the first to
appreciate that the expansion of medical science had led
doctors to specialize to such an extent that interest in the
patient as a person had become submerged. It was his
belief that a systematic study was needed to demonstrate the validity of his concepts.

In an address before the Southern Medical Association in 1924 on the influence of environment on medical
education, Robinson had put forth a program of study:

> Problems in social diagnosis and social treatment are
> constantly before us in our hospitals and dispensaries,
> and for the sake of our students' training and our patients'
> welfare they should not be ignored. But in the com-
> plexities of hospital practice, replete as it is with scientific
> problems, is not the inner man submerged? Whose duty is
> it to understand the human problems which surround but
> are apart from disease? Who is to study with a true sym-
> pathy and friendliness the troubled spirit? We all know
> that the recovery of many patients can be hastened by
> clearing away mental doubt, by relieving worry that
> may be daily wearing down courage; and yet the busy
> physician, especially when rushed by many patients in
> the dispensary or when caring for large groups of patients
> in the wards of the hospital, usually cannot extract from
> each his or her special need beyond the immediate medi-
> cal problems.

Through the help of his former associate Alan M. Chesney, who was then dean of the Johns Hopkins University
School of Medicine, Robinson was able to begin working
on this program at Johns Hopkins.

In January 1936 he submitted a plan in which he
proposed that the medical school provide an opportunity
for the study of patients at the Johns Hopkins Hospital in
order to determine the nature and extent of their personal problems that were not receiving systematic attention in relation to their medical care. The study would be
concerned with emotional disturbances, social maladjustments, faulty physical and mental hygiene and
economic difficulties, and the relation of these problems
to the physical condition, family life, occupation, and
environment of the patients. The study would aim to determine the significance of these matters in medical care
and to devise methods best suited to reveal and solve
these personal problems. The plan was approved by the
Advisory Board of the Medical Faculty and by the Medical Board of the Hospital. Through the interest of Alan
Gregg, a small grant was obtained from the Rockefeller
Foundation to support the work for five months beginning January 1, 1936. After discussing the best method of
procedure with members of the hospital staff, Robinson
selected at random 10 patients from various clinics as a
trial run. Six of these 10 patients revealed personal problems that were related to their illness. The first patient
was a woman with elevated blood pressure, symptoms of
heart disease and increased thyroid activity of four
months' duration. She worked in the hospital laundry,
said that her work was a strain and that recently she
dreaded going to work each day. It was a simple matter
to look into her working conditions; they were found to
entail an emotional strain, as she was responsible for

four assistants, young girls who were not interested in their occupation and who amused themselves by annoying their older supervisor. It was arranged to have her work alone on the other side of the ironing machine, where only one person was required. A week after this change the patient returned to the clinic and said enthusiastically: "A miracle has happened. A big burden has been lifted from me." Her symptoms had disappeared and she remained well during the three years she was followed. She gained weight, was happy and cheerful, and a significant change in personality was noted, although there had been no reduction in blood pressure.

There were many others in whom similar problems were found. By the first of May the medical school authorities agreed that "the study of the accessory factors of health," as the program had been designated, should be continued for another year on an experimental basis so that the various aspects of the subject which had been revealed might be more fully explored, and sufficient material might be collected and written up to present definite evidence of the value of the work both to the members of the faculty and to the officers of the Rockefeller Foundation. It was also arranged that Robinson would initiate a teaching program in September 1936 as part of a previously adopted plan of instruction in preventive medicine. Robinson journeyed to Boston to discuss his proposed program with Ida M. Cannon, director of the social service department of the Massachusetts General Hospital who was a pioneer in medical social work. She showed much interest in the proposed study and arranged a leave of absence for a member of her staff, Josephine C. Barbour, to work with Robinson in Baltimore. Miss Barbour was a great help in the Johns Hopkins study and later had a distinguished career as Miss Cannon's successor as director of social service at the Massachusetts General Hospital.

Robinson's program is of interest because it was among the pioneer efforts in a modern medical clinic in which a physician gave his full time to the study of the social aspects of medicine. The first contact with the patient took place in a secluded office, after the record of his medical history, examination, and provisional diagnosis had been reviewed. The first objective was to establish an intimate doctor-patient relationship by explaining the significance of the medical findings. The patient was then encouraged to talk freely about his illness and his problems by allowing him the benefit of an interested and attentive listener who had plenty of time. He was asked to tell about his daily routine and habits, his work, his family and associates, and anything else that was on his mind. Special attention was given to obtaining a detailed account of the symptoms that brought him to the hospital in order to determine whether they could all be reasonably attributed to the disease revealed by his medical study or whether they were in whole or in part attributable to an emotional reaction. Nearly every patient was visited at home after the purpose of the visit had been explained and in many instances other members of the family were interviewed. The patient was sometimes visited at his place of work and information

was gathered from various social and public health agencies to which the patient was known. Other sources that might throw light on the problem were also sought. Information thus assembled was analyzed and interpreted to the patient as a means of giving him better insight into the nature of his illness and an understanding of the relation of emotional strain or unhygienic ways of living to his state of health.

The second problem was to plan a systematic study of the social aspects of medicine as a research project from which reliable conclusions could be drawn. It was decided to center the study on patients who were admitted to the general clinics of the medical outpatient department and who resided in the Eastern Health District, and to study all of them without selection until enough data were collected to allow analysis and statistical treatment.

The third problem was to organize teaching to correlate with the clinical work of the third year students. At that time one-third of the class, a group of about 25 students, was assigned in rotation to the general medical clinics of the outpatient department for a period of eight weeks. Two hours each week was allotted to the "study of the personal, social, and sanitary background of patients." The official announcement read as follows: "Each student during his time in the medical dispensary is assigned one or more patients admitted from the Eastern Health District for the study of their personal, social and sanitary background. By means of interviews, home visits, and information gained from public health and social service sources, the student learns all he can about the patient as an individual and presents his findings at weekly conferences attended by representatives of public health, clinical medicine, and social service. Public health, hygiene, occupational, social, and economic problems are discussed as presented by the study of the individual cases." Harry S. Mustard, administrator of the Eastern Health District, and Henry M. Thomas, Jr., chief physician of one of the medical clinics, were associated with Robinson in conducting this course.

This plan of teaching was continued for three years under the original conditions, the work being supported by the Rockefeller Foundation for two years and by the John and Mary R. Markle Foundation and the Josiah Macy, Jr. Foundation during the third year. In 1939 the university received a grant from the Rockefeller Foundation to support a new department of preventive medicine. The department, which was started in the fall of that year, was headed by Perrin H. Long as professor of preventive medicine. The teaching program Robinson had organized was continued as one of the courses in this department.

In a volume entitled *The Patient as a Person: A Study of the Social Aspects of Illness*, published by the Commonwealth Fund in 1939, Robinson recounted his case studies of 174 patients subjected to detailed analysis and statistical treatment. The analysis showed that in 124 patients, or 71 percent, adverse social conditions were a significant factor in medical care. Convincing evidence was furnished that a greater knowledge of the total individual was needed in hospital practice in order to improve medical care. This problem proved especially significant in a teaching hospital where students observed for the first time the methods and standards of medical practice and where concepts and sentiments were being implanted in young developing minds. The study indicated that there was a definite need for better development of medical social work and for the cultivation of social workers as close collaborators with physicians in hospital practice. An intimate relationship between doctor and patient was seen to be a fundamental factor in medical care and it was emphasized that something had been lost in this respect by the increasing specialization of doctors in university teaching hospitals. Besides demonstrating the value of giving greater consideration to the patient as a person, both in medical care and in teaching, the study furnished a useful background for further investigation of the social aspects of illness.

Robinson developed another study in the gastrointestinal clinic of The Johns Hopkins Hospital in collaboration with Moses Paulson, a member of the staff of that clinic who was particularly interested in the relation of gastrointestinal symptoms to emotional disturbances. Fifty patients routinely assigned to Paulson were investigated, and interviews, home visits and personality studies revealed that 38 patients, or 76 percent, had emotional disturbances which were the major cause of their illness. Nearly all of these patients responded favorably when given an understanding of the true nature of their illness and were persuaded to change their attitudes towards health. This systematic study clearly demonstrated the frequency with which emotional disturbances cause digestive complaints and the necessity of investigating the personal and social problems of these patients.

In a paper on "The Study of the Patient as a Whole as Training for Medical Practice," which Robinson presented in 1938, he stated that if medical students were to understand illness and its treatment in a broad sense, they had to be taught to consider the patient as a total individual and they had to learn to appreciate the significance of social and environmental problems as a part of medical care. Robinson was an important figure in expanding interest in this problem.

In 1941 Robinson was appointed director of the blood donor service of the American Red Cross. For his accomplishments in this service as well as for his other contributions to medicine, Robinson was awarded the Medal of Merit.

At the end of World War II, Robinson retired from the Johns Hopkins faculty and became executive secretary of the Maryland Tuberculosis Association. Characteristically he was instrumental in rebuilding the program for the care of tuberculosis patients in Maryland. During this period he was particularly interested in working out a project for the improvement of the study and teaching of tuberculosis in The Johns Hopkins University School of Medicine. When this project was formulated, the Association made an annual grant to support a faculty position, a social worker, and a secretary who would devote their full time to organizing the public health aspects of the care of tuberculosis patients in the wards and the outpatient department of the Johns Hopkins Hospital and to teaching in this field. Dr. Miriam E. Brailey headed the project; she had had experience in working with tuberculosis patients, and she stimulated much interest in the disease among the students and staff.

Thus Robinson contributed to many areas of medical research and practice. Perhaps his most important contributions, however, were in medical education. The following paragraph from a letter which Robinson wrote upon his retirement from the directorship of the New York Hospital–Cornell Medical College Association reveals Robinson's view of medical education which he worked so diligently to implant in the various institutions with which he was associated:

> From the very first day the student enters the Medical College he must be exposed to those qualities of mind and heart which will teach him how to act with sincerity, courage, independence, and goodwill toward his fellows of whatever rank. The standards of professional life are largely set by the examples which are placed before the students in their plastic and formative years, and every teacher in the medical college should carry constantly in his thoughts the realization that he has about him young people whose future lives he may profoundly influence. The future medical graduate has a world to face in which there are many temptations to lower professional and spiritual standards and each one should be equipped with an armor to enable him to resist these temptations. The greatest help that can be given him comes from the example of his teachers, who will be for years the moral and intellectual guides in his professional career.

ACKNOWLEDGMENTS

I am grateful to John B. Youmans for his personal comments, to Ms. Ruth Sternfeld for the photograph from the Rockefeller University Archives, to Carol Bocchini for her editorial assistance and to Patricia King for typing the manuscript.

REFERENCES

1. Burwell CS: George Canby Robinson, 1878–1960. Trans Assoc Am Physicians 74: 40, 1961

2. Burwell CS and Dieuaide FR: Clinical experience with quinidine. Arch Intern Med 31: 518, 1923

3. Burwell CS and Robinson GC: The gases of the mixed venous blood. Proc Am Soc Clin Invest, 1923

4. Burwell CS and Robinson GC: A method for the determination of the amount of oxygen and carbon dioxide in the mixed venous blood of man. J Clin Invest 1: 47, 1924

5. Burwell CS and Robinson GC: The gaseous content of the blood and the output of the heart in normal resting adults. J Clin Invest 1: 87, 1924

6. Burwell CS and Robinson GC: The cardiac output of a single individual observed over a period of five years. J Clin Invest 6: 247, 1928

7. Burwell CS and Robinson GC: A case of coronary occlusion, associated with ventricular paroxysmal tachycardia. Med Clin North Am 12: 1435, 1929

8. Erlanger J: On the physiology of heart block in mammals, with a special reference to the causation of Stokes–Adams disease. J Exp Med 7: 676, 1905

9. Erlanger J: Part II. On the physiology of heart block in the dog. J Exp Med 8: 8, 1906

10. Erlanger J: Part III. The relation of heart block to Stokes-Adams disease. J Exp Med 8: 32, 1906

11. Robinson GC: On a cyst originating from the ductus thyreoglossus. Bull Johns Hopkins Hosp 13: 81, 1902

12. Robinson GC: The relation between congenital malformations of the heart and acute endocarditis, with report of two cases. Bull Ayer Clin Lab, Penn Hosp 1(2): 45, 1905

13. Robinson GC: The role of the typhoid bacillus in the pulmonary complications of typhoid fever. J Infect Dis 2: 498, 1905

14. Robinson GC: Bacteriological findings in fifteen cases of epidemic cerebrospinal meningitis. Bull Ayer Clin Lab, Penn Hosp 1(3): 27, 1906

15. Robinson GC: Gumma of the heart from a case presenting the symptoms of Adams–Stokes' disease. Bull Ayer Clin Lab, Penn Hosp 1(4): 1, 1907

16. Robinson GC: The presence of tubercle bacilli in the spinal fluid in tuberculosis meningitis with a series of cases from the Ayer Clinical Laboratory of the Pennsylvania Hospital. Bull Ayer Clin Lab, Penn Hosp 1(4): 42, 1907

17. Robinson GC: Gallop rhythm of the heart. Am J Med Sci 135: 670, 1908

18. Robinson GC: Blood pressure in epidemic cerebrospinal meningitis. Arch Intern Med 5: 482, 1910

19. Robinson GC: A study with the electrocardiograph of the mode of death of the human heart. J Exp Med 16: 291, 1912

20. Robinson GC: The influence of the vagus nerves on the faradized auricles in the dog's heart. J Exp Med 17: 429, 1913

21. Robinson GC: The relation of the auricular activity following faradization of the dog's auricle to abnormal auricular activity in man. J Exp Med 18: 704, 1913

22. Robinson GC: The action of the vagi on the heart in paroxysmal tachycardia. Arch Intern Med 16: 967, 1915

23. Robinson GC: The relation of changes in the form of the ventricular complex of the electrocardiogram to functional changes in the heart. Arch Intern Med 18: 830, 1916

24. Robinson GC: Auricular fibrillation; its cause and its relation to ventricular activity. Int Clin 26 (s., ii): 43, 1916

25. Robinson GC: Transient auricular fibrillation, in a healthy man following hydrogen sulphid poisoning. JAMA 66: 1611, 1916

26. Robinson GC: The influence of the vagus nerves upon conduction between auricles and ventricles in the dog during auricular fibrillation. J Exp Med 24: 605, 1916

27. Robinson GC: A case of transient auricular fibrillation following hydrogen sulphid poisoning. J Missouri Med Assoc 13: 243, 1916

28. Robinson GC: The responsibility of the profession toward the disabled soldier. J Kansas Med Soc 18: 185, 1918

29. Robinson GC: The heart in diphtheria. J Missouri Med Assoc 15: 234, 1918

30. Robinson GC: The responsibility of the medical profession to the crippled soldier. J Missouri Med Assoc 15: 250, 1918

31. Robinson GC: The significance of abnormalities in the form of the electrocardiogram. Arch Intern Med 24: 422, 1919

32. Robinson GC: The rapidity and persistence of the action of digitalis on the heart. J Missouri Med Assoc 16: 248, 1919

33. Robinson GC: Occupational therapy in civilian hospitals. Mod Med 1: 159, 1919

34. Robinson GC: The rapidity and persistence of the action of digitalis on hearts during auricular fibrillation. Trans Assoc Am Physicians 34: 118, 1919

35. Robinson GC: The rapidity and persistence of the action of digitalis on heart showing auricular fibrillation. Am J Med Sci 159: 121, 1920

36. Robinson GC: Research in clinical medicine. J Am Med Assoc 74: 910, 1920

37. Robinson GC: The value of large single doses of digitalis in the treatment of heart disease. South Med J 13: 396, 1920

38. Robinson GC: Research in clinical medicine. Am Med Assoc Bull 14: 45, 1920–21

39. Robinson GC: The use of full-time teachers in clinical medicine. South Med J 15: 1009, 1922

40. Robinson GC: The measurement of the cardiac output in man and its variations. JAMA 87: 314, 1926

41. Robinson GC: The community organization for social welfare. Methodist Q Rev 53 (Series 3): 467, 1926

42. Robinson GC: The disturbances of cardiac function leading to heart failure. South Med J 20: 222, 1927

43. Robinson GC: Mechanism and treatment of heart failure. Trans Alabama Med Assoc 60: 245, 1927

44. Robinson GC: Vanderbilt University School of Medicine, History and General Description. In Methods and Problems of Medical Education, 13th Series, pp 1–14, 1929

45. Robinson GC: Vanderbilt University School of Medicine, Department of Medicine. In Methods and Problems of Medical Education, 13th Series, pp 83–92, 1929

46. Robinson GC: The influence of the past on the present and future of medicine. Bull Johns Hopkins Hosp 58: 65, 1936

47. Robinson GC: The study of the patient as a whole as training for medical practice. J Assoc Am Med Coll 14: 65, 1939

48. Robinson GC: The Patient as a Person: A Study of the Social Aspects of Illness. New York: Commonwealth Fund; London: H. Milford, Oxford University Press, 1939

49. Robinson GC: Adventures in Medical Education. Cambridge, Mass: Commonwealth Fund, Harvard University Press, 1957

50. Robinson GC and Draper G: Studies with the electrocardiograph on the action of the vagus nerve on the human heart. I. The effect of mechanical stimulation of the vagus nerve. J Exp Med 14: 217, 1911

51. Robinson GC and Draper G: Studies with the electrocardiograph on the action of the vagus nerve on the human heart. II. The effects of vagus stimulation on the hearts of children with chronic valvular disease. J Exp Med 15: 14, 1912

52. Robinson GC and Auer J: Disturbances of the heart-beat in the dog caused by serum anaphylaxis. J Exp Med 18: 556, 1913

53. Robinson GC and Bredeck JF: Ventricular fibrillation in man with cardiac recovery. Arch Intern Med 20: 725, 1917

54. Robinson GC and Bredeck JF: Ventricular fibrillation in man with cardiac recovery. Trans Assoc Am Physicians 32: 509, 1917

55. Robinson GC and Wilson FN: A quantitative study of the effect of digitalis on the heart of the cat. J Pharmacol Exp Ther 10: 491, 1917–18

56. Robinson GC and Herrmann GR: Paroxysmal tachycardia of ventricular origin and its relation to coronary thrombosis. Trans Assoc Am Physicians 35: 155, 1920

57. Robinson GC and Herrmann GR: Paroxysmal tachycardia of ventricular origin, and its relation to coronary occlusion. Heart 8: 59, 1920–21

58. Robinson GC et al.: Behavior of certain phosphorus compounds in normal and diabetic metabolism. JAMA 78: 1753, 1922

59. Robinson GC et al.: The therapeutic use of digitalis. Medicine 1: 1, 1922

60. Robinson GC et al.: The influence of social service in the hospital. Soc Ser Q January, 1922

61. Simon S and Robinson GC: Recurrent transient complete heart-block. J Missouri Med Assoc 14: 97, 1917

62. Wilson FN and Robinson GC: Heart-block. Two cases showing unusual features. Arch Intern Med 21: 166, 1918

18.
Clinical Investigation of Chronic Diseases: Its Successful Pursuit in an Outpatient Setting

With the great discoveries made during the first decade of the 20th century in relation to syphilis—transmission to animals, identification of the spirochete, the Wassermann test and Ehrlich's introduction of Salvarsan—the clinical and experimental aspects of this disease underwent a dramatic change. Knowledge directly applicable to treatment was gained by studies of immunity and the principles of arsenical therapy in animal models of the disease. In 1915 the Johns Hopkins Hospital made a major innovation by establishing a syphilis clinic where the disease could be studied clinically and experimentally. This led to more effective care of patients and to important new knowledge of the disease. With the discovery that penicillin was treponemicidal, the prospect of eliminating syphilis as a major disease problem seemed at hand. This did not eventuate, but in the early 1950s there was such a dramatic decline in the number of new cases that the syphilis clinic at Johns Hopkins was reorganized. The clinical and epidemiologic facilities that had been created for the study and management of this single disease were utilized to investigate other chronic diseases and finally to form the base for a pioneering program in medical genetics.

THE CREATION OF 'DEPARTMENT L'

In January 1913, the Honorable Phillips Lee Goldsborough, then Governor of the State of Maryland, appointed a vice commission consisting of 14 citizens of Maryland, with Dr. George Walker as chairman. This body conducted an investigation of prostitution in Baltimore and other cities. Part of the committee's five-volume report dealt with the incidence of venereal disease in prostitutes, and doubtless the results of this particular phase of the investigation led Walker to propose to the Medical Board of the Johns Hopkins Hospital that a special clinic be established in the outpatient department for the treatment of syphilis.

The discovery of the complement-fixation reaction by Wassermann, Neisser and Bruck in 1906 and of Salvarsan (arsphenamine) by Ehrlich and Hata 3 yr later had put powerful tools for the detection and treatment of syphilis in the hands of the medical profession, so the time was ripe for mounting a concerted attack upon the disease. It was decided to organize the syphilis clinic as a subdivision of the medical clinic. In 1915, the word syphilis was taboo so the clinic had to be camouflaged under a name that meant nothing to the layman in order

Reprinted from the *Journal of Chronic Diseases* **33**: 529, 1980.

to save the patients from embarrassment. The designation chosen was 'Department L', derived from *lues venerea*, one of the older names for the disease.

From 1889 until 1915, the particular clinic in which the patient was registered when discovered to have syphilis was where treatment was administered. Thus, if he had primary syphilis with a penile chancre, he would be treated in the urology clinic; if he had a cutaneous eruption he would be cared for in the dermatology clinic; and if he had tabes dorsalis, he would be registered in the neurology clinic.

There were two major reasons for establishing 'Department L'. First, it was believed desirable to bring together in one clinic all the patients with syphilis in order that the disease might be studied from beginning to end and not as a series of unrelated episodes. Second, it was thought that the study of the disease should be placed primarily in the hands of internists, whose interests were not bounded by those of any one specialty.

The first official mention of 'Department L' in the records of the Johns Hopkins Hospital appeared in the Director's Report for the year ending 31 January 1916:

"New departments have been opened, notably a Salvarsan clinic, known as Department L, and a dental clinic. Through the generosity of the Bureau of Social Hygiene of New York and Mr. John D. Rockefeller, Jr., funds were offered to the hospital which made possible the opening of a Salvarsan clinic in September (1915). The need of such clinics is acute, not solely for the purpose of individual treatment, but from the standpoint of the welfare of the community. The work of this department has increased rapidly and as soon as it is possible to get a sufficient number of men thoroughly trained for the work of the clinic, it is expected to undertake much more than the routine examination and treatment to which, because of the small staff, the work is now limited."

This was a modest prediction for the many contributions to medicine which were to come from the work done in this outpatient facility.

WALKER—THE FIRST DIRECTOR OF 'DEPARTMENT L'

Walker made many contributions to Maryland medicine and to Johns Hopkins (Fig. 1). Born in South Carolina on 27 July 1869, he attended South Carolina College at Columbia and received his M.D. from the University of Maryland School of Medicine in 1889. He practiced in South Carolina for 6 yr before taking an internship in surgery (1895–1896) at Johns Hopkins. He then studied in a number of German universities, in-

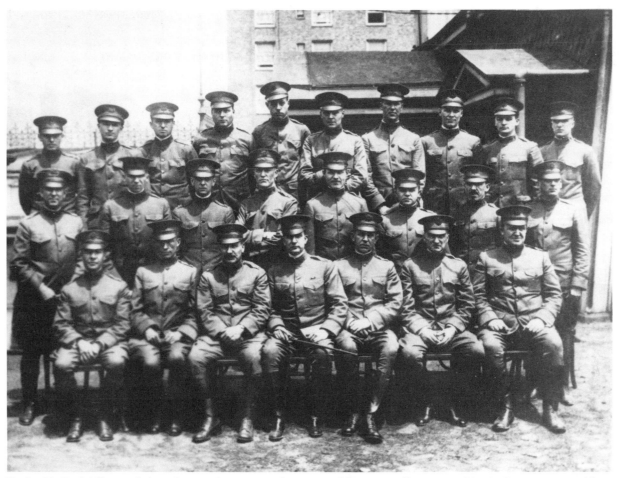

Fig 1. Medical Officers of The Johns Hopkins Hospital Unit—World War I. Walker is seated in the first row, second from the right (between Winford H. Smith and William S. Baer).
From the Alan M. Chesney Medical Archives, the Johns Hopkins Medical Institutions.

cluding those of Breslau, Leipzig and Berlin. On his return to Baltimore in 1898 he was made assistant in surgery in the outpatient department and 2 yr later became head of one of the surgical outpatient clinics. From 1907 to 1915, Walker held the title of Surgeon-in-Charge in the dispensary, and from March 1916 to September 1923 he was Assistant Visiting Surgeon in the hospital. He was associated with the Johns Hopkins School of Medicine from 1902 to 1916 as Instructor in Surgery (1902–1905) and Associate in Surgery (1905–1916).

When the U.S. entered World War I, Walker was made a member of the Advisory Commission of the Council of National Defense. He went to France with the Johns Hopkins unit in 1918. After 4 months with the unit, he joined Hugh H. Young, who was in charge of efforts to keep the American Army free of 'social' disease. Walker, who attained the rank of colonel, was given honors by the French government and the Distinguished Service Medal by the US. He was made Chief Urologist to the American Army after the Armistice.

Walker's scientific interests were related to the genitourinary system and, in later years, to the study of cancer. He contributed an excellent monograph on tuberculosis of the kidney entitled 'Studies in the experimental production of tuberculosis in the genitourinary organs', which was published in the *Johns Hopkins Hospital Reports*. Walker estabilshed a private laboratory for the study of cancer which he maintained with his own funds. He made a substantial gift to the university to establish a foundation for the study of cancer.

EARLY ORGANIZATION OF THE SYPHILIS CLINIC

Walker appointed Albert Keidel (Fig. 2) as his principal assistant in the syphilis clinic. Keidel was primarily responsible for the organization and daily operation of the clinic.

Born on 3 November 1877, Keidel was a graduate of the Johns Hopkins University (1899) and of its medical school (1903). He served on the Johns Hopkins staff as Assistant Surgeon (1913–1914), Instructor in Clinical Urology (1914–1915), Instructor in Clinical Medicine (1915–1918) and Associate in Clinical Medicine (1918–1922). He was appointed Associate Professor in 1922.

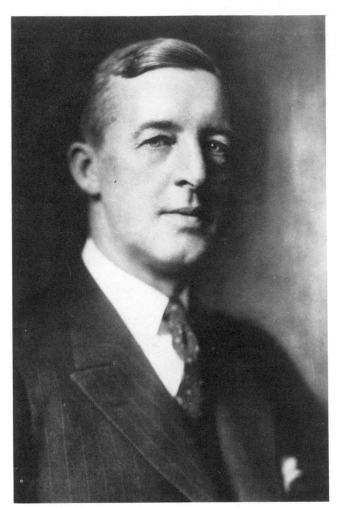

Fig 2.   Albert Keidel.
From the Alan M. Chesney Mecical Archives, the Johns Hopkins Medical Institutions.

Keidel was a pioneer in the study of syphilis in Baltimore, having introduced the Wassermann test shortly after its description in 1906 and having been the first to administer Salvarsan in Maryland (1909). In 1912, he and S. H. Hurwitz published a study entitled 'A comparison of normal and syphilitic extracts by means of the Wassermann and Epiphanin reactions'. They concluded that antibodies were present in the serum of syphilitic patients which were directed against some substance or substances found only in extracts of syphilitic tissue and that these antibodies were probably specific. At the time, there was much debate about the specificity of the Wassermann reaction. When the test was first published by Wassermann and his colleagues, the antigen was thought to be the syphilitic 'virus' and the reaction that occurred was believed to be one between mutually specific bodies, i.e., between antigen and antibody, the resulting combination having the power to fix complement. Subsequent investigation showed, however, that the Wassermann reaction could be carried out by using extracts of nonsyphilitic tissue. Whereas this discovery did not affect the reliability of the test for

diagnostic purposes, it made the test difficult to understand in terms of what was then known about the immune reaction in other infectious diseases.

Also in 1912, Keidel described a simple bleeding-tube for obtaining specimens for the Wassermann reaction that prevented contamination of the serum with foreign materials. It was not always possible or convenient to send a patient to the hospital and collection of the blood in the physician's office or in the patient's home often resulted in a worthless specimen. The essential feature of Keidel's apparatus was the substitution of a closed vacuum chamber for the cylinder and piston of the ordinary aspirating syringe. This substitution eliminated all possibility of contamination in collecting the specimen and made is possible to ship the specimen in the container in which it was originally collected.

Although Keidel was the chief architect in the organization and development of the new syphilis division of the medical clinic, Eveleth W. Bridgman of the Department of Medicine, a 1912 graduate of the Johns Hopkins University School of Medicine, was of great help in the early days of 'Department L' by bringing the viewpoint of the internist to the study and management of the patients.

The clinic grew rapidly in terms of the number of patient visits. In the first year of operation, 722 new patients were seen in the clinic for a total of 5486 visits. Over 5000 Wassermann tests were performed. A social worker was added to the clinic staff in 1917.

The activities of the clinic, however, were of necessity hampered by the exigencies of World War I. After the war, Joseph Earle Moore (Fig. 3) joined the staff of the clinic and his skill as an observer and organizer did much to fulfil the original conception of the syphilis clinic as a facility for clinical investigation. The major studies dealt with the course of the disease, with problems of diagnosis and with treatment. Particular attention was given to neurosyphilis, especially to that variety known as asymptomatic neurosyphilis, and a clearer conception of the clinical course of central-nervous-system syphilis was obtained. An intensive study of the occurrence of neurosyphilis in families was begun.

In 1921, Keidel officially succeeded Walker as director of the clinic and his principal assistants were Moore, E. L. Zimmerman and H. M. Robinson, Sr. In that year, 1000 new cases were seen in the clinic for a total of over 16,000 visits.

THE INTRODUCTION OF CONTINUOUS TREATMENT FOR EARLY SYPHILIS

Perhaps the most important of the early clinical studies were those dealing with the effects of various forms of treatment in selected groups of cases. The material of the clinic was valuable for this type of research and made possible the investigation of a number of different therapeutic problems such as the treatment of early syphilis, the prognosis and treatment of asymptomatic neurosyphilis and of cardiovascular syphilis, and

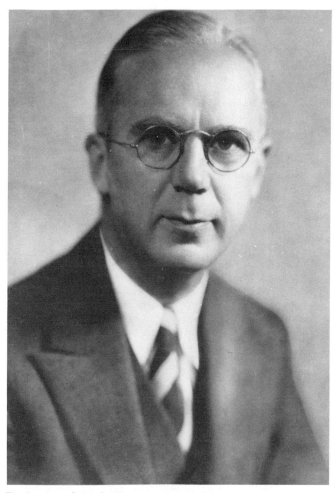

Fig 3.   Joseph Earle Moore.
From the Alan M. Chesney Medical Archives, the Johns Hopkins Medical Institutions.

the effectiveness of tryparsamide as a remedy in grave central-nervous-system syphilis.

A special form of treatment for early syphilis was instituted by Keidel, and one of the classic papers emanating from the clinic was that by Moore and Keidel entitled 'The treatment of early syphilis. I. A plan of treatment for routine use', published in 1926. At the end of the 19th century, syphilologists felt that it was important to continue treatment after clinical manifestations had disappeared in order to obtain a real cure. This feeling became a conviction when it was found that a single dose of Salvarsan did not cure the disease. When it was realized that the reversal of the Wassermann reaction was an obligatory criterion, treatment regimes grew longer and longer, and, finally, it was insisted that a full year was necessary. On this basis, innumerable treatment schedules were advocated. Moore and Keidel pointed out that full curative treatment was particularly important in early syphilis, whereas in late syphilis the objective was to control the presenting lesions. They described a definitive plan of therapy consisting of 70 weeks of continuous treatment with alternating courses of arsphenamine and bismuth. This general plan of

treatment remained in use until the advent of penicillin. They summarized the principles that they followed:

"That treatment shall be continuous, consisting of courses of arsphenamine alternating with courses of mercury by inunction (or of insoluble bismuth salts intramuscularly) plus potassium iodide; that treatment shall be carried out under detailed serologic control; that treatment shall be prolonged without intermission for one year after the blood and spinal fluid have become and have remained completely negative."

It is of interest to trace briefly the historical development of the idea of continuous vs intermittent treatment of early syphilis. Ricord was apparently the first to advocate the continuous mercurial treatment of the disease as early as 1838. Although he did not lack disciples, his greatest pupil, Fournier, abandoned continuous treatment and introduced the plan of chronic intermittent treatment with mercury for 3–5 yr. This was the system in general use until 1910. With the introduction of the arsphenamines, it was first thought that one injection of this drug, or at most a few, could cure syphilis. The experience of observers everywhere during the first few years indicated clearly that this was not the case, but rather that treatment must be prolonged, and that arsphenamines must be used in combination with a heavy metal. Most workers, clinging to Fournier's idea of chronic intermittent treatment, developed plans of therapy including the combined use of arsphenamine and mercury, courses of these two drugs being separated by rest periods. In 1916, Keidel introduced in the Johns Hopkins Syphilis Clinic the idea of continuous use of arsphenamine and a heavy metal in patients with early syphilis. His plan was based on a thorough consideration of the effects of antisyphilitic drugs and of the biology of early syphilis. Moore and Keidel, in their paper of 1926, gave the reasons that led to this decision:

"A few patients with primary or secondary syphilis may be cured by a single course of arsphenamine alone, or of arsphenamine plus mercury. In the majority, however, biologic cure does not result from a single course of treatment, and virulent treponemes remain in various foci in the body. It is of paramount importance to consider the reaction of the patient to these undestroyed organisms. Though the nature of immunity in syphilis is imperfectly understood, the course of events in an untreated infection, with gradually developing insusceptibility to reinfection, and culminating in spontaneous disappearance of the secondary outbreak, the destruction of large numbers of treponemes, and latency, indicates a considerable degree of resistance on the part of the patient. If treatment is begun in the primary or secondary stage of the disease, and the sequence of general tissue reaction, appearance of lesions and their spontaneous resolution is sharply interrupted, the development of the patient's own resistance against the treponeme is wholly or partially prevented. The patient thus enters on the first rest period without adequate resistance against the living treponemes remaining in his tissues, and must elaborate his immune reactions afresh. Depending on the location of the surviving organisms, and the length of time between treatment courses, he may repeat the process of general dissemination and tissue reaction, culminating in delayed or recurrent secondary syphilis; or he may develop that bugbear of early syphilis, a neurorecurrence.

"If on the other hand treatment is continuous, courses of arsphenamine alternating with courses of mercury, the situation is theoretically quite different.... When the first arsphenamine course had been completed, and the remaining organisms, if present, have perhaps acquired some degree of arsenic tolerance, it is possible to shift at once to mercury.

"After a few weeks of mercury therapy, it may be safely assumed that any arsphenamine tolerance acquired by the organisms in the first course has been lost, and the powerful treponemicidal attack of arsphenamine may again be utilized. This type of continuous treatment with alternating courses of the two drugs may be continued indefinitely without detriment to the patient."

In spite of the fact that this system of continuous treatment was instituted in 1916, Keidel and Moore did not describe it in the medical literature until their publication in 1926. Priority in publication, therefore, belongs to Almkvist, whose first paper on the subject appeared in 1920. Almkvist's reasons for adopting this scheme of treatment were identical to those that led Keidel to its use.

Another important study of the treatment of early syphilis was conducted by Paul Clifford Padget. His study, published in 1940, was the first in the literature with adequate long-term observation of treated patients. All of the patients were followed for at least 5 yr after termination of treatment. Sixty-five and seven-tenths per cent were cured, regardless of the type or amount of treatment given in the sense that they either experienced reinfection or at the time of their last examination showed no physical or serologic evidence of syphilis. Of the remainder, positive serologic tests were the evidence of infection in 14.9%; 12.3% had neurosyphilis and 7.1% had various late manifestations of the disease ofther than neurosyphilis. Even if one excludes from the cured group the patients in whom no examination of the spinal fluid was performed (8.7%), the ultimate satisfactory outcome in 57% is surprisingly high. This means that if the patient with early syphilis received some treatment during the first 2 yr of his infection, he had a better than even chance of becoming and remaining clinically and serologically well.

Padget received his A.B. from the University of Michigan in 1923 and his M.D. from Johns Hopkins 4 yr later. After residency training, he was Jacques Loeb Fellow in Medicine from 1931 to 1933 and Eli Lilly Fellow in 1934–1935. He was an Assistant Professor of Medicine from 1945 until his untimely death 6 yr later, at which time he was Chief of Medicine at the Fort Howard Veterans Administration Hospital.

AN ENGLISH PHYSICIAN'S DESCRIPTION OF 'DEPARTMENT L' IN THE 1920s

Sir John Conybeare of Guy's Hospital, London, while visiting the Johns Hopkins Hospital in the early 1920s, gave a vivid description of the activities in 'Department L'.*

"Dec. 8. I was taken round the department for the treatment of syphilis by Dr. Poole this afternoon. This clinic is open every afternoon of the week. On 3 days treatment is carried out and on 3 days patients are examined and lumbar punctures performed. Syphilis in all its stages is treated. The accommodation is somewhat cramped and there is more admixture of males and females than would be considered satisfactory in England. Cases are referred from other departments for treatment.

"The routine is first a general physical examination of the patient from every point of view. Blood is taken for a Wassermann, and if there is a sore, spirochetes are looked for with dark ground illumination. A lumbar puncture is done as a routine and the fluid is examined (1) for cells, (2) Wassermann, (3) colloidal gold curve. In a large proportion of primary and secondary syphilis without involvement of the central nervous system clinically abnormalities are found in the cerebrospinal fluid. When the diagnosis is established treatment is begun. Each case is dealt with on its merits, but I gather that the 606 preparations (arsphenamine) are considered more satisfactory than 914 (tryparsamide) and are usually employed at any rate in the first course of injections. A branch of the social service department works in connection with the clinic and if a patient fails to turn up for treatment he is written to. If he still fails to come one of the social service workers goes out to see him. Notices are posted on the walls to the effect that if patients fail to appear regularly they will be refused treatment in any department of the Johns Hopkins Dispensary Service.

"All fourth-year students do 3 afternoons a week for a month in the Department and practically all of them get an opportunity of doing themselves at least one or two lumbar punctures. They also do the cell counts. The Clinic has two small laboratories close at hand. In one of these spirochetes are looked for and cell counts done. In the other there are two technicians who are employed doing Wassermanns. The Department is very well patronized by patients. I was much struck by the thorough way in which the histories were taken and the general examinations of the patient. The record cards are as usual all typed by clerks at the end of the day.

"On the afternoon of Dec. 9th I again went to the Syphilis Clinic, and saw the patients being given injections. Two small adjoining rooms were used with two tables in each; one room for males and the other for females. Dr. Wassermann (no relation to the man who described the Wassermann test) was in charge and there were three fourth year students under him. On this particular afternoon only two preparations were being given: Arsphenamine (a 606 preparation) and Tryparsamide (prepared by the Powers-Weightman-Rosengarten Co. of New York). The latter preparation is used mainly for neurosyphilis and tertiary conditions.

"The patients are seen in another room and then given a small ticket on which is stated the dose they are to

---

* A copy of Conybeare's handwritten description of 'Department L' is in the Alan M. Chesney Medical Archives, the Johns Hopkins Medical Institutions. The original document is with his personal papers in the Library of the Royal College of Physicians, London.

receive. The arsenical compounds are made up in bulk and poured into a large glass cylinder graduated in 10 cc's. From the bottom of this runs a tube down to a needle with a two way tap. The needle is inserted into a vein with the tap set so that blood runs out of a side tube. When sufficient for a Wassermann test has been collected, the tap is reversed and the solution runs into the vein. The operator pinches the tube and stops the flow when the necessary amount has been given. The needle is then detached and a new one filled for the next patient. The reservoir is hung on the wall about two feet above the level of the patient's arm. A Wassermann is done every time the patient comes up for an injection.

"*Dosage. Tryparsamide* first dose 2 grams, succeeding doses 3 grams. The drug is made up in a 5% solution, i.e. 20 cc = 1 gram. *Arsphenamine* first dose 0.2 gm. succeeding doses 0.3 gm. Solution made up so that 0–1 gm. is contained in 20 cc.

"Occasionally patients have a 'nitritoid' reaction with nausea, injection of conjunctivae, swelling of face and flushing. They are at once treated with an injection (subcutaneous) of 10 minims of 1 in 1000 adrenalin.

"Each patient is given a slip giving the date on which they are to return for treatment. This is also noted on a date card kept by the social service department.

"Dr. Wassermann tells me that syphilis is a notifiable disease, not only by the doctor but by any householder or employer who may have reason to suspect anyone has syphilis. He seemed to be in doubt as to whether there is really any legal power to compel patients to have treatment, but apparently the police bring pressure to bear on any patient with contagious syphilis who refuses treatment. I gather that on the whole the patients in L Department (the polite name for the clinic) are very regular in their attendance.

"On the afternoon I was at the clinic just over 50 injections were given in about 1¾ hours. If the students got into difficulties with veins Dr. Wassermann was called in to help. The Department in spite of the somewhat cramped accommodation seemed to me to be run in a most thoroughly efficient manner, and also afforded students more practical experience than they get in most of the clinics.

"Every pregnant woman who has ever had a positive Wassermann or been treated in any department for syphilis is sent up to the clinic for a course of injections during her pregnancy."

OTHER CLINICAL STUDIES

The influence of having a careful study of the disease based on experience in well-documented cases was soon evident in the work of the clinic. Indications for lumbar puncture in the routine management of cases with syphilis were pointed out.

The importance of the plan of treatment for early syphilis described by Keidel and Moore was confirmed by their careful studies of the natural course of the illness. As indicated, one of their objectives was to prevent the late and serious results of the disease produced by involvement of the nervous system in particular and also the cardiovascular system. Outstanding in this regard were their studies in asymptomatic neurosyphilis which clearly demonstrated that early invasion of the central nervous system was common, occurring in 26% of the series of 352 patients with primary and secondary syphilis. Of 94 with early neurosyphilis, 72 were asymptomatic and were detected only by routine application of spinal puncture. They demonstrated clearly that early asymptomatic neurosyphilis was the forerunner of clinical neurosyphilis. Their plan of treatment was shown to reduce markedly the incidence of asymptomatic neurosyphilis and thus the ultimate development of the clinical disease. They could find in their material no evidence that there was a special neurotropic strain of *Treponema pallidum*.

MOORE SUCCEEDS KEIDEL AS DIRECTOR

Upon Keidel's retirement in 1929, Moore was placed in charge of the clinic and was responsible for its increasing success. Under his aggressive leadership, it became the foremost center in the world for the study of syphilis, and Moore himself became an international authority.

Moore obtained his premedical education at the University of Kansas where he also took the first 2 yr of his medical course before transferring in 1914 to the Johns Hopkins University School of Medicine. After receiving his M.D. in 1916, he served as a resident house officer in the Johns Hopkins Hospital for a year, and then entered the United States Army as a first lieutenant. He served in France where he was associated with Young and developed his first interest in venereal disease. After the war, he identified himself at once with the Syphilis Division of the Department of Medicine. Moore also became associated with Keidel in private practice and their partnership lasted until Keidel retired in 1939.

Among Moore's valuable contributions were his elucidation of the natural history of neurosyphilis and the recognition of the occurrence of false-positive serologic tests for syphilis in certain chronic diseases. He was a strong supporter of Thomas Parran in the latter's move to bring the problem of syphilis before the public. Perhaps his major accomplishment was the demonstration at Johns Hopkins of the feasibility of using an outpatient clinic as a productive clinical research facility.

Moore was effective in communicating to students and young physicians his enthusiasm for the discovery of better methods for the prevention and treatment of syphilis, as evidenced by the following recollections of Paul W. Spear of the class of 1934:

"My first association with Medicine I was in the summer of 1932 after the end of my second year. I subsequently served my required out-patient clerkship there and after completing my house staff training, returned to work in the clinic as a voluntary Assistant Dispensary Physician and later as Instructor in Medicine on the Medical School faculty.

"The students were welcomed as full-fledged participants in the activities of a very busy clinic. Earle Moore was everywhere. His personality dominated Medicine I completely, whether it was teaching students or discussing investigative problems with staff, or telling the latest jokes.

"My earliest recollection of that first summer was

being introduced to the 'treatment room' where Harry Robinson, Sr. held sway. Students were expected to administer all the drugs when available—Salvarsan, bismuth, Neosalvarsan, etc.

"On my first attempt at doing a lumbar puncture, my hand shook so violently that the test tube into which the spinal fluid dropped rattled uncontrollably against the needle. Later, it became just another routine procedure done without benefit of gloves. Hands were carefully scrubbed and other sterile techniques were employed but, in contrast to what was done in other treatment clinics, gloves were scorned. We never saw infections.

"After a short rest, patients were allowed to get up and go home—usually by street car. It was later shown that the incidence of post-lumbar puncture headache did not depend on keeping patients flat in bed for longer periods but rather using small caliber needles to minimize leakage of spinal fluid.

"At that time arsphenamine (Salvarsan), Ehrlich's 'magic bullet', was widely used. It had to be dissolved in acid solution and then carefully neutralized with alkali to a pH of 7.4. On one notorious and unfortunate occasion during that summer, by error, two patients received unneutralized arsphenamine after which they walked to the stairway outside the treatment room and dropped dead. The strongly acid solution produced intravascular denaturation of protein with obstruction of the microcirculation from the precipitated protein. In the next few years, neoarsphenamine gradually replaced arsphenamine as the drug of choice making such accidents impossible.

"Dr. Moore, of course, had a special flare for exciting student interst and for cultivating their powers of observation. On one occasion, he gathered all the students and offered a 'quarter' to the one who made the pertinent observation regarding a patient whom he had brought in. No one of us noted that the man's hair looked a little 'moth-eaten'. He had the 'spotty alopecia' seen in secondary syphilis. Incidentally, we were not permitted to use the term 'lues'. It was a 'pet peeve' of Dr. Moore's. He would always point out that 'lues' was the Latin word for plague and that if you wished to use the word correctly you would have to say 'lues venerea' (venereal plague).

"A sign of acceptance as a junior staff member was being assigned to 'The Book', which meant that you were the triage physician for the morning, who saw all new patients assigning them for work-up to students and staff, deciding which patients required emergency care and entering all of this in the clinic roster ('The Book'). It was a job requiring quick decisions, spot decisions, spot diagnoses and keeping everyone happy, not always easy.

"A number of patients developed jaundice of varying intensity following treatment. This was called 'arsphenamine jaundice'. Recovery was usually uneventful after which treatment was cautiously resumed. A few developed 'acute yellow atrophy'. It seems obvious, of course, now that it was serum hepatitis that was responsible and that the fatal cases were the result of acute hepatic necrosis secondary to overwhelming doses of the virus.

"We worked in the treatment room, as students, two mornings. On the other three, we were assigned a new case to work-up, as well as follow-up cases. The faculty involved in the review of student work-ups included the entire staff from the most senior to the most junior. It was always exciting to have Dr. Moore as your instructor for the morning but there were many others, including 'Tommy' Turner, Max Wintrobe and Harry Eagle, all of whom were able clinicians as well as distinguished investigators.

"At the end of the morning, Dr. Longcope, attended by his house staff retinue, made rounds of all the medical clinics looking at unusual cases and deciding which ones might warrant admission to the ward.

"One of the dividends of being a member of the Medicine I staff was the monthly meeting of the Journal Club which met in the evening at Dr. Moore's home or another of the senior staff. Aside from the stimulating interchange of the latest information from the literature, there was good food and drink and an equally stimulating interchange of the latest humor, mostly ribald, which Oscar Block, one of the junior staff, duly recorded in the notebook he always carried for that purpose.

"Above all, Medicine I was a place where physicians, young and old, worked in extraordinary harmony held together by Earle Moore's strong hand. There was a combination of clinical concern and intellectual curiosity which produced a steady stream of important papers in the field of syphilology as well as empathetic treatment of patients.

"It was an exciting experience which has not been dulled by the passage of almost forty years since I worked there."

Many of the young men who trained under Moore later became leaders in the venereal disease control programs of their home states and countries.

Moore was the first practicing physician to be made a full professor in the Johns Hopkins University School of Medicine and for many years he was in charge of the private inpatient clinic, the Marburg, at the Johns Hopkins Hospital. He established the *American Journal of Syphilis* (now the *Journal of Chronic Diseases*), of which he was co-editor. From 1944 to 1946, he was Assistant Division Chief of the Committee on Medical Research and Chairman of the Syphilis Study Section. From 1940 to 1954, he was Chairman of the Subcommittee on Venereal Diseases of the National Research Council, and during the latter 4 yr of his tenure he was also a member of the Committee on Medicine. After the war, he continued to serve as a consultant to the surgeon-general of the U.S. Army from 1943 to 1950. He was a special consultant to the U.S. Public Health Service from 1938 until the time of his death, a consultant to the Maryland and New York State Health Departments, and a member of a special advisory committee to the Secretary of the Navy.

So great was the affection and respect in which he was held by his colleagues that on Moore's 60th birthday, in 1952, a dinner was held in Washington, D.C., under the chairmanship of Parran to commemorate the event. More than 100 distinguished colleagues attended to do him honor. Moore was the recipient of many honors, including the Medal of Merit for his work in venereal disease control during World War II. The outpatient clinic for clinical research at Johns Hopkins is named after him. Moore's estate was bequeathed to Johns Hopkins as an endowment for the William Osler Chair of Medicine, which is currently held by Victor A. McKusick, Chairman of the Department of Medicine.

There were many physicians who gave devoted

service to the syphilis clinic and without their enthusiastic support the program could not have achieved what it did in the advance of our scientific knowledge of the disease. Among those who contributed to the success of Medicine I were: Robinson, Sr., Zimmerman, Jarold E. Kemp, Harry L. Wassermann, Frank R. Smith, Jr., Charles F. Mohr, Conrad Acton, Bowman J. Hood, H. M. Robinson, Jr., Vail Robinson, Frank Reynolds, Ernest S. Cross, Jr., Ralph J. Young and C. Walter Sherrington. One deserves special mention. Richard D. Hahn (Fig. 4), born in Baltimore, Maryland, in 1912, received his undergraduate and medical training at Johns Hopkins. His residency training was taken at the Cincinnati General Hospital and from 1939 to 1941 he had a fellowship in the Department of Medicine at Johns Hopkins. From that time on, he was associated with the syphilis clinic and after the clinic's activities were reoriented he continued to follow patients with syphilis in the Subdepartment of Dermatology, which was then headed by Dr. E. W. Smith. Hahn is the author of 26 articles dealing with various aspects of syphilis and its treatment. He rose to the rank of Associate Professor of Chronic Disease in the School of Hygiene and Public Health and achieved the same academic rank in the School of Medicine.

EXPERIMENTAL SYPHILIS

Before World War I, it was not possible to organize an experimental laboratory because of insufficient funds.

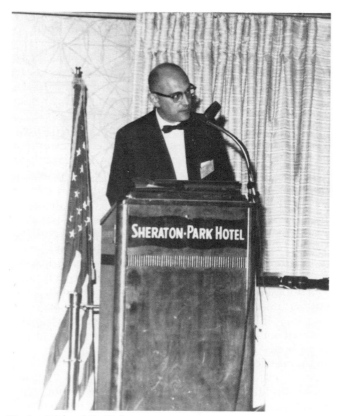

Fig 4.   Richard D. Hahn.

After the war, however, with the increased emphasis on venereal disease, funds were attracted to the clinic from a number of sources, including the Interdepartmental Social Hygiene Board and the Carnegie Corporation. Steps were first taken in 1921 to develop research and teaching in syphilis on a full-time basis within the department of medicine. Wade H. Brown, a graduate of the Johns Hopkins University School of Medicine, then working at the Rockefeller Institute, was invited to come to Johns Hopkins but he declined. Alan M. Chesney accepted the post with the titles of Associate Professor of Medicine, Associate Physician to the Hospital and Co-director (with Keidel) of the Syphilis Clinic. From that time on, the study of syphilis was approached along two different lines: one using observations on patients and the other observations on experimental animals. These two lines of research overlapped in many phases so that no sharp distinction should be drawn between them. The participation of the laboratory investigators in the work of the clinic constituted a valuable feature of the division because it was essential that these investigators be familiar with the course of syphilis in human beings as well as in animals.

IMMUNITY IN SYPHILIS—THE WORK OF CHESNEY

Chesney (Fig. 5) was born on 17 January 1888. He graduated from the Johns Hopkins University, where he had a distinguished career, both academically and athletically. He entered the Johns Hopkins medical school in 1908 and graduated 4 yr later with such other distinguished contributors to American medicine as Ernest Goodpasture, Maurice Pincoffs, Mont Reid and Lewis Weed. Following an internship and assistant residency in medicine at Johns Hopkins, Chesney went to the Rockfeller Institute for 3 yr to work on pneumonia with Rufus Cole and O. T. Avery. While there, he conducted a classic study of the growth curve of the pneumococcus in broth culture. In 1917, he was commissioned a first lieutenant in the medical corps. He served in France, first with the British Army and later with the AEF. In 1919, he joined the medical faculty of Washington University in St. Louis, heading the Infectious Disease Division in the Department of Medicine under G. Canby Robinson. One of Chesney's contempories on that faculty was E. K. Marshall, Jr., with whom he formed an enduring friendship. When Canby Robinson became Temporary Director of the Department of Medicine at Johns Hopkins in 1921, he brought Chesney to Baltimore as Associate Professor to direct the newly created syphilis division. In preparation, Chesney returned to the Rockefeller Institute for Medical Research, where he worked for the better part of a year with Brown and Louise Pearce (a Johns Hopkins medical school graduate) who were conducting classic studies on experimental rabbit syphilis.

In their studies, Brown and Pearce used the method of testicular inoculation that had been described by Parodi in 1907. Parodi had inserted a small piece of a syphilitic papule under the tunica vaginalis of the testes

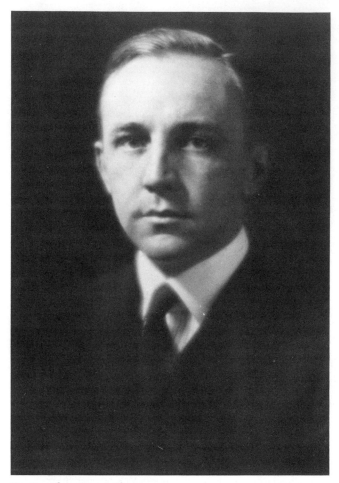

Fig 5.   Alan Mason Chesney.
From the Alan M. Chesney Medical Archives, the Johns Hopkins Medical Institutions.

of a rabbit. When he examined the testes 1 month later, he found round-cell infiltration as well as numerous spirochetes. Brown and Pearce's original paper in a long series on experimental infection and immunity appeared in 1920. By excising at various intervals after scrotal inoculation the inguinal lymph nodes of rabbits and testing for the presence of spirochetes by injecting these excised nodes into other animals, Brown and Pearce demonstrated how quickly the treponemes spread. They concluded that for all practical purposes there was no appreciable time during which a syphilitic lesion could be regarded as confined to the focus of entry. Having demonstrated the wide dissemination of spirochetes in rabbits before clinical signs appeared, Brown and Pearce then found that rabbits who had recovered from clinical syphilis harbored virulent spirochetes almost indefinitely even though there were no further overt manifestations of infection. In another of their articles entitled 'Superinfection in experimental syphilis following the administration of subcurative doses of arsphenamine or neoarsphenamine', they concluded that subcurative treatment of animals with marked primary lesions of the testicles altered the animals' resistance to such an extent as to render them susceptible to a second cutaneous in-

fection without having effected a cure of the original infection. When the experimenters modified the course of the infection by suppressing the initial lesion, as, for example, by castration or subcurative therapy, they found that while the syphilitic lesions as a rule remained localized in the controls, almost all the 'treated' animals showed generalized lesions involving the eye, mucous membranes and so forth. The conclusion seemed justified that the natural progress of syphilis is bound up with immune reactions which are capable of modification by spontaneous or by externally regulated influences. Such considerations were obviously most important in the treatment of the human disease.

For 10 yr after his return to Baltimore, Chesney's energies were in large measure devoted to the syphilis division; time being spent in the outpatient clinic, on the wards and in the experimental laboratory. His studies of immunity in syphilis quickly established him as an imaginative investigator of infectious diseases and he soon shared, with Brown and Pearce, leadership in the field of investigative syphilology. Among his contributions were the demonstration by animal inoculation of *T. pallidum* in blood, spinal fluid and joint fluid of patients with early syphilis, and the demonstration of the tendency of *T. pallidum* to localize in traumatized areas in both man and animals. Most important were his experiments covering more than a decade on the basic mechanisms of immunity in syphilis in which the slow evolution of immunity in the experimental disease was demonstrated and the fact established that immunity persisted long after presumed elimination of the causative agent by specific treatment. These experiments were summarized in his monograph 'Immunity in syphilis' which appeared in *Medicine* in 1926.

Chesney *et al.* found that syphilitic rabbits could be treated with arsphenamine in such a manner as to render the lymph nodes incapable of transmitting the infection to normal rabbits, even if treatment was begun late in the course of the disease. Those treated late, in spite of apparent cure, were almost uniformly refractory to a second infection. Chesney concluded, contrary to earlier ideas, that this refractory state could be explained by the existence of acquired immunity which persisted after abolition of the disease rather than by the persistence of the first infection.

One important and difficult question was whether or not treatment, when given late in the course of the disease, was effective in completely eliminating the infection from the rabbit's body. In a series of experiments in which emulsions of lymph nodes and internal organs from untreated and later treated rabbits were inoculated into normal animals, Chesney and Kemp obtained evidence that in a large majority of the animals treatment rendered noninfectious those organs tested as well as the lymph nodes. In all their experiments, care was taken to maintain strictly comparable relations regarding dosage of drug and time of administration. Kemp and Chesney obtained additional evidence which threw doubt upon the validity of the reinoculation method as a criterion of cure. They found that, whereas rabbits which were originally inoculated in the testes and treated late in the course of the disease were almost uniformly refractory to a second intratesticular inoculation, other syphilitic rabbits similarly treated and reinoculated by a different method (deposition of spirochetes upon a granulating wound on the back) were susceptible to a second infection in 50% of the cases. Since markedly divergent results, depending upon the particular method selected for reinoculation, were obtained in otherwise comparable groups, it was apparent that no conclusion could be drawn as to the presence or absence of the first infection from the response of an animal to reinoculation. Chesney and Kemp assembled evidence indicating that it was possible to reinfect a treated rabbit without producing any lesion whatsoever at the site of reinoculation. Nevertheless, in their experiments, such animals gave evidence of systemic invasion by the treponemes as demonstrated by lymph node transfer, and in a large proportion of the cases a positive Wassermann reaction appeared in the blood. Thus, it appeared that at least two factors might be involved in bringing about such an altered response to a second inoculation: one, the time at which treatment was begun, and two, the manner in which the second inoculation was made. On the basis of their observations, Chesney and Kemp suggested that some of the relapsing Wassermann reactions occurring in patients with early syphilis who had been well treated did not represent a relapse of their first infection as was generally held, but a true reinfection in which no lesion occurred at the portal of entry but in which systemic distribution of the organisms took place and was accompanied by the reappearance of a positive Wassermann reaction. In other words, in such individuals, a second infection may have taken place and undergone an unusual course by reason of the fact that it was introduced into a patient still under the influence of an immunologic change brought about by the first infection. Such individuals might be regarded as partially refractory to a second infection. They concluded that in dealing with human beings it seemed best to rely on the safer criterion of reinfection and demand a characteristic primary lesion followed by the evolution of secondary manifestations since in clinical practice there were no means of differentiating such patients from those in whom the subsequent reappearance of a positive Wassermann reaction represented a true serological relapse. Chesney and Kemp emphasized the method of inoculating rabbits with lymph nodes from human patients as a test for a cure.

Chesney summarized his views on immunity in syphilis as follows: "I think of acquired immunity in syphilis as a state of resistance which evolves comparatively slowly and at its best is not always complete, general in its distribution but imported to some tissues more than to others . . . but not necessarily dependent upon the persistence of infection for its maintenance."

Both Chesney and W. Kolle (the latter working in Germany) showed that, one established, the state of resistance to reinfection persisted during the lifetime of the animal. The development of resistance could be prevented by treatment given early in the infection and making possible the successful reinfection with an homologous strain of spirochetes (before the 45th day in rabbits, and before, during or shortly after the secondary outbreak in man). If treatment was delayed until after the 90th day in the rabbit or until after the completion of the secondary period in man, however, these immune relationships were established and were not alterable by further treatment.

By ingenious experiments, Chesney et al. demonstrated that in the rabbit the eye does not share to the some extent as other tissues in the general resistant state which develops during the course of syphilitic infection, and suggested that this phenomenon may be a partial explanation for the repeated relapses of interstitial keratitis in congenital syphilis.

At the time Chesney's monograph was written, experimentalists were divided into two schools regarding the existence of acquired immunity. Chesney's experiments indicated that a true acquired immunity developed during the course of experimental syphilis. In summarizing his own and earlier experiments, he concluded that the determining factor in the development of such immunity was the duration of the primary or immunizing infection prior to its termination by treatment. If the immunizing infection lasted less than 3 months, reinoculation of the homologous strain by the same route as the original inoculation was usually followed by clinical reinfection. If the immunizing infection was terminated by treatment after 3 months, similar reinoculation with the homologous strain usually did not result in symptomatic reinfection. The experimentalists agreed on these observations but differed as to whether this failure to react to the second infection represented a true immunity or whether it represented an altered reactivity of the animal due to the persistence of the original infection. Numerous studies substantiating Chesney's conclusions appeared after his review.

Arnold Rich, Chesney and Thomas B. Turner showed that allergy in the sense of hyperreactivity to the organism is not an essential part of the immune process in syphilis. Indeed, animals that are immune to a second inoculation are extraordinarily passive to the presence of the organism.

One of Chesney's closest collaborators was Kemp, who received his A.B. from Western Maryland College in 1917 and his M.D. from Johns Hopkins in 1921. From 1922 to 1926, he worked closely with Chesney in the laboratory and also participated in many excellent clinical studies with Keidel and Moore. Kemp was assistant professor of dermatology under Stokes at the University of Pennsylvania from 1926 to 1928. He returned to Baltimore in 1928 and entered practice with J. W. Lord, serving as instructor in clinical dermatology at Johns Hopkins. In 1932, he became a member of the staff of the Public Health Institute in Chicago and later was Chief of the Medical Division and director of the research department there. In 1938, he had a myocardial infarction but recovered sufficiently to return to limited clinical and research activities. In 1940, he returned to Johns

Hopkins to take over the training program in venereal disease control in the School of Medicine and the School of Hygiene and Public Health. He had just returned to Baltimore from a field trip when he died suddenly on 19 October 1941 at the age of 43.

HARRY EAGLE'S RESEARCH LABORATORY

One of the outstanding experimental laboratories associated with the syphilis division was directed by Eagle (Fig. 6). Eagle received his M.D. from Johns Hopkins in 1927. In 1928, he became associated with the serologic laboratory of the syphilis division where he remained for 4 yr with the title of assistant and then instructor in the department of medicine. In 1932–1933, he was a National Research Council fellow at the Harvard Medical School and for the ensuing 3 yr an Assistant Professor of Microbiology at the University of Pennsylvania School of Medicine. In 1936, he returned to the Johns Hopkins School of Hygiene and Public Health as director of a special laboratory for experimental therapeutics under the auspices of the U.S. Public Health Service and remained there until 1946. From 1946 to 1948, he was Adjunct Professor of Bacteriology in the Johns Hopkins School of Hygiene and Public Health. He

remained a commissioned officer in the U.S. Public Health Service until 1961.

After the introduction of the Wassermann test and later the flocculation tests, a myriad of technical procedures for the diagnosis of syphilis were proposed which led to considerable confusion on the part of the physician. Eagle's laboratory, in which the serological reactions in syphilis were the subject of intensive study in the years between 1928 and 1933, did much to alleviate this confusion.

Michaelis first observed that a precipitate sometimes forms when the aqueous liver extract used in the Wassermann reaction is added to syphilitic serum. Jacobsthal *et al.* found that when an alcoholic extract of either syphilitic liver or guinea pig heart is diluted with salt solution and added to syphilitic serum, microscopically visible aggregates of lipoid particles are formed. A period of 10 yr passed before this precipitation phenomenon was made sufficiently delicate to be used as a reliable diagnostic procedure. Soon, however, a number of precipitation tests appeared, most of them identified by the name of the person responsible for their development. It was not generally recognized that all of these reactions involved exactly the same phenomenon, the combination of reagin-globulin with the lipoid particles

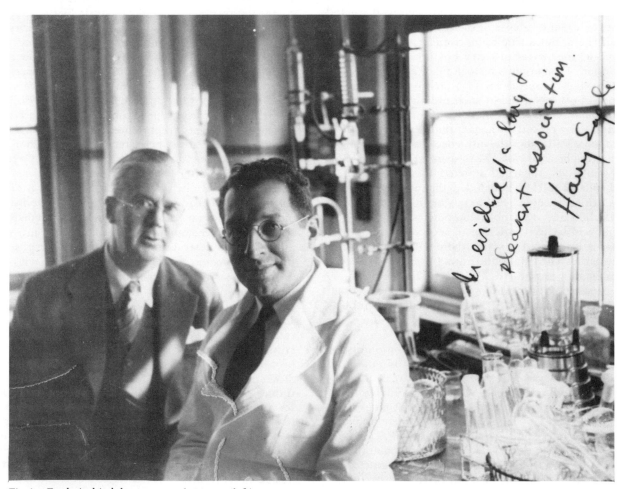

Fig 6.   Eagle in his laboratory with Moore (left).

of the antigen and the flocculation of this combination; and that the same reagin determines both complement-fixation (Wassermann reaction) and precipitation. Eagle emphasized that all of these tests were based on the precipitation phenomenon described by Michaelis and by Jacobsthal, and that they differed chiefly in the physical conditions of the tests, the physical state of the lipoid suspension and the quantitative relationships of the reagents. He analyzed these phenomena in a series of perceptive studies and offered a step-by-step explanation of their mechanisms which more satisfactorily fitted the observed facts than any theretofore proposed. He did much to advance the arrival at a standardization of serum tests by indicating clearly which of the various steps in their performance deserved discarding as antiquated relics of custom, which of them were generally acceptable to modern serologists, as well as which of them were still unsettled points of controversy. He showed that in the state of knowledge at that time no flocculation test could entirely replace the Wassermann test. He discussed with clarity the meaning of the laboratory report to the practitioner. Eagle's work was included in an important monograph entitled *The Laboratory Diagnosis of Syphilis: The Theory, Technique and Clinical Interpretation of the Wassermann and Flocculation Tests with Serum and Spinal Fluid;* his original investigations were presented with modest regard to their importance in relation to the studies of others. Eagle made adequate use of the enormous bibliography of the subject and succeeded in presenting its most complex and technical aspects in language intelligible to any well-trained physician. Eagle's contributions improved the technique of the Wassermann reaction with better understanding of the principles involved. His studies explained the fortifying effect of cholesterol upon the antigen as used in the Wassermann and flocculation tests, and he discovered other substances with similar sensitizing properties. Although Eagle himself developed an improvement in the flocculation test, he pointed out that there was no basis in fact for the occasionally acrimonious disputes as to priority in this field of research.

Beginning in 1936, important studies on the chemotherapy of syphilis were carried out by Eagle in collaboration with George Doak and H. G. Steinman. A major aspect was the synthesis of a large series of phenylarsenoxides in an attempt to arrive at better agents for the treatment of syphilis. Although that work was aborted with the discovery of the therapeutic activity of penicillin, interesting correlations were observed between chemical structure and biological activity. One of those compounds proved to be highly effective in the treatment of early African trypanosomiasis; this discovery led to studies on the pharmacologic basis of arsenic resistance in trypanosomes. During World War II, Eagle worked extensively on the usefulness of 2,3-dimercaptopropanol (BAL) in the treatmemt of arsenic poisoning. He developed a formulation suitable for systemic administration, in which BAL was incorporated into peanut oil and benzyl benzoate, and demonstrated its effectiveness in promoting the excretion of arsenic. This found an important application in the treatment of acute arsenic poisoning in man, which was later extended to the treatment of lead, mercury and antimony poisoning.

Beginning in 1944 and continuing until Eagle's move to the National Institutes of Health in 1947 to become Scientific Director of the Cancer Institute, his laboratory was heavily engaged in an analysis of the pharmacologic parameters determining penicillin activity, including the relative activity of penicillins F, G, K and X, the effect of the method of administration on therapeutic efficacy and the clear demonstration that the primary determinant of its therapeutic activity was the total time for which it remained at effective levels. The wide sensitivity of various species of bacteria to penicillin was shown to be related to their varying combining affinity for penicillin. At the concentration lethal for any particular species, whether 0.01 or 100 μg/ml, all the organisms examined were found to have bound essentially the same amount of penicillin (approx. 1000 molecules per organism). This finding was corroborated many years later by Strominger in his classic studies on the mode of action of penicillin in preventing cell wall synthesis.

Eagle's later studies on the use of cultured treponemes in diagnostic tests for syphilis led to his delineation of their complete growth requirements, and these studies in turn served as a take-off point for Eagle's studies 20 yr later on the detailed growth requirements of cultured mammalian cells.

In 1947, Eagle became Scientific Director of the Research Branch of the National Cancer Institute; from 1949 to 1959, he served as Chief of the Section on Experimental Therapeutics of the National Microbiological Institute (NIH) and for the next 2 yr as Chief, Laboratory of Cell Biology, National Institute for Allergy and Infectious Diseases. In 1961, he was appointed professor in the department of cell biology at Albert Einstein College of Medicine. His outstanding research contributions led to his election to the National Academy of Sciences and the American Academy of Arts and Sciences. He received the Presidential Certificate of Merit in 1948 and has been honored by many other important awards and prizes. Among his research interests are bacterial physiology, blood coagulation, detoxification of metal poisoning, mode of action of antibiotics and the serodiagnosis and chemotherapy of syphilis. Since 1974, he has been Associate Dean for Scientific Affairs at Albert Einstein and, since 1975, the director of its Cancer Research Center.

CONGENITAL SYPHILIS

The staffs of the obstetrical and syphilis clinics at the Johns Hopkins Hospital were among the pioneer workers in the study of syphilis complicated by pregnancy and in the antenatal prevention of congenital syphilis. The early work was done under the direction of J. Whitridge Williams, Professor of Obstetrics, and Keidel. The results of these studies, published by Williams, have since been confirmed by many investigators in various countries. Later studies were reviewed in 1934 by John McKelvey and Turner.

In 1922, Williams reported that of 109 infants born to seronegative syphilitic women, 43 were certainly, and seven others questionably, syphilitic; of the 50 mothers of these infected infants, 46 had never received any antisyphilitic treatment. A clinical cooperative group in 1934 recorded 13 presumably certain or probable instances of syphilis among live newborns and 45 dead-born babies among 182 seronegative mothers, all but 18 of whom had had some previous treatment. In practically every instance in which a seronegative mother was delivered of a syphilitic infant, there was some mention of syphilis in the mother's history. McKelvey and Turner (1934) analyzed 943 pregnancies occurring in syphilitic women with regard to the presence or absence of congenital syphilis in the offspring, particular attention being paid to the effect of maternal antisyphilitic treatment on the outcome of pregnancy. In addition, the relative value in the diagnosis of congenital syphilis of such signs as the cord Wassermann test, placental histology and roentgen examination of the infant's bones for syphilitic epiphysitis were considered. Among cases showing a negative cord Wassermann reaction, the infant was nonsyphilitic in 86.2%, and among those giving a positive reaction, the infant was normal in only 18.6%. Among cases in which the placenta was normal on macroscopic and microscopic examination, the infant proved to be nonsyphilitic in 79.9%, while among cases showing syphilitic changes in the placenta the offspring was syphilitic in all but 12.1%. When these two diagnostic aids were considered together, the information was more valuable than when each was considered alone. Infants presenting evidence of syphilitic epiphysitis invariably exhibited other evidence of congenital syphilis. However, among children showing no abnormalities on roentgen examination, 20.5% were subsequently shown to have congenital syphilis.

The striking beneficial effect of antenatal arsphenamine therapy was shown by the fact that among pregnancies occurring in untreated syphilitic mothers the infant was born alive in only 54.1%, and 64.5% of living offspring were syphilitic; the administration of as little as 1 g or less of arsphenamine changed these figures to 89 and 27%, respectively. Administration of larger amounts of arsphenamine or related products brought about a further reduction in fetal mortality and in the percentage of syphilitic offspring; when as much as 4 g (from 12 to 14 injections) was given, no syphilitic offspring was observed. The administration of heavy metals, mercury or bismuth compounds, in addition to arsphenamine, enhanced the good results achieved with the latter alone. Better results were obtained when maternal treatment was started in the first half of pregnancy than when begun in the latter half. It was found particularly important, however, that the arsenicals be given in the 2 months immediately preceding delivery.

The results in cases treated before pregnancy and not during pregnancy were, in general, as good as when the mother was treated during pregnancy only. Here, however, the status of the syphilitic infection in the mother was probably the important factor. Antisyphilitic treatment both before and during pregnancy yielded results superior to treatment during either period alone.

McKelvey and Turner's conclusions were:

1. The Wassermann test on the blood of the umbilical cord and study of the placental histology are important aids in the diagnosis of congenital syphilis and should be carried out on all patients not proved during pregnancy to be free from syphilis. Of the two, the former is the more reliable.

"2. The presence of characteristic changes in the epiphyses of the long bones during the first two weeks of life is diagnostic of congenital syphilis, but the absence of epiphyseal abnormalities does not rule out congenital infection.

"3. Antenatal treatment of pregnant syphilitic patients with arsphenamine reduces the percentage of fetal deaths and the percentage of syphilitic infants in a striking manner. The good results are roughly proportional to the amount of treatment given and the time at which it is started; even a few treatments in the last weeks of pregnancy, however, will materially alter the outcome."

THE FAMILY SYPHILIS CLINIC

In 1939, a family syphilis clinic was established within the Syphilis Division under the combined auspices of the Departments of Pediatrics, Obstetrics and Medicine. Attendance in the clinic was limited to syphilitic pregnant women and their offspring, children under 14 yr of age with syphilis and contacts under 14 yr of adult patients with syphilis. The care of the children in the group was entrusted to a pediatrician, Mary Hooke Goodwin, since in infants and younger children it was felt that pediatric care was often more important than specific antisyphilitic measures. This clinic proved extraordinarily successful in the management of patients falling into this category.

THE TRAINING PROGRAM OF THE SYPHILIS DIVISION

The first course in venereal disease control was offered in 1930 in conjunction with a similar one in tuberculosis control. The syphilis program was under the direction of Turner. When Turner left to go to the International Health Division of the Rockefeller Foundation in 1932, H. Hanford Hopkins (Fig. 7) took charge. Hopkins received his A.B. from Johns Hopkins in 1923 and his M.D. in 1927. Following an internship at the Henry Ford Hospital in Detroit, he returned to Johns Hopkins as Jacques Loeb Fellow in Medicine under Keidel and Moore. During the first year of his fellowship, he introduced the Kolmer modification of the Wassermann reaction. The first paper he wrote was on the juxta-articular nodules of Jeanselme. Rich helped him with the pathologic changes pointing out that rheumatic nodules contained Aschoff bodies which were absent in the syphilitic nodules. Other papers were on the prognosis of asymptomatic neurosyphilis and the association of tertiary skin lesions with neurosyphilis. He appointed Assistant in Medicine in 1929 and instructor the following year, reaching the rank of associate professor prior to his retirement in

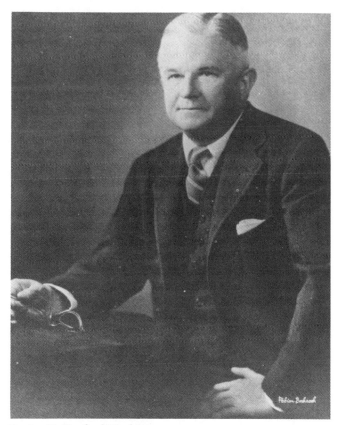

Fig 7.   H. Hanford Hopkins.

1967. For many years, Hopkins served as the admitting officer in 'Department L'. The admitting officer examined quickly all new patients, made a presumptive diagnosis, by darkfield examination or otherwise, initiated treatment at once if indicated, or if it was a late case performed a lumbar puncture and made an appointment for a complete physical examination. Hopkins remembers 'Department L' as a veritable pathologic museum with every manifestation of syphilis including huge aneurysms pounding through the sternum, advanced aortic insufficiency, general paresis, tabes dorsalis, Charcot joints, Hutchinson's triad and all the lesions of the eye and eigth nerve. The test question for suspected paretics was to require the patient to say: "Around the rugged rock the ragged rascal ran." Hopkins was an outstanding member of the Subdepartment of Dermatology. During the 1930s, he was Consultant to the State Department of Health in venereal disease control, visiting syphilis clinics scattered over the state. He was on the staff of the syphilis clinic for 15 yr.

A short time after the training course in syphilis began, the interest in veneral disease control was fostered by the vigorous national program instituted by Parran, then Surgeon-General of the U.S. Public Health Service. Moore proposed to the Public Health Service in 1936 that Johns Hopkins offer extended training activities in venereal disease control for public health officers and other physicians who had responsibility for municipal, state or national programs. The Rockefeller

Foundation was asked, and agreed to assign, Turner to Johns Hopkins to develop these expanded training activities which were undertaken jointly by the School of Hygiene and the hospital. This venture was highly successful and over the next 10 yr a succession of outstanding members of the U.S. Public Health Serivce as well as a large number of health officers from all over the country were sent to Johns Hopkins for this special training. This was the first coopcrative effort among the three Johns Hopkins Medical Institutions in an academic activity. As a result, many excellent people were trained who later had distinguished careers in the U.S. Public Health Service and in the affairs of the National Institutes of Health. These activities continued into the World War II period. Many men on the faculty at Johns Hopkins were able assistants to Moore in these activities of Medicine I, including Bowman J. Hood, Hahn, Padget, Mohr, Robinson, Sr. and Wassermann among others.

THE CONTRIBUTIONS OF TURNER

Moore chose wisely when he selected Turner (Fig. 8) to direct the first syphilis training program. Turner

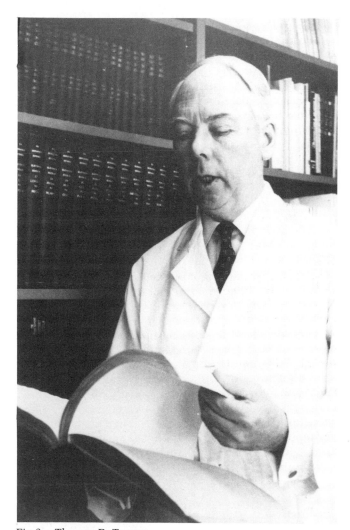

Fig 8.   Thomas B. Turner.
From the Alan M. Chesney Medical Archives, the Johns Hopkins Medical Institutions.

received his M.D. from the University of Maryland School of Medicine in 1925 and interned at the Hospital for the Women of Maryland the following year. In 1926–1927, he was Resident in Medicine at the Mercy Hospital and the following year was a Jacques Loeb Fellow in Medicine at the Johns Hopkins University School of Medicine. From 1928 to 1932, he was an instructor and associate in medicine at Johns Hopkins and from 1930 to 1932 a lecturer in public health administration. He became a staff member of the International Health Division of the Rockefeller Foundation in 1932, a position he held for 7 yr. Turner was Professor of Microbiology at the Johns Hopkins School of Hygiene and Public Health from 1939 until 1957, when he became Dean of the Medical Faculty at Johns Hopkins.

Turner made many important research contributions to syphilis and the treponematoses. In 1936, he presented an important paper entitled 'The preservation of virulent *Treponema pallidum* and *Treponema pertenue* in the frozen state' before the American Society for Clinical Investigation at its annual meeting in Atlantic City. Hitherto, it had not been possible regularly to maintain the spirochetes of yaws or syphilis in a virulent state outside an animal or human host for longer than a few days. These organisms lose pathogenicity for laboratory animals when grown on artificial media. When, however, *T. pallidum* and *T. pertenue* are frozen at temperatures approximating $-78°C$. and maintained at this temperature, they retain normal morphology and motility, and their virulence for rabbits is essentially unchanged after at least 4 months.

Infectious material from rabbits was stored in a thermos jug containing dry ice (solid CO_2) and 95₃ alcohol. Eight specimens of syphilis treponemes (Nichols strain) and six specimens of yaws spirochetes were tested before freezing and at intervals of 2 weeks, 1, 2 and 4 months after freezing. After these intervals, the appearance of the organisms was unchanged and upon inoculation of rabbits the incubation period and the character of the initial lesion did not vary significantly from that produced by the same lot of material before freezing. Material from seven additional strains of yaws spirochetes and lymph node material from five different strains of *T. pallidum* were tested after 2 months with similar results.

This work was extended to filterable viruses with similar favorable results. In a later paper, titration experiments made with the spirochetes of relapsing fever before and after freezing showed the following:

"1. With each freezing and thawing there is a slight but regular decrease in virulence, which decrease bears no relation to the duration of storage at $-78°C$. Ordinarily infectivity is destroyed by more than four refreezings.

"2. There is not always close correlation between motility and infectivity.

"3. Cooling spirochetes from $0°C$ to $-78°C$ over a 2- to 6-hour period damages them only slightly more than does rapid cooling, but warming from $-78°C$ to $0°C$ over a 2- to 6-hour period kills most of the organisms. Rapid thawing, as in a water bath, damages the spirochetes less than thawing more slowly, as at room temperature.

"4. At storage temperatures of [$12°C$ and $-20°C$ there is a gradual decrease in virulence over a period of days or weeks, and by the 6th week the infectivity of the material was markedly reduced. Thus, optimum conditions for the preservation of spirochetes, and probably other microorganisms, in the frozen state are afforded by rapid cooling, storage at $-78°C$, and rapid thawing. These organisms are severely damaged by storage at temperatures of $-20°C$ or higher, and by slow thawing."

Over a number of years, Turner *et al.* made important contributions on the biological relationships between *T. pallidum*, *T. pertenue* and *T. cuniculi*. The first studies were published in 1938. In an important study carried out 8 yr later, three groups of 20 rabbits each were simultaneously inoculated, respectively, with the causative agent of syphilis (*T. pallidum*), yaws (*T. pertenue*) and venereal spirochetosis of rabbits (*T. cuniculi*). Each species of spirochete had been maintained under laboratory conditions for a number of years. A fourth group of 20 rabbits was maintained as uninfected controls.

Rabbits employed in the experiment were all from an inbred stock and were approximately the same age and weight. They were maintained under the same laboratory conditions throughout the experiment, which covered a period of 6 months.

In general, the clinical course in experimental syphilis, yaws and cuniculi infection was similar. While the lesions observed in each disease exhibited certain similarities, they were, on the whole, sufficiently distinctive to permit easy differentiation of the experimental diseases. When all the animals of one group were compared with all those of another, the differences were quite pronounced. The tissue reaction among the syphilis animals as a group was more intense and more extensive than among either the yaws or cuniculi rabbits.

The serologic response to infection, as tested by one of the well-known serologic tests for syphilis, was similar among the three groups of rabbits, although among the syphilis animals as a group the serologic titer tended to rise more rapidly, to reach a higher level and to decline more rapidly than it did among the animals of the other two groups.

Thus, when tested years after original isolation from their natural hosts, the causative agents of syphilis, yaws and venereal spirochetosis of rabbits produced in rabbits a disease picture which exhibited certain similarities, but also characteristic differences, confirming previous observations made in this same laboratory using other strains of these three treponemes.

Because under the conditions of the experiments the environment to which both host and parasite were subjected was similar, it was concluded that the differences noted in the host-parasite reaction were due to substantial biologic differences between *T. pallidum*, *T. pertenue* and *T. cuniculi*.

In 1939, Turner addressed the question as to whether immunity in syphilis is cellular or humoral, and showed conclusively that the serum of syphilitic animals or man contains an antibody that combines directly with virulent *T. pallidum*. He incubated emulsions of the living organisms, derived from rabbit syphilomas, with syphilitic and normal serum; and after an interval, inoculated the mixture intradermally in the skin of rabbits' backs. When normal serum was used, typical chancres appeared at the sites of inoculation after the usual incubation period, just as when the treponemes were suspended in isotonic sodium chloride. When syphilitic sera were employed, on the contrary, there was either no lesion at the portal of entry or its appearance was greatly modified and the incubation period delayed. This phenomenon, indicating the presence in syphilitic sera of an antibody that destroyed *T. pallidum* organisms or at least interfered with their virulence, was not, however, utilizable in any practical manner.

Some 10 yr later, Robert A. Nelson, Jr., working in Turner's laboratory, undertook a study of the unsolved problem of growth of *T. pallidum* on artificial media. Although neither he nor others have as yet solved this problem, he was successful in maintaining the organisms alive, motile and virulent for 5–10 days on an artificial medium largely free of tissue components. This having been accomplished, Nelson and Manfred Mayer conceived the simple idea of mixing an emulsion of motile treponemes in this medium with syphilitic or normal serum plus complement, and observing the result directly under the microscope. When the mixture consisted of normal serum plus treponemes plus complement, nothing happened within 15–8 hr; the organisms remained motile and virulent. On the other hand, if syphilitic sera (from animals or man) were employed, the treponemes were immobilized and killed. By appropriate absorption experiments, it was next demonstrated that the antibody responsible for this phenomenon is distinct from reagin.

Further studies which originated at Johns Hopkins provided additional information about this treponemal immobilizing antibody:

(1) It does not occur in the serum of normal persons or of those suffering from nontreponemal diseases.

(2) It occurs uniformly in syphilis and the closely related treponematoses of yaws, pinta and bejel, but not in other spirochetal diseases such as leptospirosis, relapsing fever, rat bite fever or Vincent infections.

(3) In untreated syphilitic infection, its rate of appearance in the serum approximately parallels that of reagin; it is first detectable when the primary lesion is from 5 to 15 days old and rapidly increases in titer for the first few weeks reaching a plateau at about the second or third month of infection. However, in syphilitic rabbits, it does not decline or disappear from the serum following the spontaneous healing of the chancre as does reagin and it is probable that in humans with untreated infection it does not spontaneously decrease in titer with the passage of years.

(4) In treated early syphilis, treponemal immobilizing antibody disappears from the serum as does reagin but at a slower rate and not necessarily in a parallel manner. Thus, patients treated for early syphilis are usually found years later to be seronegative with both tests, although sometimes they are positive for treponemal immobilizing antibody and negative for reagin.

(5) In treated late syphilis, treponemal immobilizing antibody usually does not disappear from the serum, though reagin may do so. These and other data permit the conclusion that the treponemal immobilization (TPI) test detects an antibody specific for syphilis and the related treponematoses.

These studies of Turner *et al.*, covering two decades, were summarized in 1957 in a monograph entitled *Biology of the Treponematoses* by Turner and David H. Hollander.

MOORE'S CLASSIC MONOGRAPHS ON SYPHILIS

In 1933, Moore published a monumental work entitled *The Modern Treatment of Syphilis* and in 1941 a second edition of this book appeared. In this second edition of nearly 700 pages, Moore discussed authoritatively and in detail every facet of the treatment of syphilis in the pre-penicillin era. The book is a landmark in the history of the subject.

John F. Mahoney, R. C. Arnold and A. Harris first tried penicillin in syphilis "after limited animal experimentation indicated that penicillin possesses some spirocheticidal activity". Four patients with primary lesions were treated with 25,000 units intramuscularly at 4-hr intervals for 8 days. The chancres all became darkfield negative within 16 hr and various serological tests rapidly became negative also. During the first 8 hr of therapy, the patients complained of malaise and headache, and had slight elevations of temperature. The lesions became painful and the regional lymph nodes were enlarged and tender. These results were described in a preliminary report entitled 'Penicillin treatment of early syphilis' published in *Venereal Disease Information* in 1943. Mahoney's observations were promptly confirmed by C. W. Barnet who reported similar results in seven cases of early syphilis. Mahoney *et al.* soon reported a follow-up study of their original patients and in 1946 the U.S. Public Health Service issued a statement in which it was pointed out that there were some treatment failures especially in those treated late and in those treated with a total of only 600,000 units as against 2.4 million units. Moore and his colleagues gained enormous experience with the use of this antibiotic in various stages of the disease. These early reports were followed by a flood of studies of such magnitude that in 1946 Moore felt impelled to summarize them together with his own conclusions in book form. This volume was a definitive compilation of the experience up to that date and dealt with the use of penicillin in every stage of syphilis. By 1953, Moore was able to state that penicillin, first introduced into the treatment of syphilis in 1943, had completely replaced arsenic, bismuth and mercury in all stages of the disease.

FURTHER STUDIES WITH PENICILLIN

The introduction of penicillin created the need for evaluation of immunity factors in relation to penicillin therapy. In an important study, Hollander, Turner and Nell found that subcurative doses of penicillin prolonged the incubation period. In some rabbits, the incubation period was prolonged to several weeks by means of sub-clinical infection, but then "the evolution of the syphilitic infection after termination of treatment was in general similar to that observed in untreated animals. . . . Wholly symptomless infection was not observed. Rabbits were either cured or subsequently developed clinically recognizable lesions." The implication was clear that in man it was better to waste some penicillin than to give too little in both prophylaxis and therapy.

In 1955, Hardy and Nell succeeded in preparing suspensions of *T. pallidum* suitable for specific agglutination studies and capable of being stored for months. By means of such studies, they demonstrated true syphilitic antibodies different from 'nonspecific Wassermann antibody'. This test, like the TPI test, is highly specific, although certain technical problems have limited its use.

THE CHRONIC BIOLOGIC FALSE-POSITIVE (BFP) TEST FOR SYPHILIS

Ever since the early days of the Wassermann test, it was known that false-positive tests might be obtained. Moore *et al.* made systematic studies of this phenomenon and designated as BFP those tests which were not due to technical errors. The first paper describing these studies was published in 1940 by Moore, Eagle and Mohr and was entitled 'A suggested approach to the clinical study of biologic false positive tests for syphilis'. Later results were described by Moore and Mohr in an article in the *Journal of the American Medical Association* entitled 'Biologically false positive serologic tests for syphilis: type, incidence and cause'. The authors distinguished between acute and chronic BFP reactors. The acute variety, they pointed out, was a temporary phenomenon which occurred most often in connection with various acute infectious diseases and usually disappeared spontaneously within 6 months. The chronic variety, on the other hand, was not associated with any evident acute cause and the standard serodiagnostic tests remained positive for long periods of time. In a later study, Moore and Lutz dealt comprehensively with the chronic biologic false-positive test for syphilis.

CHANGE TO THE STUDY OF OTHER CHRONIC DISEASES

The Syphilis Division of the Medical Clinic, with its dual facilities and organization—a clinic and a laboratory side by side, the one attempting to study syphilis in the human being, the other approaching the study of the disease in the experimental laboratory—was probably, during the four decades of its existence, the most active center for research in syphilis in this country. Its contribution was threefold:

(1) It brought to bear upon the diagnosis and treatment of all phases of syphilis the point of view of the internist, and not that of the specialist in a more restricted field.

(2) It provided an opportunity for the instruction of students and physicians in the management of patients with syphilis.

(3) It conducted investigations of the disease as it occurs in man and as it is experimentally produced in rabbits.

All of these things had been done previously, but never before by a group of men working closely together in the same clinic. It was a unique development and is an outstanding example of the application of epidemiologic, clinical and laboratory research techniques to the study and treatment of an important disease.

When the advent of penicillin suddenly changed the character of the syphilis clinic, Moore, with his characteristic drive and initiative, turned his attention to other chronic diseases. He realized clearly that the organization and the methods he had developed for long-term follow-up and study of syphilis could be ideally applied to other chronic diseases. Thus, he organized a chronic-disease clinic, proposing as a start to study the natural history of three classes of patients that had accumulated in the long years of his attention to syphilis and its various manifestations. First, as pointed out earlier, he had Mohr were interested in those patients who had a positive serologic test for syphilis but turned out not to have the disease; the so-called false-positive serologic test for syphilis. He developed the idea that since patients with systemic lupus erythematosus were known to have a false-positive serologic test for syphilis, the myriad of patients that he accumulated with this serologic abnormality could form the base of a long-term prospective study of the pathogenesis of the connective-tissue diseases. The study, of course, was made possible by the development of the TPI test. It proved a very fertile field for clinical investigation. Second, he proposed to study the natural history of hypertensive vascular disease since a mass of clinical data had been gathered over many years on these patients, including the serial recording of their blood pressure. Third, he saw the opportunity to make observations on the natural history of serum hepatitis, as many such cases had accumulated in the clinic files as a result of the use of arsenicals in the treatment of syphilis.

Working with Moore in the operation of this multifaceted chronic-disease clinic was Ernest W. Smith, who was later Director of the Subdepartment of Dermatology for several years. Other participants conducted follow-up clinics: Albert H. Owens, in oncology; Lawrence E. Shulman, in connective-tissue disease; and W. Gordon Walker, in renal disease. Moore obtained a training grant for these activities from the National Heart Institute.

After Moore developed prostatic cancer in 1954, Smith became associate director of the clinic to provide for a smooth transition in leadership. Smith became the director and discharged his duties with distinction until 1957.

THE DIVISION OF MEDICAL GENETICS

Dr. Victor A. McKusick (Fig. 9) became the director of the clinic on 1 July 1957, at which time he developed a Division of Medical Genetics in the Department of Medicine. Moore had published serially McKusick's classic monograph *Heritable Diseases of Connective Tissue* in successive issues of the *Journal of Chronic Diseases* beginning in 1955. The name of the clinic was changed to the Joseph Earle Moore Clinic.

McKusick received his medical degree from Johns Hopkins in 1946. After an internship and assistant residency on the Osler Medical Service, he obtained research training in the cardiovascular field from 1948 to 1950 at the U.S. Public Health Service Hospital in Baltimore. He was Chief Resident Physician at the Johns Hopkins Hospital in 1951–1952. McKusick has been a member of the faculty of the Department of Medicine at Johns Hopkins continuously since 1947. He was appointed a professor in 1960 and became Chairman of the Department of Medicine in 1973.

McKusick's contributions to the field of cardiovascular sound were largely descriptive and were incorporated in his monograph *Cardiovascular Sound in Health and Disease.* He adapted the sound spectrography method of the Bell Telephone Laboratory. He used the method, which he called spectral phonocardiography, in describing heart sounds and murmurs as well as respiratory sounds. Also in the cardiovascular field, McKusick, through comparative epidemiologic studies in the U.S. and the Orient, and through clinical investigations in both areas, re-established Buerger's disease as a valid

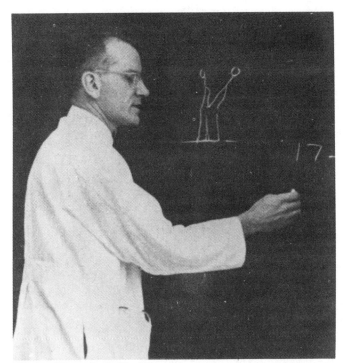

Fig 9. Victor A. McKusick.
From the Alan M. Chesney Medical Archives, the Johns Hopkins Medical Institutions. Courtesy of Dr. Michael Criley.

entity. McKusick is a member of the American Society for Clinical Investigation, the Association of American Physicians, the American Society of Human Genetics (president, 1974) and other scientific and professional societies. He is a member of the National Academy of Sciences and of the American Philosophical Society. In 1977, he received the Gairdner Award and is also a recipient of the John Phillips Award of the American College of Physicians and the William A. Allan Award of the American Society of Human Genetics.

FELLOWS IN THE JOSEPH EARLE MOORE CLINIC

From Moore's clinic, McKusick inherited a tradition for long-term follow-up, an important link with the School of Hygiene and an ongoing fellowship program that had external funding. Moore had many contacts in England, and at a time when it was not easy to recruit fellows in this country, many were sent to him from England for training. Those who were already working in the Joseph Earle Moore Clinic when McKusick assumed the directorship included Edmund A. Murphy, Thomas Scott and R. H. Bannerman, McKusick continued the practice of recruiting fellows from abroad, and while he was the director, more than 100 able young men and women from abroad were trained in the Joseph Earle Moore Clinic.

Dr. Samuel H. Boyer, IV, was McKusick's first fellow. Boyer graduated from the Stanford Medical School in 1954. After an internship at Stanford, he went to Downstate Medical Center in Brooklyn to work on heart sounds under William Dock. Boyer came to Baltimore in 1956. He first worked in phonocardiography, but soon transferred his interest to medical genetics. He undertook a study of the genetics and cardiovascular features of Friedreich's ataxia in collaboration with Arthur Chisholm, of Toronto, a fellow in cardiology at the time. In the summer of 1958, Boyer spent several months with James V. Neel in the Department of Human Genetics at Ann Arbor and the remainder of the year at the Galton Laboratory in London. He returned to the Division of Medical Genetics in September of 1959 and has been there uninterruptedly since that time. In 1971, he was appointed Professor of Medicine and, in 1972, Professor of Biology in the Department of Biology of the Johns Hopkins University School of Arts and Sciences. From July 1973 to November 1975, he served as Co-chief of the Division of Medical Genetics with Murphy. In 1975, he became a Howard Hughes Investigator. Since 1975, he has been editor of the *Johns Hopkins Medical Journal.*

Among the early foreign fellows were Malcolm Ferguson Smith and Ian Porter from England, Alan Skyring and Barry Smithurst from Sydney, Australia, and Hymie Gordon from South Africa.

David Price Evans and David Weatherall were the first of more than a dozen fellows from the University of Liverpool. Indeed, an important aspect of the fellowship program was the relationship which was established with the Department of Medicine at the University of

Liverpool. A project involving the Rh problem was a joint one between the department in Liverpool and the staff of the Medical Genetics Division, particularly Julius R. Krevans. Many studies were conducted on prisoner volunteers (it is noteworthy that such studies would be impossible now).

Dr. Wilma Bias was also involved with the program for developing a prevention for Rh disease. She, and David Bolling, subsequently members of the faculty of the Division of Medical Genetics in immunogenetics, and statistical genetics, respectively, started out as fellows in the division. Diagamlier S. Borgoankar was appointed in 1964 as director of the cytogenetics laboratory.

A Ph.D. program in human genetics was initiated early in the 1960s. This program gave degrees under the aegis of a university-wide committee. Alan E. H. Emery was the first recipient of the Ph.D. under this program in 1963. Emery is now Professor of Human Genetics in Edinburgh University. David Rimoin, a Canadian who had graduated from McGill University School of Medicine, worked for a Ph.D. in human genetics from 1964 to 1967, his thesis being on genetic disorders of the endocrine system with particular reference to pituitary dwarfism and diabetes. Samia Temtamy, a fellow from Egypt from 1961 to 1966, completed a thesis for the Ph.D. in human genetics on the genetics of hand malformations. Claude M. Laberge, a Canadian from Laval University in Quebec City, earned a Ph.D. by performing genetic studies on French Canadian populations. In 1968, Dr. William McElroy, who was then Chairman of the Department of Biology, established a section of human genetics in the Department of Biology and gave all members of the then existing university-wide committee appointments in the Department of Biology at the same level as they held in their primary departments.

Irene Hussels (later Maumenee) came to the Joseph Earle Moore Clinic from Franceschetti in Geneva as a fellow in 1969. She subsequently continued her genetic work as a member of the faculty of the Department of Ophthalmology. G. S. Mutalik, later Dean of the Medical School at Poona, India, collaborated with Murphy in one of the early formalistic papers on genetic counseling.

Among the fellows in medical genetics from abroad, several have settled in the United States: Ian Porter, who was until recently chairman of the Department of Pediatrics at Albany; Hymie Gordon, who is in charge of medical genetics at the Mayo Clinic; Rimoin, who is chief of medical genetics at the Harbor General Hospital (of UCLA) in Torrance, California; and Bannerman, now in the Department of Medicine in Buffalo. Fellows from the U.S. have included Roswell Eldridge, who is at the National Institute of Neurological Diseases at Bethesda; Judith G. Hall at the University of Washington in Seattle; R. Neil Schimke at the University of Kansas School of Medicine in Kansas City; Charles I. Scott at the University of Texas in Galveston; Thaddeus E. Kelly in the Department of Pediatrics at the University of Virginia in Charlottesville; and Richard Goodman, a graduate of Ohio State University School of Medicine, who has subsequently settled in Israel where he is Professor of Medical Genetics in Tel Aviv.

In addition to the United Kingdom and other countries mentioned, Joseph Earle Moore Clinic fellows have come from Norway, Finland, Denmark, Italy, Japan, Thailand, Iran, Iraq, France, Germany, Argentina, Venezuela, Mexico and several other countries.

A major contribution of the program of training in medical genetics in the Joseph Earle Moore Clinic came from McKusick's directing a large number of previously largely undifferentiated young clinicians into medical genetics as an academic clinical discipline. He showed them that hereditary diseases constitute an exciting area for investigation and a satisfying area for clinical service. The Joseph Earle Moore Clinic program, situated as it has been in a large general hospital, brought genetics into the mainstream of clinical medicine.

Although the largest number of the fellows, particularly at the beginning, came from backgrounds in internal medicine, many had had special training in areas such as rheumatology, endocrinology, cardiology (many in this area because of McKusick's earlier interests) and gastroenterology. There were also fellows from neurology, orthopedic surgery, dermatology, dentistry, psychiatry, opthalmology and obstetrics−gynecology. Pediatrics was a particularly stong area with Hall, Scott, Kelly and David Danks (now Professor of Pediatrics at Melbourne) as outstanding representatives. The great strides in pediatrics came at a time when genetics was not an administratively organized unit in the Department of Pediatrics at Johns Hopkins, notwithstanding the excellent work of Barton Childs.

Several of the fellows were launched in special areas of medical genetics in which they have since achieved particular eminence. For example, David Price Evans performed a classic study of the genetics of isoniazid metabolism (1958−1959) and has had a continuing interest in pharmacogenetics, a field to which he is a major contributor. He is now Professor of Medicine at Liverpool, England.

AREAS OF RESEARCH INTEREST

The research interests of the division of medical genetics have covered all areas of human genetics. The division has developed competence in biochemical genetics, immunogenetics, statistical genetics, cytogenetics and clinical genetics, with laboratories in all of these areas.

Murphy (Fig. 10), originally brought to Johns Hopkins as a fellow by Moore to pursue studies of hypertension in 1956, developed the statistical and biomathematical aspects of the genetics program. After training elsewhere, Murphy has worked continuously in the Joseph Earle Moore Clinic since 1968. He served as Co-chief of the Division of Medical Genetics from July 1973 to November 1975, at which time he became the sole chief of the division.

Murphy's interest in peripheral vascular disease,

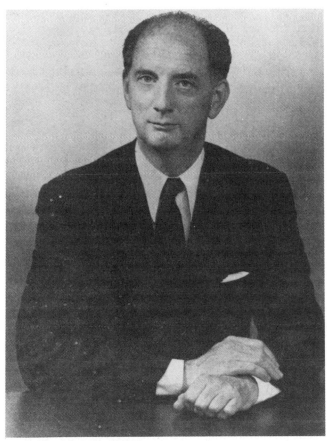

Fig 10.   Edmond A. Murphy.

genetics and statistics has led to a series of papers, both practical and theoretical, on the physiology and pathology of platelet survival, the adaptation of target theory to platelets, longevity and carcinogenesis (with Bolling and two graduate students, Mildred Francis and Ann Zauber) and to interpretations of the genetics of the vascular disease with Caroline Bedell Thomas (a former mentor of Murphy's) and Peter Kwiterovich. Murphy has contributed to the theoretical (logical) basis of medicine in general and genetic counseling, in particular, with several monographs on these subjects.

When the division began in 1957, the primary research areas included heritable disorders of connective tissue and the genetics of cardiovascular disease. McKusick soon turned attention to linkage and chromosome mapping in man. Dr. James Renwick, who with Sylvia Lawler had been responsible for identifying the nail—patella/ABO linkage (one of the first clearly established autosomal linkages in man), was persuaded to come to Baltimore in November 1958 for a sojourn of several months. Over the next 10 yr, Renwick retained a relationship with the division, making two or three trips a year to Baltimore. With the help first of Jane Schulze and later of Bolling, Renwick developed computer methods for analyzing pedigree data for linkage.

In 1958, McKusick became interested in the analysis of the linkage between the glucose 6-phosphate dehydrogenase (G6PD) and colorblindness loci on the X-chromosome and devised the Grandfather Method for analyzing linkage. Porter found that these two loci are only about 5 centimorgans apart. Further studies on the X-chromosome eventuated in the publication of a monograph entitled 'On the X-chromosome of man' which appeared first in the *Quarterly Review of Biology* in 1962.

Another important discovery in the area of linkage was R. P. Donahue's assignment of the Duffy blood group locus to chromosome No. 1 in 1968. This was the first specific autosomal assignment in man. Donahue was a Ph.D. candidate studying fertilization and early (preimplantation) stages of development. He determined his own karyotype and found a chromosomal variant not well known at that time. He was heterozygous for what is now termed $1qh$, an extended segment of heterochromatin adjacent to the centromere on the long arm of chromosome 1. At the time it was called 'uncoiler' (unc. No. 1) because in the preparations of that day it looked like a spirally uncoiled segment. Donahue had the enterprise to check as many relatives as possible for the same chromosome variant and at the same time to check all available genetic-marker traits, mainly blood groups. When the data were laid out, it was clear that a particular Duffy blood type was transmitted through the family along with $1qh$. The discovery, together with the introduction of the method of somatic-cell hybridization, ushered in an era of rapid advance in mapping the autosomes and by 1976 each of the 22 autosomes had at least one locus assigned to it.

Boyer, as a result of his contacts with Harry Harris at the Galton Laboratory, had developed an interest in genetic polymorphism. Using starch gel electrophoresis, he began, in 1959, to search for polymorphisms and discovered the first genetically variant myoglobins, and the A—B electrophoretic polymorphism of G6PD. Acquiring an interest in hemoglobins, he restudied a previously described family, segregating both hemoglobin Hopkins-2 and sickle hemoglobin. He investigated the switch in adult hemoglobin type that occurs in sheep and has for many years examined the distribution of fetal hemoglobins in adults. In recent years, he has turned from a study of protein gene products to the study of the gene itself. This work has been done with a graduate student, Louis Kunkel, and an associate, Kirby Smith, among others. They have studied unique DNA components of the Y-chromosome and carried the same techniques over to the study of other chromosomes such as the X-chromosome.

McKusick's division continued to study heritable disorders of connective tissue. Editions of *Heritable Disorders of Connective Tissue* were published in 1956, 1960, 1966 and 1972. Studies in homocystinuria in 1964—1965 led to the separation of this condition from the Marfan syndrome. In the 1966 edition, the development of the nosology of the mucopolysaccharidoses was particularly noteworthy. In the late 1960s and early 1970s, McKusick's collaboration with Elizabeth Neufeld and George Martin, both of the National Institutes of Health, was highly rewarding in terms of elucidating the mucopolysaccharidoses and the Ehlers-Danlos syndromes, respectively, at a molecular level.

STUDIES OF THE AMISH

Beginning in 1962, extensive studies have been carried out in the Amish. In 1962, McKusick read an article about a physician in Paradise, Pennsylvania, who had many Amish patients; it was noted that chondrodystrophies were particulary frequent among the Amish. McKusick was interested in skeletal dysplasias as a natural outgrowth of his work on heritable disorders of connective tissue. Later in 1962, he received from the Johns Hopkins Press the manuscript of John Hostetler's book *Amish Society* (McKusick was then a member of the faculty advisory committee to the Press). He was immediately impressed that the Amish people were precisely the type of population that would be valuable to a geneticist interested in recessive disorders. By teaming up with Hostetler, McKusick was able to get his studies underway rather quickly. Janice England, a Ph.D. candidate in medical sociology who was already working in Lancaster County on health attitudes, became a fellow and assisted in early studies, particularly of the Ellis–van Creveld syndrome. Hostetler and McKusick collaborated with Bowman of Harrisburg in the study of pyruvate kinase deficiency hemolytic anemia in the Mifflin County (PA) Amish. They extended their studies of cartilage–hair hypoplasia, the new form of dwarfism first described in the Amish, to all Amish because it was found to be widespread. Dr. Hostetler obtained entry for McKusick's group to Amish communities throughout the country and in Ontario. This involved trips to Holmes county and neighboring areas of Ohio, to Adams, Allan, Elkhart and LaGrange Counties in Indiana as well as the neighboring area of southern Michigan, and to Ontario. In all of these areas, other genetic diseases besides dwarfism were investigated. McKusick would write to doctors practicing in each area requesting information about genetic disorders they might have observed among the Amish and enclosing a check list of categories of hereditary diseases and some specific disorders.

The Joseph Earle Moore Clinic did not serve simply as a base from which studies of the Amish were launched. Success in studying Amish came in large part from the fact that staff members of the Joseph Earle Moore Clinic went to the Amish as doctors—and as doctors genuinely interested in helping them. That they were prepared to give the Amish medical attention in the Joseph Earle Moore Clinic, to mobilize specialty resources of the Johns Hopkins Hospital to treat them and even in some cases to provide transportation to and from the hospital did much to gain their full cooperation. Since the Amish do not approve of Blue Shield/Blue Cross or other health insurance, medical care can be unusually burdensome.

The computer facilities of the Moore Clinic were put to extensive use in the Amish studies. Complete censuses organized by nuclear families and including basic demographic information were assembled for Lancaster County (Pennsylvania), Holmes County (Ohio), Geauga County (Ohio), Elkhart–LaGrange Counties (Indiana). A complete genealogy of the Lancaster County Amish, i.e. the tracing of all individuals back to the immigrant founders, was also assembled on the computer. These files were the basis for several publications done by photo-offset of the computer printout: directories, genealogies and an index to published genealogies. The Amish had no problem with making use of these products of modern technology. Providing these publications was the *quid pro quo* that allowed collection of genealogic information.

In August 1964, an article describing the studies of dwarfism in the Lancaster County Amish appeared in the Medicine section of *Time*. After reading this article, Eleanor Jones, an achondroplastic woman in charge of planning the program for the annual national convention of Little People of America, Inc. to be held in Gloucester City, New Jersey, in July 1965, invited McKusick to speak on genetics in relation to dwarfism. McKusick quickly accepted because of his interest in skeletal dysplasias and because of his recognition of this organization as another useful base for genetic study. Roswell Eldridge attended the meeting with McKusick and together they were able to identify 12 or 13 varieties of dwarfism. That meeting initiated a continuing relationship between the Joseph Earle Mogre Clinic and the Little People of America, Inc., which has been mutually highly productive. The Joseph Earle Moore Clinic became identified as a national center for medical problems of little people, just as it has been for the Amish. In return for the opportunity to investigate little-peoples' genetic diseases, the clinic physicians had to be prepared to do all they could to treat diseases as well as to treat nongenetic illnesses the little people might develop. Steven Kopits, with the help of David Hungerford and Vernon T. Tolo, developed a strong program in the orthopedic management of skeletal dysplasias. A program in rehabilitation was developed by Arthur Siebens, one in special neurosurgical problems by George Udvarhelyi, and another in hearing and other otolaryngological problems by Ernest Kopstein. A competent staff was organized for dietary, psychologic, vocational and genetic counseling. John P. Dorst, Chief of Pediatric Radiology, provided expert aid in the differential diagnosis of the many chondrodysplasias by radiologic means.

Genetic nosology, that is, the delineation and classification of genetic disease, was another compelling interest of the Joseph Earle Moore Clinic. From the studies he had carried out on the X-chromosome, McKusick assembled a list of all X-linked traits as an indication of what genetic information is carried by the human X-chromosome. The catalogue of X-linked loci was published in the monograph on the X-chromosome referred to earlier. When McKusick undertook studies of the Amish, he expected to find 'new' recessive diseases and, therefore, it was important to know what recessive diseases were already known; he thus assembled a similar catalogue of autosomal recessives. Then, for the sake of completeness, he compiled a catalogue of autosomal dominant traits.

Bolling, who was in charge of computational aspects of the Joseph Earle Moore Clinic's programs, persuaded McKusick to put this material on the computer for ease of updating and corrections. The three catalogues, together with indices, were first published in 1966 under the title *Mendelian Inheritance in Man*. The editions of 1966, 1968 and 1971 were photo-offset publications of the computer printout and were all in upper-case lettering. Beginning with the fourth edition in 1975 and continuing with the fifth in 1978, the computer tapes were used to drive an automatic typesetter and thereby obtain a book of conventional style.

An additional nosologic effort was a series of conferences entitled 'The clinical delineation of birth defects' which the Joseph Earle Moore Clinic sponsored jointly with the National Foundation–March of Dimes for five successive years (1968–1972). These were 1-week conferences during which the nosology of genetic diseases in various areas was discussed. The conferences resulted in the publication of 18 books containing a wealth of clinical information from Johns Hopkins and elsewhere. The books were published as part of the Birth Defects Original Article Series of the National Foundation–March of Dimes under the general editorship of Daniel Bergsma.

Another interest of McKusick's, hemophilia in the royal houses of Europe, led to a paper in the *Scientific American* (Sci. Am. 213: 88, 1965) which had unexpected repercussions. The paper contained some comments about the possibility that the gene which had done so much damage was still extant. The attempts to solve the problem to everyone's satisfaction resulted in the development of a formal system of genetic counseling to which Murphy, Gary Chase, Bolling and several fellows contributed and which culminated in a text by Murphy and Chase. This continues an active interest in the clinic, and one intimately related to linkage analysis, the detection of the carrier state and the peculiar problems of age-dependent genetic disease. The last are illustrated by ongoing studies by Murphy, Anne Krush and Francis Milligan of familial polyposis coli. Susan Folstein and Reed Pyeritz are pursuing similar studies of Huntington's chorea and the Marfan syndrome, respectively.

The field of genetic counseling is a sensitive one, both personally and politically. Inevitably all who practice it must sooner or later become concerned with the modern version of an old problem, eugenic impact. Problems of normality and disease, classification and formal taxonomy suddenly acquire vital importance and have loomed large in Murphy's writings in the last 10 yr or more. The more explicitly practical questions of the impact of counseling have been the subject of collaborative studies with Childs and Claire Leonard in the department of pediatrics. McKusick has repeatedly pointed out the important function of inheritance in identifying those at risk of genetic disease ('practicing preventive medicine at the family level'). The extensive file of disorders in pedigrees that Margaret Hawkins Abbott has maintained in the Moore Clinic for over 20 yr is a rich resource of which only a small fraction has been tapped. The practical value of looking at the relatives of patients with heritable disorders has been admirably illustrated

by studies of polyposis coli, which in recent years have uncovered many latent victims.

Interest in isolated growth hormone deficiency as the basic defect in midgets of the General-Tom-Thumb type was stimulated by a patient with mitral stenosis who was admitted to the inpatient clinic research unit under Dr. J. O'Neal Humphries. The woman was normally developed sexually, and, in fact, had had a daughter of normal stature whom she had breast-fed. Thomas Merimee measured growth hormone in this woman by the radioimmunoassay method. The conventional wisdom at that time was that *asexual* ateleiotic dwarfs had hypopituitarism (and hypogonadism) as the basis of their growth problem, but that *sexual* ateleiotic dwarfs (such as this woman) had some constitutional problem, perhaps end-organ unresponsiveness, and had normal growth hormone. The work that was subsequently done by Rimoin, Merimee and McKusick established that many of the General-Tom-Thumb-type sexual ateleiotic dwarfs had isolated growth hormone deficiency inherited as an autosomal recessive trait. This work and Rimoin's comparison of diabetes mellitus in the Amish and in Indians of the southwest stimulated further studies in the genetics of endocrine diseases and led to the publication of a monograph entitled *Genetic Disorders of the Endocrine System* by Rimoin and R. Neil Schimke.

Other large-scale studies were conducted in the Joseph Earle Moore Clinic on familial dysautonomia, familial Mediterranean fever, amyloid neuropathy, diastrophic dwarfism and the TAR (thrombocytopenia-absent radius) syndrome.

McKusick acquired much experience in assembling cases of hereditary diseases through studies of heritable disorders of connective tissue. Patients were traced through the files of ophthalmology, dermatology, cardiology, orthopedic surgery and many other specialties that deal with various manifestations of these pleiotropic syndromes such as the Marfan syndrome, Ehlers–Danlos syndrome and pseudoxanthoma elasticum. The study of homocystinuria also illustrates a special approach taken by the Joseph Earle Moore Clinic in the 1960s. While Charles Dent of the University College, London, was at Johns Hopkins in 1964 to give the Thayer Lecture, he informed McKusick of his experience with cases of homocystinuria simulating the Marfan syndrome. With the cooperation of the Wilmer Ophthalmologic Institute and eye clinics all over the country, Schimke, working with McKusick, had urine samples mailed to Baltimore on cases of presumed Marfan syndrome and/or ectopia lentis. It was found that nontraumatic ectopia lentis is due to homocystinuria in about 5% of cases. Homocystinuria had been identified as a disorder usually accompanied by moderate or severe mental retardation, because it was first discovered in the course of a urine chromatography survey in institutions for the mentally retarded in Northern Ireland. Study of cases ascertained through ectopia lentis showed that the disease is consistent with superior intelligence as illustrated by the Ph.D. degree held by at least one subject. The studies of dysautonomia, skeletal dysplasias, amyloid neuropathy, limb anomalies, intestinal polyposis and other disorders likewise illustrated the need to use special means of assembling representative groups for study. Studies in the Joseph Earle Moore Clinic also showed the usefulness, indeed necessity, in genetic studies, of encompassing the full age range, and that the unit of study in medical genetics is the family as much or more than the individual patient. The children of families under study were investigated and many children with genetic disorders seen in the Joseph Earle Moore Clinic were admitted to the pediatric clinical research unit under the care of the Joseph Earle Moore Clinic staff. The genetic muco-polysaccharidoses, starting with the prototype Hurler syndrome, a disorder of children under age 10, exemplifie a group of conditions, some of which are present only in young children, others mainly in adults.

An important contributor to the programs of the Joseph Earle Moore Clinic and the Division of Medical Genetics has always been the case assistant. It was found that the best type of person for this position was an individual with college education and a lot of common sense, often a person who had raised a family to the point where the children were in school. The case workers in the Joseph Earle Moore Clinic are a direct outgrowth of the case workers in the syphilis clinic. They work not only in the genetics clinic but in other aspects of the program.

The other clinical units of the Joseph Earle Moore Clinic thrived. The Oncology Clinic under Albert Owens split off as the Grant Ward Clinic and moved to a separate facility in Carnegie 3. Eventually this clinic became a part of the Oncology Center. The Hypertension Clinic was directed by several different persons; one of them was Nemat Borhani, an Iranian American who was a fellow in genetics and previously interested in hypertension. He subsequently received training and a doctorate with Dr. Abraham Lilienfeld in the School of Hygiene and Public Health. Borhani is presently professor of preventive medicine at the University of California, Davis. R. Patterson Russell, a former student and medical resident at Johns Hopkins who had spent a year with Sir George Pickering at Oxford, is now director of the Hypertension Clinic. The Connective Tissue Clinic, which originated from Moore's interest in the chronic BFP test for syphilis, has always been one of the leading clinics at Johns Hopkins. The Sarcoid Clinic, now under the guidance of Carol J. Johns, has been another outstanding one.

Soon after the development of the General Clinical Research Centers Program of the National Institutes of Health, the staff of the Joseph Earle Moore Clinic felt that an outpatient general clinical research center had much to recommend it. Many chronic diseases can be best studied, and perhaps in some instances only studied, on an ambulatory basis. In addition, it is less expensive to conduct studies in ambulatory patients. Several applications were made during the early 1960s for a general outpatient clinical research center in the Moore Clinic. These applications came to naught. One of them had been scheduled for a project site visit which was cancelled the day before the arranged visit, and a second

application was approved by the study section with high priority but was vetoed at the highest level in the NIH; namely, by the director James Shannon. Shannon had qualms about general clinical research centers in the ambulatory setting because he feared that such a program would open a Pandora's box. Finally, however, with the contraction of research funding from Congress in the early 1970s, the economic argument became a compelling one and the Johns Hopkins application for support was at last approved. The grant was activated in 1973. Remodeling of the Joseph Earle Moore Clinic was completed in 1974 with a rededication of the clinic in May of that year. Dr. William Hillis became the director of the Outpatient Clinical Research Center (OPD-CRC), which is a unique facility. Although many general clinical research centers (GCRCS) see outpatients in conjunction with their inpatient programs, the Joseph Earle Moore Clinic is the only free-standing OPD-CRC. Johns Hopkins, therefore, has three general clinical research centers: the adult GCRC, the pediatric GCRC and the OPD-CRC.

Many noteworthy nongenetic studies are being conducted in the Joseph Earle Moore Clinic OPD-CRC illustrating the appropriateness of this setting for clinical investigation of certain types. These studies have included those by Mackenzie Walser on ketoacid analogs in uremia and liver failure and those by Phillip Reid on antiarrhythmic agents. Family studies by groups other than the Division of Medical Genetics included those by Stephen Baylin of the Endocrinology and Oncology Division on multiple endocrine adenomatosis and those of Frank Arnett on the genetics of rheumatic diseases.

The relationship with the School of Hygiene, which was particularly strong in biostatistics and epidemiology, also involved the Department of Public Health Administration where venereal disease control was taught in the past. Lilienfeld was responsible for this relationship with the School of Hygiene and Public Health. He had been in the Department of Epidemiology in the early 1950s and had been a member of the Galton–Garrod Society, composed of a small group of faculty sharing an interest in human genetics. Lilienfeld spent 1954–1958 in Buffalo as epidemiologist at the Roswell Park Cancer Institute. Ernest Stebbins, Dean of the School of Hygiene and Public Health, recruited him back to Baltimore to serve as a physician in the Joseph Earle Moore Clinic and as the director of the chronic-disease program in the School of Hygiene. He had a joint appointment in medicine and for a number of years his office was in the Joseph Earle Moore Clinic. He then acquired facilities in the School of Hygiene and developed a sizable division of chronic diseases in the Department of Epidemiology. For a time, there was a separate Department of Chronic Diseases, but when Philip Sartwell, Professor of Epidemiology, retired, chronic diseases was combined with the Department of Epidemiology with Lilienfeld as its head.

A history of the Joseph Earle Moore Clinic and the Division of Medical Genetics would be incomplete without reference to the Bar Harbor Course. In February

1959, during a site visit for a program project grant application, Dr. Earl Green, director of the Jackson Laboratory (Bar Harbor, Maine), visited the Joseph Earle Moore Clinic. McKusick was invited to visit the Jackson Laboratory which he did the following July (1959). The Bar Harbor Course was conceived in Testa's Restuarant in Bar Harbor on a warm July day over lunch with Dr. John Fuller, who was assistant director for training at the Jackson Laboratory. McKusick believed it would be appropriate for the Jackson Laboratory and the Johns Hopkins University, with a group of guest lecturers, to collaborate in the course because the scientists at the Jackson Laboratory functioned like medical geneticists in that they investigated mutations, searching for basic defects and how these are inherited. They had, of course, some techniques available to them which were not at the disposal of the human geneticist, and McKusick thought it would be useful for medical geneticists to be informed about the many mouse models. McKusick approached Mr. Basil O'Connor and Bergsma of the National Foundation—March of Dimes for support of the course. This fitted in well with the Foundation's new thrust in the area of birth defects, undertaken in 1958. The first 2-week course was given in August 1960 and the pattern has been consistently followed since that time. Lectures are held in the morning and evening, and the afternoons are kept for recreational activities or for optional workshops. The staff of the course has usually comprised at least six lecturers from other institutions, about 12 faculty members from the Johns Hopkins, and about 12 staff members from the Jackson Laboratory.

Beginning in 1967, a mammalian genetics course alternated yearly with the human course. This course had much greater emphasis on experimental mammalian genetics, but had a good deal of the same orientation as the medical genetics course. Between 1967 and 1979, a steady convergence of mouse genetics and human genetics occurred. The bodies of genetic information concerning the two species are now about on a par, and many of the same investigative tools are used. Comparative genetics of the two species is a useful approach as illustrated particularly with the X-chromosome, which has identical genetic content in the two species (Ohno's law), and the major histocompatibility complexes of the two species (H2 and HLA). The 20th annual course, in 1979, was a joint course (man and mouse) and the same pattern is planned for future years.

Thus, for over half a century, a unit which began as a special clinic for the treatment of patients with syphilis has been a successful outpatient facility for clinical investigation of chronic diseases. It is still a flourishing facility for patient care, teaching and research in medical genetics and other areas of clinical medicine.

ACKNOWLEDGEMENTS

I am deeply indebted to the following colleagues who have given me invaluable assistance in the preparation of this vignette: Richard Hahn, H. Hanford Hopkins, Victor McKusick, Edmund Murphy, Ernest Smith, Paul Spear and Thomas B. Turner. I wish to thank Carol Bocchini and Patricia King for their editorial work and typing, respectively.

REFERENCES

1. Bloomfield AL, Rantz LA and Kirby WMM: The clinical use of penicillin. J Am Med Ass 124: 627, 1944
2. Borgaonkar DS, Tryps L, Krush AJ and Murphy EA: The identification of individuals at high risk for large bowel cancer and the application of preventive measures in their management. Cancer 40: 2531, 1977
3. Boyer SH, Fainer DC and Naughton MA: Myoglobin: inherited structural variation in man. Science 140: 1228, 1963
4. Boyer SH, Porter IH and Weilbaecher RG: Electrophoretic heterogeneity of glucose-6-phosphate dehydrogenase and its relationship to enzyme deficiency in man. Proc Natn Acad Sci 48: 1868, 1962
5. Brown WH and Pearce L: A note on the dissemination of spirocheta pallida from the primary focus of infection. Arch Derm Syph 2: 470, 1920
6. Brown WH and Pearce L: Experimental syphilis in the rabbit—I. Primary infection of the testicle. J Exp Med 20: 475, 1920
7. Brown WH and Pearce L: Experimental production of clinical types of syphilis in the rabbit. Arch Derm Syph 3: 254, 1921
8. Brown WH and Pearce L: Superinfection in experimental syphilis following the administration of subcurative doses of arsphenamine or neoarsphenamine. J Exp Med 33: 553, 1921
9. Brunt PW and McKusick VA: Familial dysautonomia. A report of genetic and clinical studies, with a review of the literature. Medicine 49: 343, 1970
10. Chesney AM: Immunity in syphilis. Medicine 5: 459, 1926
11. Chesney AM: Acquired immunity in syphilis. Am J Syph 14: 289, 1930
12. Chesney AM, Halley CRL and Kemp JE: Studies in experimental syphilis—VII. Reinoculation of treated and untreated syphilitic rabbits with heterologous strains of Treponema pallidum. J Exp Med 46: 223, 1927
13. Chesney AM and Kemp JE: Incidence of spirocheta pallidum in cerebrospinal fluid during early stage of syphilis. J Am Med Ass 83: 1725, 1924
14. Chesney AM and Kemp JE: Experimental observations on the 'cure' of syphilis in the rabbit with arsphenamine. J Exp Med 39: 553, 1924
15. Chesney AM and Kemp JE: Studies in experimental syphilis—III. Further observations on the possibility of cure of syphilis in the rabbit with arsphenamine. J Exp Med 42: 17, 1925
16. Chesney AM and Kemp JE: Studies in experimental syphilis—IV. The survival of Treponema pallidum in the internal organs of treated and untreated rabbits. J Exp Med 42: 33, 1925
17. Chesney AM and Kemp JE: Observations on the possibility of cure of experimental syphilis in the rabbit. Trans Ass Am Physns 40: 189, 1925
18. Chesney AM and Kemp JE: Studies in experimental syphilis—VI. On variations in the response of treated rabbits to reinoculation. J Exp Med 44: 589, 1926
19. Chesney AM and Kemp JE: The curability of syphilis. J Am Med Ass 88: 905, 1927
20. Chesney AM, Turner TB and Grauer FH: Studies in experimental syphilis—X. Observations on cross-inoculations with heterologous strains of syphilitic virus. Bull Johns Hopkins Hosp 52: 145, 1933
21. Chesney AM, Woods AC and Campbell AD: Observations on the relation of the eye to immunity in experimental syphilis. J Exp Med 69: 163, 1939

22. Committee on Medical Research and the United States Public Health Service: The treatment of early syphilis with penicillin. J Am Med Ass 131: 265, 1946

23. Doak GO and Eagle H: Correlations between the Chemical Structure and Biological Activity of Arsenosobenzenes. First Symposium on Chemical–Biological Correlation, Chemical–Biological Coordination Center, National Research Council, National Academy of Sciences, Publication 206, pp. 7–43, 1951

24. Doak GO, Eagle H and Steinman HG: The preparation of phenylarsenoxides in relation to a projected study of their chemotherapeutic activity—I. Monosubstituted derivatives. J Am Chem Soc 62: 168, 1940

25. Doak GO, Eagle H and Steinman HG: The preparation of phenylarsenoxides—II. Derivatives of amino- and hydroxyphenylarsenoxides. J Am Chem Soc 62: 3010, 1940

26. Donahue RP, Bias WB, Renwick JH and McKusick VA: Probable assignment of the Duffy blood group locus to chromosome 1 in man. Proc Natn Acad Sci 61: 949, 1968

27. Eagle H: The mechanism of complement fixation. J Gen Physiol 12: 825, 1929

28. Eagle H: An explanation of the Wassermann and precipitation tests for syphilis. Bull Johns Hopkins Hosp 47: 292, 1930

29. Eagle H: Specific agglutination and precipitation—I. The mechanism of the reaction. J Immun 18: 393, 1930

30. Eagle H: Studies in the serology of syphilis—I. Mechanism of the flocculation reactions. J Exp Med 52: 717, 1930

31. Eagle H: Studies in the serology of syphilis—II. The physical basis of the Wassermann reaction. J Exp Med 52: 739, 1930

32. Eagle H: Studies in the serology of syphilis—III. Explanation of the fortifying effect of cholesterol upon the antigen as used in the Wassermann and flocculation tests. J Exp Med 52: 747, 1930

33. Eagle H: Studies in the serology of syphilis—IV. A more sensitive antigen for use in the Wassermann test. J Exp Med 53: 605, 1931

34. Eagle H: Studies in the serology of syphilis—V. The cause of the greater sensitivity of the icebox Wassermann; the zone phenomenon and complement fixation. J Exp Med 53: 615, 1931

35. Eagle H: Studies in the serology of syphilis—VI. The induction of antibody to tissue lipoids (a positive Wassermann reaction) in normal rabbits. J Exp Med 55: 667, 1932

36. Eagle H: Studies in the serology of syphilis—VIII. A new flocculation test for the serum diagnosis of syphilis. J Lab Clin Med 17: 787, 1932

37. Eagle H: Some applications of colloid chemistry in the serum diagnosis of syphilis. J Phys Chem 36: 259, 1932

38. Eagle H: Studies in the serology of syphilis—XIII. The use of the same antigen for the Wassermann reaction and the author's flocculation test; and a recommended Wassermann technic. J Lab Clin Med 19: 621, 1934

39. Eagle H: The Laboratory Diagnosis of Syphilis: The Theory, Technique and Clinical Interpretation of the Wassermann and Flocculation Tests with Serum and Spinal Fluid. St. Louis: C. V. Mosby, 1937

40. Eagle H: On the spirocheticidal action of the arsphenamines on Spirocheta pallida in vitro. J Pharmac Exp Ther 64: 164, 1938

41. Eagle H: The minimal effective concentrations of arsenic and bismuth compounds on T. pallidum in vitro in relation to the therapeutic dose. Am J Syph Gonorrhea Vener Dis 23: 310, 1939

42. Eagle H: The effects of molecular oxygen and sulfhydryl compounds on the antispirochetal action of arsenic, bismuth and mercury compounds in vitro. J Pharmac Exp Ther 66: 10, 1939

43. Eagle H: The role of molecular oxygen in the antispirochetal activity of arsenic and bismuth compounds in vitro. J Pharmac Exp Ther 66: 423, 1939

44. Eagle H: On the specificity of serologic tests for syphilis as determined by 40,545 tests in a college student population. Am J Syph Gonorrhea Vener Dis 25: 7, 1941

45. Eagle H: The relative activity of penicillins F, G, K and X against spirochetes and streptococci in vitro. J Bact 52: 81, 1946

46. Eagle H: The systemic treatment of arsenic poisoning with BAL (2,3-dimercaptopropanol). Vener Dis Inf 27: 114, 1946

47. Eagle H: Speculations as to the therapeutic significance of the penicillin blood level. Ann Int Med 28: 260, 1948

48. Eagle H: Blood levels, renal clearance and chemotherapeutic activity, with particular reference to arsenicals and penicillin. In: Evaluation of Chemotherapeutic Agents. New York Academy of Medicine, Section on Microbiology, Symposium No. 2. New York: Columbia University Press, pp. 25–43, 1949

49. Eagle H: Host, drug and parasite factors that modify the therapeutic activity of penicillin. In: Advances in Internal Medicine. New York: Interscience Press, 1949

50. Eagle H and Doak GO: The biological activity of arsenosobenzenes in relation of their structure. Pharmac Rev 3: 107, 1951

51. Eagle H and Hogan RB: On the presence in syphilitic serum of antibodies to spirochetes; their relation to so-called Wassermann reagin and their significance for the serodiagnosis of syphilis. J Exp Med 71: 215, 1940

52. Eagle H, Hogan RB, Doak GO and Steinman HG: The effect of multiple substituents on the toxicity and treponemicidal activity of phenylarsenoxides. J Pharmac Exp Ther 74: 210, 1942

53. Eagle H, Magnuson HJ and Fleischman R: Clinical uses of 2,3-dimercaptopropanol (BAL)—I. The systemic treatment of experimental arsenic poisoning (mapharsen, lewisite, phenylarsenoxide) with BAL. J Clin Invest 25: 451, 1946

54. Eagle H, Magnuson HJ and Fleischman R: Relation of the size of the inoculum and the age of the infection to the curative dose of penicillin in experimental syphilis, with particular reference to the feasibility of its prophylactic use. J Exp Med 85: 423, 1947

55. Eagle H and Mendelsohn W: On the spirocheticidal action of the arsphenamines on Spirocheta pallida in vitro. Science 87: 194, 1938

56. Eagle H and Saz AK: Antibiotics. A Rev Microbiol 9: 173, 1955

57. Erickson PT and Eagle H: Evaluation of spirochete complement fixation reaction in comparison with the Eagle flocculation and Wassermann procedures. Vener Dis Inf 21: 31, 1940

58. Evans DAP, Manley KA and McKusick VA: Genetic control of isoniazid metabolism in man. Br Med J 2: 485, 1960

59. Evans DAP and White TA: Human acetylation polymorphism. J Lab Clin Med 63: 394, 1964

60. Finney JMT: A Surgeon's Life. New York: G. P. Putnam's, 1940

61. Hahn RD: Reinfection in congenital syphilis. Am J Syph Gonorrhea Vener Dis 25: 200, 1941

62. Hall JG, Levin J, Kuhn HP, Ottenheimer EJ, Van Berkum KAP and McKusick VA: Thrombocytopenia with absent radius (TAR). Medicine 48: 411, 1969

63. Hardy PH, Jr and Nell EE: Specific agglutination of Treponema pallidum by sera from rabbits and human beings with treponema infections. J Exp Med 101: 367, 1955

64. Hollander DH, Turner TB and Nell EE: The effect of long continued subcurative doses of penicillin during the incubation period of experimental syphilis. Bull Johns Hopkins Hosp 90: 105, 1952

65. Hopkins HH: Prognostic import of a negative spinal fluid in early and latent syphilis. Arch Derm Syph 24: 404, 1931

66. Hopkins HH: Incubation period of clinical neurosyphilis. Arch Neurol Psychol 29: 158, 1933

67. Kahn AS, Nelson RA Jr and Turner TB: Immunological relationships among species and strains of virulent treponemes as determined by the treponemal immobilization test. Am J Hyg 53: 296, 1951

68. Keidel A: Studies in asymptomatic neurosyphilis—IV. The apparent role of immunity in the genesis of neurosyphilis. J Am Med Ass 79: 874, 1922

69. Keidel A and Hurwitz SH: A comparison of normal and syphilitic extracts by means of the Wassermann and epiphanin reactions. J Am Med Ass 59: 1257, 1912

70. Keidel A and Moore JE: Studies in asymptomatic neurosyphilis—I. A tentative classification of early asymptomatic neurosyphilis. Arch Neurol Psychol 6: 286, 1921

71. Kemp JE and Menninger WC: The influence of inadequate treatment of early syphilis on the incidence and incubation period of neurosyphilis. Bull Johns Hopkins Hosp 58: 24, 1936

72. Kemp JE and Poole AK: Familial neurosyphilis—IV. Incidence of neurosyphilis among the parents of congenitally neurosyphilitic children. J Am Med Ass 84: 1395, 1925

73. Luetscher JA Jr, Eagle H and Longcope WT: The effect of BAL on the excretion of arsenic in arsenical intoxication. J Clin Invest 25: 535, 1946

74. Magnusen HJ: Current concepts of immunity in syphilis. Am J Med 5: 641, 1948

75. Mahloudji M, Teasdall RD, Adamkiewicz JJ, Hartmann WH, Lambird PA and McKusick VA: The genetic amyloidoses with particular reference to hereditary neuropathic amyloidosis, type II (Indiana or Rukavina type). Medicine 48: 1, 1969

76. Mahoney JF, Arnold RC and Harris A: Penicillin treatment of early syphilis: a preliminary report. Am J Pub Hlth 33: 1387, 1943

77. Mahoney JF, Arnold RC and Harris A: Penicillin treatment of early syphilis; a preliminary report. Vener Dis Inf 24: 355, 1943

78. Mahoney JF, Arnold RC, Sterner BL, Harris A and Zwally MR: Penicillin treatment of early syphilis—II. J Am Med Ass 126: 63, 1944

79. McKelvey JL and Turner TB: Syphilis and pregnancy. Analysis of outcome of pregnancy in relation to treatment in 943 cases. J Am Med Ass 102: 503, 1934

80. McKusick VA: On the X chromosome of man. Q Rev Biol 37: 69, 1962

81. McKusick VA: Heritable Disorders of Connective Tissue. 4th ed. St. Louis: C. V. Mosby, 1972

82. McKusick VA: Bar Harbor course in medical genetics. Science 176: 820, 1972

83. McKusick VA: The growth and development of human genetics as a clinical discipline. Am J Hum Genet 27: 261, 1975

84. McKusick VA (ed.): Medical Genetic Studies of the Amish. Selected Papers. Baltimore: Johns Hopkins University Press, 1978

85. McKusick VA: Mendelian Inheritance in Man. 5th ed. Baltimore: Johns Hopkins University Press, 1978

86. McKusick VA: Genetic nosology—three approaches. Am J Hum Genet 30: 105, 1978

87. McKusick VA, Egeland JA, Eldridge R and Drusen DE: Dwarfism in the Amish—I. The Ellis–Van Creveld syndrome. Bull Johns Hopkins Hosp 115: 306, 1964

88. McKusick VA, Eldridge R, Hostetler JA, Egeland JA and Ruangwit U: Dwarfism in the Amish—II. Cartilage–hair hypoplasia. Bull Johns Hopkins Hosp 116: 285, 1965

89. McKusick VA and Ruddle FH: The status of the gene map of the human chromosomes. Science 196: 390, 1977

90. Michaelis L: Die Wassermannsche syphilis reaktion. Berl Klin Wschr 44: 1103, 1907

91. Michaelis L: Präcipitin reaktion bei syphilis. Berl Klin Wschr 44: 1477, 1907

92. Moore JE: Studies in asymptomatic neurosyphilis—II. The classification, treatment and prognosis of early asymptomatic neurosyphilis. Bull Johns Hopkins Hosp 33: 231, 1922

93. Moore JE: Studies in asymptomatic neurosyphilis—III. The apparent influence of pregnancy on the incidence of neurosyphilis in women. Arch Int Med 30: 548, 1922

94. Moore JE: The relation of neurorecurrences to late syphilis. Arch Neurol Psychiat 21: 117, 1929

95. Moore JE: The Modern Treatment of Syphilis. 2nd ed. Springfield, Illinois: Charles C Thomas, 1941

96. Moore JE: Penicillin in Syphilis. Springfield, Illinois: Charles C Thomas, 1946

97. Moore JE: The changing pattern of syphilis, 1941–1953. Ann Int Med 39: 644, 1953

98. Moore JE and Eagle H: The Treatment and Prophylaxis of Syphilis. New York: Oxford University Press, 1939

99. Moore JE and Eagle H: The quantitative serologic test for syphilis: its variability, usefulness in routine diagnosis and possible significance. A study of 1665 cases. Ann Int Med 14: 1801, 1941

100. Moore JE, Eagle H and Mohr CF: A suggested approach to the clinical study of biologic false positive tests for syphilis. J Am Med Ass 115: 1602, 1940

101. Moore JE and Faupel M: Asymptomatic neurosyphilis—V. A comparison of early and late symptomatic neurosyphilis. Arch Derm Syph 18: 99, 1928

102. Moore JE and Hopkins HH: Asymptomatic neurosyphilis—VI. The prognosis of early and late asymptomatic neurosyphilis. J Am Med Ass 95: 1637, 1930

103. Moore JE and Keidel A: The treatment of early syphilis—I. A plan of treatment for routine use. Bull Johns Hopkins Hosp 39: 1, 1926

104. Moore JE and Kemp JE: Studies in familial neurosyphilis—III. Conjugal neurosyphilis. Arch Int Med 32: 464, 1923

105. Moore JE and Kemp JE: The treatment of early syphilis—III. The Wassermann reaction in treated early syphilis. Bull Johns Hopkins Hosp 39: 36, 1926

106. Moore JE and Lutz WB: The natural history of systemic lupus erythematosus: an approach to its study through chronic biologic false positive reactors. J Chron Dis 1: 297, 1955

107. Moore JE and Mohr CF: Biologically false positive serologic tests for syphilis: type, incidence and cause. J Am Med Ass 150: 467, 1952

108. Moore JE and Padget P: The problem of seroresistant syphilis. J Am Med Ass 110: 96, 1938

109. Moore JE and Woods AC: Syphilitic primary optic atrophy—II. General considerations and the results of treatment by standard methods (especially subdural treatment and induced fever): a critical review. Am J Ophthal 23: 145, 1940

110. Moore JE and Woods AC: The pathology and pathogenesis of syphilitic primary optic atrophy. Am J Syph Gonorrhea Vener Dis 24: 59, 1940

111. Murphy EA: The Logic of Medicine. Baltimore: Johns Hopkins University Press, 1976

112. Murphy EA: Probability in Medicine. Baltimore: Johns Hopkins University Press, 1979

113. Murphy EA and Bolling DR: Testing of single locus hypotheses where there is incomplete separation of the phenotypes. Am J Hum Genet 19: 322, 1967

114. Murphy EA and Chase GA: Principles of Genetic Counseling. Chicago: Yearbook, 1975

115. Nelson RA Jr: Factors affecting the survival of *Treponema pallidum in vitro*. Am J Hyg 48: 120, 1948

116. Nelson RA Jr and Diesendruck JA: Studies on treponemal immobilization antibodies in syphilis—I. Techniques of measurement and factors influencing immobilization. J Immun 66: 667, 1951

117. Nelson RA Jr and Mayer MN: The mobilization of *Treponema pallidum in vitro* by antibody produced in syphilitic infection. J Exp Med 89: 369, 1949

118. Nelson RA Jr, Zheutlin HEC, Austin PGN and Hill JH: Applications of the treponemal immobilization test to problems of clinical syphilis. Presented before the Symposium on the Latest Advances in the Study of the Venereal Diseases, Washington, D.C.: 27–28 April 1950

119. Nelson RA Jr, Zheutlin HEC, Diesendruck JA and Austin PGN: Studies on treponemal immobilizing antibodies in syphilis; incidence in serum and cerebrospinal fluid in human beings and absence in "biologic false positive" reactors. Am J Syph 34: 101, 1950

120. Padget PC: Long-term results in the treatment of early syphilis. Am J Syph Gonorrhea Vener Dis 24: 692, 1940

121. Parodi U: Ueber die uebertragung der syphilis auf den hoden des kaninchens. Centralbl F Bakt 44: 428, 1907

122. Pearce L and Brown WH: A study of the relation of *Treponema pallidum* to lymphoid tissues in experimental syphilis. J Exp Med 35: 39, 1922

123. Pearl R and Pearl RD: The Ancestry of the Long-lived. Baltimore: Johns Hopkins University Press, 1934

124. Rich AR, Chesney AM and Turner TB: Experiments demonstrating that acquired immunity in syphilis is not dependent upon allergic inflammation. Bull Johns Hopkins Hosp 52: 179, 1933

125. Rimoin DL, Merimee TJ and McKusick VA: Growth-hormone deficiency in man: an isolated, recessively inherited defect. Science 152: 1635, 1966

126. Rimoin DL and Schimke RN: Genetic Disorders of the Endocrine Glands. St. Louis: C. V. Mosby, 1971

127. Schimke RN, McKusick VA, Huang T and Pollack AD: Homocystinuria: studies of 20 families with 38 affected members. J Am Med Ass 193: 711, 1965

128. Smith FR Jr: Late congenital syphilis; study of the results of treatment of 267 patients. Bull Johns Hopkins Hops 53: 231, 1933

129. Sternberg TH and Turner TB: The treatment of sulfonamide resistant gonorrhea with penicillin sodium. Results in 1686 cases. J Am Med Ass 126: 157, 1944

130. Thomas CB and Murphy EA: The circulatory response to smoking. J Chron Dis 8: 202, 1958

131. Thomas CB and Murphy EA: Further studies on cholesterol levels in the Johns Hopkins medical students. The effect of stress at examinations. J Chron Dis 8: 661, 1958

132. Thomas CB, Murphy EA and Bolling DR: The precursors of hypertension and coronary disease: statistical consideration of distributions in a population of medical students—I. Total serum cholesterol. Bull Johns Hopkins Hosp 114: 290, 1964

133. Turner TB: The preservation of virulent *Treponema pallidum* and *Treponema pertenue* in the frozen state. J Clin Invest 15: 470, 1936

134. Turner TB: Protective antibodies in the serum of syphilitic rabbits. J Exp Med 69: 867, 1939

135. Turner TB and Chesney AM: Experimental yaws—II. Comparison of the infection with experimental syphilis. Bull Johns Hopkins Hosp 54: 174, 1934

136. Turner TB, Cumberland MC and Li HY: Comparative effectiveness of penicillins G, F, K and X in experimental syphilis as determined by a short *in vivo* method. Am J Syph Gonorrhea Vener Dis 31: 476, 1947

137. Turner TB and Fleming WL: Prolonged maintenance of spirochetes and filterable viruses in the frozen state. J Exp Med 70: 629, 1939

138. Turner TB, Fleming WL and Brayton NL: Protective antibodies in the serum of human syphilitics. J Clin Invest 18: 471, 1939

139. Turner TB and Hollander DH: Biology of the Treponematoses. Monograph. Geneva: World Health Organization, 1957

140. Turner TB and MacLeod C: Cross immunity in experimental syphilis, yaws and venereal spirochetosis of rabbits. Trans Ass Am Physns 57: 265, 1942

141. Turner TB, MacLeod C and Updyke EL: Cross immunity in experimental syphilis, yuws and venereal spirochetosis of rabbits. Am J Hyg 46: 287, 1947

142. Turner TB and (by invitation) Nelson RA Jr: The relationship of treponemal immobilizing antibody to immunity in syphilis. Trans Ass Am Physns 63: 112, 1950

143. Turner TB and Saunders GM: Yaws in Jamaica—I. Epidemiological study of two rural communities. Am J Hyg 21: 483, 1935

144. Walker G: Studies in the experimental production of tuberculosis in the genitourinary organs. Johns Hopkins Hosp Rep 16: 1, 1911

145. Walker G: Venereal Disease in the American Expeditionary Forces. Baltimore, Maryland: Medical Standard, 1922

146. Wassermann H and Goodman MJ: The results of treatment in late mucocutaneous and osseous (benign late) syphilis. Am J Syph Neurol 18: 458, 1934

147. Weatherall DJ: Thalassaemia in a Gurkha family. Br Med J 1: 1711, 1960

148. Weatherall DJ: Enzyme deficiency in haemolytic disease of the newborn. Lancet 2: 835, 1960

149. Weatherall DJ and Clegg JB: The Thalassaemia Syndromes. 2nd ed. Oxford: Blackwell Science, 1972

150. Wexler J, Eagle H, Tatum HJ, Magnuson HJ and Watson EB: Clinical uses of 2,3-dimercaptopropanol (BAL)—II. The effect of BAL on the excretion of arsenic in normal subjects and after minimal exposure to arsenical smoke. J Clin Invest 25: 467, 1946

151. Williams JW: The significance of syphilis in prenatal care and in the causation of fetal death. Johns Hopkins Hosp Bull 31: 141, 1920

152. Williams JW: The value of the Wassermann reaction in obstetrics, based upon the study of 4547 consecutive cases. Johns Hopkins Hosp Bull 31: 335, 1920

153. Williams JW: Influence of the treatment of syphilitic pregnant women on the instance of congenital syphilis. Johns Hopkins Hosp Bull 33: 383, 1922

154. Young HH: Hugh Young, A Surgeon's Autobiography. New York: Harcourt, Brace, 1941

155. Zellmann HE and Nelson RA Jr: The effect of penicillin therapy on the titer of treponemal immobilizing antibody in human syphilitic patients. Presented before the Symposium on Recent Advances in the Study of Venereal Disease, Washington, D.C., 24–25 April 1951

19.
Albion Walter Hewlett: Pioneer Clinical Physiologist

INTRODUCTION

The modern practice of medicine is to a large extent applied physiology. In the decades since 1900 physicians have remolded the major concepts upon which the care of the sick is based. During this period the science of medicine at times pushed the art of medicine into a secondary position. One of those who successfully combined the two was Albion Walter Hewlett, a trained physiologist who developed into a skillful practitioner. Throughout his career he was orderly, thorough, scientific and appreciative of the needs of the patient; he was a brilliant teacher, a sound medical statesman and an outstanding example of the contributions made by graduates of The Johns Hopkins School of Medicine to the growth and development of other medical institutions.

Hewlett, the son of Frederick and Cleora Melissa Whitney Hewlett, was born on November 27, 1874 at Petaluma, California. We learn something of his early schooling from the reminiscences of Joseph Erlanger (a Nobel Prize winner for his work on single nerve fibers) who was a friend and classmate of Hewlett's. They both were enrolled in the "classical" course at the San Francisco Boys High School (despite its name it was co-educational). Those satisfactorily completing this course could be recommended for admission to the University of California without an examination. Hewlett suggested to Erlanger that the two of them try to gain admission to the University after completion of the second year at high school. They were both admitted, Hewlett without conditions, Erlanger with a condition in Latin, with the understanding that the condition would have to be removed by the end of the first year.

The University of California was a land grant college, and three years of military training was required. Commissioned officers served a fourth year but neither Hewlett nor Erlanger took the examination for that rank. It is well in retrospect that they did not for in their senior year they had to decide where they would pursue their medical studies. In San Francisco, at that time, there were two medical schools—the Troland Medical School and the Cooper Medical College. The latter was the better one and was located just around the corner from Erlanger's home. Erlanger recalled that but for a happy circumstance it would have been the school of his choice. Hewlett had met Herbert Moffitt, then a senior student at the Harvard

Medical School. (Subsequently, Moffitt became the dean and professor of medicine at the University of California Medical School in San Francisco and one of the city's and nation's most honored practitioners.) Moffitt told Hewlett about The Johns Hopkins University, which had recently started a medical school which he believed would be better than Harvard's. This was, indeed, a strong recommendation. So Erlanger and Hewlett decided to apply for admission there. Perusal of the catalogue indicated that they could meet all the entrance requirements except that for a reading knowledge of French. Erlanger arranged to acquire this skill during the summer months and without further formalities he was accepted for admission. According to Erlanger, Hewlett was also accepted, but at the eleventh hour he decided to attend the Cooper Medical College. However, after completion of the first year there, he applied for admission to the second year class at Johns Hopkins.

JOHNS HOPKINS SCHOOL OF MEDICINE

In a letter to William H. Welch, dean of The Johns Hopkins University School of Medicine, on January 11, 1897 Hewlett requested acceptance with second year standing. He pointed out that he had graduated from the University of California with the B.S. degree in 1895 and that he was at present an instructor in physics and chemistry at Cooper Medical College. At the medical college he studied osteology, dissected the lower parts and passed an examination in this subject. He indicated that he would be prepared for an examination on the head and upper parts which would complete his work in gross anatomy. In histology he took the term course at Berkeley after which he purchased a microscope and studied on his own, using slides which his friend Erlanger kindly lent him. In physiology he had been examined on the first third of Michael Foster's textbook and expected to be prepared for an examination on the whole. In laboratory work on that subject he had done the muscle-nerve experiment and a few pulse and cardiac tracings. He indicated that in physiological chemistry he would have to accept a condition, for with the exception of urine analysis, he had done no work in this area. Having the highest average in a class of 50 or more at Cooper Medical College, he offered his scholarship as his main selling point. Of his work at the University of California, he wrote that Mr. Erlanger could testify for him.

At a meeting of the medical faculty on January 28, 1897, Welch presented Hewlett's application. The opin-

Reprinted from the *Johns Hopkins Medical Journal* **144**: 202, 1979.

ion was expressed that Mr. Hewlett would hardly be able to meet the standards in histology, physiology and anatomy. He could enter only after examination in histology and good evidence of satisfactory work in physiology and anatomy. Welch therefore informed Hewlett that it was very doubtful that he could enter the second year in October 1897. (Welch had apparently written an earlier letter encouraging him to make the attempt.)

In his reply to Welch on March 22, Hewlett expressed his disappointment in the medical faculty's decision and hoped that a fuller statement of his case might change their verdict. He enclosed special letters from his teachers of anatomy, histology and physiology, which discussed his fitness for advanced standing. These letters from Martin Kellogg, president of the University of California, Joseph Le Conte, professor of natural history, and Drs. Ritter and Johnson, assistant professors in zoology, were all very laudatory. In Dr. Johnson's letter there was a comparison between Erlanger and Hewlett which read as follows: "I may say that Mr. Joseph Erlanger, who is now attending your institution, is a classmate of Mr. Hewlett's. The two gentlemen were nearly equal in scholarship at graduation. So far as zoology was concerned if there was any advantage it was on the side of Mr. Hewlett." Hewlett indicated that he had not requested this comparison but stated that with Mr. Erlanger's excellent showing at Johns Hopkins, he was certain that it would help him (Hewlett). "Outside of zoology, my marks, as I remember, were considerably better than his."

A note in the Johns Hopkins records dated April 20, 1897 signed by William Henry Welch reads as follows: "Brought Mr. Hewlett's application with these letters a second time before faculty at the meeting of April 1, 1897. A more encouraging view was taken, and it was noted that he may be allowed to try to enter second year. Answered his letter April 2 telling him of this decision and suggesting that he would have to pass examinations in normal histology and physiological chemistry and give evidence that his work in anatomy and physiology has been reasonably equivalent to that given here. Knowledge of normal histology especially emphasized. Said that if he takes the summer course at University of Chicago his chance of entering will be improved."

Hewlett took this advice and on October 6, 1897 he paid the registration fee and deposit required by The Johns Hopkins University School of Medicine at that time—$100 (Figs 1 and 2).

Hewlett's interest in scientific work began early and, according to Ray Lyman Wilbur, he did volunteer work in Walter E. Garrey's physiology laboratory, with which Wilbur was connected, during his student period at the Cooper Medical College. However, his first real scientific study was conducted in collaboration with Erlanger during his second year at Johns Hopkins. This resulted in a paper entitled "A Study of the Metabolism in Dogs with Shortened Small Intestines" which was published in the *American Journal of Physiology* in 1901.

Erlanger recalled that these were the dogs that the noted surgeon William Stewart Halsted and his col-

laborator (F. P. Mall) had used in their search for reliable intestinal sutures. The experiments he did with Hewlett were carried out to determine the permissible excision lengths of small intestine in surgical situations. Joseph H. Flint (a member of Hewlett's class and his fraternity brother at the Pithotomy Club) also was working in Mall's laboratory. Flint told Hewlett that metabolism observations on these dogs were wanted and Hewlett asked Erlanger to join him in the study.[1]

The results of the studies by Erlanger and Hewlett were definite but not earth-shaking. Dogs from which 70 to 83% of the combined jejunum and ileum had been removed lived indefinitely after recovery from the operation. Their nutrition was either perfectly normal or so poor that even when eating ravenously they were unable to keep well nourished. Such dogs tended to have diarrhea, particularly with a diet rich in fat or containing too much inert, nondigestible material. The diarrhea was serious and could cause death. On a diet poor in fat the dog with a shortened small intestine absorbed the fat as well, or almost as well, as a normal dog. As the fat in the diet was increased the fall in the percentage eliminated in the feces which occurs in the normal animal either occurred to a lesser extent or not at all in dogs deprived of small intestine. With a high-fat diet 25% of the ingested fat appeared in the feces, whereas in normal dogs only about 4.5% appeared.

COOPER MEDICAL COLLEGE

After Hewlett's graduation from The Johns Hopkins University School of Medicine in 1900 he became an intern on the medical service at the New York Hospital. He then went to Tubingen, Germany (1902–03), where he was attracted to Ludolf Krehl. Krehl was one of the first to emphasize abnormal function (pathological physiology) as contrasted to pathological anatomy which at that time was in its zenith under Rudolph Virchow.[2]

---

[1] Erlanger's recollection of this event appears to be somewhat erroneous. On page 5 of the paper in the *American Journal of Physiology* this statement appears: "In the early part of 1900 Flint and Rand conducted a series of experiments in the anatomical laboratory of the Johns Hopkins University to determine the limits to which intestinal resection could be carried in dogs and to study the anatomical results of such resections. Of the dogs operated upon by them, three were alive in the autumn of 1900, and through the kindness of Mr. Flint and Mr. Rand the authors of this paper were allowed to use these dogs in the metabolism experiments which will be described below." The work which Halsted did with Mall while the two were in Welch's laboratory was done much earlier; Mall at that time was a fellow in the laboratory, as was Halsted. Mall had just returned from Germany and after two years with Welch, he went to Clark University as professor of anatomy, and then to Chicago; he did not return to Hopkins until 1893 when he was made the first professor of anatomy.

[2] Ludolf Krehl, famous for his clinical contributions and especially for a treatise on pathologic physiology, received his clinical training under H. Curschmann and L. Wagner and studied

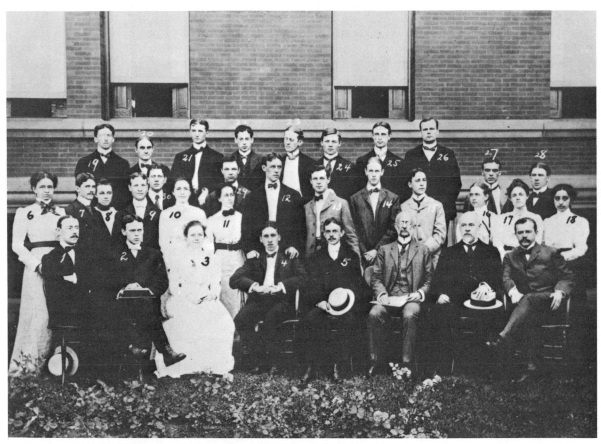

Fig 1.   The Class of 1900 of The Johns Hopkins University School of Medicine.

1. W. P. Healy 2. P. G. Woolley 3. R. Fairbank 4. J. B. MacCallum 5. W. C. Kellogg 6. F. R. Sabin 7. H. W. Little 8. E. L. Lowell 9. W. A. Fisher, Jr. 10. D. M. Reed 11. E. A. Stone 12. M. Warren 13. W. H. Lewis 14. H. A. Christian 15. M. Bettman 16. E. Briggs 17. M. W. Marvell 18. C. Meltzer 19. P. Keyes 20. W. F. Hendrickson 21. H. C. Evans 22. A. L. Fisher 23. G. Y. Rusk 24. A. W. Hewlett 25. W. R. Dancy 26. J. Akerman 27. A. H. Eggers 28. A. S. Chittenden 29. H. W. Allen 30. R. F. Rand

Faculty members, first row, l. to r., Dr. Hurd, Dr. Welch, Dr. Kelly

pathologic anatomy with Cohnheim. But it was probably Carl Ludwig, director of the Physiological Institute in Leipzig, then developing his interpretation of normal and abnormal function of natural processes, who was more influential on Krehl's career than any of these. Krehl served as Ludwig's assistant. He became a great skeptic in his search for truth among natural phenomena. Krehl examined and reexamined, leaving with his students an intentional impression of uncertainty; persisting even after a thorough exploration of all paths leading to the conclusion. In such a role he proved an excellent teacher in the amphitheater and at the bedside, an inspiration to his pupils, and an exemplary clinician in caring for the sick.

In 1892, Krehl answered the first of several academic calls and became chief of the Polyclinic in Jena. In turn, he was chief and professor of medicine at Marburg, Greifswald, and Tubingen, and successor to Naunyn in Strasbourg. At his final post in Heidelberg, he succeeded Erb in 1906 as professor of medicine and chief of the medical service in the university hospital. Krehl's great monograph, *Fundamentals of General Clinical Pathology*, was published in 1893. Five years later the title was changed to *Pathological Physiology*. This text went through many German editions and was translated into other languages, including the third edition which was translated into English in 1905 by Hewlett; this last volume went through three American revisions.

Early in Krehl's career, systematic investigations centered about the heart and included discussions of failure of the heart valves, idiopathic myocardial disease, coronary occlusion, the beer drinker's heart, and fatty degeneration of the heart muscle—studies which were based upon anatomy, physiology, and chemistry, each with relevance to specific clinical cases. The gitalin part of digitalis (Verodigen) and of strophanthin was introduced in his clinic, and the influence of digitalis on urine excretion was demonstrated.

In coronary disease Krehl pointed out several clinical-pathologic phenomena. He noted that survival was possible with asymptomatic, complete occlusion of an artery or of a large branch. Another type of coronary patient may die suddenly, without apparent pain and without terminal respiratory agony.

Krehl's interest in investigation began with the patient, and a fundamental requirement of a lecture hall was a door wide enough to admit a bed patient for demonstration.

Other outstanding Americans studied in Krehl's clinic, including J. H. Pratt and T. R. Boggs.

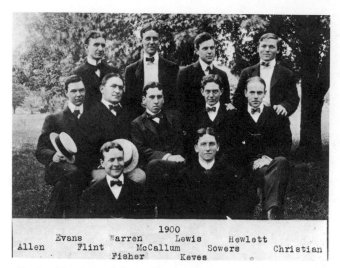

Fig 2.   Members of the Pithotomy Club in the Class of 1900.

Hewlett pursued that interest vigorously throughout his career. His first major contribution was to translate Krehl's book on clinical pathology (1905). In so doing, he rewrote the section dealing with cardiac arrhythmias based on his own observations and graphic records which were responsible for the correct explanation of the nature of auricular fibrillation. Sir William Osler, in his introduction to this work, said: "In this book, disease is studied as a perversion of physiological function. The title, 'Clinical Physiology,' expresses well the attempt which is made in it to fill the gap between empirical and scientific medicine. Every few years the laboratories seem to run ahead of the clinics and it takes time before the facts of one are fully appreciated by the other."

From Europe Hewlett returned to Cooper Medical College. Here he was strongly influenced by two members of the faculty. One was Joseph Oakland Hirschfelder, a graduate of the University of Leipzig, who was an expert clinician and investigator, working experimentally for years in an attempt to find a cure for tuberculosis. The other was Walter E. Garrey, professor of physiology, under whom Hewlett conducted much of his research.

While at Johns Hopkins Hewlett had learned of Flexner's work on the occurrence of a fat-splitting ferment in peritoneal fat necroses. It seemed reasonable to assume that this ferment was the fat-splitting enzyme of the pancreas, which, as a result of the pancreatic disease, escaped in considerable quantity. By what path the ferment reached the fat cells, however, had been largely a matter of conjecture. Working on this problem in Garrey's laboratory, Hewlett showed the presence of lipase in the urine and roughly estimated the quantity present in dogs in whom pancreatic disease had been experimentally produced. The lipase was found in the greatest amount as a result of experimental acute hemorrhagic pancreatitis. It was found over a period of from three to five days after obstruction of the pancreatic duct. He concluded that severe pancreatic trauma may cause the appearance of lipase in the urine. His paper on this subject, "On the Occurrence of Lipase in the Urine as a Result of Experimental Pancreatic Disease," appeared in the *Journal of Medical Research*. It was read before the California Academy of Medicine on February 23, 1904.

Hewlett's next study, "On the Effect of the Bile Upon the Ester-splitting Action of Pancreatic Juice," was carried out at Garrey's suggestion and with the aid of a grant from the Rockefeller Institute for Medical Research. Hewlett tried to determine the effect of bile upon the ester-splitting action of pure pancreatic juice obtained from dogs by means of secretin injections or by injections of both secretin and pilocarpine. He concluded that it seemed more probable that the bile acted as an accelerator upon the fat-splitting ferment and that this zymoexcitor was at least in part lecithin. A preliminary communication of this work was published in *The Johns Hopkins Hospital Bulletin*.

After these first three papers, Hewlett's interest shifted to the study of various aspects of cardiovascular physiology. One of his most impressive studies was "The Effect of Amyl Nitrite Inhalations Upon the Blood Pressure in Man." He found that in man there was an immediate fall of maximal pressure, averaging 13 mmHg and lasting less than 40 seconds, which was accompanied by a smaller fall of minimal pressure and an increased pulse rate. These changes were followed by a secondary rise (about 28 mmHg) of maximal pressure to considerably above the original height, accompanied by a less marked rise of the minimum pressure and by a return of the pulse rate to normal. These changes in blood pressure corresponded to an increased systolic output and increased force of the heartbeat (augmentor effect). With the assistance of Dr. Lehmann, Hewlett was able to see with the fluoroscope that "as the action of the heart slowed down the excursion of the left ventricle became wider by 1/2 centimeter but soon returned to normal." In other words, besides being a vasodilator, amyl nitrite was an active cardiac stimulant, more rapid than any except adrenalin. Relaxation of the peripheral blood vessels under the influence of the amyl nitrite, as shown by the plethysmographic studies, was present in all of Hewlett's experiments, in spite of the peculiar variations in blood pressure. The vasodilatation reached its maximum within the first minute and gradually subsided after the second; a definite effect was still noticeable 10 to 12 minutes afterwards. In older persons Hewlett found that the pulse rate often did not change, probably owing to the absence of the tonic activity of the vagus.

In 1907 C. I. Young and A. W. Hewlett studied the normal pulsations within the esophagus. Minkowski had recently shown that the movements of the left "auricle" could be recorded from within the esophagus. He introduced a stomach tube which had a small rubber balloon fastened over the end. Young and Hewlett obtained an exceptionally good set of normal esophageal tracings which differed in some important particulars from those published as normal by Minkowski. They also studied heart action by this method in abnormal states. In the same year Hewlett made a careful study of the heart block seen in patients receiving digitalis. All of these early studies on the circulation were done before any electrocardiograms had been taken in the United States.

Hewlett's study entitled "The Interpretation of the Positive Venous Pulse" was also published in 1907 in the *Journal of Medical Research*. The term "positive venous pulse" was used by some to indicate a regurgitant venous pulsation caused when a stream of blood was forced back into the veins from the heart. It was contrasted with the venous pulsations caused by an intermittent interruption of the flow toward the heart, the so-called negative venous pulse. In his paper, Hewlett described three conditions which could give rise to a positive venous wave in early ventricular systole and called attention to some of their differential characteristics. The conditions were: (a) the simultaneous contraction of auricles and ventricles, (b) tricuspid insufficiency, and (c) paralysis of the auricles.

In 1908 Hewlett published his last two papers from the Cooper Medical College. The first, entitled "Clinical Observations on Absolutely Irregular Hearts," appeared in the *Journal of the American Medical Association*. Hewlett noted that the distinguishing characteristics of the absolutely irregular heart were: (1) absence of normal auricular contractions; (2) the total irregularity itself; and (3) its permanency. Hewlett pointed out that Mackenzie had established several criteria as evidence of auricular contractions: (a) an auricular wave in the apex tracing just preceding the ventricular wave; (b) an auricular wave on the jugular and liver pulsations; and (c) the presystolic accentuation of the murmur of mitral or tricuspid stenosis. To these he added: (1) the presence of an auricular wave on the cardiogram obtained from within the esophagus, and (2) the auricular wave on the electrocardiogram. None of these methods of examination had made it possible to demonstrate that the auricles contract before the ventricles in absolutely irregular hearts. Hewlett analyzed a large number of cases and found that the heart lesion most frequently encountered was mitral insufficiency, which occurred in ten cases and was associated with mitral stenosis in five more. Mitral stenosis alone was present in two cases, aortic lesions in three and adhesive pericarditis in one. The remaining 11 cases showed no definite signs of valvular disease and were designated as myocardial disease. Among the etiologic factors rheumatism stood preeminent. Other factors were abuse of alcohol and hyperthyroidism. In the discussion of this paper Arthur D. Hirschfelder (son of J. O. Hirschfelder), who was at the time head of the cardiac laboratory at Johns Hopkins, pointed out that paralysis of the auricles was first demonstrated experimentally in animals by von Frey and Krehl in 1890 and subsequently in man by Mackenzie (1894) by means of the venous tracings. The absolute determination, however, was not decisive until Hewlett demonstrated it by means of a tracing from the esophagus. Prior to this, it might have been possible for a weak auricular contraction to go on without notice on the venous pulse. Now comparatively small contractions could be recorded in these excellent esophageal tracings.

The second paper, entitled "Heart Block in the Ventricular Walls," appeared in the *Archives of Internal Medicine*. Hewlett's conclusions were that ventricular contractions could cause waves on the jugular pulse with little or no effect on the apex beat. Such contractions may be followed immediately by normal contractions without a diastolic period. The right ventricle may begin its contraction distinctly later than the left. In Hewlett's study, these were largely effects produced by strophanthin and were probably to be interpreted as instances of intraventricular heart block.

THE MICHIGAN PERIOD

Hewlett had attained the rank of assistant professor of medicine when he accepted the position of professor of medicine at the University of Michigan School of Medicine in 1908, succeeding George Dock, who had accepted a similar post at Tulane.[3]

At Michigan, Hewlett continued his studies of the circulation, but his interest shifted from the heart itself to the peripheral circulation. He and J. G. Van Zwaluwenburg devised a method for estimating the blood flow in the arm, a preliminary report of which appeared in the *Archives of Internal Medicine*. They noted that of the various factors entering into the problem of circulatory dynamics the most important was the rate of blood flow. Earlier T. G. Brodie had estimated the blood flow in an organ in the dog by suddenly occluding its efferent vein and measuring the change of volume by an oncometer. Under these circumstances the arterial blood entered the organ with undiminished speed at first, but soon the flow was retarded by the rise of pressure in the veins and capillaries. The organ therefore swelled rapidly at first and then progressively more slowly. The earliest portion of this curve represented the rate at which the blood entered under normal conditions. The method was applicable only to organs from which all efferent blood could be collected by a single vein. Hewlett and his collaborator used Brodie's principle in order to determine the rate of flow in the arm of man. A distensible cuff similar to that used for determining arterial pressure was placed about the upper arm and an attempt was made to adjust the pressure in the cuff so that the veins would be occluded and the arteries left opened. The resulting changes in the volume of the arm were recorded by a plethysmograph and a Brodie volume recorder. By this method the rate of flow was found to vary considerably in different individuals and to vary to a lesser extent in the same individual under different circumstances. Up to that time the only similar methods recorded for estimating the rate of flow in the arm were those suggested by O. Muller and A. Muller. Both these authors, however, stopped the circulation in the arm before measuring the rate at which the blood entered the

---

[3] The position as Dock's successor was first offered to Rufus Cole, who had graduated from the University of Michigan and attended its medical school for one year before transferring to Johns Hopkins. When Cole decided instead to accept the directorship of the newly established Hospital of the Rockefeller Institute, the professorship was offered to Hewlett.

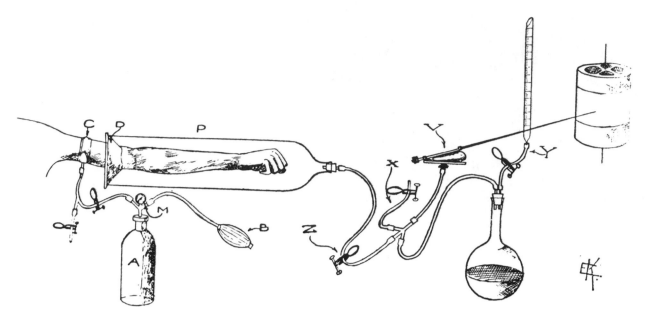

Fig 3.   Diagram of apparatus for determining the rate of blood flow through the arm. The arm is placed in the plethysmograph, P, the opening of which is closed by a piece of rubber dam, D, and the connection with the skin made tight with soap-suds. The narrow pressure cuff, C, is placed around the arm about 3 cm. above the opening into the plethysmograph. The pressure cuff is inflated by opening the stop-cock connecting it with the large bottle, A, in which the pressure has previously been raised by the rubber bulb, B. Pressures are read by the spring manometer, M. The plethysmograph is connected with the volume recorder, V, which writes upon a moving drum. Air can be let out of the system by the stop-cock, X, and water can be introduced from the burette, Y, so that the writing point of the volume recorder can be adjusted at will. The stop-cock, Z, serves to disconnect the plethysmograph from the recording apparatus during adjustments of the former. The recording apparatus is graduated by allowing 5 cc of fluid at a time to flow in from the burette, and marking the elevation of the volume recorder thus produced (79).

plethysmograph; consequently, normal conditions were not approximated (Figs 3 and 4).

Hewlett and Van Zwaluwenburg found that application of heat to the body as a whole was an effective and certain method of increasing the rate of flow through the arm. The most striking results were obtained in an individual who was placed in a very hot tub bath and left there about 10 minutes. They also studied unusually slow and unusually rapid rates. Those below 2.0 cc per 100

gram of arm substance per minute they placed in the former category. Eleven patients with rates in this category were recorded. Two were severe diabetics, two had had advanced gastric carcinoma, one an advanced nodular sclerosis of the radial arteries, one had valvular heart disease with absolutely irregular rhythm and one had partial heart block. The main factors possessed in common by these patients were moderate emaciation, asthenia and a cool, dry skin. The more rapid rate, over 5

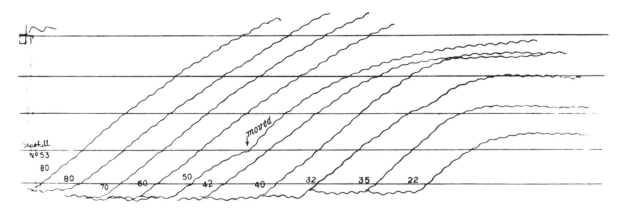

Fig 4.   × ½ linear. Tracings showing the effect of different cuff-pressures. The first are parallel, the later ones tend to become horizontal, owing to the escape of venous blood beneath the cuff. The numerals represent the pressures applied by the pressure cuff. Each space between the straight horizontal lines represents 5 cc increase in arm volume. The time record was inadvertently omitted (79).

cc of blood flow per 100 gram of arm substance per minute, was more numerous, occurring in 23 of their observations on 18 patients. The fastest rate was in a severe form of exophthalmic goiter.

On March 13, 1973 William Dock, a former member of Hewlett's department at Stanford, wrote to Hewlett's son William in reference to Hewlett and Van Zwaluwenburg's article published in *Heart* in 1909:

Perhaps you have a bound copy of your father's reprints, but I thought you might like to see a few pages from his classic paper—'The First Quantitative Measurements of Blood Flow in a Limb.' In 1970 Eugene Braunwald, now head of medicine at the Peter Bent Brigham Hospital, reported using that method to demonstrate that arteriosclerotic narrowing could be reversed, flow to the leg increased and symptoms relieved by regimens which greatly lowered levels of blood cholesterol and triglyceride. I enclose xerox copies of that report, since Figure 7 is almost identical with Figure 4 in your father's paper. The changes in limb volume are now measured with a strain-gauge, introduced by Whitney in 1953. A late application is pulse measurement in the finger and in the penis of normal and impotent men. Because our diabetic, two pack a day veteran smokers have leg problems and impotence at an early age, we became concerned about vascular disease causing both disabilities. This led me back to the 1909 paper.

Your father's selection of cases for study was as astute as his ingenuity in devising a method still in use. He found that in anemia the flow to the arm rose very little, and we now know blood is shunted to more vital areas. In the hyperthyroid patient, as shown on one of the sheets enclosed, flow is greatly increased, and we know this is needed to radiate the excessive heat produced by this disease. In 1925 I saw this method being used by Sir Thomas Lewis, the editor of *Heart*, and a very old friend of your father, to study flow in the hands of ladies with Raynaud's disease, characterized by white, aching hands in cold weather.

In the few weeks I was with your father, as resident, he showed me the Frank capsule he had just obtained for recording pulses with a synchronous electrocardiogram. He never had a chance to use it, but I put it to work, devised a way to record heart sounds with it, and thus set out on a path I still follow.

In his reply Mr. William Hewlett recalled meeting Sir Thomas Lewis when Lewis visited California during the early 1920s. Although he was a youngster at the time, Hewlett had a vivid memory that "Lewis was most fascinated with our humming birds, the like of which he had never seen."

In a paper published in *Heart* in 1911, Hewlett studied the "Effect of Room Temperature Upon the Blood Flow in the Arm, with a Few Observations on the Effect of Fever." These studies were undertaken with the hope of defining more accurately the degree to which variations in room temperature might affect the peripheral blood flow in man. The conclusions he reached were: (1) ordinary variations in the external room temperature produced marked effects upon the rate of blood flow in the arm, (2) the rate of flow when external warmth caused perspiration was often five or more times the rate when the person felt chilly, (3) perspiration caused by a warm room was usually preceded or accompanied by a sudden acceleration of the flow, (4) the previous state of warmth or chilliness influenced the flow at a given external temperature, and (5) the flow was exceptionally slow when the temperature rose during fever and was moderately accelerated when the temperature fell during fever.

In a paper published in 1911 in the *Transactions of the Association of American Physicians*, Hewlett, Van Zwaluwenburg and Mark Marshall reported "The Effect of Some Hydrotherapeutic Procedures Upon the Blood Flow in the Arm." When hot water was applied to the arm, the local blood flow rate increased from four to eight times, and when cold was applied, the local rate fell to one-half or one-fourth of the original. These variations were often associated with similar, though less marked, changes in the blood flow in the opposite arm, the latter also being influenced by the room temperature and the chilliness or warmth of the individual. The authors believed that acceleration of blood flow in an arm not directly exposed to the hot procedure was due in the main to reflexes excited by thermic stimulation of the cutaneous sense organs.

In 1912 Hewlett, Van Zwaluwenburg and J. H. Agnew discussed "A New Method for Studying the Brachial Pulse of Man." For some time Hewlett and his colleagues had been using the method suggested by Brodie and Russell for the study of blood flow in the arm. The venous outflow from the arm was obstructed by suddenly inflating a circular cuff to a pressure somewhat below that which prevailed in the arteries. Since the chief inflow to the portion of arm studied was through the brachial artery, they obtained by this means an approximate record of the volume flow in the brachial artery during each portion of the pulse cycle. A single normal individual was studied under varying conditions which affected the blood flow in the arm and the form of the pulse. A limited number of observations were also made on individuals with abnormal forms of pulse. The normal individual was first studied during varying room temperatures in order to determine the effect of local variations of blood flow upon the form of the pulse as recorded in this manner. During agreeable room temperatures the major portion of the blood entered the plethysmograph during each primary systolic pulse wave. Thereafter, to the next systolic wave, little if any blood entered. At that point the blood flow in the brachial artery was merely at a standstill, save for slight oscillations. Without nitroglycerine, the height of the pulse waves varied with the rate of blood flow, whereas with nitroglycerine, they remained nearly constant and maximal. The chief inflow continued to take place during the primary pulse waves, and little or no inflow occurred during the remainder of the pulse period. In some tracings from this individual, as well as from others studied, there was a slight backflow in the brachial artery during the period following the primary pulse wave. When the room temperature was raised sufficiently to cause uncomfortable warmth, the blood flow in the arm increased. At this time the primary wave was not materially increased over that seen at the upper limit of the usual flow, but in place of an almost stationary stream following the primary wave there was now a continued influx of blood through this portion of the pulse period. In order to explain these observations, the authors considered: (1) the factors which influenced the size of the primary pulse wave, and (2) those which determined the general rate of blood flow in the arm. The primary pulse wave was produced by the systolic output from the heart and was modified by the arteries which conducted this wave to the arm. In their opinion its size depended chiefly upon the size of the brachial artery, being larger when the artery was relaxed and smaller when it was contracted. The average blood flow in the arm, however, depended in part upon the average blood pressure, but chiefly upon the degree of constriction of the finer arterioles controlling the escape of blood from the arterial reservoirs to the capillaries and veins. In the individual studied the primary pulse waves in the brachial artery supplied almost as much blood to the arm as could escape into the capillaries during a complete pulse period. Consequently, the flow in the brachial artery was almost nil except at the time of the primary wave.

Nitroglycerine in medicinal doses of 1 or 2 drops (1% solution) produced characteristic changes in the pulse form as studied by their method. The primary wave was increased in height and the smaller secondary waves were obliterated, leaving only the well-marked dicrotic wave. At the same time the blood flow through the arm was not materially affected. They interpreted these changes as being due to a relaxation of the larger arteries of the arm without a corresponding effect upon the arterioles. The large primary wave of the nitroglycerine pulse was nearly always followed by a marked negative wave and this in turn by the dicrotic wave. They believed that the negative wave was due to a reflux of blood which had entered the relaxed artery in excessive quantity and found no immediate egress through the arterioles.

It is now well known that in most tracings from the peripheral arteries various secondary waves follow the principal or primary wave on the descending limb of the pulse. The chief of these is usually spoken of as the dicrotic wave; when this wave can be distinctly felt by the palpating finger on the radial artery, the pulse is described as dicrotic. The typical dicrotic pulse is relatively common in typhoid fever, but it occurs not infrequently in all types of infections and may be encountered in other conditions such as congestive heart failure. From a study of the pulse flow in the brachial artery Hewlett concluded that in febrile patients showing palpable types of dicrotic pulse, characteristic changes occurred in the brachial flow, consisting in a marked back flow in the brachial artery just after the entrance of the primary pulse wave and in an inflow and outflow with the dicrotic wave.

Hewlett later studied the effect of posterior pituitary substance upon the pulse form of febrile patients. He found that, with the injection of 1½ cc of pituitrin in-

tramuscularly, this type of pulse could be converted into a normal form. Following such an injection the pulse form usually showed a definite change in 10 to 15 minutes, the maximum effect being reached in about an hour, after which it continued for the next 2 or 3 hours. The change in form was regularly accompanied by a diminution in the size of the volume pulse in the arm. Hewlett's explanation assumed a constriction of the larger arteries in the arm or a constriction of vascular areas elsewhere in the body, particularly in the head and splanchnic regions. These pulse changes produced by pituitary substance were opposite to those that he had described following a therapeutic dose of nitroglycerine.

During the period in which Hewlett held the chair of medicine at Michigan there was widespread interest in the irregularities of the heartbeat, and knowledge in this field was expanding rapidly. Hewlett himself had made important contributions to this subject. As soon as the necessary funds could be obtained Hewlett purchased an Einthoven string galvanometer, and electrocardiograms were taken for the first time at the University Hospital in the spring of 1914.

Frank N. Wilson, who had been appointed assistant in the department upon his graduation from Michigan in 1913, was assigned the task of installing and operating this instrument. Since no other space was available it was placed in Hewlett's private office, a small room separated by a thin wooden partition extending halfway to the ceiling from the general office of the department, which was on the second floor of the medical wing of the old University Hospital. The electrocardiographic tracings were carried downstairs, where a tiny darkroom was available for their development. In spite of these meager and inconvenient facilities, many interesting observations were made and a number of papers were published. With Hewlett's help a method for recording the venous pulse, taken with a Frank capsule, simultaneously with the electrocardiogram was developed, which added greatly to the value of the tracings. One of the most important studies carried out dealt with the production of atrioventricular rhythm in normal subjects after the administration of atropine.

In 1916 Hewlett was offered the position of professor of medicine at Leland Stanford University. Before he assumed this responsibility, he wrote a summary of the course of developments during his eight years in the department of medicine at Michigan which was published in the *Transactions of the Clinical Society of the University of Michigan*. He pointed out that in 1908 the University Hospital had already reached dimensions which justified the hopes of those who looked forward to a clinical center in Ann Arbor. The growth of the combined departments of internal medicine, pediatrics and infectious diseases had kept pace with that of the hospital and approximately one-fourth of all patients coming to the hospital were seen at some time by the staff of those departments. He believed that the service to be rendered in internal medicine at a university hospital should be based in large part upon the special examinations then possible in any good medical center but which could be obtained elsewhere only with considerable difficulty and expense. The examinations to which he referred included microscopic and chemical examinations of the blood, the stomach contents and the excreta; cardiographic records; bacteriologic and serologic examinations; and x-rays. (These, of course, are rather primitive examinations compared to the complex technical procedures now available in general hospitals.)

Hewlett stated that a university clinic should also be a center for testing new methods of diagnosis and treatment and for the scientific study of disease:

> The clinic which is not adding to the sum total of medical knowledge is already falling in the rear. Members of the clinical staff must devote a portion of their time to research, and facilities for such research must be furnished by the hospital or by the university. It seems evident that men who are willing to devote their best years to the university side of medicine should be provided with adequate facilities for study and research. The problems confronting internal medicine at the present day involve not alone the usual clinical observations of patients but the study of these patients by the various methods that have been developed in biochemistry, physiology, bacteriology and immunology. These methods are often costly both in time and money and they require laboratory space, special apparatus and the services of technical assistants. Without these facilities such work can be carried on only under considerable difficulty. Our facilities for the study of cardiovascular disease have been excellent but only beginnings have been made along other lines. In the leading clinics, new ideas are being originated or having originated elsewhere, are being tested; and at the present day, so far as internal medicine is concerned, this means work in a clinical laboratory equipped for chemical, bacteriologic and physiologic work. The University Hospital has reached a size that is adequate or nearly adequate for its university purposes and it seems to me that the time is at hand when more effort should be made toward its development as a center for clinical research. In the appointment of my successor a step in this direction has been made. Dr. Foster (Nellis Foster) has made important contributions in applying the methods and data of biochemistry to the solution of clinical problems and he is to have a chemical laboratory connected with his service. It seems to me that further encouragement to this and to similar lines of development must be given if Michigan is to keep pace with the leaders in clinical medicine.

Albion W. Hewlett was truly at the forefront of those who assumed leadership in creating medicine's scientific base through the development of clinical investigation.

It was also just as Hewlett was leaving Michigan in 1916 that the first edition of his book *The Pathological Physiology of Internal Diseases*, a volume of over 700 pages, appeared. This monograph was based in large part on his own clinical observations and experimental work and was the definitive medical treatise of the day dealing with the functional aspects of disease. It went through several editions and a revision was in preparation at the time of Hewlett's death. His colleagues took the responsibility of finishing this final 1928 revision. Among those participating were Thomas Addis, George DeForest Barnett, Walter Whitney Boardman, Ernest Charles Dickson, Henry George Mehrtens, Williams Ophuls, Jay Marion Read, Howard Frank West, and Harry Alphonso Wyckoff. The editorial supervision was under the direction of George DeForest Barnett and an appreciation was written by Ray Lyman Wilbur.

At Michigan, Hewlett had maintained an almost incredible schedule. In addition to his voluminous research, writing, and other activities, including a modest private practice, he scrupulously maintained his schedule of class lectures, ward rounds and personal contact with his students and house staff. The latter believed him to possess to an extraordinary degree the gift of the great teacher in being able to make complex subjects appear simple and understandable.

WAR SERVICE

During World War 1 Hewlett served as a Lieutenant Commander in the Stanford Navy Base Hospital Unit. During this period he was stationed for a time in Scotland and came to know the University of Edinburgh well. Here he learned of the legendary reasoning powers of Dr. Bell of that institution, the man who gave rise in the mind of A. Conan Doyle to that incomparable detective of fiction, Sherlock Holmes. This undoubtedly interested him greatly. Diagnosis, the supreme art of the physician, requires sound deductive reasoning especially when not all of the available information needed to solve the nature of the ailment in question is necessarily at hand, and where every clue must be carefully followed and weighed before a final conclusion can be arrived at. Hewlett himself possessed extraordinary reasoning powers.

Hewlett also served with the Base Hospital in France at a time when influenza was prevalent. He and W. M. Alberty later wrote an excellent description of their experience with influenza at that time.

STANFORD UNIVERSITY

After assuming the professorship of medicine at Stanford, Hewlett performed research on the action of tyramin on the normal circulation of man, the results of which were published in 1918. He found that after the subcutaneous injection of 60–80 mg, the systolic pressure rose to levels of from 150 to 200 mmHg. This increase in pressure began within five minutes after injection, attained its maximum in about 10 minutes, and subsided more gradually to its previous level, which was usually reached in from 15 to 30 minutes. The diastolic pressure frequently rose also but never to any great extent. The volume pulse in the arm became larger and more sustained; the heart rate slowed and extrasystoles occasionally occurred. These circulatory changes, except for being more prolonged, resembled those which followed the intravenous injection of epinephrine in moderate doses. Subcutaneous injection of epinephrine, on the other hand, rarely caused any marked rise of systolic pressure and not infrequently lowered the diastolic pressure. In a subsequent paper Hewlett and W. E. Kay studied the effects of tyramin on the circulation during infections and during or after operations. Repeated injections of tyramin were given to four patients who showed evidence of circulatory failure during the course of infectious disease. These usually caused a transient rise of blood pressure and an increase in the size of the pulse. These effects were less marked than those produced when the drug was given in similar doses to persons with a normal circulation. In none of the cases did a permanent improvement occur.

Repeated injections of tyramin were also given to seven patients who showed evidence of circulatory failure during or after operations. These usually caused a transient rise of blood pressure and an increase in the size of the pulse. Striking improvements in the general condition of some of these patients occurred. Five of the seven patients recovered and in three of these the drug benefited a condition which appeared, at the time, to be desperate. In five other patients tyramin failed to abort asthmatic paroxysms although other drugs (epinephrine and atropine) were subsequently used with benefit.

One of Hewlett's students with whom he did a number of studies was John K. Lewis. In 1922 Lewis and Hewlett investigated the cause of increased vascular sounds after epinephrine injections. It was well known that certain individuals showed a definite reaction after the subcutaneous or intramuscular injection of epinephrine with increased pulse pressure, increased pulse rate, tremor, palpitation and a feeling of apprehension. In addition the arterial pulse in the arm became larger and the vascular sounds heard during the auscultatory determinations of blood pressure became louder. The cause of this increase in vascular sounds was not known. Besides confirming the increase in loudness of the sounds, Lewis and Hewlett found a correlation between the changes in the sound and the changes in pulse pressure, which appeared to be better than the correlation between the changes in sounds and the changes in the pulse volume. A comparison of the effects produced by epinephrine, nitroglycerine and tyramine also showed that the correlation of changes in vascular sounds with changes in pulse pressure was more exact than the correlation with changes in pulse form or pulse volume. From this they inferred that these drugs influence the vascular sounds more through their effect on the systolic output from the heart than through their effect on the blood vessels.

At Stanford, Hewlett continued his functional studies on the cardiovascular and respiratory system. A series of experiments were carried out on the response to exercise, the ultimate purpose being a better understanding of dyspnea. In 1923 he and J. R. Nakada studied recovery from the hyperpnea of moderate exercise. After muscular exercise, the excessive pulmonary ventilation lessens rapidly at first and then more slowly. The promptness of recovery is obviously one of the factors which indicate the individual's reaction to exercise. It is difficult to measure the total duration of dyspnea because the final approach to the resting level is very gradual with no sharp end point. In this paper they sought a numerical expression for the earlier and more rapid stages of recovery.

In 1924 Hewlett studied the vital capacities of patients with cardiac complaints. He noted that in heart disease vital capacity measurements had proved valuable both in estimating the gravity of the lesion, especially as regards pulmonary congestion, and in following the progress of the disease over longer or shorter periods. This paper was a statistical study of the vital capacity in a group of patients, most of whom complained of symptoms suggesting heart disease. Particular attention was paid to the association of diminished vital capacity with other objective evidences of cardiac disease. The vital capacity records utilized in this paper were obtained from patients who had been referred to the electrocardiograph laboratory of the Stanford Medical School. Since May 1922 it had been customary in that laboratory to measure the vital capacities of all patients sent for electrocardiograms and to express these capacities as percentages of the average normal according to height standards. It was found that the vital capacity of college students based on a height standard was considerably higher than the vital capacity of patients with cardiac complaints and without objective evidence of thoracic disease. This difference was greater for women than for men. Vital capacity readings between 60 and 75% of the college standard were suspiciously low; those less than 60% were almost uniformly abnormal. In this series of patients with cardiac complaints serious lesions were more common among the men than the women. The symptoms most commonly associated with low vital capacity were cough and dyspnea. The seriousness of the various tabulated manifestations of heart disease as judged by vital capacity averages was, in descending order: extrasystoles, hypertension, left ventricular preponderance as expressed electrocardiographically, enlarged heart, T negative in lead 1, auricular fibrillation, and, lastly, a widened QRS complex. If cases of evident aortic insufficiency and of aortic aneurysm were omitted, a positive Wassermann reaction in his patients was not associated with any reduction of vital capacity. He inferred that syphilis was on the average a small factor in the production of serious cardiac failure except when it involved the aorta or the aortic valves.

That dyspnea may occur during exercise and that it is more apt to occur under certain pathological conditions are now commonplace observations, but in 1924 the physiological mechanisms involved were largely obscure. The effects of exercise had been studied mainly on normal individuals and relatively few observations had been made on patients or on normal individuals subjected to abnormal conditions. In a paper published in 1924 Hewlett, Lewis and Franklin studied the effect of artificial stenosis upon dyspnea produced by exercise. Artificial obstruction to respiration was produced by having the subject breathe through bored corks, the bores being 8 mm and 6 mm in diameter. Under resting conditions the 8 mm bore produced but little subjective and no demonstrable objective effects. The 6 mm bore caused slight subjective discomfort and invariably slowed the respiratory rate. In one series of experiments it lessened the average minute volume of respired air.

During exercise both bores reduced the respiratory rate and lessened the minute volume of respired air. With the smaller bore a maximum minute volume of approximately 30 L was attained but the rapidly increasing distress indicated that this amount of ventilation was insufficient for the establishment of a steady state. With the larger bore, a steady state could be established with a minute volume of approximately 44 L, in contrast with the minute volume of approximately 53 L when breathing was not obstructed. With the 6 mm bore, oxygen absorption during the first one and one-quarter minutes was definitely lessened and lack of oxygen contributed to the early discontinuance of the exercise. If a mixture rich in oxygen was breathed, the early distress was less marked and exercise could be continued longer.

Hewlett's last paper, "The Effect of Breathing Oxygen-enriched Air During Exercise Upon Pulmonary Ventilation and Upon the Lactic Acid Content of Blood and Urine," with G. D. Barnett and J. K. Lewis as his collaborators, was published posthumously. They determined the increase in lactic acid in blood and urine resulting from measured treadmill exercise. A smaller rise of blood lactic acid and a smaller excretion of lactic acid were found when oxygen-enriched air was breathed. Excess excretion of lactic acid over the resting level was only demonstrated in experiments in which the blood lactic acid rose to 30 or 40 mg/dl. Earlier this group had also published a paper on "The Effect of Training on Lactic Acid Excretion."

From the presented sample of Hewlett's research, it is evident that he was first and foremost a clinical investigator, studying the effects of disease upon the function of the cardiovascular and pulmonary system in man. In 1908, Hewlett was elected a charter member of the American Society for Clinical Investigation and was one of three members of its original council. It was fitting that in the year of his death, 1925, he was president of the society.

At the eighteenth annual meeting of the Society in Atlantic City, New Jersey, in 1926, the following resolution on his death was presented by Rufus Cole and David M. Cowie, both of whom were also charter members:

> During the past year we have lost by death one of the small group of men to whom the foundation of this society was due and one who later became its president, Dr. Albion Walter Hewlett.
>
> While still a medical student his intellectual ability, his industry and his power of clear thinking and accurate expression marked him as one who was destined to become an important figure in his profession. He very early began to exhibit an interest in the fundamental processes concerned in disease and was not content merely to observe and describe the superficial and obvious. This interest led him to the study of normal physiologic processes and to apply the methods of this study to the sick.
>
> These interests, which 20 years ago were not so common as they are now, led him and others of like mind to gravitate together, and as a result there came into being this organization of men bound together for searching out the underlying secrets of disease.
>
> But Dr. Hewlett was also interested in men, in sick individuals, in the classification of disease, in diagnosis and in treatment. He was a skillful clinician. These qualities were the ideal ones for the successful teacher and leader, and it was not surprising therefore that he was called while very young, to become the professor of medicine at one of the important universities, the University of Michigan.
>
> While at Ann Arbor Dr. Hewlett endeared himself to faculty and student body alike. His sincerity and the thoroughness with which he executed the trust placed in him as head of the department of medicine was an inspiration and stimulation to all: particularly to the young men who were fortunate enough to become intimately associated with him.
>
> Under Dr. Hewlett's direction the department of medicine at Michigan continued to grow and made marked and well-recognized advancement. Under his leadership valuable contributions to scientific medicine were made.
>
> Later he was called to the home of his boyhood, to become professor of medicine at Leland Stanford University. Here he continued his valuable work as a physician, teacher and investigator.
>
> Dr. Hewlett possessed not only unusual intellectual equipment and ability as an investigator, as teacher and physician, he was possessed of a most attractive personality. Quiet and thoughtful and giving the impression of much reserve power and force, yet he was a most interesting and agreeable companion. All the members of the early group comprising this society were his personal friends. He was always interested in the younger members of this society and many of them became greatly influenced in their later careers by his writings and by his personal influence.
>
> The profession of medicine has lost in Dr. Hewlett one of its ablest and most valuable colleagues; this society has lost one of its wisest and most capable members.
>
> But we have lost much more, we have all lost a sincere and true friend.
>
> It is therefore especially fitting for this society to record our admiration for Dr. Hewlett as an able scientist, our appreciation of him as a wise and successful physician, and at the same time express the personal affection which all of us had for him as a fellow worker and a friend.

After Hewlett's death, a "Hewlett Club" was formed by former students to honor and perpetuate his memory. At the Club's first anniversary meeting, the following comments about Hewlett were made by one of his students (unfortunately, the student's name is unknown):

> Although he was best known to physicians in general as a scientific worker, those of us who were privileged to have him for a teacher appreciated him more as a clinician. His clear and logical discussions in the wards, the clinics, and classrooms have been of irreplaceable benefit to all of us. When he pointed out the solution of a difficult problem in diagnosis it was never with an air of mysticism or a matter of opinion, but always in a logical, orderly fashion which often surprised one with its simplicity and left one chagrined that he had not arrived at the same conclusion himself. One naturally looks for the source of such skill. As nearly as one can analyze such a thing, I should say that it came from a naturally keen, alert mind which was able to

absorb a great deal of information logically and concisely excluding useless or unimportant material and a refusal to allow prejudice or emotions to interfere with his judgment. Dr. Hewlett's personality was a puzzle to many. Many were closely associated with him for a number of years but felt that they never really knew him. I'm sure this was due to an innate modesty and reserve and not to a cold, unsympathetic nature. No greater proof of this can be had than observation of his keen interest in the welfare of all of the students and their problems. He was willing to listen patiently to anything we wished to discuss with him and we often took advantage of his good nature to accomplish something which we had no right to expect at all. His interns were given a free hand in the wards and he obtained a good position for everyone who ever served as his senior or resident . . . One had only to be with him away from the atmosphere of the hospital to appreciate his sense of humor and interest in general things . . . Truly he was a rare combination of investigator, clinician and man. No better name could have been chosen to stand for all that is desirable in a physician.

Another of his students, Gunther W. Nagel, recorded the following telling memory of Hewlett: "Dr. Albion W. Hewlett walked briskly down the center aisle, hardly glancing at the patients lying or half sitting in the white iron framed beds arranged on either side of the medical ward in the aging brick hospital at Clay and Webster Streets. I followed in starched intern whites. Dr. Hewlett had been away and wished to select a patient or two for presentation in class later that morning. Without a pause or moment's hesitation, he said, 'We'll demonstrate the man with the stomach trouble in bed 7, and the one in bed 3 who has gout.' Noting my astonishment, with what must be considered understandable satisfaction that he should know so much about patients he had never seen before, much less talk to, he explained: 'The man in 7 has a thick rim of barium around his lips. He has obviously just had x-ray films of his stomach. Number 3 has a small tophus on his left ear, which is typical of gout.'" Nagel's experience abundantly documents Hewlett's abilities in clinical medicine.

ACKNOWLEDGMENTS

I am indebted to Dr. Robert J. Glaser and Ms. Claire Still for information from the Archives of the Leland Stanford School of Medicine. I wish to thank Ms. Carol Bocchini for her editorial assistance and Ms. Patricia King for typing the manuscript. My particular thanks go to Dr. David Rytand for sharing his rich knowledge of the past accomplishments of the Department of Medicine at the Leland Stanford School of Medicine.

REFERENCES

1. Britt DB, Kemmerer WT and Robison JR: Penile blood flow determination by mercury strain gauge plethysmography. Invest Urol 8: 673, 1971

2. Brodie TG: The determination of the rate of the blood flow through an organ. Reported at the 7th International Physiological Congress, August 1907

3. Flexner S: On the occurrence of the fat-splitting ferment in peritoneal fat necroses and the histology of these lesions. J Exp Med 2: 413, 1897

4. Hewlett AW: The superficial glands of the oesophagus. J Exp Med 5: 319, 1901

5. Hewlett AW: Report of a case of paratyphoid fever. Am J Med Sci 124: 200, 1902

6. Hewlett AW: Ueber die Einwirkung des Peptonblutes auf Hamolyse und Baktericidie; Bemerkungen uber die Gerinnung des Blutes. Arch f Exp Path u Pharmakol 49: 307, 1903

7. Hewlett AW: On the occurrence of lipase in the urine as a result of experimental pancreatic disease. J Med Res 11: 377, 1904

8. Hewlett AW: The effect of the bile upon the ester-splitting action of pancreatic juice: A preliminary communication. Johns Hopkins Hosp Bull 16: 20, 1905

9. Hewlett AW: A unilateral paradoxical pulse. JAMA 45: 1405, 1905

10. Hewlett AW: The motor complications of herpes zoster. Calif State J Med 4: 119, 1906

11. Hewlett AW: Doubling of the cardiac rhythm and its relation to paroxysmal tachycardia. JAMA 46: 941, 1906

12. Hewlett AW: The effect of amyl nitrite inhalations upon the blood pressure of man. J Med Res 15: 383, 1906

13. Hewlett AW: Theophyllin as a diuretic. Calif State J Med 5: 221, 1907

14. Hewlett AW: Digitalis heart block. JAMA 48: 47, 1907

15. Hewlett AW: The blocking of auricular extrasystoles. JAMA 48: 1597, 1907

16. Hewlett AW: The interpretation of the positive venous pulse. J Med Res 17: 119, 1907

17. Hewlett AW: Heart block in the ventricular walls. Arch Intern Med 2: 139, 1908

18. Hewlett AW: The common cardiac arrhythmias and their clinical significance. Int Clinics 17: 47, 1908.

19. Hewlett AW: Clinical observations on absolutely irregular hearts. JAMA 51: 655, 1908

20. Hewlett AW: A patient with extreme cyanosis. Physician and Surgeon 31: 509, 1909

21. Hewlett AW: The relation of hospitals to medical schools of the U.S. Physician and Surgeon 21: 481, 1910

22. Hewlett AW: The effect of varying room temperatures upon the peripheral blood flow. Proc Am Physiol Soc p. 18, 1910

23. Hewlett AW: Angina pectoris. Physician and Surgeon 32: 165, 1910

24. Hewlett AW: Circulatory changes in exophthalmic goitre. Ohio Med J 6: 525, 1910

25. Hewlett AW: Auricular fibrillation associated with auricular extrasystoles. Heart 2: 107, 1910

26. Hewlett AW: Effect of room temperature upon the blood flow in the arm, with a few observations on the effect of fever. Heart 2: 230, 1911

27. Hewlett AW: The relation of cardiac irregularities to treatment. JAMA 57: 1512, 1911

28. Hewlett AW: Infantilism with pituitary disease. Physician and Surgeon, 33: 17, 1911

29. Hewlett AW: The history of some famous quacks. Detroit Med J 11: 388, 1912

30. Hewlett AW: Infantilism in pituitary disease. Arch Intern Med 9: 32, 1912

31. Hewlett AW: The clinical study of high blood pressure. Bull Med Chir Fac 4: 211, 1911–12

32. Hewlett AW: A case of tracheal tug in a supposed mediastinal tumor. Physician and Surgeon 34: 230, 1912

33. Hewlett AW: A case of strychnine poisoning. Physician and Surgeon 34: 183, 1912

34. Hewlett AW: A case of pernicious malaria complicated with suppurative parotitis. Physician and Surgeon 34: 522, 1912

35. Hewlett AW: A case of chronic uremia with bilateral

swelling of the submaxillary glands. Physician and Surgeon 34: 523, 1912

36. Hewlett AW: A case of diabetic coma. Physician and Surgeon 35: 129, 1913

37. Hewlett AW: The circulation in the arm of man. Am J Med Sci 145: 656, 1913

38. Hewlett AW: Active hyperemia following local exposure to cold. Arch Intern Med 11: 507, 1913

39. Hewlett AW: Clinical effects of "natural" and "synthetic" sodium salicylate. JAMA 61: 319, 1913

40. Hewlett AW: A case of strychnine poisoning. Am J Med Sci 146: 536, 1913

41. Hewlett AW: The relation of pathologic physiology to internal medicine. JAMA 61: 1583, 1913

42. Hewlett AW: Bilateral intermittent swellings of the parotid glands due to the infection of Steno's ducts (sialodochitis). J Mich Med Soc 12: 664, 1913

43. Hewlett AW: Reflexionen der primaren Pulswelle im menschlichen Arme. Deut Arch f klin Med 116: 237, 1914

44. Hewlett AW: Bilateral intermittent swelling of the parotid glands due to infection of Steno's ducts (sialodochitis). Trans Clin Soc Univ Mich 5: 16, 1914

45. Hewlett AW: The pulse-flow in the brachial artery. IV. Reflections of the primary wave in dicrotic and monocrotic pulse forms. Arch Intern Med 14: 609, 1914

46. Hewlett AW: The effect of pituitary substance upon the pulse form of febrile patients. Proc Soc Exp Biol Med 12: 61, 1914

47. Hewlett AW: The effect of pituitary substances upon the fever pulse. Trans Clin Soc Univ Mich 6: 63, 1915

48. Hewlett AW: The Pathological Physiology of Internal Diseases. New York and London: D. Appleton and Company, 1916

49. Hewlett AW: Eight years in the department of internal medicine. Trans Clin Soc Univ Mich 7: 146, 1916

50. Hewlett AW: The significance of pulse form. JAMA 67: 1134, 1916

51. Hewlett AW: The clinical features of spontaneous pneumothorax. Int Clinics 3: 95, 1916

52. Hewlett AW: The pulse flow in the brachial artery. V. The influence of certain drugs. Arch Intern Med 20: 1, 1916

53. Hewlett AW: Cooperation between pharmacology and therapeutics. JAMA 69: 1123, 1917

54. Hewlett AW: The action of tyramin on the circulation of man. Arch Intern Med 21: 411, 1918

55. Hewlett AW: Pathological physiology and its relation to internal medicine. Oxford Loose-leaf Medicine, 1: 109, 1919

56. Hewlett AW: Recent advances in the diagnosis of heart disease. Northwest Med 19: 224, 1920

57. Hewlett AW: Case showing bundle branch block with extrasystoles originating in ventricular septum. Heart 9: 1, 1922

58. Hewlett AW: Effect of massage, heat and exercise on the local circulation. Calif State J Med 20: 276, 1922

59. Hewlett AW: Paroxysmal tachycardia. Case where quinidin lessened the frequency of attacks. Med Clin North Am 6: 205, 1922

60. Hewlett AW: Quinidin in auricular fibrillation, indications for the administration of. Calif State J Med 20: 395, 1922

61. Hewlett AW: A case showing rapid ventricular rhythm with periods of auriculoventricular dissociation. Heart 10: 9, 1923

62. Hewlett AW: Clinical aspects of auricular fibrillation. Calif West Med 22: 479, 1924

63. Hewlett AW: The vital capacities of patients with cardiac complaints. Heart 11: 195, 1924

64. Hewlett AW and Alberty WM: Influenza at the Navy Base Hospital in France. JAMA 71: 1056, 1918

65. Hewlett AW, Barnett GD and Lewis JK: The effect of breathing oxygen-enriched air during exercise upon pulmonary ventilation and upon the lactic acid content of blood and urine. J Clin Invest 3: 317, 1926

66. Hewlett AW, Barnett GD and Lewis JK: The effect of breathing oxygen-enriched air upon the excretion of lactic acid. Proc Soc Exp Biol Med 22: 538, 1925

67. Hewlett AW and Barringer TB Jr: The effect of digitalis on the ventricular rate in men. Arch Intern Med 5: 93, 1910

68. Hewlett AW and Clark WRP: The symptoms of descending thoracic aneurysm. Am J Med Sci 87: 792, 1909

69. Hewlett AW and Erlanger J: A study of the metabolism in dogs with shortened small intestines. Am J Physiol 6: 1, 1901

70. Hewlett AW, Gilbert QO and Wickett AD: The toxic effects of urea on normal individuals. Arch Intern Med 18: 636, 1916

71. Hewlett AW, Gilbert QO and Wickett AD: The toxic effects of urea on normal individuals. Trans Assoc Am Physicians 31: 311, 1916

72. Hewlett AW and Jackson NR: The vital capacity in a group of college students. Arch Intern Med 29: 515, 1922

73. Hewlett AW and Kay WE: The effect of tyramin on circulatory failure during infections and during or after operations. JAMA 70: 1810, 1918

74. Hewlett AW, Lewis JK and Franklin A: The effect of some pathological conditions upon dyspnea during exercise. I. Artificial stenosis. J Clin Invest 1: 483, 1925

75. Hewlett AW, Lewis JK and Franklin A: An experimental study of the effect of stenosis upon the respiratory changes induced by muscular exercise. Proc Soc Exp Biol Med 22: 64, 1925

76. Hewlett AW and Sweeney JP: The quinidin treatment of auricular fibrillation. JAMA 77: 1793, 1921

77. Hewlett AW and Van Zwaluwenburg JG: Method for estimating the blood flow in the arm: A preliminary report. Arch Intern Med 3: 254, 1909

78. Hewlett AW and Van Zwaluwenburg JG: The pulse flow in the brachial artery. Arch Intern Med 12: 1, 1913

79. Hewlett AW and Van Zwaluwenburg JG: The rate of blood flow in the arm. Heart 1: 87, 1910

80. Hewlett AW and Van Zwaluwenburg JG: Comparison between the blood-flow in the arm and in the hand. Proc Soc Exp Biol Med 8: 111, 1910−11

81. Hewlett AW, Van Zwaluwenburg JG and Agnew JH: A new method for studying the brachial pulse of man. Trans Assoc Am Physicians 27: 188, 1912

82. Hewlett AW, Van Zwaluwenburg JG and Marshall M: The effect of some hydrotherapeutic procedures on the blood-flow in the arm. Arch Intern Med 8: 591, 1911

83. Hewlett AW, Van Zwaluwenburg JG and Marshall M: The effect of some hydrotherapeutic procedures upon the blood flow in the arm. Trans Assoc Am Physicians 26: 357, 1911

84. Hewlett AW and Wilson FN: Coarse auricular fibrillation in man. Arch Intern Med 15: 786, 1915

85. Krehl L and Hewlett AW: Chemical correlations in the organism. Am J Clin Med 14: 1105, 1907

86. Lewis JK and Hewlett AW: The cause of increased vascular sounds after epinephrin injections. Heart 10: 1, 1923

87. Lewis JK, Hewlett AW and Barnett GD: The effect of training on lactic acid excretion. Proc Soc Exp Biol Med 22: 537, 1925

88. Muller A: Methoden zur Bestimmung von Schlagvolumen und Herzarbeit und deren Ergebnisse. Bed ii d Verhandl d Kong f inn Med 25: 325, 1908

89. Muller O: Das absolute Plethysmogram. Munchen Med Wchnschr 55: 1819, 1908

90. Young CI and Hewlett, AW: The normal pulsations within the esophagus. J Med Res 16: 427, 1907

20.

Applying the Methods of Science to the Study of Tropical Diseases—The Story of Andrew Watson Sellards

Many medical scientists who received their early training at Johns Hopkins have completed a successful career on the faculty of another medical institution. Andrew Watson Sellards received his M.D. from The Johns Hopkins University School of Medicine, finished his residency training in medicine in Baltimore and then made distinguished contributions to tropical medicine while a member of the faculty of the Harvard Medical School.

Sellards was born in Scranton, Kansas in 1884. He obtained his A.B. from Kansas University in 1903 at the age of 19 and his M.A. the next year. He entered The Johns Hopkins University School of Medicine in 1905 (Fig 1). The following letter was written by one of his teachers in support of his application:

To the Dean,
Johns Hopkins Medical School
Baltimore, Maryland

August 7, 1905

Dear Sir:

I write this letter to introduce Mr. Watson Sellards who plans to attend Johns Hopkins Medical School this fall. Mr. Sellards, M.A., University of Kansas, 1904, was a student in my department for several years and assistant in bacteriology for two terms. He has been a very excellent student and has shown considerable aptitude for research. An article written by him on a subject worked out here appeared in the "Centralblatt für Bakteriologie und Parasitenkunde" of last December. He has an excellent foundation for both continued student life and for research work in either bacteriology or chemistry. I have not the slightest doubt that his work with you will continue the success he has had here.

Very respectfully,
M. A. Barber
Associate Professor, Bacteriology
and Cryptogamic Botany
University of Kansas

In his application, Sellards amplified the record of his extensive course work in bacteriology and in chemistry: "Under 'Length of Course' those marked 1 are 20-week courses and those marked ½ are 10-week courses. Six hours per week throughout the term (20 weeks) was the amount of laboratory work required in the physical

Reprinted from the *Johns Hopkins Medical Journal* **144:** 45, 1979.

chemistry course. The work was under the direction of Dr. E. C. Franklin and consisted in such experiments as the demonstration of Boyle's law for gases, various methods of determining the specific gravity of gases, liquids, and solids, molecular weight determinations, measurements of the electrical conductivity of salts in solution and so forth." William Henry Welch, who was then dean, made the following note on Sellards's application: "Question of acceptance of physical chemistry in place of laboratory physics (recommended). Otherwise satisfactory." This special work in chemistry and bacteriology was obviously excellent preparation for Sellards as illustrated by his subsequent research career.

RESEARCH AS A MEDICAL SCHOOL UNDERGRADUATE

Soon after his arrival at The Johns Hopkins University School of Medicine, Sellards sought an opportunity to continue his interest in research. He found a stimulating home in the biological division of the department of medicine which was under the direction of Rufus I. Cole, soon to become director of the new Hospital of the Rockefeller Institute for Medical Research. Cole also headed one of the several full-time research laboratories in the medical clinic of The Johns Hopkins Hospital which had been organized by Lewellys F. Barker in 1905 when he became professor of medicine at Johns Hopkins. The *Bulletin of the Johns Hopkins Hospital* for June–July 1907 contains 18 research reports from these laboratories. Among them was an article by P. C. Jeans and A. W. Sellards entitled "The Tuberculoopsonic Index and Treatment by Tuberculin." In spite of their careful work in preparing the proper emulsion, using as sources of the tubercle bacilli strains obtained from Dr. Baldwin of the Saranac Laboratory and a glycerine agar-agar culture obtained from Dr. Ford of the bacteriological laboratory of The Johns Hopkins Hospital and said to be directly descended on artificial cultivation from an original culture obtained from Robert Koch "many years ago," their results with the opsonic index in terms of its diagnostic value were disappointing. The authors thought, however, that the results obtained by the administration of tuberculin in small infrequent doses were encouraging. They believed that the method of vaccination may be a correct one, even though the control of

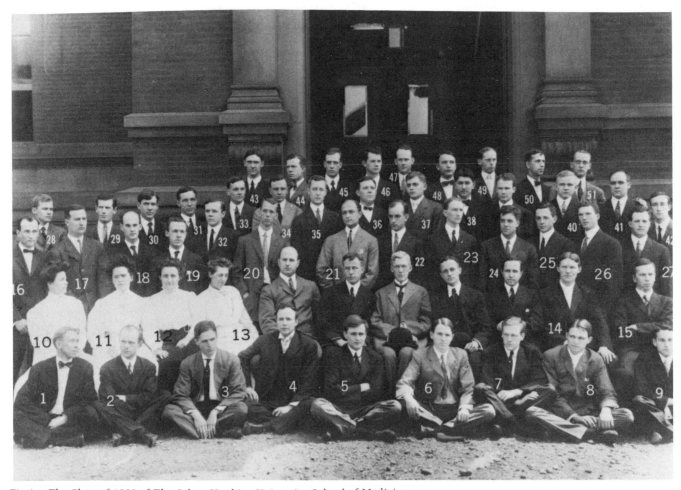

Fig 1.   The Class of 1909 of The Johns Hopkins University School of Medicine.
1. J. L. Birdsong 2. R. L. Waite 3. W. S. Wyatt 4. W. E. Hart 5. H. S. Thomson 6. P. I. Nixon 7. J. B. Murphy 8. P. C. Jeans
9. S. W. Schaefer 10. E. M. Girdwood (Mrs. George Peirce) 11. F. C. Child 12. I. C. Youmans 13. J. M. Torrey 14. J. R. Elliott 15. T. W. Harvey, Jr. 16. E. Cooper 17. P. B. Moss 18. B. Z. Cashman 19. G. H. Woltereck 20. J. A. Bass 21. C. R. Austrian 22. W. F. Cole 23. Not identified 24. F. B. Mann 25. W. L. Estes, Jr. 26. E. R. Gentry 27. T. L. Ferenbaugh 28. J. W. W. Dimon 29. H. L. Connett 30. E. Goetsch 31. A. W. Sellards 32. W. G. Wallace 33. I. C. Walker 34. S. W. Budd 35. M. Emmert 36. E. W. Stick 37. A. O. Fisher 38. G. R. Pretz 39. C. R. Kingsley, Jr. 40. A. B. Cecil 41. J. Crawford 42. C. R. Essick 43. L. H. Watkins 44. C. W. Webb 45. A. J. Wiesender 46. J. R. Stewart 47. H. Q. Fletcher 48. M. T. Burrows 49. T. P. Sprunt 50. F. M. Meader 51. W. A. Baetjer
Faculty members, second row, left to right, DeWitt B. Casler, Thomas R. Boggs, Lewellys F. Barker, Harvey Cushing, John W. Churchman
From the Alan M. Chesney Medical Archives, The Johns Hopkins Medical Institutions

the administration by the opsonic index was inadequate. Needless to say, the use of tuberculin in treatment as well as the intense interest in Wright's opsonic index died down quickly.

The following year Sellards reported his study on the hemolytic action of bile and its inhibition by blood serum. Bile and bile salts are active hemolytic agents *in vitro*. Sellards demonstrated that normal serum protects effectively against the hemolytic action of bile. In serum dilutions as high as 1:3,000 a trace of this protective action still persisted. Precipitation of the proteids by heat did not affect this inhibitory property of the serum. Sellards believed that these facts had a direct bearing on the explanation of the etiology of acute hemorrhagic pancreatitis. Following the injection of bile, there is a necrosis of the pancreas, caused by the bile, and the hemor-

rhage would presumably neutralize the action of the bile. Except for the protection afforded by the blood serum, a simple catarrhal jaundice might perhaps be followed by serious consequences such as the development of a severe secondary anemia.

Another of Sellards's papers published while he was a medical student dealt with the effect of heated serum on rouleaux formation of red blood corpuscles. His experiments concerned auto-rouleaux formation and the artificial production of a serum causing rouleaux formation. In an emulsion of red blood corpuscles in salt solution, microscopic examination showed that the corpuscles were very evenly distributed. In a control preparation consisting of equal volumes of washed corpuscles and unheated serum, only a very slight change was seen. The corpuscles were somewhat less uniformly distributed throughout the field and a very few short rouleaux were present. If, however, a volume of washed corpuscles was mixed with an equal volume of serum, which had been heated to 60°C, a very definite change occurred at once. Practically no free corpuscles were seen but they were arranged in long symmetrical rouleaux, which formed a rather coarse network throughout the preparation. Sellards concluded that heated serum developed a property of causing human erythrocytes to collect in rouleaux and that this property was not due to the destruction of an antibody by heat, but to a definite increase of a normal property of serum.

At the end of each of his papers Sellards acknowledged the assistance and suggestions of Dr. Rufus Cole during the course of the investigations. Working in Cole's laboratory, or visiting there, were many individuals who were associated with the Army Medical Corps and were involved in studies in the field of tropical medicine. Perhaps it was contact with one or more of these individuals that led to Sellards's first period of work in the Philippines.

EXPERIENCE IN THE PHILIPPINES

After his graduation from Johns Hopkins in 1909, Sellards worked in the Philippines as an instructor in tropical medicine, an assistant resident physician in the Philippine General Hospital, and as an assistant to the Bureau of Science in Manila. His training in chemistry came to the fore in his studies of Asiatic cholera. He noted immediately that the symptoms of Asiatic cholera were different from those of other acute bacterial infections in that the body temperature was usually normal or subnormal during the stage of collapse and that there was a pronounced disproportion between temperature and pulse rate. He concluded that the various features of the disease such as the short course, the abrupt onset, and the low body temperature resembled more closely acute intoxications of chemical origin than ordinary "infectious fevers." It was clear to Sellards that in addition to the hypothetical toxin of the cholera vibrio, the sudden loss of large quantities of fluid from the body gave rise to a considerable mechanical disturbance in the circulation of the blood, which in turn might be responsible for all of the symptoms of the disease. The principal evidence indicating serious metabolic disorder was the rather high percentage of cases which died in uremia. Sellards thus considered the possible relation between uremia and certain symptoms of acid intoxication occurring in Asiatic cholera. In looking for evidence of acid intoxication, his attention was directed especially to the examination of the urine in regard to 1) acetone and acetoacetic acid; 2) the ammonia coefficient; and 3) tolerance of the body to alkalies, i.e., the amount of alkali required by the body to render the urine alkaline. No examinations of the blood were attempted. The methods for determination of the carbon dioxide content of the blood at that time were not satisfactory. The results of his studies were clearcut. Examination of the urine in cholera showed an almost constant increase in the excretion of ammonia. Cholera

patients showed a definite tolerance to alkalies, a considerable excess of sodium bicarbonate being required to render the urine alkaline as compared with normal individuals. Following the injection of alkalies, there was sometimes a sudden and marked increase in the excretion of urea; the early administration of alkalies practically eliminated death from uremia. He thought that his studies would be more important if a similar condition proved to be present in uremia from other causes rather than if it were specific for cholera. Thus, this work led him to study the acidosis of nephritis when he returned to Johns Hopkins.

In a paper written with A. O. Shaklee, "Indications of Acid Intoxication in Asiatic Cholera," Sellards noted that the theory of acid intoxication in clinical medicine rested almost entirely upon the investigation of diabetes; he suggested that the opportunities were great for extending such studies to patients with cholera. In their investigations, Sellards and Shaklee observed that the stage of uremia in cholera and the acid intoxication of diabetes had the following features in common: 1) there was a well-marked tolerance for alkali; 2) the relative and absolute amounts of ammonia in the urine were considerably increased in both diseases. The administration of alkalies even in large amounts sometimes failed to reduce the excretion of ammonia. In cholera the urine frequently showed a pronounced diminution in the amount and percentage of urea; 3) there might be a definite reduction in the carbon dioxide content of the blood in the uremia of cholera as well as in diabetic coma; and 4) in both diseases a diminished alkalinity of the blood was reported.

RETURN TO RESIDENCY TRAINING AT JOHNS HOPKINS

In 1911 Sellards returned to the United States, becoming an assistant resident physician (December 1911–December 1914) and instructor in medicine at The Johns Hopkins University School of Medicine. He was also assigned to the chemical division of the medical clinic and was made its temporary director. Sellards continued his studies on the tolerance of the body toward fixed bases by determining the amount of sodium bicarbonate which must be introduced into the body in order to render the urine alkaline. In his first paper, published in the Bulletin of the Johns Hopkins Hospital of October 1912, he reported his results in normal individuals following the ingestion of sodium bicarbonate and the tolerance to sodium bicarbonate in artificially produced acidoses, in five cases of diabetes, in an obscure uremia accompanied by an increased excretion of ammonia, and in a group of 13 nephropathies.

In his study of 13 patients representing several types of nephropathies evidence was obtained which indicated that the tissues of the body, even in the early stages of an acidosis, could take up sodium bicarbonate readily. Sellards thought that a slight increase in the acid metabolism was compensated for, in part, by the fixed bases of the body and not wholly by an increase in the excretion of ammonia and of acid. He noted that during pathologic processes when the body was becoming impoverished in certain constituents, the composition of the blood may have been maintained in a relatively normal condition at the expense of the other tissues. He felt that the determination of the tolerance to bicarbonates afforded some information concerning any deficiency which may exist in the content of the tissues in fixed bases; this evidence was of a different nature from that obtained by the determination of the reaction of the blood.

One of Sellards's objectives was to develop a better clinical method for studying titratable alkalinity of the blood and its application to acidosis. He described the method which he developed in an article which appeared in the *Bulletin of the Johns Hopkins Hospital* of April 1914. Sellards found that changes in the titratable alkalinity of the blood occurred which gave rise to distinct qualitative differences in the reaction of normal and pathologic sera to phenolphthalein. Experimental conditions were readily obtained under which the blood serum during an acidosis was neutral or acid, whereas under the same conditions all normal sera were strongly alkaline. The less severe grades of diminished alkalinity could be detected in a qualitative way from the behavior of sera before and after the removal of protein and by the selection of a solvent, such as alcohol, in which the ionization and hydrolysis of carbonates was diminished. The effect of protein and of the solvent upon the reaction permitted a variety of combinations of these factors for detecting varying grades of diminished alkalinity. Definite changes occurred in the titratable alkalinity in experimental and spontaneous acidosis, in certain nephropathies, and in some anemias. The method also afforded valuable information in the differentiation of certain obscure comas. Sellards found cases of diabetes in which the excretion of ammonia and of acetone and related substances was normal, but in which the titratable alkalinity was decreased and the tolerance to bases was increased. This afforded proof of impoverishment in bases in these cases.

Changes in the titratable alkalinity were accompanied by corresponding changes in the tolerance of the body to fixed bases. The titratable alkalinity was found to be of important biological significance. The available evidence indicated that the physico-chemical reaction of the blood was maintained at a fairly constant value, even in outspoken grades of acidosis. Sellards was one of the pioneers in recognizing the importance of acidosis as a manifestation of disease but the techniques at the time were primitive and the important advances came only after Van Slyke introduced his method for the study of the acid-base equilibrium.

In a paper published in the *Bulletin of the Johns Hopkins Hospital* of May 1914, Sellards discussed the essential features of acidosis and their occurrence in chronic renal disease. The theory of acidosis was at that time in a developmental stage and there were many obstacles to determining whether acidosis developed in the course of nephritis. Sellards expressed the belief that the underlying principle of acidosis was a general impoverishment of the body in bases, which might be brought about by a variety of methods, such as: 1) simple starvation, i.e., the withholding of bases from the food; 2) disturbances of acid formation and elimination; and 3) loss of alkali as such during successive purgation. In a study of the acidity of the urine, Henderson and Palmer had come to the conclusion that acidosis was an important symptom in cardiorenal cases. The method used by them consisted in the measurement of the concentration of hydrogen ions in the urine by a series of indicators. The average acidity in a group of cardiorenal cases was higher than the average acidity in a group of normals.

In Sellards's view acidosis was the effect rather than the cause of the renal lesion and thus constituted a condition of only secondary importance. He listed the characteristics of the acidosis as: a) increase in tolerance to bases; b) decrease in titratable alkalinity of the blood; c) decrease in the carbon dioxide content of the blood; d) normal excretion of ammonia; and e) absence of any disturbance of carbohydrate or fat metabolism, and absence of the salts of any abnormal organic acids. Changes in the titratable alkalinity of the blood which could be detected by the use of phenolphthalein afforded a ready means for the prompt diagnosis of acidosis, and the method was particularly applicable in renal disease. An important conclusion was that symptoms of uremia are due not to the presence of a toxin (as widely believed at the time), but to the absence of a normal constituent of the blood, namely, the carbonates. Therefore, therapeutic bleeding for the removal of any circulating toxins would result in a still further diminution of a substance in which the blood was already seriously depleted. This disadvantage could be readily obviated by the injection of bicarbonate. Sellards felt that the acidosis was produced by defective function of the kidney in the excretion of acid salts.

In a "popular" address on the bonds between tropical and general medicine delivered at the School of Tropical Medicine of the University of Puerto Rico on February 22, 1927, Sellards spoke of these early studies on acidosis:

Biochemistry has also made its contributions. Some years ago there was a small outbreak of Asiatic cholera in Manila. At that time it fell to my lot to be on duty in the cholera wards. Some of the patients in the stage of reaction showed unmistakable clinical signs of air-hunger, an almost typical Kussmaul's coma. Obviously these cases were not associated with diabetes, and the urine, as a rule, was free from acetone. However, the clinical signs of acidosis were characteristic and it seemed advisable to look for some method other than the tests for acetone bodies for the recognition of acidosis. Accordingly these patients were injected with sodium bicarbonate. Enormous quantities—90 or 100 grams—were often required to render the urine alkaline, whereas if a healthy person takes a teaspoonful of soda the urine changes promptly from an acid to an alkaline reaction. Formerly, a large proportion of all cases of Asiatic cholera, roughly 15%, died of uremia. Now it was found that early treatment of cholera patients with bicarbonate practically eliminated the complication of uremia. Therefore it seemed probable that a similar lack of alkali might occur in patients developing uremia in the terminal stages of Bright's disease as we see it in cold climates. Accordingly, in Baltimore I examined such patients. They showed an even more intense degree of acidosis than the cholera patients, but obviously they were in the end stages of a long-standing disease and no lasting benefit could be expected from treatment with alkali. For our understanding of nephritis it is important for us to know that acidosis is one of the factors which is responsible for the symptoms of uremia. This fact is now generally accepted, for it has been confirmed by many observers using chiefly the method of direct chemical analyses of the blood—a method that in my opinion is rather less delicate than the test of tolerance to alkali.

STUDIES ON AMEBIASIS

Another disease in which Sellards developed a lasting interest during his stay in the Philippines was amebic dysentery. He and E. L. Walker set about to prove, by reproducing the disease experimentally, that amebae really were the cause of "amebic" dysentery. First, they re-emphasized the necessity in practice of distinguishing the harmless *Entamoeba coli* from the pathogenic *Entamoeba histolytica* in the stools of patients. Volunteers were then fed cysts of the various strains. Those who ingested *E. coli* developed no disease, whereas dysentery was produced in some of those who received *E. histolytica* cysts. Furthermore, many of those who did not develop clinical dysentery became "carriers." Walker and Sellards drew the important conclusion that *E. histolytica* was, to all intents and purposes, the sole cause of amebic dysentery and that exact diagnosis was of the utmost importance. They also emphasized that vegetative forms did not survive outside the body but that cysts were the important element in transmission of the disease. Consequently, the recognition of "carriers" of cysts was the key to intelligent public health preventive measures.

As to treatment, they made the important statement: "The evidence . . . points to the conclusion that the ordinary routine treatment with ipecac, while efficient in relieving attacks of dysentery and in causing the entamoeba to disappear temporarily from the stools, frequently does not kill all of the entamoeba in the intestine; consequently the patient is liable to a relapse of the dysentery."

Sellards continued his work on amebiasis after his return to Baltimore and in November 1914 published with Walter A. Baetjer, a medical school classmate, a study of the experimental production of amebic dysentery by direct inoculation into the cecum. The inoculation of kittens per rectum and the feeding of dysenteric stools rich in amebae were used for the production of dysentery with widely varying degrees of success; in general, however, infections were obtained in about 50 percent. It was not possible by either of these methods to propagate a strain of pathogenic amebae beyond a limited number of passages. Inoculation of eight strains of dysentery, some of which were from distinctly atypical cases, directly into the cecum in ten kittens produced an infection in all instances. Definite evidence was obtained

that the amebae were able to injure and penetrate the healthy mucosa.

Sellards continued his work in amebic dysentery during a second stay in the Philippines and also in 1923 did a series of investigations concerning amebic dysentery in collaboration with Max Theiler. They first demonstrated that kittens could be readily infected with *E. histolytica* by the injection of cysts directly into the large bowel, providing strong evidence that excystation occurred in the colon. Additional evidence was obtained that stasis is an important factor in producing an infection of the intestine with *E. histolytica*.

Kittens were infected with *E. histolytica* and the large intestine was then deprived of its normal supply of water by placing a ligature around the gut. The amebae disappeared early in the course of the infection in three animals in which this procedure was carried out. According to their conception, the cysts of *E. histolytica*, when ingested by mouth, are carried rapidly by peristalsis through the small bowel and set up lesions at points of stasis in the large intestine. In three kittens amebic infection of the colon readily invaded the ileum when the ileo-colic sphincter was rendered functionless. Under the conditions of these experiments, the sphincter was an important factor in the mechanical protection of the ileum.

THE MOVE TO HARVARD

In the summer of 1913 Sellards joined Richard P. Strong, E. E. Tyzzer, C. T. Brus and others on an expedition to the West Coast of South America to study verruga peruana (Oroya fever) as well as other diseases seen in Columbia and Ecuador and in the Peruvian Andes. A year later Richard P. Strong, under whom Sellards had worked in the Philippines, offered him a position as his assistant at the School of Public Health at Harvard. (Strong was a member of the first class to graduate from The Johns Hopkins University School of Medicine.)

On July 14, 1914, Strong wrote to Sellards:

I'm glad to have your letter and to hear of your plans. As I wrote you, we are prepared to open a small clinic here in the near future. I'm writing to ask whether you would care to accept the position here, provided I can arrange it for you to look after this clinic and to do some teaching, the rest of the time to be spent in research here or upon work largely in Central America for the present at the station we hope to have there. I think I could arrange for a salary of $2,500.

On July 18 George C. Shattuck[1] wrote to Strong:

You are quite right. It was a clear understanding that you should have an assistant and the funds can be furnished. Get Sellards by all means if you can.

---

[1] George Cheever Shattuck was the last of five generations of notable Boston physicians. In 1907, two years after graduation from Harvard Medical School, he worked for several months in Richard Strong's laboratory in the Philippines which resulted in a paper on tropical ulcer. In 1908 Shattuck became alumni assistant in clinical medicine at Harvard. There can be little doubt

On August 20 Sellards replied to Strong's July 14 letter:

Many thanks, indeed, for your letter which came a day or two ago from Santiago. I have just come back from a visit in the Adirondacks where I went to see Dr. Janeway, for developments were proceeding rather slowly by correspondence. [Evidently Sellards was negotiating with Theodore C. Janeway for a position in Janeway's new full-time department of medicine at Johns Hopkins.] There really is a very attractive field here for work but it is not clear yet that this is the time to take it up. I want to come to see you when it is convenient for you after your return, for then it will be very easy to decide after a short talk about it.

There are many reasons why I would like to be at Harvard but on the other hand I am right in the midst of some work in regard to the transmission of leukemia to monkeys and I would want to be perfectly sure that you are satisfied with the details of the work that I am planning. I will look forward to seeing you soon and will probably send a note to Harvard in case this should miss you.

Strong wrote on October 2, 1914:

Your letter has just been received and I note that you are ready to leave Baltimore at almost any time. I am writing to offer you a position here at a salary of $2,500.

In regard to teaching I should like to have you give the course in clinical laboratory work, which begins in December in the School of Tropical Medicine. It may be necessary to include some instruction in helminthology in this course for the present year. I am writing to offer you the post now as I should like to print your name in the schedule for this course if practicable. The schedule is about to go to press. The clinic I wrote you about last spring is not yet established, and Dr. Warren [the Dean] who has had the matter in hand is still out of town and will not be back until some time next week. A great deal of work here, you understand, is in the developmental stage. This I can talk all over with you when I come to Baltimore.

Sellards accepted the position as associate in tropical medicine at Harvard in 1914. At Harvard, Sellards gradually advanced through the various academic grades, being appointed associate professor in 1932. Although Sellards's forte was research, it may be seen in Strong's recommendation of Sellards for promotion to associate professor that Sellards also excelled as a teacher:

I may say that he is a man who has always, but especially in the past few years had the best interest of the school at

heart and the highest opinion with respect to ethical matters. He has an excellent appreciation of high standards of scientific work, and his own scientific work has been performed with great care, accuracy, patience and conservatism.

He has traveled extensively and come into contact with the study of diseases in foreign and tropical countries and his vision in connection with both medical teaching and research has thus been greatly broadened, as well as his experience with men.

Perhaps what may not be known to all the members of the committee is that Dr. Sellards has an excellent influence upon the students in this medical school. This influence is a quiet and unobtrusive one and the students have found it of advantage to come to him for assistance, information and especially for advice in connection with their problems. Moreover he apparently has special ability in finding out the needs of the medical students and in assisting them in their work. In addition to his ability in research Dr. Sellards has special ability as a teacher.[2]

While serving in World War I as a major in the medical corps, Sellards developed an interest in the pathogenesis of measles. He inoculated monkeys and then man with the blood of measles patients but did not succeed in transferring the disease. This was accomplished later by Blake and Trask at the Rockefeller Institute for Medical Research; it was shown that monkeys developed the disease spontaneously and for this reason Sellards and others failed in their attempt to transmit the virus to monkeys that were probably naturally immune.

Sellards spent the winter of 1921–22 working with Ernest W. Goodpasture in the Philippines. They were interested in the investigation of three diseases: amebic

[2] Dr. Sellards's ability as a teacher is also attested to by the reminiscences of one of his former students, Thomas H. Weller, who is now Richard Pearson Strong Professor of Tropical Public Health at Harvard:

My contact with Watson Sellards began in 1938, when as a second year medical student, I undertook elective research in the Department of Comparative Pathology and Tropical Medicine. Sellards, a bachelor, lived what seemed to me to be a lonely existence in a room at the Harvard Club, but belonged to a small club of contemporary scientists and businessmen that owned a converted farmhouse in Dover on the upper Charles River. Characteristically, he befriended one or two medical students each year; I was fortunately selected. Thus, there were intermittent dinners together at the Harvard Club, and occasional weekends of canoeing and hiking along the upper Charles River. When Sellards hosted a formal dinner for his friend, Dr. Ernest Goodpasture who was lecturing at Harvard, the guest list consisted of Dean Burwell, five professorial heads of Departments, and three medical students. His relationships with his student surrogate sons were ever considerate. In retrospect, it was a mutually supportive relationship.

Sellards was a heavily built individual with an almost disproportionately large balding head. He moved slowly and spoke softly, often with a half-smile. There were no flashes of anger, but he harbored deep resentments. His relationships with other groups working on yellow fever were expressed indirectly, as when he would emphasize that no accidental infections with yellow fever had occurred in *his* laboratory.

In the fall of 1940, we engaged in collaborative work that involved implantation of embryonic rabbit tissues in the anterior chamber of the eye of the rabbit, and the subsequent introduction of Variola virus. A former Navy corpsman, Byron Bennett, carried out the mechanical operations in the laboratory for Sellards. Bennett's relationship was that of a co-worker. On October 8, 1940, as we were preparing the customary informal lunch in the laboratory, Sellards had a cerebrovascular episode and was unconscious for an hour. This episode left no overt residua, and Sellards resumed work after a brief period of hospitalization. However, Sellards was not well and later that winter went on sick leave, ending our pleasant association.

that the warm relationship that developed between Strong and Shattuck played a considerable part in the decision to initiate a School of Tropical Medicine at Harvard. Strong became professor and head of the department of tropical medicine in 1913.

In the winter of 1914–15 typhus fever broke out in the prison camps of Serbia. Within six months the epidemic had resulted in 150,000 deaths from the disease. The American Red Cross organized a commission charged with the development of methods for controlling the epidemic. The membership was: George Shattuck, Richard Strong, A. W. Sellards, S. Burt Wolbach and Hans Zinsser.

dysentery, Tsutsugamushi fever and yaws. The study of yaws turned out to be particularly interesting as the disease proved susceptible to intravenous injections of arsenic (salvarsan).

While working with Goodpasture, Sellards maintained an active correspondence with Strong about their work as illustrated by the following letter from Sellards to Strong on February 13, 1922.

Your letter has just come and I will start in on yaws . . . From a public health standpoint, it seems to me the most interesting question is whether cases cured with salvarsan have any immunity against reinfection. Secondly, it would be a God-send in field work to have some simple safe way of administering salvarsan other than by injection . . .

Goodpasture could obtain no confirmation of Castellani's and of Bowman's work on the differentiation of the two diseases (syphilis and yaws) by complement fixation tests; approximately 18 cases were completely cured of clinical manifestations (by several injections of neosalvarsan) but the Wassermann did not even diminish in its titer. There is no truth in the statement . . . that the serum of a recently cured case is curative on injection into a yaws patient and that the serum of the patient cured with serum is also curative . . .

Salvarsan treatment of yaws is certainly the most dramatic in medicine. It constitutes the best method (at present unused) of gaining the confidence and enthusiasm of the masses of the people in public health measures (in the tropics). The cured cases will likely show no immunity on re-inoculation but I am sure that it is feasible to eradicate the disease anyhow . . .

Goodpasture has some good sections of fresh cholera intestines and something on the toxemia. He isolated something, (maybe a proteose) from cholera stools which killed dogs in a few hours with intestinal lesions. He will not commit himself yet but it is goodbye to Kraus' cholera toxine . . .

Governor General Wood thought highly of Sellards's work in the Philippines as indicated by a letter written to Strong on August 12, 1925.

Dear Strong,
A. W. Sellards is anxious to have another detail here. He has been doing extremely good work. He is thoroughly in touch with the medical situation, which, as you know, is a difficult one to become familiar with, and I am anxious that he should have another detail here. His research work is as you know very valuable to the Harvard School of Tropical Medicine, and I know it is very valuable to our people here. Permitting him to return will be a distinct aid to us and I am sure will be of value to the home school. Please see that he gets back here if it is possible to do so.
Sincerely yours,
Governor General Wood
P.S. We are right on the verge of big things in our leprosy problem and the work the doctor has been doing has a very important bearing upon our future handling of this disease.

YELLOW FEVER STUDIES

In 1926 Sellards went to Parahyba, Brazil, to study yellow fever under the auspices of the Rockefeller Foun-

dation. This marked the beginning of his most important scientific contributions. In 1886 Weil had described infectious jaundice due to a spirochete. Sellards showed 1) that the fomites of Weil's disease were dangerous, whereas the fomites of yellow fever were not; 2) that the serum of patients convalescent from Weil's disease could protect a guinea pig inoculated with *Leptospira* organisms, but convalescent serum from yellow fever had no such power; and 3) that the Pfeiffer reaction was positive in Weil's disease, but negative in yellow fever. Thus Sellards contributed materially to the demonstration that the two diseases represented separate entities.

Sellards's next contribution followed the epoch-making discovery by Stokes, Bauer and Hudson that certain species of monkeys, *Macacus rhesus* and *sinicus*, are susceptible to yellow fever and are suitable as experimental animals. Wilbur A. Sawyer has given a vivid account of this discovery by members of the West African Yellow Fever Commission of the International Health Division of the Rockefeller Foundation, working under Dr. Henry Beeuwkes. The isolation of the organism causing yellow fever had been considered an essential early step in the program of the commission and every effort was made during the first two years to find leptospirae or other organisms in the blood of patients, in cultures inoculated with their blood, or in inoculated experimental animals. At that time it had become generally accepted that *Leptospira icteroides* was the cause of yellow fever, for in several yellow fever epidemics in South and Central America, Noguchi and other experienced investigators had isolated this pathogenic organism from the blood of patients who had symptoms similar to those of yellow fever. However, the results of the West African Commission had been uniformly negative (as Sellards's results had been).

During 1926 and 1927, a series of epidemics of yellow fever occurred, beginning in Nsawam, about 20 miles inland from Accra, and spreading to five towns in the region and to the city of Accra itself. It was in one of these towns, Larteh, that the first successful transfer of yellow fever from patients to monkeys took place in May 1927. Confirmation of the discovery of the susceptibility of monkeys to yellow fever followed promptly.

At Dakar, in December 1927, Mathis, Sellards and Laigret isolated a virus strain from a case of yellow fever in a young Syrian. After commencement of the fever 16 mosquitoes were fed on the patient and blood collected and inoculated into a rhesus monkey. The monkey developed yellow fever. Twenty-four days after feeding on the patient the mosquitoes were allowed to feed on a rhesus monkey which also developed yellow fever. This strain was maintained in monkeys either by the bites of infected monkeys or by direct passage for a period of nearly three months.

In the winter of 1927–28 Sellards gathered additional material in Dakar and showed that virus maintained by inoculation of infected material into the brains of mice could produce encephalitis in a monkey and that such a monkey was protected from yellow fever even though there was no evidence of hepatitis.

The study of yellow fever was, of course, greatly facilitated by the important discovery of Stokes and his collaborators. However, the cost of transporting monkeys from India to the West Coast of Africa, which necessitated transshipment in Europe, was considerable. Apart from financial considerations, the study of the yellow fever virus could be conducted far more readily in countries where the natural carrier of the infection was absent. Experiments in localities where *Aedes aegypti* was present involved keeping all infected animals under mosquito netting to prevent the chance of their being bitten by any mosquito and possibly starting an epidemic. In temperate countries such difficulties did not arise as even in the presence of *Aedes*, the temperature conditions were such that the mosquitoes could never become infective.

Prior to 1928, unlike the majority of human infections which could be investigated in the main laboratories of Europe and America, the study of yellow fever had been confined to the regions in which it occurred. Although the French Yellow Fever Commission in 1903 had carried infected mosquitoes back to Paris from Brazil, no method of maintaining the virus was then known.

With all of these problems in mind and in view of the fact that yellow fever seemed clearly to be caused by a filterable virus, Sellards and Hindle attempted to transport the infected material in a new way. Sellards gave an account of his successful transportation of the yellow fever virus from Africa to the United States in a talk presented before the Southern Medical Association in 1929.

It is a little more than two years since Stokes and his associates made the discovery that the ordinary Indian monkey is extremely susceptible to yellow fever. So it is feasible and altogether desirable now to carry out laboratory studies on this disease in a Northern climate where conditions are much safer for everyone concerned. For my own work with yellow fever patients I had the good fortune to be associated with French physicians in West Africa, taking with me some rhesus monkeys to Senegal and also a strain of stegomyia mosquitoes that came originally from Havana. Mathis, Laigret and I infected these monkeys and mosquitoes with yellow fever. Having secured the virus there remained the problem of getting it home safely. The journey to Africa is a long one, the route ordinarily traveled being by way of England. On my way out I stopped in London where Dr. Wenyon, the director of the Wellcome Bureau, was extraordinarily helpful and very stimulating in his friendly encouragement. He said: "Yes, you will be sure to find some yellow fever patients and you'll bring the virus home in a little tube." Later on, in Senegal, with the virus in hand, this remark of Dr. Wenyon came back to me and it seemed as though there ought to be some simple way of preserving it for a few weeks. Of the procedures available for field work mere freezing of some infective tissue is often an efficient means of preservation. Even the poorest steamers have freezing compartments. So in addition to other material, some infected liver and blood were frozen under aerobic conditions, the vials being sealed to exclude the freezing mixture. These specimens were carried to London, where

Dr. Hindle (a Beit Memorial Research Fellow in tropical medicine) very kindly arranged for the testing of the material. The first monkey inoculated died in seven days of typical yellow fever.

On March 25, 1928, Sellards wrote the following letter from the Hotel Russell in London to his chief, Professor Richard Strong, in Boston: "I have stopped off here at Wenyon's laboratory to get my material into shape. It is a temptation to hurry home and take a chance on everything, but in the long run it is probably a case of doing the sensible thing.

"It is possible that I may need Theiler's[3] help in New York in handling things there. If I do I will cable you on leaving here. I have made no reservations yet but may be able to catch the Leviathan on April 4 . . . "

The results of this work in the preservation of yellow fever virus were published by Sellards and Hindle in 1928. They had shown that the virus could maintain its virulence for at least 12 days when frozen.

After his return to Boston, Sellards continued his work in yellow fever. In 1930 he published a paper in the *Proceedings of the National Academy of Sciences* entitled "The Cultivation of Treponemata from the Blood of Normal Monkeys (*Macacus rhesus*) and from the Blood of Monkeys Infected with Yellow Fever." Blood cultures were made from 22 normal monkeys and growth of a treponema occurred in the blood of one animal. Similar cultures from monkeys infected with yellow fever resulted in growth of treponemata in 9 of 26 animals. Some of the strains obtained from yellow fever sources on injection in large amounts into monkeys produced a rapidly fatal intoxication characterized by jaundice and a fatty liver. Thorough immunization of five monkeys with cultures of treponemata obtained from yellow fever sources resulted in partial to complete protection against the "virus" of yellow fever. The designation *Treponema xanthogenes* appeared to Sellards appropriate for the organism which produced jaundice and a yellow fatty liver on injection into normal monkeys. The immunological data were sufficiently striking to require a reconsideration of treponemata in the study of the etiology of yellow fever. Sellards realized that the observations were incomplete, especially in regard to pathology, mosquito transmission and immunological work, particularly with human convalescent serum.

In another paper published in 1931 Sellards described the behavior of the virus of yellow fever in monkeys and mice. A strain of virus from a yellow fever monkey maintained by repeated passage from brain to brain of mice until it no longer infected monkeys (*M. rhesus*) by ordinary routes of injection was compared with the original strain of yellow fever maintained in monkeys and mosquitoes. Monkeys inoculated into the brain with a suspension of infective mouse brains developed regularly a fatal encephalitis but without characteristic changes in

---

[3] Much of the experimental work on yellow fever performed in this country by Theiler, which led to the development of an effective yellow fever vaccine, was done using Sellards's strain.

the liver. Blood of such animals proved noninfectious for monkeys. Direct inoculation from brain to brain through a series of four monkeys failed to restore the virulence of the strain; obviously this experiment by no means exhausted the possibilities of restoring the mouse strain of virus to its original condition in which it produced a fatal infection in monkeys after intraperitoneal injection with extensive necrosis of the liver. Tests for cross-immunity were carried out by injecting normal monkeys intraperitoneally with mouse virus and subsequently testing them with the typical virus of yellow fever. Also, monkeys immunized to typical yellow fever were injected intracerebrally with infective mouse brains. Cross-protection was very well marked though it was not complete. The results of these cross-immunity tests were entirely consistent with the interpretation that the virus in mice was yellow fever, and there was no indication that it was contaminated by any secondary virus.[4]

While working in Tunis in 1931 in Nicolle's laboratory, Sellards injected his mouse brain virus into man, hoping to produce immunity with material comparable to the "fixed" rabbit virus of rabies. The experiment was successful, showing that neurotropic virus was immunizing.

On December 4, 1935, Andrew Watson Sellards was awarded the "Medaille d'Or of the Societé de Pathologie Exotique in honor of A. Laveran" for his work on yellow fever. This medal is the principal prize of the Society.

After receiving this medal Sellards wrote the following letter to the Society:[5]

> My dear Colleague,
>
> Let me convey to you something of the pleasure and the honor which I enjoy in having before me today the gold medal of your society bearing the likeness of Laveran, the Founder of Exotic Pathology. This fine distinction from your society gives me a keen sense of responsibility for I can receive it only as a representative of a large group of your colleagues with whom it has been my happy privilege to work during the past decade.
>
> In October 1927 on a rainy afternoon in Paris I came unacquainted to your Institute and I recall vividly today, the constant and kindly courtesies accorded by your colleagues to the stranger in their midst. On that afternoon your distinguished President, Professor Roubaud, offered every encouragement for a visit to Senegal and in his own handwriting gave me a kindly note of introduction to General Mathis, the Director of the Pasteur Institute of French West Africa. Subsequently on the African coast the energetic efforts of Docteur Bouet were successful in arranging transportation on a freighter for me from Liberia to Senegal. Arriving in Dakar in the

early morning, I was filled with wonder and with pleasure to see General Mathis coming on board by ascending easily and successfully a rope ladder which was thrown over the side of the boat. We soon found Docteur Laigret, a mission was formed for our work, and we spent a very busy day in the hospital and at the Institute. It has often taxed my strength to keep pace with the indefatigable energy of Docteur Mathis . . .

> In September 1931, at the Gare St. Lazare, General Mathis was at the station and it soon developed in conversation that he had travelled throughout the night from Marseilles to meet my boat train. In our work at the Pasteur Institute, it is always pleasant to recall the generosity of Professor Pettit and the hospitality which he extended in his laboratory and in his home. Professor Calmette gave his time and thought to a careful consideration of our problems. The wise counsel and the sympathetic understanding of the beloved Professor Roux proves to be an influence that must endure throughout one's lifetime.
>
> Another master, Charles Nicolle arranged for some additional studies in Tunis. There I met my friend Laigret for the second time on the soil of Africa; together we made some preliminary observations. These were carried forward with skill and patience by Laigret in the succeeding years. Looking back to Senegal in 1927 no one could have imagined that the very active virus which we isolated then would be brought back seven years later to Senegal in a greatly modified form to be used by Laigret for vaccination against yellow fever . . .
>
> It is inspiring to note that all have been actuated by a disinterested desire to advance our scientific knowledge. The privilege of taking part in this work has given me the most fascinating opportunities that I have ever experienced in medicine.
>
> You can well understand that it is a stimulating sensation to have before one, the likeness of the distinguished Professor Laveran.
>
> A. Watson Sellards

During his undergraduate training at Kansas, Sellards developed a consuming interest in applying the methods of science to the study of human disease. This desire to unravel nature's secrets was reinforced during his student days at Johns Hopkins and remained with him throughout his long career at Harvard. His studies in tropical disease took him all over the world and created a wide appreciation of the global interests of American science.

In 1942 Sellards's difficulties with hypertension increased; he had a series of strokes ending with a cerebral hemorrhage from which he died on December 1, 1942.

ACKNOWLEDGMENTS

I am indebted to Dr. Thomas Weller for his reminiscences of Sellards and to Richard J. Wolfe of the Francis A. Countway Library of Medicine, Harvard University, for permission to use the material from the papers of Dr. Richard P. Strong.

My deep gratitude goes to Carol Bocchini for her editorial assistance and to Patricia King for the typing of the manuscript.

REFERENCES

1. Baetjer WA and Sellards AW: Continuous propagation of

---

[4] It is interesting that the technique of intracerebral injection for transference of the virus in mice was first suggested to Theiler by the work of Andervont to whom in turn it was first suggested by Charles E. Simon of Baltimore. Andervont used it in his work on herpes virus and Theiler gives him full credit for the suggestion in the introduction to his original paper (Theiler's) on this subject.

[5] Bull Soc Pathol Exot 29: 815, 1936

amoebic dysentery in animals. Bull Johns Hopkins Hosp 25: 165, 1914

2. Baetjer WA and Sellards AW: The behavior of amoebic dysentery in lower animals and its bearing upon the interpretation of the clinical symptoms of the disease in man. Bull Johns Hopkins Hosp 25: 237, 1914

3. Beecher HK and Altschule MD: Medicine at Harvard: The First 300 Years. Hanover, New Hampshire: University Press of New England, p 310, 1977

4. Bennett BL, Baker FC and Sellards AW: The susceptibility of the mosquito *Aedes triseriatus* to the virus of yellow fever under experimental conditions. Ann Trop Med Parasitol 33: 101, 1939

5. Henderson LJ and Palmer WW: On the intensity of urinary acidity in normal and pathological conditions. J Biol Chem 13: 393, 1912–13

6. Jeans PC and Sellards AW: The tuberculo-opsonic index and treatment by tuberculin. Bull Johns Hopkins Hosp 18: 232, 1907

7. Lacy GR and Sellards AW: Investigation of immunity in yaws. Philippine J Sci 30: 453, 1926

8. Lopez-Rizal L and Sellards AW: A clinical modification of yaws observed in patients living in mountainous districts. Philippine J Sci 30: 497, 1926

9. Mathis C, Sellards AW and Laigret J: Medécine expérimentale—Sensibilité du Macacus rhesus au virus de la fièvre jaune. Comptes Rendus De L'Académie de Sciences 186: 604, 1928

10. Minot GR and Sellards AW: The antagonistic action of negative sera upon the Wasserman reaction. J Med Res 34: 131, 1916

11. Minot GR and Sellards AW: Injection of hemoglobin in man and its relation to blood destination with special reference to the anemias. J Med Res 34: 469, 1916

12. Minot GR and Sellards AW: The preparation of hemoglobin for clinical investigations. J Med Res 37: 161, 1917

13. Noguchi H: Yellow fever research, 1918–1924: A summary. J Trop Med Hyg 28: 185, 1925

14. Rackemann FM: Andrew Watson Sellards, 1884–1942. Trans Assoc Am Physicians 59: 34, 1946

15. Sawyer WA: Recent progress in yellow fever research. Medicine 10: 509, 1931

16. Schobl O, Sellards AW and Lacy GR: Some protean manifestations of the skin lesions of yaws. Philippine J Sci 30: 475, 1926

17. Sellards AW: The haemolytic action of bile and its inhibition by blood-serum. Bull Johns Hopkins Hosp 19: 268, 1908

18. Sellards AW: The effect of heated serum on rouleaux formation of red-blood corpuscles. Bull Johns Hopkins Hosp 19: 271, 1908

19. Sellards AW: Tolerance for alkalies in Asiatic cholera. Philippine J Sci 5: 363, 1910. [In this paper he emphasized the increased tolerance for alkali in cholera patients, especially those who were anuric, and he pushed the intravenous injection of solutions of sodium bicarbonate with what he thought were good therapeutic results.]

20. Sellards AW: The determination of the equilibrium in the human body between acids and bases with especial reference to acidosis and nephropathies. Bull Johns Hopkins Hosp 23: 289, 1912

21. Sellards AW: A clinical method for studying titratable alkalinity of the blood and its application to acidosis. Bull Johns Hopkins Hosp 25: 101, 1914

22. Sellards AW: The essential features of acidosis and their occurrence in chronic renal disease. Bull Johns Hopkins Hosp 25: 141, 1914

23. Sellards AW: Further observations on the relationship of the renal lesions of Asiatic cholera to the ordinary nephrites with special reference to acidosis. Am J Trop Dis Prev Med 2: 104, 1914–15

24. Sellards AW: The principles of acidosis and clinical methods for its study. Cambridge Mass.: Harvard University Press, 1917

25. Sellards AW: Bacterial cultures of human spleens removed by surgical operation. N Orl Med Surg J 69: 502, 1917

26. Sellards AW: Sensitive action of dilute sodium hydroxid on certain races of the pneumococcus. J Am Med Assoc 71: 1301, 1918

27. Sellards AW: Investigations of tropical sunlight with special reference to photodynamic action. J Med Res 38: 293, 1918

28. Sellards AW: Insusceptibility of man to inoculation with blood from measles patients. Bull Johns Hopkins Hosp 30: 257, 1919

29. Sellards AW: The reaction of monkeys to the inoculation of measles blood. Bull Johns Hopkins Hosp 30: 311, 1919

30. Sellards AW: Asiatic cholera: Survey of Literature from September 1, 1920 to March 1, 1921. Nelson Loose-Leaf Med, London and NY 2: 104, 1921

31. Sellards AW: Bacillary dysentery. Oxford Med 4: 767, 1921

32. Sellards AW: Amebiasis. Oxford Med 5: 799, 1921

33. Sellards AW: The cultivation of a rickettsia-like microorganism from Tsutsugamushi disease. Am J Trop Med 3: 529, 1923

34. Sellards AW: A review of the investigations concerning the etiology of measles. Medicine 3: 99, 1924

35. Sellards AW: The Pfeiffer reaction with Leptospira in yellow fever. Am J Trop Med 7: 71, 1927

36. Sellards AW: The relation between Weil's disease and yellow fever. Ann Trop Med Parasitol 21: 245, 1927

37. Sellards AW: Bonds of union between tropical medicine and general medicine. Science 66: 93, 1927

38. Sellards AW: La lutte contre la fièvre jaune. Bull Soc Pathol Exot 21: 70, 1928

39. Sellards AW: Observations on yellow fever. South Med J 23: 121, 1930

40. Sellards AW: The cultivation of treponemata from the blood of normal monkeys (Macacus rhesus) and from the blood of monkeys infected with yellow fever. Proc Natl Acad Sci 16: 223, 1930

41. Sellards AW: The behavior of the virus of yellow fever in monkeys and mice. Proc Natl Acad Sci 17: 339, 1931

42. Sellards AW: Technical precautions employed in maintaining the virus of yellow fever in monkeys and mosquitoes. Am J Trop Med 12: 79, 1932

43. Sellards AW: The interpretation of the incubation of the virus of yellow fever in the mosquito (Aedes Aegypti). Ann Trop Med Parasitol 29: 49, 1935

44. Sellards AW: The infection and immunization of mice by intraperitoneal and subcutaneous infection of the virus of yellow fever. Ann Trop Med Parasitol 29: 55, 1935

45. Sellards AW: Immunization in yellow fever and other virus diseases. N Engl J Med 216: 455, 1937

46. Sellards AW: Immunization against yellow fever with a consideration of the effects of a virulent neurotropic strain on the central nervous system of monkeys. Am J Trop Med 21: 385, 1941

47. Sellards AW and McLaughlin AJ: Effect of the concentration of the solution in the treatment of collapse in Asiatic cholera. Philippine J Sci 5: 391, 1910

48. Sellards AW and Shaklee AO: Indications of acid intoxication in Asiatic cholera. Philippine J Sci 6: 53, 1911

49. Sellards AW and Baetjer WA: The propagation of amoebic dysentery in animals and the recognition and reproduction in animals of atypical forms of the disease. Am J Trop Dis 2: 231, 1914

50. Sellards AW and Baetjer WA: The experimental production of amoebic dysentery by direct inoculation into the caecum. Bull Johns Hopkins Hosp 25: 323, 1914

51. Sellards AW and Baetjer WA: The recognition of atypical forms of intestinal amoebiasis. Bull Johns Hopkins Hosp 26: 45, 1915

52. Sellards AW and Baetjer WA: Bacterial cultures of human spleens removed by surgical operation. N Orl Med Surg J 69: 502, 1917

53. Sellards AW and Baetjer WA: Amoebic dysentery and associated conditions. Med Clin North Am 1: 1125, 1918

54. Sellards AW: Investigation of tropical sunlight with special reference to photodynamic action. J Med Res 38: 293, 1918

55. Sellards AW and Baetjer WA: The clinical significance of the irregular distribution of various cells and parasites in the blood stream and the production of abortive leukaemic changes and of splenomegaly in the Macacus rhesus. Bull Johns Hopkins Hosp 29: 135, 1918

56. Sellards AW and McIver MA: The treatment of amoebic dysentery with Chaparro Amargosa (Castela Nicholsoni of the family Simarubaceae). J Pharmacol Exp Ther 11: 331, 1918

57. Sellards AW and Wentworth JA: Insusceptibility of monkeys to inoculation with blood from measles patients. Bull Johns Hopkins Hosp 30: 57, 1919

58. Sellards AW and Sturm E: The occurrence of the Pfeiffer bacillus in measles. Bull Johns Hopkins Hosp 30: 331, 1919

59. Sellards AW and Bigelow GH: Investigation of the virus of measles. J Med Res 42: 241, 1921

60. Sellards AW and Leiva L: Investigations concerning the treatment of amoebic dysentery. Philippine J Sci 22: 1, 1923

61. Sellards AW and Leiva L: The effect of stasis on the development of amoebic dysentery in the cat. Philippine J Sci 22: 39, 1923

62. Sellards AW, Goodpasture EW and deLeon W: Investigations concerning yaws. Philippine J Sci 22: 219, 1923

63. Sellards AW and Theiler M: Investigations concerning amoebic dysentery. Am J Trop Med 4: 309, 320, 326, 1924

64. Sellards AW and Leiva L: The experimental therapy of amoebic dysentery. J Pharmacol Exp Ther 22: 467, 1924

65. Sellards AW and French GRW: The effects of Castela Nicholsoni in the treatment of chronic amoebic dysentery. US Naval Med Bull 21: 184, 1924

66. Sellards AW and Theiler M: The relationship of L. icterohaemorrhagiae and L. icteroides as determined by the Pfeiffer phenomenon in guinea pigs. Am J Trop Med 6: 383, 1926

67. Sellards AW, Lacy GR and Schobl O: Superinfection in yaws. Philippine J Sci 30: 463, 1926

68. Sellards AW and Schobl O: Experimental pneumonia in monkeys. Philippine J Sci 31: 1, 1926

69. Sellards AW and Theiler M: Pfeiffer reaction and protection tests in Leptospiral jaundice (Weil's disease) with Leptospira icterohaemorrhagiae and Leptospira icteroides. Am J Trop Med 7: 369, 1927

70. Sellards AW and Gay DM: The fate of Leptospira icteroides and L. icterohaemorrhagiae in the mosquito, Aedes aegypti. Ann Trop Med Parasitol 21: 32, 1927

71. Sellards AW and Baetjer WA: The occurrence of atypical amoebiasis. Parasitology 19: 48, 1927

72. Sellards AW and Siler JF: The occurrence of rickettsia in mosquitoes (Aedes aegypti) infected with the virus of Dengue fever. Am J Trop Med 8: 299, 1928

73. Sellards AW and Theiler M: The immunological relationship of yellow fever as it occurs in West Africa and in South America. Ann Trop Med Parasitol 22: 449, 1928

74. Sellards AW and Hindle E: The preservation of yellow fever virus. Br Med J 1: 713, 1928

75. Sellards AW and Laigret J: Médecine expérimentale—Vaccination de l'homme contre la fièvre jaune. Comptes rendus des séances de l' Académie des Sciences t. 194, p. 2175 (seánce du 13 juin 1932) Paris.

76. Sellards AW and Bennett BL: Vaccination in yellow fever with noninfective virus. Ann Trop Med Parasitol 31: 373, 1937

77. Sellards AW and Pinkerton H: The behavior of murine and human leprosy in foreign hosts. Am J Pathol 14: 421, 1938

78. Spooner LH, Sellards AW and Wyman JH: Serum treatment of type I pneumonia. JAMA 71: 1310, 1918

79. Stokes A, Bauer JH and Hudson NP: Experimental transmission of yellow fever to laboratory animals. Am J Trop Med 8: 103, 1928

80. Strong RP et al.: Verruga peruana, Oroya fever and uta: Preliminary report of the first expedition to South America from the department of tropical medicine at Harvard University. JAMA 61: 1713, 1913

81. Tyzzer EE, Sellards AW and Bennett BL: The occurrence in nature of "Equine Encephalomyelitis" in the ring-necked pheasant. Science 88: 505, 1938

82. Tyzzer EE and Sellards AW: The pathology of equine encephalomyelitis in young children. Am J Hyg 33: 69, 1941

83. Walker EL and Sellards AW: Experimental amoebic dysentery. Philippine J Sci 8: 253, 1913

84. Weller TH: Personal communication, 1978

85. Yellow fever; A compilation of various publications, Senate documents 61, number 822, Washington, D.C., 1911

21.

W. Horsley Gantt—A Legend in His Time

Horsley Gantt, still a productive scientist in the laboratory at the age of 83, is a legend in his own time. One of Adolf Meyer's significant contributions to Johns Hopkins, Gantt has been for almost half a century the most distinguished American disciple of the famous Russian physiologist, Pavlov.

The grandson of a prominent physician and a direct descendant of Pocahontas, Gantt was born on October 24, 1892 at Wingina, Virginia and was raised in an atmosphere rich in intellectual and moral stimulation. He received his B.S. at the University of North Carolina, with a major in psychology and philosophy. His first faculty appointment was as Instructor in Chemistry and Anatomy at the University of Virginia in 1918. He received his M.D. from that institution in 1920.

Gantt first came to Baltimore during World War I to intern at Union Protestant Hospital which later became Union Memorial Hospital. He returned to Baltimore in 1920 to the Church Home and then moved to the University of Maryland Hospital when Dr. Maurice Pincoffs was made head of its Department of Medicine. There Gantt worked on the so-called Lyon's method of "draining the gall bladder

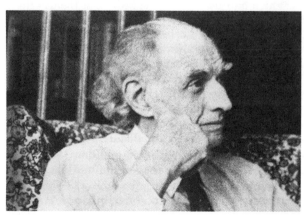

Fig 1. W. Horsley Gantt, 1974.
(Photograph courtesy of David White)

Reprinted from the *Johns Hopkins Medical Journal* **139**: 121, 1976.

by magnesium sulfate." This procedure was based on work by S. J. Meltzer at the Rockefeller Institute which showed that magnesium sulfate caused relaxation of the sphincter of the biliary duct and contraction of the gall bladder. Although this procedure was widely used, Gantt felt that the evidence for its effectiveness was insufficient; however, he was unable to resolve his doubts about it until he worked on the problem in Pavlov's laboratory in Russia.

THE RUSSIAN EXPERIENCE

Gantt embarked for Russia on June 10, 1922 when Dr. Pincoffs agreed to give him a three-month leave of absence to work with the American Relief Administration there under Herbert Hoover. He first visited the center of the famine area on the Volga where people were dying of cholera, smallpox, and typhus. He was then dispatched to the former capital city of Tsarist Russia, Petrograd. On October 29, 1922, described by Gantt as "the happiest day of my professional life in Europe," his interpreter, Dr. Zellheim, took him to visit Pavlov's laboratory. Gantt knew of Pavlov's work on digestion for which he had received the Nobel Prize for Medicine and Physiology in 1904, but thought he had been dead for years. Pavlov's obituary had been published in the 1918 edition of the Encyclopaedia Britannica, stating that he had died in 1916. Thus, Pavlov had the distinction of rereading his obituary at intervals for some 20 years. When they first met, Gantt was unaware of Pavlov's research on the conditional reflex. Pavlov explained it to Gantt in German and also through his interpreter. The demonstration of "reducing the complex 'psychical function' to drops of saliva, to a quantitative measure," stirred Gantt greatly, for he saw it clearly as a way to study mentality and its disorders. Mental phenomena—at least certain of them—could be reduced to the level of a simple experiment. Psychiatry could be studied by the use of objective scientific methods.

Gantt's plans and his entire life were profoundly altered by his chance meeting with Pavlov. Until the end of his stay with the Relief Mission, Gantt worked with Pavlov and his assistant, Volborth, first on the problem of the Lyon's drainage technique. He then spent a year doing research on pathology of the liver at the University College Medical School in London. While he was working in London, the new Communist government in Russia, having rejected further American aid, refused Gantt permission to return to work with Pavlov. For more than a year Gantt struggled with the Russian authorities, finally getting as close as Finland and chiding them by publicly implying that conditions must be so bad in Russia that they did not want him to return and observe them. Eventually, the government gave in and Gantt returned to Pavlov's laboratory at the Institute of Experimental Medicine in Petrograd where he was to spend the next five years.

Who was this legendary Russian physiologist who had such a determining influence on the career of Horsley Gantt? Pavlov was born on September 26, 1849 in the village of Ryazan in Central Russia. In 1870 he abandoned his theological studies to enter the University of St. Petersburg (Leningrad), where he studied chemistry and physiology. After graduation with an M.D. from the Imperial Medical Academy at St. Petersburg in 1879 and completion of his dissertation in 1883, he studied for two years (1884–1886) in Germany in the laboratory of the famous cardiovascular physiologist Carl Ludwig (in Leipzig), where he met William Welch (later of Johns Hopkins) who was also working with Ludwig. Later Pavlov worked with the gastrointestinal physiologist Rudolf Heidenhain.

Pavlov's first independent research was on the physiology of the circulation including regulation of blood pressure (1888–1890). His surgical skills were developed to such a degree that he was able to introduce a catheter into the femoral artery of a dog and to record without anesthesia the influence on blood pressure of various pharmacological and emotional stimuli. In 1890 he became Professor of Physiology in the Imperial Medical Academy where he remained until his resignation in 1924. From 1890 to 1900 Pavlov studied the secretory activity accompanying the digestive process. While working with Heidenhain, he had devised an operative procedure for the preparation of a miniature stomach pouch which isolated that organ from the salivary and pancreatic secretions while preserving its nerve supply from the vagus. This technique enabled Pavlov to study the secretions of the gastrointestinal tract in the normal animal over its life span. His cumulative studies were published in a book entitled *Lectures on the Work of the Principal Digestive Glands* in 1897. It was primarily for this work on the physiology of digestion that he was awarded the Nobel Prize for Medicine and Physiology in 1904.

It was during these studies that Pavlov developed the concept of the conditional reflex. In a classic experiment, he trained a hungry dog to salivate at the sound of a bell, which was previously associated with the sight of food. He thus used the salivary secretion as a quantitative measure of the psychical, or subjective, activity of the animal in order to emphasize the advantage of objective, physiological measures of mental phenomena and higher nervous activities. These were pioneering studies relating human behavior to the nervous system.

It was Sir Charles Sherrington, an English physiologist, who recognized that the spinal reflex is composed of integrated actions of the nervous system involving the excitation and inhibition of many nerves. To these components, Pavlov added cortical and subcortical influences and postulated the origin of neurotic disturbances principally through a collision or conflict between cortical excitation and inhibition.

Before returning to America in 1929, Gantt learned Pavlov's techniques, he learned Pavlov's language, and he learned to live as a Russian during a very dramatic period in the life of that nation. Fortunately, most young scientists, while they work hard and make important sacrifices in the pursuit of a career in medical research, do not have to endure the privations which Gantt faced in Russia. Although he did not suffer from obvious malnutrition, he knew on frequent occasions the pangs of hunger after going several days without food. For a period of two years, after having pneumonia in 1924 followed by poor nutrition, he was coughing blood and may well have had tuberculosis. His only available therapy appeared to be exercise, so he forced himself to walk one and a half hours daily regardless of the weather. Essentially everything in Russia was in short supply in 1927–1928, and he had to stand in line for two hours to buy four sheets of paper (the ration) on which to record his experiments. One of very few Americans in Russia at the time, Gantt served somewhat as an "unofficial ambassador." It was during this time that he met John Dos Passos. They walked across the wilds of the Caucasian Mountains where there were no roads, discussing the pros and cons of Marxism, and while they seldom, then or later, agreed on politics, they remained the best of friends until Dos Passos' death in 1970. One of Gantt's most important contributions while in Europe was his assessment of the effects of war, famine, revolution, and national influence on disease incidence, which he published in his first book, *Medical Review of Soviet Russia*. The medical historian Fielding H. Garrison has referred to this work as an opening chapter in "geo-medicine."

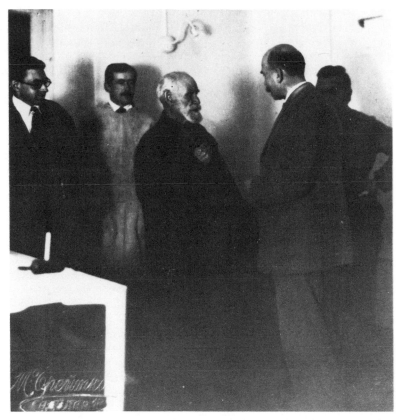

Fig 2. Gantt, Bykov, Pavlov, conversing with Selheim, 1923. As there was no electricity in the laboratory, note candle on the table. Because of the cold in the building, overcoats were worn.
(Photograph courtesy of W. H. Gantt)

RETURN TO BALTIMORE

Upon Gantt's return to the U.S. in 1929, Adolf Meyer brought him to Hopkins as head of a newly formed Pavlovian laboratory. As Gantt has related the incident, his appointment by Meyer was so obtrusely subtle that he (Gantt) did not realize that he had been offered the position until he was in the process of exploring the offer of another post.

What Gantt accomplished in the ensuing years in the Pavlovian Laboratory has been recorded in his nomination in 1970 by William G. Reese, J. E. Peters, and R. A. Dykman for the Nobel Prize in Medicine and Physiology:

"We nominate Gantt for his outstanding accomplishments in probing the inner biological universe and extending man's knowledge of comparative and human psychobiology and psychopathology . . .

" . . . His first research in America in his own laboratory at the Johns Hopkins, explored the anatomy of conditional reflexes. By direct stimulation of brain tissue, he found that the central nervous system, separated from its peripheral receptors and effectors, could elaborate conditional reflexes. This success depended upon his invention, with Loucks, of the methodology of exciting tiny coils in the brain substance by an external induction coil. This pioneering endeavor paved the way for increasingly refined, but no more ingenious, studies by many scientists. In subsequent extensive work on the peripheral and central effects of drugs, Gantt found the centrally-evoked effects could be conditioned, whereas peripherally-evoked effects could not. This work has done much to stimulate the development of psychopharmacology.

"He showed the effects of food deprivation upon salivary conditional reflexes and established a mathematical relation describing the magnitude of the conditional reflex as related to the intensity of conditional and unconditional stimuli. Pioneering in the important domain of conditional heart rate and blood pressure changes, he and his collaborators demonstrated similar, though less precise, mathematical relations. His early work on the autonomic components of the orienting or investigating reflex antedated by some 20 years the recent intensive interest in this field.

"In a beautiful but very simple experiment in which vestibular mechanisms were conditioned, he found that reflexes elicited by galvanic stimulation (loss of balance, vomiting, etc.) could also be elicited (after a suitable number of pairings) in much the same form by conditional stimuli. This experiment along with others led him to emphasize the shortcomings of teleology . . .

"He made significant contributions to the long-term vicissitudes of experimental neurosis and the factors which ameliorate or intensify its manifestations. He contributed much toward establishing an objective approach to psychopathology in man and demonstrated the clinical use of the conditional reflex method in the diagnosis of organic and functional psychopathology. He showed that the cretin could form conditional reflexes only after thyroid replacement therapy. His work stimulated the development of the standard conditioning test for deafness.

"From his extensive studies over time of various motor and autonomic components of conditional reflex in normal and abnormal dogs, he adduced and formulated the general principles of autokinesis and schizokinesis. These principles may be important to the understanding of long-term psychophysiological adjustments and maladjustments as is the principle of homeostasis to the understanding of short-term adjustments. They have great, though yet largely unexplored, power in explicating neurosis and psychosomatic illnesses of man."

One of the principal additions to Pavlov's studies that Gantt initiated was his use of cardiovascular measures of the conditional reflex. With the use of such measures, accurate relations are seen that are not evident when only the motor or the motor and secretory responses are included. Cardiovascular changes, like salivary and gastric changes, are autonomic responses; but unlike digestive secretions, the cardiovascular response is a general, supporting activity, preparing the body for an emergency, quickly supplying blood to activated organs involved in the emergency. In 1939, Hoffman and Gantt established that the heart rate in the cardiac conditional reflex is parallel in intensity to the quantitative salivary conditional reflex. The cardiac conditional reflex, however, differs from the specific conditional reflexes in two important respects: it is the first to form and the last to disappear. It sometimes forms with a single pairing of the conditional stimulus with the unconditional stimulus. However, when the salivary conditional reflex or the motor conditional reflex is extinguished and the dog appears to be completely inhibited and quiescent, his

cardiac conditional reflex may be as active as if there were no extinction of the other conditional reflex. The persistence of the heart rate in the conditional reflex and its resistance to adaptation through extinction is what Gantt terms schizokinesis. There is not only a schism between cardiac function and observable behavior but schizokinesis reproduces a maladaptation or lack of harmonious activity of the various physiological systems. The organism may be quiet and adjusted in one function and violently agitated in another. This could be related to hypertension and other cardiac diseases—the body reacting to old and long-forgotten episodes with the heart but not with the somatic system.

Since 1939, Gantt and his collaborators, including Hoffman, Dykman, Robinson, Teitelbaum, Stephens, Lynch, Reese, Gliedman, Newton, Perez-Cruet, Andrus and others, using heart rate measures have been able to observe the influence of the experimenter, the "Effect of Person." This term Gantt uses to cover "all effects of one individual on another, whether man on dog, dog on dog, etc., whether this effect be inborn or acquired." The influence of the individual, seen in his experiments by recording heart rate, may act as an acquired signal for what has been his relation to the subject in the past, or as the result of inborn relationships. The inborn "Effect of Person" is evident throughout the animal kingdom, though its mechanism remains a mystery.

It appears from Gantt's studies that if an excitation involves the central nervous system, such as food in a hungry dog, or such as pain, the reaction can be conditioned. But if one produces a change in heart rate, e.g., by the injection of acetylcholine (slowing), or by the injection of atropine (acceleration), these changes cannot be conditioned. It was impossible in Gantt's experiments on heart rate to form a conditional reflex because the stimulus acted at the peripheral nerve ending; it did not produce its effect through the central nervous system.

One of Gantt's important studies begun over a decade ago was his attempt to reproduce the development of a renal diuresis as a result of a conditional stimulus. Bykov stated that this could be done and that it had a double control—if one took out the hypophysis one would still get the conditional diuresis; if one left the hypophysis and cut the renal nerves, one would still get it; but if one took away both controls, one would not get any renal conditional reflex. Gantt set out to confirm Bykov's work. One kidney in each dog was transplanted to the neck of the dog, and the other was extirpated so that one kidney which had no nerves going to it would do the whole work for the dog. It had only the blood supply from the connected carotid artery to the renal artery and the jugular vein to the renal vein. Gantt was unable to get any conditional diuresis in these dogs. He then studied dogs with a normal kidney *in situ*, taking out the other kidney and bringing the ureter from the kidney to the surface of the abdomen so that he could collect the urine without its going through the bladder. For a number of years, he and various collaborators measured electrolytes, specific gravity, creatinine, protein, osmolality, volume, and so forth, but were not able to see a single element become a conditional reflex. There was no evidence whatever of any conditional reflex diuresis. Also, using phloridzin, which causes sugar to appear in the urine, Livingston and Gantt (1968) found no evidence of any conditioning. Using pitressin, which inhibits diuresis, they were unable to get any conditional reflex, although one had been reported by Bykov. If they measured heart rate, however, the heart rate became conditioned to administration of water to the thirsty dog. Here was another evidence of schizokinesis—one organ being conditioned, the other not.

With these results, Gantt began to think more deeply about the function of the kidney. The function of this organ is to balance and maintain the body fluids. If one compares its function with that of the gastrointestinal secretions, there is a marked difference. The saliva, the gastric juice, and the pancreatic juice in the human can amount to as much as several gallons of fluid in one day. But if one does not get the food that has been suggested by the appearance of a signal, no damage is done to the body because all of the fluid in the intestine is reabsorbed. There is no loss of electrolytes or water from the body. However, if the kidney began secreting in response to a signal for water and then did not get the water and a conditional diuresis appeared, the kidney would be throwing off substances of which there is great need in the preservation of body economy. When urine reaches the pelvis of the kidney it does not enter the system anymore. Thus, it is an entirely different physiological situation whether the kidney will form a diuresis as a conditional reflex and whether there is a motor conditional reflex to a signal for pain. This brought Gantt to the idea of the conditional reflex as a stereotyped mechanistic reaction—the idea that teleology for the physiological functions of the body is maintained by the organ which you are working with. The cardiovascular reactions and the gastrointestinal reactions prepare the system for what is to come. But the kidney does not need that kind of preparation for the ingestion of water because it is a slow acting organ which can take hours to throw out the excess water necessary. Its function is entirely different from that of the heart or the salivary gland. It was Gantt's final conclusion "that a physiological system is conditionable if the conditional reflex usu-

ally serves some end or purpose in the economy of the organ," the principle of organ-system responsibility. The kidney is not very responsive to the external universe; it is concerned primarily with the internal universe.

In summing up Gantt's contributions, Reese, Peters, and Dykman contended: "Gantt has been and remains a continuing link between international scientists, never bending to the shifting political winds or tides in his own or other countries, never sacrificing integrity for expediency .... Through his translations of Pavlov and Luria, Gantt introduced the English-speaking world to a highly scientific body of theory and experimentation. In pleading for realistic understanding of Russia and Russian science, Gantt maintained an objective position over the years.[1] Once condemned in the U.S. for being pro-Russian and simultaneously in the U.S.S.R. for being capitalistic and anti-Russian, he is now favorably recognized in both countries.

"His laboratory work, for over half a century of continuing productivity, is characterized by painstaking, methodical, objective questioning of nature and cautious reporting of her answers only after verification and reverification. From personally collected data, he has adduced and explicated significant principles which have illuminated many aspects of physiology, medicine, and psychology. It is no easy matter to single out Gantt's most significant contributions to clinical medicine, pathophysiology, psychopathology, neurophysiology, neuropharmacology, psychology, comparative psychobiology and psychiatry."

"RETIREMENT"

Gantt is an example of the fact that often universities reward their faculty members "more with love and less with remuneration." His laboratory in the old Physiology Building of the Medical School was only air-conditioned after the S.P.C.A. objected to the environment for the dogs in the suite they

---

[1]Gantt's attitude toward Communism and politics has been attested to by an eyewitness meeting him in Russia in 1927. Writing in his autobiography, "The Best Times," 1966, Dos Passos records from conversations during their trek across the Caucasian Mountains in 1927:

Horsley himself lacked interest in politics. At home he had never even registered to vote. He agreed with me that as an experiment in human organization communism was of interest; but all his thoughts were for science. In your lab you could perform your experiment, report the findings. Other men could repeat your experiment to check the results. You were on firm ground there. (John Dos Passos: The Best Times. New York: The New American Library, 1966, p. 191) shared with Gantt. The Pavlovian Laboratory was supported by the Rockefeller Foundation for 15 years due to the faith which Alan Gregg had in the importance of Gantt's work. (It was Gregg who had recommended Gantt to Adolf Meyer.) Lewis Weed, the dean of the Medical School, at one time wanted to drop Gantt because of a paucity of publication, but Gregg persuaded him not to, saying that "Gantt is a long distance runner." Fortunately, Gantt was supported in his work by others, including Drs. Thomas Turner and E. C. Andrus, who maintained an appreciation of his studies for a period of over 40 years.

Since "retiring" from Hopkins as Emeritus Associate Professor of Psychology in 1958, Gantt, at the invitation of Drs. Middleton and Casey, founded the Pavlovian Laboratory of the Veterans Administration Hospital at Perry Point and has worked there full-time as chief scientist. From 1958 until 1968 the Veterans Hospital donated his time for simultaneous directorship of the Pavlovian Laboratory at Johns Hopkins when Dr. Joseph V. Brady was appointed to succeed him in this position.

In addition to his full-time duties at the V.A. Hospital, Gantt has guided the continuing development of the Pavlovian Society, which he co-founded in 1955, and continues to edit the *Pavlovian Journal for Biological Science* (formerly *Conditional Reflex*), which he also established. He travels extensively, and has lectured throughout the U.S. as well as in many areas abroad. Besides writing and translating seven books and editing fifteen others, he has published over 400 research articles, one-fourth of which have appeared since his so-called retirement in 1958. He is now working primarily on an ambitious project to apply behavioral prophylaxis for humans. The development of a rational prophylactic psychiatry has long been a vision for Gantt. His studies of dogs as well as patients by the Pavlovian methods suggest that one may be able to predict to some extent (by examination of motor, cardiovascular, respiratory conditional reflexes) which individuals are susceptible to stress. This might in turn open the way to helping such individuals before they develop mental illness.

During his career Gantt has been an active member of many professional societies, including the Purkinje Medical Society (Prague, Honorary), the American Neurological Association, the American Physiological Society, the Collegium Internationale Activitates Nervousae Superiores (President), the Royal Society of Medicine (London), the American College of Psychiatrists, and the International Collegium of Psychosomatic Medicine. He was president of the Society of Biological Psychiatry, the American Psychopathological Association (1961) and the Pavlovian Society (1955–1965).

Among many awards which Gantt has received are the Lasker Award in 1944 for the work in his volume, *Experimental Basis for Neurotic Behavior*, the American Heart Association Award in 1950 for his investigations on hypertension, the Gold Medal Award from the Society of Biological Psychiatry in 1972, and the van Giesen Award from the New York Psychiatric Institute in 1975. On a very memorable occasion in 1974 the Pavlovian Society presented a handsome bronze bust of William Horsley Gantt to the Johns Hopkins University School of Medicine. Along with this went the "prayer that your great medical Olympus will remain as durable as this bronze."

REFERENCES

1. DeGast E: The life and times of Dr. Horsley Gantt. Baltimore, 68: 16, 1975
2. Gantt WH: Reminiscences of Pavlov. J Exp Anal Behav 20: 131, 1973
3. Gantt WH: Does teleology have a place in conditioning? *In* Contemporary Issues in Conditioning and Learning. McGuigan FJ, Ed. Washington, D.C.: V. H. Winston & Sons, 1973, pp. 111–126
4. Gantt WH: Ivan Petrovich Pavlov. Encyclopaedia Britannica. 15th ed. Helen Hemingway Benton, publ., 1974, p. 1095
5. Gantt WH: A scientist's last words. *In* Legacies in the Study of Behavior. Cullen JW, Ed. Springfield, Ill.: Charles C Thomas, 1974, pp. 46–61
6. Reese WG: Presentation of presentation. Pavlovian Journal 10: 125, 1975